# Computational Immunology: Models and Tools

# Computational Immunology: Models and Tools

Editor: Lacy Beckett

AMERICAN
MEDICAL PUBLISHERS
www.americanmedicalpublishers.com

AMERICAN
MEDICAL PUBLISHERS
www.americanmedicalpublishers.com

**Cataloging-in-Publication Data**

Computational immunology : models and tools / edited by Lacy Beckett.
p. cm.
Includes bibliographical references and index.
ISBN 979-8-88740-017-4
1. Immunoinformatics. 2. Immunology--Data processing. 3. Bioinformatics.
4. Immune system. 5. Computational biology. I. Beckett, Lacy.
QR182.2.I46 C66 2023
616.079 028 5--dc23



American Medical Publishers,
41 Flatbush Avenue,
1st Floor, New York,
NY 11217, USA

ISBN 979-8-88740-017-4 (Hardback)

# Contents

# Preface

The main aim of this book is to educate learners and enhance their research focus by presenting diverse topics covering this vast field. This is an advanced book which compiles significant studies by distinguished experts in the area of analysis. This book addresses successive solutions to the challenges arising in the area of application, along with it; the book provides scope for future developments.

Computational immunology refers to a field of science, which includes high-throughput bioinformatics and genomic approaches to immunology. The primary goal of this field is to transform immunological data into computational problems, solving such problems by utilizing computational and mathematical methods and then converting the results into immunologically relevant interpretations. Computational immunology is a subfield of bioinformatics that uses similar concepts and tools, such as sequence alignment and protein structure prediction. The other fundamental tools used in this field include ClustalW, TreeView and BLAST. It also makes use of special immunoinformatics tools like Collier-de-Perles and StructuralQuery for conducting variable domain structure analysis, and V-QUEST for conducting TR and IG sequence analysis. Computational immunology uses the immunological data for identifying infectious diseases, allergies and host responses. It is also helpful in understanding the type of specificity in immunogenicity and immune network. This book provides significant information of computational immunology to help develop a good understanding of its models and tools. It is appropriate for students seeking detailed information in this area of study as well as for experts.

It was a great honour to edit this book, though there were challenges, as it involved a lot of communication and networking between me and the editorial team. However, the end result was this all-inclusive book covering diverse themes in the field.

Finally, it is important to acknowledge the efforts of the contributors for their excellent chapters, through which a wide variety of issues have been addressed. I would also like to thank my colleagues for their valuable feedback during the making of this book.

**Editor**

# 1

# Evidence for Shaping of Light Chain Repertoire by Structural Selection

*Adar Toledano[1†], Yuval Elhanati[2†], Jennifer I. C. Benichou[1], Aleksandra M. Walczak[3], Thierry Mora[4] and Yoram Louzoun[1*]*

[1] Department of Mathematics, Gonda Brain Research Center, Bar Ilan University, Ramat Gan, Israel, [2] Joseph Henry Laboratories, Princeton University, Princeton, NJ, United States, [3] Laboratoire de Physique Théorique, UMR8549, CNRS and Ecole Normale Supérieure, Paris, France, [4] Laboratoire de physique statistique, UMR8550, CNRS, UPMC and Ecole normale supérieure, Paris, France

***Correspondence:**
*Yoram Louzoun*
*louzouy@math.biu.ac.il*

*†These authors have contributed equally to this work.*

The naïve immunoglobulin (IG) repertoire in the blood differs from the direct output of the rearrangement process. These differences stem from selection that affects the germline gene usage and the junctional nucleotides. A major complication obscuring the details of the selection mechanism in the heavy chain is the failure to properly identify the D germline and determine the nucleotide addition and deletion in the junction region. The selection affecting junctional diversity can, however, be studied in the light chain that has no D gene. We use probabilistic and deterministic models to infer and disentangle generation and selection of the light chain, using large samples of light chains sequenced from healthy donors and transgenic mice. We have previously used similar models for the beta chain of T-cell receptors and the heavy chain of IGs. Selection is observed mainly in the CDR3. The CDR3 length and mass distributions are narrower after selection than before, indicating stabilizing selection for mid-range values. Within the CDR3, proline and cysteine undergo negative selection, while glycine undergoes positive selection. The results presented here suggest structural selection maintaining the size of the CDR3 within a limited range, and preventing turns in the CDR3 region.

**Keywords: deep sequencing, B cell receptor, light chain, selection, rearrangement**

## INTRODUCTION

The diversity of immunoglobulins (IGs) is essential for the function of the adaptive immune system. The IG repertoire is shaped first by the V(D)J recombination processes, and then by selection forces. The rearrangement mechanism determines which genes are combined, as well as the makeup of the junction. Bone marrow and peripheral selection alter this initial repertoire to produce the naïve repertoire observed in the peripheral blood. The repertoire is then further shaped by antigen driven selection to produce the memory repertoire.

The diversity of the IG heavy chain has been studied extensively, like that of the T cell beta chain [see Ref. (1) for review]. It has been shown that much of the diversity originates from the V–D and D–J junctions (2). Current methods to estimate the identity and position of DH are inaccurate for short DH genes (3). Errors in the identification of DH can be erroneously considered as nucleotide addition or deletion. Moreover, in short D genes, the V–D and D–J junctions can overlap and introduce another layer of ambiguity. Here, we focus on the less studied IG light chain to study the roles generation and selection have in establishing functional diversity. An added benefit of studying light chain diversity is that with no D gene inside the CDR3, the junction diversity is more readily separated into contributions from gene selection, and from N insertions (4, 5).

We analyze here the kappa light chain locus (IGK), as the Lambda locus (IGL) has fewer germline genes, and as such has a more limited variability.

Counting all possible V and J choices, deletions, and insertions leads to a vast potential diversity. However, multiple lines of evidence now support that the repertoire is limited:

- The choice of IGKV and IGKJ genes in IGK rearrangement is not completely uniform and preferential use of several genes has been shown (5).
- The IGK polymorphism across individuals has been shown to be much lower than the heavy chain IGH in humans (5, 6).
- Recent results have shown that surprisingly over 20% of light chains CDR3 peptide sequences (out of 700,000 IGL sequences) were "public" (i.e., shared by two or more individuals). Moreover, full length IGL protein sequences (VJ recombinants) are also frequently shared. In a recent study, public rearrangements made up of 60.2% of the total sequenced IGK rearrangement (7).

These results together suggest that non-uniform rearrangement, biased junction formation, structural selection, and functional selection can shape the repertoire (5, 8–12). However, the relative contribution of these different mechanisms in the light chain repertoire has never been studied. We here study the extent and origin of IGK diversity using sequences of the recombined gene obtained from blood samples for humans and mice. This observed recombined repertoire is shaped by the rearrangement mechanism and by selection (either positive or negative). To understand how the repertoire is selected, these two processes must be separated.

We do not delve here on the V and J usage and their correlation. Those have been argued based on both theoretical and experimental results to be induced by the receptor editing mechanism (13–16).

The generation and the selection processes are stochastic in nature, with different recombined peptides having different likelihoods of being generated and selected. We use statistical models, where the probability of assigning each observed sequence to appropriate germline genes and junction sequences are computed, to infer and disentangle the two processes. We find that structural selection strongly shapes the observed light chain repertoire.

We have used similar models on T cells and heavy chain B cells (17, 18). Here, these models enable us to study the variability of the IGK light chain during the generation and initial selection stage of B cells. The IGK samples, sequenced from healthy donors and from transgenic mice, are first divided into functional and non-functional recombined genes. The functional sequences are in-frame (IF) and with no stop codon, and as such code for a peptide that can potentially be the light chain of the IG. Out-of-frame (OF) sequences, on the other hand, underwent recombination that resulted in some of the conserved codons of the J template to be out of their normal reading frames and thus lack essential conserved amino acids when translated. They sometimes also have stop codons, which prevent them from being fully translated. These OF sequences, having never coded for any protein, did not undergo selection and represent the results of the raw generation process. By comparing the statistics of the OF sequences (the generation process statistics), to the IF sequences, selection can be inferred (see Materials and Methods). We have studied Rapid Amplification of cDNA Ends (RACE)-based cDNA sequences of human and mouse light chains. The human light chains were taken from peripheral blood and were separated into naïve and memory cells. The mouse cells were separated into blood and bone marrow cells (see Table S1 in Supplementary Material for details).

## MATERIALS AND METHODS

### Generation Model

The V(D)J recombination process involves a random number of insertions and deletions, and often produces OF sequences. These sequences code for non-functional proteins and can still appear in a blood sample, if the second chromosome in the cell underwent a successful recombination. In such cases, the sequences experienced no selection and owe their survival to the receptor expressed by the other chromosome. Thus, they provide us a glimpse into the pure generation process. We used these OF sequences to infer the statistics of the V(D)J recombination process.

Each observed sequence can be the result of a number of scenarios that include different initial gene choices, followed by a variable number of deleted and inserted base pairs. Estimating the probability of a sequence can be done by summing over all the different possible scenarios for producing a given sequence, weighting each scenario by its probability. Each scenario's probability (Pgen) is calculated using a probabilistic generation model of the form P(V,J)P(delV\V)P(delJ\J)P(ins). In brief, the various factors account for the probabilities of uncorrelated events leading to a specific VJ rearrangement: choice of which gene segments to recombine P(V,J), probability of the number of deletions from the ends of the V and J genes at the junctions P(delV|V) and P(delJ|J), choice of number of nucleotides to insert P(ins), as well as factors to account for unequal nucleotide preference in the inserted sequences. This type of model was used before to infer the generation process of heavy chain in B cells and beta chain in T cells.

Here, we used the Baum–Welch algorithm to efficiently infer the parameters of the generation model (18). In short, by reformatting the generation model as a Markov model, we used the forward–backward algorithm once per sequence, then summing over all sequences to update the model parameters. This is a dynamic programming approach that bypasses the need to enumerate all possible recombination scenarios.

### Selection Model—Probabilistic Model

The naïve productive sequences (IF and with no stop codon), unlike the non-productive ones, have passed an initial selection process before being admitted to the periphery. We used the productive sequences to learn the selective forces acting on amino acids by comparing how their statistics differ from the raw product of V(D)J recombination learned from the OF sequences.

Using the generation model as a starting point, we infer selection factors $Q$ acting on each sequence in the naive repertoire, where $Q$ is defined as the fold increase of the probability to see a sequence in the functional repertoire (naive, productive) compared with the previously learned generation probability: $Q = P_{post}/P_{pre}$. To infer those factors, we use a factorized model $Q = q(V,J)q_L\Pi q_{i;L}(a_i)$, where we assume that selection acts independently on the V,J gene choice [through factor $q(V,J)$], the length $L$ of the CDR3 sequence (through factor $q_L$), and on each of the amino acids $a_i$ at positions $1 \leq i \leq L$ between the conserved cysteine near the end of the V gene and the conserved tryptophan within the J gene [through factors $Q_{i;L}(a_i)$]. We use an expectation–maximization procedure to update the selection factors until convergence (1).

## Study Subjects

For the human data, 12 apparently healthy adult subjects (3) were recruited for high-throughput sequencing using the 454 platform. Two 45-ml blood draws were collected in heparin tubes from each subject at a single time point. Mononuclear cells were isolated using Ficoll-Paque Plus (GE Healthcare), and then sorted by flow cytometry into naïve (CD20+, CD27−) and memory (CD20+, CD27+) populations. Informed consent was obtained from all donors. This work was performed in accordance with an IRB-approved protocol at Pfizer, Inc.

For the mouse data, blood and bone marrow RNA was extracted from healthy C57BL/6J mice using Qiagen RNAeasy Mini (19). RNA was provided as input to Clonetech SMARTer 5′RACE reactions, using murine IgK specific primers. Amplicons received Roche 454 adaptors with DNA barcode multiplex identifiers, and then sequenced with Titanium chemistry. The human and mouse data used here are based on previous publications (3, 20).

## Target Amplification and 454 Sequencing

Unbiased amplification of repertoires was performed by 25 cycles of 5′RACE, using individual isotype-specific reverse primers. Primers were optimized for efficiency, fidelity, and completeness of repertoire recovery by informatics screening, gel-analysis, and high-throughput sequencing of recovered products. The degree of germline-dependent amplification bias was assessed by comparing amplified products of stimulated naïve B cell pools to direct sequencing of the same pools. Cycle-dependent effects on diversity estimates were evaluated by high-throughput sequencing. All products received multiplex identifiers (barcodes) to allow unambiguous identification of all products by sequence analysis in subsequent processing steps. Multiplex identifiers differed by at least three base pairs from any other multiplex identifier sequence, and only reads with exact-matches were included in the analysis. Products were sequenced with 454 Titanium. Sequencing quality was assessed by keypass control. Sample QC was confirmed by demultiplexing and VK segment genotype. Sequencing depth was determined by diversity estimate rarefaction and simulations of germline-profile stabilization as a function of sequencing depth. A detailed validation of the sequencing methodology has been provided previously (12).

## V–J and Clone Detection Pipeline—Deterministic Model

We detected clones by clustering together sequences with similar CDR3 sequences (further explained below), to minimize the effect of potential biases in sequence copy numbers.

Specifically, sequences were grouped into clones using a two-step approach. First, we assigned each sequence V and J germline genes by running the IgBLAST tool (21) against human and mouse germline sequence databases (appropriately). Next, to count the clones, we grouped all sequences according to their V and J usage as well as the distance between V and J, since SHMs usually do not produce insertions or deletions of nucleotides (22). Thus, every clone emerging from the same founder cell should have the same distance between V and J. We then took all of the sequences with the same V–J and the same distance between V and J and grouped them using a phylogenic approach. All the sequences with an identical V–J and an identical distance were aligned together, using an artificial sequence composed of the germline sequences and gaps between them. The beginning and the end of all sequences of each dataset were trimmed so that all the sequences have same length V and J segments. The sequences of each group are thus already aligned and a phylogenetic tree was built using maximum parsimony (23) and/or neighbor joining (24) methods (from the PHYLIP 3.69 program package). We then parsed this tree with a cutoff distance of four mutations into clones. Thus, a clone was defined as a set of sequences similar to one another, up to a distance of four mutations. These methods were extensively validated in previous studies (1–3, 25–27).

## Sequence Analysis

### CDR3 Length

We calculate CDR3 length according to the number of amino acids between the conserved cysteine and phenylalanine. We then used the same sequence to compute the total CDR3 molecular mass (MW) using the "peptides" R package (values are rounded up to two digits). We then computed the distribution of CDR3 lengths in AA and in MW, and compared the SD of these distributions in different sets. For the MW relative difference, we calculate the SD of the MW in the IF sequence divided by the SD of the MW in the OF sequence minus 1 (to have 0 represent a state of no selection). The AA length SD ratio was calculated similarly. We did the same thing for the relative difference average of the MW and length.

### Selection vs. Generation Probabilities

In the $p - q$ plot, we present the log of the selection factor $q$ vs. the log of the generation probability $p$. We computed the Spearman correlation between these two values for the generation probability of VJ pairs and for the probability of a given amino acid in each position and CDR3 length. Formally, we calculated the correlation between the generation probability and selection factors across amino acids where $P_{i;L}(a_i)$ is the generation probability for amino acid $(a_i)$ in position $i$ for length $L$ (for maximum length 19, this can be coded with 20*19*19 parameters, some of which are zeros). The $Q_{i;L}(a_i)$ is the selection factors of the same amino acid, length, and position.

### Average Selection Factor

To present the selection factors of the different amino acids in the different positions, we averaged all the $q$-values over CDR3 lengths for each codon. Then, we present the results of the log values on a heat map. We also computed the log of the average of the selection affecting all codons translated to the same amino acid as presented in **Figures 2** and **3**.

## RESULTS

### CDR3 Are Selected to Have a Narrower Distribution

Naive B cells have undergone light chain-dependent selection (28). To study this selection, we first investigated the difference in the light chain CDR3 length distribution before and after selection in naïve and memory repertoires (the naïve pool in the peripheral blood, and the memory pool resulting from germinal center driven selection). The length of CDR3, defined as the number of nucleotides between the cysteine and phenylalanine surrounding the CDR3 [see Ref. (29) for CDRs positions definitions], was analyzed in samples from peripheral human blood that contains naïve and memory cells and mice B cell samples in the blood and bone marrow (see Table S1 in Supplementary Material and Materials and Methods for details).

We used deterministic and probabilistic generation model to compare the OF and IF repertoires. The probabilistic generation model was developed to best fit the OF human light chain samples, and the model was then applied to evaluate the generation probability of the IF naïve light chain repertoire. The validity of this method has been extensively tested (17, 18). For the other human and mice samples (mouse blood, mouse bone marrow, and human memory B cells), where the data were more limited, we only used the deterministic model, where each sequence is assigned the most probable V and J genes and the most probable alignment as estimated by our clone detection pipeline, which was also validated in multiple studies (1, 3, 25). The general features, such as V and J genes, are similar in the deterministic and probabilistic models. Note that we here study generic properties of the B cell receptor repertoire, and our results do not require an extreme sequencing depth or a very low-sequencing error level. Thus, the 454 sequencing used here is precise enough for the current analysis.

For each observed clone, only one sequence (the ancestor of the clone) was analyzed. Multiples conditions were compared. We used the OF sequences as representative the output of the rearrangement process, and compared those to naive cells to study the selection taking place in the bone marrow, or in the periphery prior to antigen exposure. We also used memory cells to test the effect of antigen exposure on the L chain repertoire. Finally, we analyzed mouse bone marrow and peripheral B cells and compared them with mouse OF cells to test again selection within the bone marrow and in the transition to the naive repertoire in the periphery. The probabilistic model was applied to the human naive cells and it thus represents again the selection affecting the naive repertoire, probably prior to antigen exposure.

A comparison between the OF-based stochastic model and the length distribution in the IF naïve human sequences indicates that there is a very weak change in the average length of the CDR3 (**Figure 1C**). The slightly longer CDR3s in functional sequences are in contrast with previously reported shortening of the heavy chain during development (30). This increase is accompanied by a parallel increase in the total molecular mass.

A more drastic change between the IF and the OF rearrangements is the reduction in the length variance (**Figure 1B**), indicating selection against short or long CDR3 sequences. A similar result can be observed when comparing the results of the deterministic model (full vs. dashed lines in **Figure 1A** and appropriate bars in **Figures 1B,C**). The reduction in the length

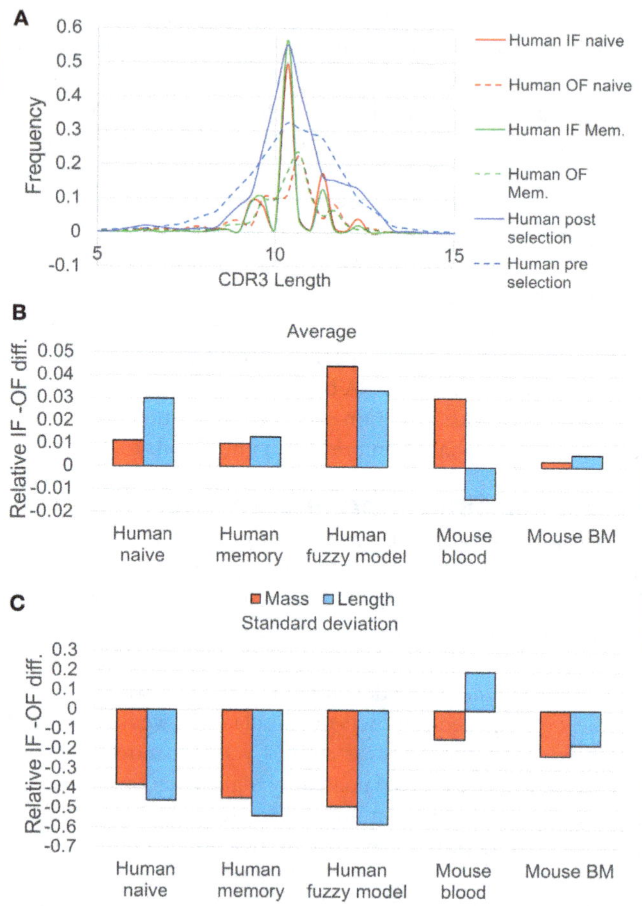


**FIGURE 1** | **(A)** Comparison of CDR3 length distribution in human in-frame (IF) and out-of-frame (OF) sequences. The continuous lines represent the IF reads, while the dashed lines represent the OF reads. Pre-selection (IF) and post selection (OF) curves (blue) correspond to human naive sequences analyzed using the probabilistic model, whereas the red curves correspond to the same human naive sequences analyzed using the deterministic model. The CDR3 length distribution is narrower after selection, indicating selection against too long or too short sequences. **(B)** The relative difference between the SD of CDR3 length/mass between IF sequences and OF sequences (the ratio minus 1), for different samples of human and mice. The blue bars represent the CDR3 length ratio, and the red bars represent the calculation of CDR3 mass ratio (the *p* values of the *F*-test are less than 0.001 except from the mouse blood sample which are less than 0.01). **(C)** The same for the average over length/mass of the CDR3, for different samples of human and mice (the *p* values of the *T*-test are less than 0.001 except from the mouse BM and the mouse blood which are less than 0.1).

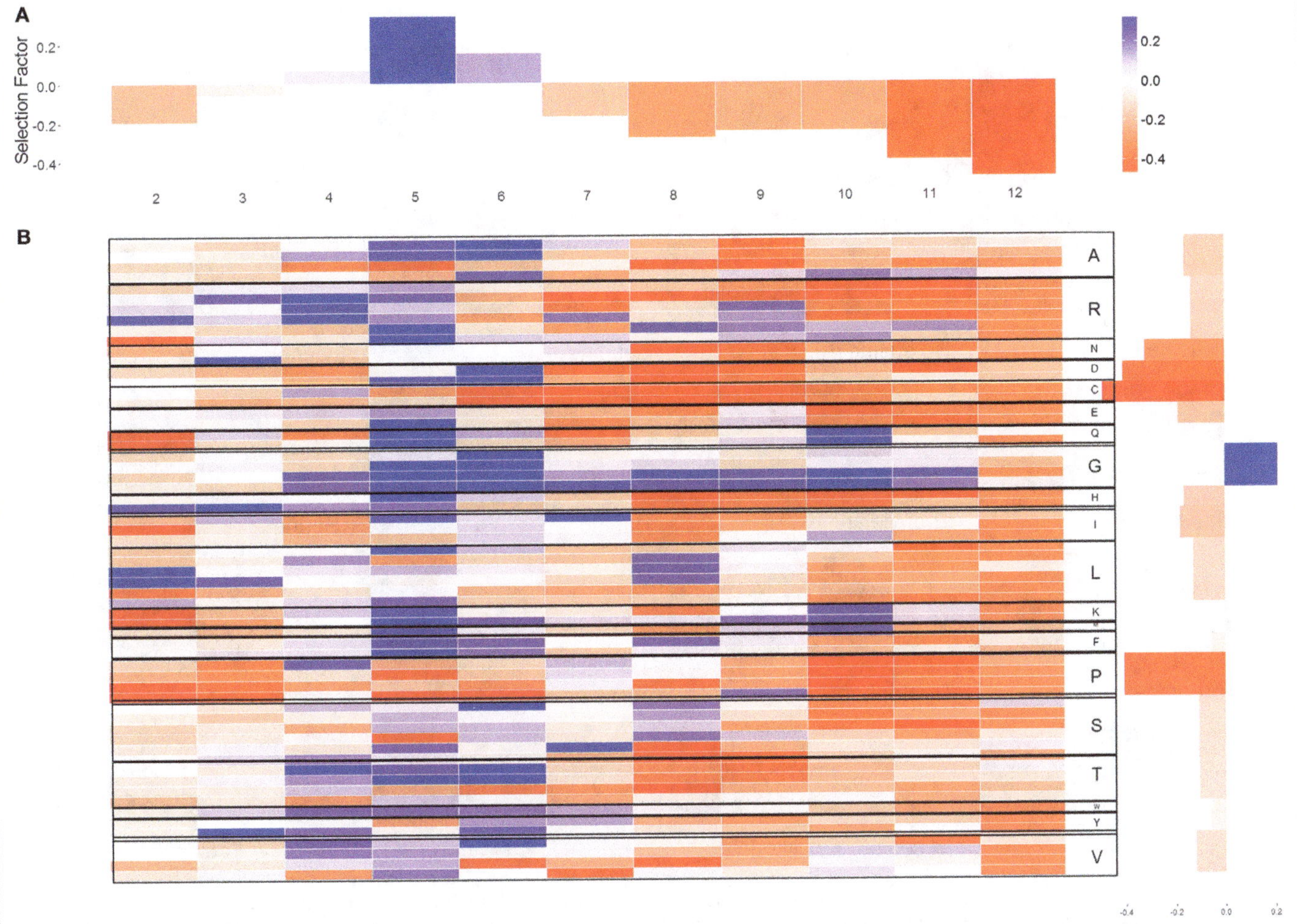


**FIGURE 2** | Selection factors for sequences. **(A)** The average of the $q$-values for each location in CDR3 in log scale [positive selection represented by positive values $\log(q) > 0$ and negative selection represented by negative values $\log(q) < 0$]. **(B)** The $x$-axis represents the different location in CDR3; the $y$-axis represents the different codons. In the right side of the figure, each codon is translated to its amino acid. The blue cells represent $\log(q)$ values larger than 0 for codon in a certain position. The red cells represent $\log(q)$ values lower than 0. The white cells indicate that there was no selection.

distribution width is highly significant. The length distribution for mice shows the same trends ($F$ test $p <$ 1.e−3 for all tests, except for mouse blood where the IF CDR3 lengths are slightly more diverse than OF).

The difference in the human repertoire CDR3 length variance is much larger than in the mouse repertoire. The main reduction in the CDR3 length variability occurs in the human repertoires between the OF and naïve, and not between the naïve and memory, suggesting a pathogen-independent selection for intermediate CDR3 length. While in the mouse repertoire the SD of the length measured in nucleotides did not decrease significantly in the blood, the SD of the total molecular mass of the CDR3 did decrease significantly ($F$ test, $p < 0.01$). The difference suggests that in humans, the total mass of the CDR3 is maintained by limiting the CDR3 length variability, in mouse the result is obtained by balancing large and small amino acids within the CDR3. The simplest explanation for the reduction in the light chain mass variability would be structural selection of the shape of the light chain, where too large or small total mass would prevent the binding to the heavy chain or to potential antigens.

## Selection Is Not Sensitive to Codon Identity

Beyond the length and size of the CDR3 region, the specific composition of the CDR3 affects its selection and production scores. We have used the human kappa chain probabilistic generation and selection models to estimate selection pressures for amino acids and individual codons (**Figures 2** and **3**). This is done using selection factors that measure the selection pressures on the different codons or amino acids, for every position and CDR3 length. These are learned from IF data, such that their combined effect amounts to the difference in amino acid usage from the OF sequences (see Materials and Methods for details). For presentation, the factors were averaged over CDR3 lengths (**Figures 2A,B**), and over codons for the same amino acid (**Figure 3**). We present the log of the selection factor. Selection factors higher than 1 (log

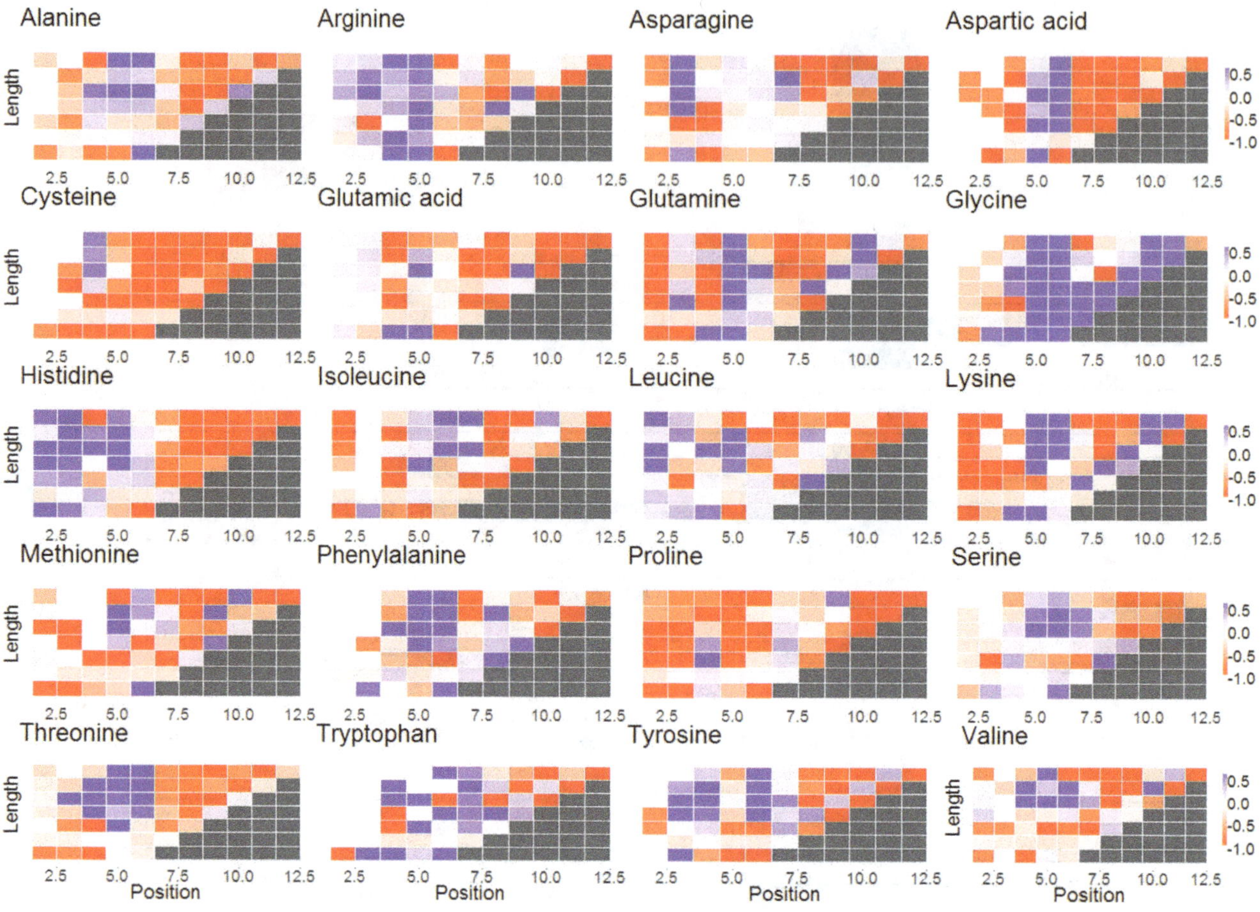


**FIGURE 3** | Subplots of selection factors of different lengths for each amino acid. The *x*-axis represents the different locations in CDR3; the *y*-axis represents the different lengths of the CDR3. The blue cells represent log(*q*) values larger than 0 for codon in a certain position. The red cells represent log(*q*) values lower than 0. The white cells indicate that there was no selection.

higher than 0—blue values in **Figures 2** and **3**) represent positive selection (i.e., sequences containing this codon/AA at this specific position are over-represented compared with the expected from the OF sequences), while factors lower than 1 (log lower than 0—red values in **Figures 2** and **3**) correspond to negative selection.

Different codons coding for the same amino acid have highly similar selection patterns (**Figure 2B**), suggesting that the selection affecting naïve B cell acts on amino acids, and not on codons. Such selection would agree with structural selection on the formed light chain, instead of a genetic mechanism favoring some specific nucleotides in the junctions (the variance of the log selection factors between the codons coding for the same amino acid is 0.154 and the variance between amino acid is 0.372).

## Selection Favoring Glycine and Against Proline, Cysteine, and Aspartic Acid

Selection patterns differ between amino acids. Cysteine (Wilcoxon test, $V = 203$, $p$-value = 4.618e−15), proline ($V = 645$, $p$-value = 1.746e−13), and aspartic acid ($V = 773$, $p$-value = 2.955e−08) clearly undergo negative selection, whereas glycine ($V = 4206$, $p$-value = 1.168e−06) is under positive selection (in almost all locations along the CDR3) (**Figures 2** and **3**). In addition, some amino acids such as histidine and arginine have a positive selection in the beginning of the CDR3 and negative selection on the other side. Proline is unique as an amino acid, since its residue (R) is attached to NH atoms. This special structure breaks (spatially) long-peptide chains. Therefore, it is sometimes used in points of sharp folding of proteins (31). Proline may thus undergo negative selection to avoid the curvature and folding. Similar results were observed in the heavy chain (3).

A similar argument may explain selection against cysteine to prevent disulfide bonds, as is also observed in heavy chain (17). The selection in favor of glycine is the precise opposite with a selection for a tiny (the smallest) AA that has very limited interactions with other AA and a limited effect on the shape of the light chain CDR3 region. We currently have no clear model for the negative selection that observed in the aspartic acid, since its properties are highly Ph sensitive, and we cannot determine in which conditions selection shapes the repertoire.

## Selection Is Mainly Positive in Positions 5–6 of CDR3 and Mainly Negative in the Following Positions

Selection is not uniform along the CDR3. The log of the selection factors are close to 0 in the third amino acid of the CDR3 that is outside the binding site of the antigen ($-0.032 \pm 0.4868$). For most amino acids, positions 5 and 6 undergo a significant positive selection, showing a clear deviation in favor of rare amino acids (correlation between the log of the selection factor of position 5 with the AA frequency is 0.329, correlation with position 6 is 0.249), exactly at the beginning of the antigen binding site [5th position—(29)]. From positions 7 to 12, on the opposite site of the binding site, a significant negative selection can be observed for most amino acids apart from glycine and in specific positions also alanine, lysine, and glutamine, suggesting that long sequences are quite restrictive in this area, which ties in with the fact that long CDR3 are generally selected against as discussed above (these positions only exist in long CDR3 that are selected against).

For some amino acids, selection is length and position dependent, while for others, it is almost constant. Specifically, certain amino acids undergo different selection when close to the ends of the CDRs, in contrast to the middle (see, for example, alanine or aspartic acid in **Figure 3**). Other amino acids have positive or negative selection in almost all lengths and positions (glycine and cysteine and proline, respectively) in agreement with previous results (17). Note that this selection occurs in the naive repertoire, and it is thus probably not driven by pathogens.

## DISCUSSION

Immunoglobulin genes are created in a stochastic V(D)J recombination process that is function independent. The distribution of possible receptors is not uniform; there is large variability in the generation probability of different elements of the rearrangement [e.g., V(D)J choice, junctional composition]. Beyond these differences, there are differences between the naïve repertoire and the one directly emerging from the rearrangement process.

A possible reason for this last difference may be the relation between the biochemical properties of the receptor and its potential binding to antigens. Such binding is mainly associated with the properties of the variable peptide chain of the CDR3. Many of the sequences generated might not code for receptor proteins that could potentially bind antigen. Some form of selection could then act to purify the generated repertoire into the functional one, observed in the naïve pool in the periphery. For example, there could be positive selection for binding self-antigens.

Here, we explored this notion of initial selection by analyzing the difference between the properties of IF and OF light chain rearrangements in naïve and memory repertoires, in human and mouse cells using probabilistic and deterministic generation models. An important advantage of the light chain repertoire analysis is the absence of the D gene, drastically simplifying the rearrangement process.

We have shown that selection acts mainly on the CDR3 rather than on the templated part of the V and J genes. Within the CDR3, selection tends to limit the variance of the CDR3 size in both human and murine repertoires in the transition from the direct rearrangement process to the naïve repertoire. These variances decrease by more than 45% during this transition. Interestingly, while in human light chains, the variance reduction is mainly through the removal of light chains with a low or high number of nucleotides in the CDR3, in mice the reduction is through a change in the distribution of amino acids in the CDR3, making it more restrictive. The reduction in CDR3 length variance was mainly observed between the repertoire emerging from the rearrangement and the naïve repertoire and not between the latter and memory, suggesting the vast majority of the structural selection occurs in the bone marrow, and is not pathogen driven.

In humans, amino acids affecting the structure of the CDR3 region, such as proline, are selected against, while tiny amino acids such as glycine are favored. Similar preferences have been observed in the heavy chain (18).

A correlation has been observed between the production probability of each amino acid and its selection in the transition from rearrangement to the naïve pool, suggesting a long-term evolutionary process favoring some junctional amino acids, which are later further selected within a host. Such a behavior has been previously reported in the heavy chain and T cell beta repertoires (17, 18). Selection does not seem to be affected by the codon used, but it is both position and CDR3 length dependent, for some amino acids. Among most amino acids, 5′ regions have higher selection scores than 3′ regions.

All of these elements strongly suggest structural selection where the proper structure of the light chain, and possibly its binding to the heavy chain are selected for. The main selection step has been reported between the OF and the IF naïve repertoire.

The V and J composition of the light chain are not independent. However, this dependence could be the direct result of light chain editing (replacement of non-functional rearrangement by new rearrangements) (14–16). Moreover, differences in the VJ pairing of IF and OF are expected even in the absence of selection, since IF rearrangement are typically made after OF rearrangement, due to repeated light chain rearrangement in the same chromosome, and as such favor more distal VJ combinations (13).

The difference between IF and OF B cell receptor repertoire was argued to highlight properties of B cell receptors associated with diseases or pathogenic challenges. However, current and other recent results (2, 3, 17, 18, 25, 26, 30, 32–37) highlight that the observed naïve repertoire is very different from the direct result of the rearrangement process. Thus, three different repertoires should be defined:

(1) A repertoire produced from rearrangement during the early pro- and pre-B cells stages in the bone marrow.
(2) A naïve repertoire, which is the result of bone marrow selection mechanisms that may be either antigen dependent or independent, and
(3) A memory and plasma-blast repertoire shaped by antigen and possibly pathogen driven selection.

The difference between the last two repertoires seems to be more limited than the difference between the first two. The next challenge will be to develop models to detect within the structurally selected naïve repertoire, BCRs with a potential functional CDR3. Using statistical models of the naïve repertoire that went through the initial structural selection step, we will be able to detect minute differences that indicate selection by exposure to pathogens.

## AUTHOR CONTRIBUTIONS

AM performed analysis, wrote part of manuscript, and produced figures. YE designed and performed probabilistic analysis, and wrote part of manuscript. YL designed analysis and wrote part of manuscript. AW and TM helped writing the analysis and designing the probabilistic model. JB performed the BCR bioinformatics.

## FUNDING

YE, TM, and AW were supported by grant ERCStG no. 306312. YE was supported in part by The V Foundation for Cancer Research Grant D2015-032. YL and AT were supported by ISF grant 98315.

## SUPPLEMENTARY MATERIAL

**TABLE S1** | The samples that were used for each model and their quantity. In subsets of both the mouse data and of the human data, we perform the analysis only on the deterministic model because of small sample sizes.

## REFERENCES


1. Benichou J, Ben-Hamo R, Louzoun Y, Efroni S. Rep-seq: uncovering the immunological repertoire through next-generation sequencing. *Immunology* (2012) 135:183–91. doi:10.1111/j.1365-2567.2011.03527.x
2. Cohen JI, Heijst J, Glanville J, Louzoun Y. Converging evolution leads to near maximal junction diversity through parallel mechanisms in B and T cell receptors. *Phys Biol* (2017) 14(4):045003. doi:10.1088/1478-3975/aa7366
3. Benichou J, Glanville J, Prak ETL, Azran R, Kuo TC, Pons J, et al. The restricted DH gene reading frame usage in the expressed human antibody repertoire is selected based upon its amino acid content. *J Immunol* (2013) 190:5567–77. doi:10.4049/jimmunol.1201929
4. Pallarès N, Frippiat J-P, Giudicelli V, Lefranc M-P. The human immunoglobulin lambda variable (IGLV) genes and joining (IGLJ) segments. *Exp Clin Immunogenet* (1998) 15:8–18. doi:10.1159/000019054
5. Jackson KJL, Wang Y, Gaeta BA, Pomat W, Siba P, Rimmer J, et al. Divergent human populations show extensive shared IGK rearrangements in peripheral blood B cells. *Immunogenetics* (2012) 64:3–14. doi:10.1007/s00251-011-0559-z
6. Watson CT, Steinberg KM, Graves TA, Warren RL, Malig M, Schein J, et al. Sequencing of the human IG light chain loci from a hydatidiform mole BAC library reveals locus-specific signatures of genetic diversity. *Genes Immun* (2015) 16:24–34. doi:10.1038/gene.2014.56
7. Hoi K, Ippolito G. Intrinsic bias and public rearrangements in the human immunoglobulin Vλ light chain repertoire. *Genes Immun* (2013) 14:271–6. doi:10.1038/gene.2013.10
8. Brezinschek HP, Brezinschek RI, Lipsky PE. Analysis of the heavy chain repertoire of human peripheral B cells using single-cell polymerase chain reaction. *J Immunol* (1995) 155:190–202.
9. Schelonka RL, Tanner J, Zhuang Y, Gartland GL, Zemlin M, Schroeder HW. Categorical selection of the antibody repertoire in splenic B cells. *Eur J Immunol* (2007) 37:1010–21. doi:10.1002/eji.200636569
10. Cox JP, Tomlinson IM, Winter G. A directory of human germ-line Vχ segments reveals a strong bias in their usage. *Eur J Immunol* (1994) 24:827–36. doi:10.1002/eji.1830240409
11. Yamada M, Wasserman R, Reichard BA, Shane S, Caton AJ, Rovera G. Preferential utilization of specific immunoglobulin heavy chain diversity and joining segments in adult human peripheral blood B lymphocytes. *J Exp Med* (1991) 173:395–407. doi:10.1084/jem.173.2.395
12. Glanville J, Zhai W, Berka J, Telman D, Huerta G, Mehta GR, et al. Precise determination of the diversity of a combinatorial antibody library gives insight into the human immunoglobulin repertoire. *Proc Natl Acad Sci U S A* (2009) 106:20216–21. doi:10.1073/pnas.0909775106
13. Louzoun Y, Friedman T, Luning Prak E, Litwin S, Weigert M. Analysis of B cell receptor production and rearrangement: part I. Light chain rearrangement. *Semin Immunol* (2002) 14(3):169–90. doi:10.1016/S1044-5323(02)00041-6
14. Luning Prak ET, Monestier M, Eisenberg RA. B cell receptor editing in tolerance and autoimmunity. *Ann N Y Acad Sci* (2011) 1217:96–121. doi:10.1111/j.1749-6632.2010.05877.x
15. Tiegs SL, Russell DM, Nemazee D. Receptor editing in self-reactive bone marrow B cells. *J Exp Med* (1993) 177:1009–20. doi:10.1084/jem.177.4.1009
16. Li Y, Louzoun Y, Weigert M. Editing anti-DNA B cells by Vλx. *J Exp Med* (2004) 199:337–46. doi:10.1084/jem.20031712
17. Elhanati Y, Sethna Z, Marcou Q, Callan CG, Mora T, Walczak AM. Inferring processes underlying B-cell repertoire diversity. *Philos Trans R Soc Lond B Biol Sci* (2015) 370:20140243. doi:10.1098/rstb.2014.0243
18. Elhanati Y, Murugan A, Callan CG, Mora T, Walczak AM. Quantifying selection in immune receptor repertoires. *Proc Natl Acad Sci U S A* (2014) 111:9875–80. doi:10.1073/pnas.1409572111
19. Available from: https://www.ncbi.nlm.nih.gov/bioproject/PRJNA212030
20. Wesemann DR, Portuguese AJ, Meyers RM, Gallagher MP, Cluff-Jones K, Magee JM, et al. Microbial colonization influences early B-lineage development in the gut lamina propria. *Nature* (2013) 501(7465):112–5. doi:10.1038/nature12496
21. Ye J, Ma N, Madden TL, Ostell JM. IgBLAST: an immunoglobulin variable domain sequence analysis tool. *Nucleic Acids Res* (2013) 41:W34–40. doi:10.1093/nar/gkt382
22. Odegard VH, Schatz DG. Targeting of somatic hypermutation. *Nat Rev Immunol* (2006) 6:573–83. doi:10.1038/nri1896
23. Kolaczkowski B, Thornton JW. Performance of maximum parsimony and likelihood phylogenetics when evolution is heterogeneous. *Nature* (2004) 431:980–4. doi:10.1038/nature02917
24. Saitou N, Nei M. The neighbor-joining method: a new method for reconstructing phylogenetic trees. *Mol Biol Evol* (1987) 4:406–25.
25. Liberman G, Benichou J, Tsaban L, Glanville J, Louzoun Y. Multi step selection in Ig H chains is initially focused on CDR3 and then on other CDR regions. *Front Immunol* (2013) 4:274. doi:10.3389/fimmu.2013.00274
26. Yaari G, Benichou JI, Vander Heiden JA, Kleinstein SH, Louzoun Y. The mutation patterns in B-cell immunoglobulin receptors reflect the influence of selection acting at multiple time-scales. *Philos Trans R Soc Lond B Biol Sci* (2015) 370:20140242. doi:10.1098/rstb.2014.0242
27. Liberman G, Benichou JI, Maman Y, Glanville J, Alter I, Louzoun Y. Estimate of within population incremental selection through branch imbalance in lineage trees. *Nucleic Acids Res* (2015) 44:e46–46. doi:10.1093/nar/gkv1198
28. LeBien TW, Tedder TF. B lymphocytes: how they develop and function. *Blood* (2008) 112:1570–80. doi:10.1182/blood-2008-02-078071
29. Available from: https://www.imgt.org/IMGTrepertoire/2D-3Dstruct/FClength/human/Hu_FRlength.html
30. Martin VG, Wu Y-CB, Townsend CL, Lu GH, O'Hare JS, Mozeika A, et al. Transitional B cells in early human B cell development—time to revisit the paradigm? *Front Immunol* (2016) 7:546. doi:10.3389/fimmu.2016.00546
31. MacArthur MW, Thornton JM. Influence of proline residues on protein conformation. *J Mol Biol* (1991) 218:397–412. doi:10.1016/0022-2836(91)90721-H
32. Boyd SD, Marshall EL, Merker JD, Maniar JM, Zhang LN, Sahaf B, et al. Measurement and clinical monitoring of human lymphocyte clonality by massively parallel VDJ pyrosequencing. *Sci Transl Med* (2009) 1:12ra23. doi:10.1126/scitranslmed.3000540

33. Levine MH, Haberman AM, Sant'Angelo DB, Hannum LG, Cancro MP, Janeway CA, et al. A B-cell receptor-specific selection step governs immature to mature B cell differentiation. *Proc Natl Acad Sci U S A* (2000) 97:2743–8. doi:10.1073/pnas.050552997
34. Briney B, Willis J, McKinney B, Crowe J Jr. High-throughput antibody sequencing reveals genetic evidence of global regulation of the naive and memory repertoires that extends across individuals. *Genes Immun* (2012) 13:469. doi:10.1038/gene.2012.20
35. Dunn-Walters DK, Ademokun AA. B cell repertoire and ageing. *Curr Opin Immunol* (2010) 22:514–20. doi:10.1016/j.coi.2010.04.009
36. Wang C, Liu Y, Xu LT, Jackson KJ, Roskin KM, Pham TD, et al. Effects of aging, cytomegalovirus infection, and EBV infection on human B cell repertoires. *J Immunol* (2014) 192:603–11. doi:10.4049/jimmunol.1301384
37. Boyd SD, Gaëta BA, Jackson KJ, Fire AZ, Marshall EL, Merker JD, et al. Individual variation in the germline Ig gene repertoire inferred from variable region gene rearrangements. *J Immunol* (2010) 184:6986–92. doi:10.4049/jimmunol.1000445

# 2

# Predicting Antigen Presentation—What Could we Learn From a Million Peptides?

***David Gfeller*** [1,2]* **and** ***Michal Bassani-Sternberg*** [1,3]*

[1] *Department of Oncology, Ludwig Institute for Cancer Research, University of Lausanne, Lausanne, Switzerland,* [2] *Swiss Institute of Bioinformatics (SIB), Lausanne, Switzerland,* [3] *Department of Oncology, Ludwig Institute for Cancer Research, University Hospital of Lausanne, Lausanne, Switzerland*

***Correspondence:**
*David Gfeller*
*david.gfeller@unil.ch;*
*Michal Bassani-Sternberg*
*michal.bassani@chuv.ch*

Antigen presentation lies at the heart of immune recognition of infected or malignant cells. For this reason, important efforts have been made to predict which peptides are more likely to bind and be presented by the human leukocyte antigen (HLA) complex at the surface of cells. These predictions have become even more important with the advent of next-generation sequencing technologies that enable researchers and clinicians to rapidly determine the sequences of pathogens (and their multiple variants) or identify non-synonymous genetic alterations in cancer cells. Here, we review recent advances in predicting HLA binding and antigen presentation in human cells. We argue that the very large amount of high-quality mass spectrometry data of eluted (mainly self) HLA ligands generated in the last few years provides unprecedented opportunities to improve our ability to predict antigen presentation and learn new properties of HLA molecules, as demonstrated in many recent studies of naturally presented HLA-I ligands. Although major challenges still lie on the road toward the ultimate goal of predicting immunogenicity, these experimental and computational developments will facilitate screening of putative epitopes, which may eventually help decipher the rules governing T cell recognition.

**Keywords: human leukocyte antigen peptidomics, human leukocyte antigen ligand prediction, antigen presentation, T cell epitope, computational immunology**

## INTRODUCTION

Recognition of infected or malignant cells by T cells relies on the presentation of immunogenic self and non-self peptides at the cell surface. Two main pathways have been identified for antigen presentation and processing (1–3).

In the class I pathway, intracellular proteins are degraded into small peptides by the proteasome. These peptides are transported into the endoplasmic reticulum by the transporter associated with antigen processing (TAP) protein complex. There, they can bind to human leukocyte antigen class I (HLA-I) molecules in complex with beta2-microglobulin (β2m). After trafficking to the cell surface, the complexes may be recognized by CD8 T cells. HLA-I proteins are primarily encoded by three genes (HLA-A, HLA-B, and HLA-C), which are widely expressed in most cell types in human. In addition, specialized cell types can express HLA-E, HLA-F, or HLA-G genes. HLA-A, -B, and -C genes (hereafter referred to as HLA-I) are the most polymorphic genes in the human genome and over 12,000 distinct alleles are documented in the human population (4). Humans have in general different combinations of HLA-I alleles and, therefore, express up to six different HLA-I proteins (two for each gene). HLA-I molecules bind short peptides, mainly 9–11 amino acids, and different HLA-I alleles have distinct binding specificities, which implies that a broad spectrum of peptides can be displayed across different individuals.

In the class II pathway, peptides coming from the degradation of phagocytosed extracellular proteins are presented on HLA-II molecules for recognition by CD4 T cells (5). In addition, endogenous proteins can be presented on HLA-II molecules when degraded through autophagy (6). HLA-II proteins are encoded by several genes (HLA-DRA, HLA-DRB1,3,4,5, HLA-DPA1, HLA-DPB1, HLA-DQA1, HLA-DQB1) and also show a very high level of polymorphism in the humans (except for HLA-DRA). HLA-II form heterodimers (HLA-DRA/HLA-DRB1,3,4,5; HLA-DPA1/HLA-DPB1 and HLA-DQA1/HLA-DQB1). These dimers bind longer peptides (12–20 amino acids) within an open-ended peptide-binding site. Several other steps are involved in presentation of class II epitopes, such as loading on HLA-II molecules catalyzed by HLA-DM, peptide exchange catalyzed by HLA-DO, the presence of other enzymes such as cathepsins or pH gradients (7–10). Unlike HLA-I, HLA-II molecules are mainly expressed on specific professional antigen-presenting cells (pAPCs) such as dendritic cells or B cells (1), and rarely also by cancer cells such as melanoma (11). pAPCs can also uptake exogenous antigens and present them on HLA-I (12). This process is called cross-presentation, and it is crucial for priming of naïve T cells (13, 14). Altogether, the cellular antigen processing and presentation machinery ensures that the restrictive loading of either intracellular (class I) or extracellular (class II) peptides of the right length will take place in specialized cellular compartments.

The set of peptides presented on HLA molecules is called the HLA peptidome, also referred to as immunopeptidome or HLA ligandome. The HLA peptidome is a rich and complex repertoire of peptides that inform T cells about abnormalities in the genome, transcriptome, and proteome of infected or malignant cells (15–17). It is constantly modulated by HLA or peptides' source protein expression levels, by posttranslational modifications and by the many enzymes, chaperones, and transporters that comprise the antigen processing and presentation machinery (7, 18–20). In particular, the catalytic subunits of the constitutive proteasome, the immunoproteasome, and the thymic proteasome are tightly regulated, leading to the production of distinct repertoires of presented peptides in different cell types and under different conditions (21–24).

Historically, the study and predictions of class I and class II T cell epitopes have mainly developed in the field of infectious diseases, and large datasets of peptides displayed at the surface of infected cells and recognized by T cells are available from HIV, dengue, or influenza (25, 26). In the field of cancer immunology, tumor-associated antigens (defined here as genes expressed in cancer cells and not, or very poorly, in normal cells) have received much attention for almost 30 years (27). For instance, T cell recognizing specific epitopes of NY-ESO or MAGE-1 proteins can be found in melanoma patients, indicating that the immune system can mount a response against tumor-specific antigens (27–29). More recently, many evidences have been accumulated indicating that cancer cells express unique mutated antigens, the so-called neoantigens, which can be recognized by the patients' own (autologous) T cells (15, 30–35). The total number of somatic mutations in some tumors has been shown to correlate with the therapeutic efficacy of checkpoint blockade antibodies (36–39), suggesting that neoantigens could play an important role in tumor immune recognition. Moreover, several studies demonstrated clinical benefit mediated by the administration of highly enriched populations of neoantigen-reactive $CD4^+$ and $CD8^+$ T cells (34, 40) and by neoantigen-based vaccines (41, 42). Potential neoantigens are typically predicted first by identifying non-synonymous alterations from next generation sequencing data and second by predicting the binding to HLA molecules of peptides encompassing these non-synonymous genetic alterations (43). For these reasons, predictions of peptides presented on HLA-I and HLA-II molecules have gained renewed interest in the field of tumor immunology. Predicted neoantigens need to be then experimentally validated for HLA binding and immune recognition *in vitro* (44–47).

Here, we review approaches developed for predicting antigen presentation in human cells, with a focus on the latest experimental and computational developments to take advantage of in-depth and accurate mass spectrometry (MS) data of HLA peptidomics. Our aim is to describe the main steps of antigen presentation that proved to be successful in making quantitative predictions of antigens. The more biological aspects of antigen presentation and processing are covered in many other reviews (1–3, 8).

## MAIN SOURCES OF HLA LIGAND DATA

A cornerstone in our ability to understand and predict antigen presentation has been the experimental identification of specific peptides interacting with HLA molecules. First, from an experimental point of view, HLA-I molecules do not fold stably in the absence of a ligand and, therefore, all biochemical, structural, and functional studies of HLA-I molecules rely on the availability of known HLA-I ligands. Second, all computational methods to predict HLA ligands at a large-scale use data-driven approaches based on sequence patterns identified within known ligands.

Two main classes of experimental assays have been developed to identify HLA ligands. The first class of assays consists of *in vitro* assays. For HLA-I molecules, refolding assays use conformational pan HLA-I antibodies to test whether the HLA-I complex is properly folded in the presence of a peptide (48–52). Peptide-rescuing assays consist of a photo-cleavable peptide that is stripped by UV radiation in the presence of another peptide (53–55). Competitive assays with radiolabeled peptides have been used to determine relative affinity (IC50) (56). Dissociation assays based on radiolabeled β2m have been used to probe the stability of peptide–HLA-I complexes (57, 58). Surface plasmon resonance techniques can be used to measure actual Kd values (59). *In vitro* binding assays have also been used for HLA-II ligands (60–62). Compared to class I ligands, screening of class II ligands at high throughput is facilitated since HLA-II molecules have an open-ended peptide-binding site. Therefore, peptides can be fixed on plates, which allow for the use of peptide microarrays (63), or directly encoded in different display systems such as phage or yeast display (64, 65).

*In vitro* binding assays play a central role in our ability to identify T cell epitopes from viral or cancer-specific antigens (66, 67). When used in combination with state-of-the art predictions tools, they enable rapid validation of predicted targets and are currently key to most neoantigen discovery approaches in cancer immunotherapy (30, 31, 68, 69). The main caveat of *in vitro* assays for HLA-I ligands is that the peptides have to be determined *a priori* and chemically synthesized, since both the C- and N-terminus of most HLA-I ligands need to be free in most cases. This limits the use of high-throughput and unbiased peptide screening technologies. Furthermore, the involvement of the components of the antigen-loading complex is missing in *in vitro* binding assays and, therefore, signals related to antigen loading *in vivo* cannot be captured.

The second type of experimental assays for HLA ligand identification is based on MS measurement of eluted HLA-binding peptides. This approach is the only methodology to comprehensively interrogate the repertoire of HLA ligands presented naturally *in vivo* (16, 18, 70, 71). The best-established HLA peptidomics methodology is based on immunoaffinity purification (IP) of HLA complexes from detergent solubilized lysates, followed by extraction and purification of the peptides. Typically, either anti-pan-HLA class I, anti-HLA-DR, or anti-pan-HLA class II monoclonal antibodies are used. The extracted peptides are then separated by high-pressure liquid chromatography and directly injected into a mass spectrometer. The resulting spectra obtained from the fragmentation of the peptides are compared with *in silico* generated spectra of peptides from protein sequence databases with MS search tools. Therefore, this search is limited to the available databases, usually the annotated human proteome. Moreover, peptides that have features that make them incompatible with ionization, those that are too hydrophobic or too hydrophilic, might not be detected with standards methods. With the new generation of mass spectrometers, thousands of HLA ligands can be identified per sample (15, 18, 72, 73). Cell lines, including human cancer cell lines, tumors, healthy tissues, and body fluids such as plasma have been subjected to HLA peptidomics analyses (18, 70–84). However, MS-based HLA peptidomics approaches have limited sensitivity and require a relatively large amount of biological sample (~1 $cm^3$ of tissue or $1 \times 10^8$ cells) (21). Furthermore, despite major improvement in the quality of HLA peptidomics data, one can never exclude small residual contaminations from co-eluted peptides or wrong annotation of spectra depending on the false discovery rate threshold used in spectral searches.

Dedicated proteogenomics computational pipelines for customized reference databases have been developed to expand the search space beyond the canonical human proteome. Customizing references to include somatic alterations observed in tumors have been used for direct identification of neoantigens by MS in murine and human cancer cell line models (31, 35, 80, 85), B cell lymphomas (86), and melanoma tissues (15). Similar approaches were also used for other cryptic peptides resulting from unconventional coding sequences in the genome (87) and new open reading frames (88) (see Non-Canonical HLA-I Ligands).

Historically, the first HLA-I motifs (e.g., HLA-A02:01) were found by looking at peptide sequences of eluted ligands identified by MS (89, 90). To overcome the fact that eluted peptides come from up to six HLA-I alleles in unmodified cell lines or tissue samples, two experimental approaches have been developed. The first approach consists of transfecting a soluble HLA allele into a cell line and pulling down only the soluble HLA-I molecules in complex with their ligands (91, 92). While it has been shown that the repertoire of peptides presented on transfected soluble HLA-I and the endogenous membranal HLA-I molecules are highly similar (93), the non-physiological expression level of the soluble HLA-I molecules and the potential different environment in the loading compartment could affect the overall peptide repertoire. Furthermore, endogenous HLA-I alleles can be shaded or naturally secreted from cells in culture (94) and could contaminate the secreted peptidome (75). Nevertheless, this approach proved very powerful to identify HLA-I motifs (77, 78, 95–97). Of particular interest is the study by Di Marco and co-authors where the motifs of 15 HLA-C alleles could be determined, together with motif for HLA-G01:01 (75). This detailed view of HLA-C alleles binding specificities enabled the authors of this study to identify for the first time specificity determinant residues in the HLA-C-binding site that provide likely molecular mechanisms explaining the differences observed between HLA-C binding motifs. The second experimental approach consists of using genetically modified cell lines that express only one allele (98, 99) and was used to study binding motifs of highly similar alleles, like HLA-B27:02 to HLA-B27:09 (100). This approach was also recently used to screen 16 HLA-A and HLA-B alleles, and this work confirmed that predictors trained on MS data could improve predictions of naturally presented HLA-I ligands (70). One advantage of this approach is that theoretically all peptides come from one single allele (see above for potential sources of contaminations). In parallel, we and others introduced computational techniques based on motif deconvolution (72, 101) and peptide clustering (102, 103) to accurately determine HLA-I restriction of eluted ligands from pooled samples without requiring to experimentally isolate each HLA-I allele and without relying on HLA-I ligand predictors (see below for a detailed description of these approaches).

## Comparison of MS and *In Vitro* Data

Until 2012, the number of MS datasets was significantly lower than *in vitro* data (**Figure 1**), which partly explains why *in vitro* binding data were mainly used for training HLA-I ligand predictors. However, the situation has changed quite dramatically over the last 4 years. Combining data from IEDB (25) together with recent HLA peptidomics studies (see Supplementary Material), we can observe that roughly 10 times more unique HLA-I ligands and three times more unique HLA-I–peptide interactions are currently available from MS studies (**Figure 1**, the lower number of interactions than peptides for MS data comes from the fact that several MS samples did not have HLA typing information or allele restriction could not be determined with motif deconvolution). The coverage of HLA-I alleles is also larger in HLA peptidomics samples compared to *in vitro* binding data (**Figure 1**). Moreover, all curves for MS data do not show signs of saturation, suggesting that these numbers are likely to further increase in the coming years, especially with the growing interest in HLA peptidomics profiling of cancer samples from patients with diverse ethnic

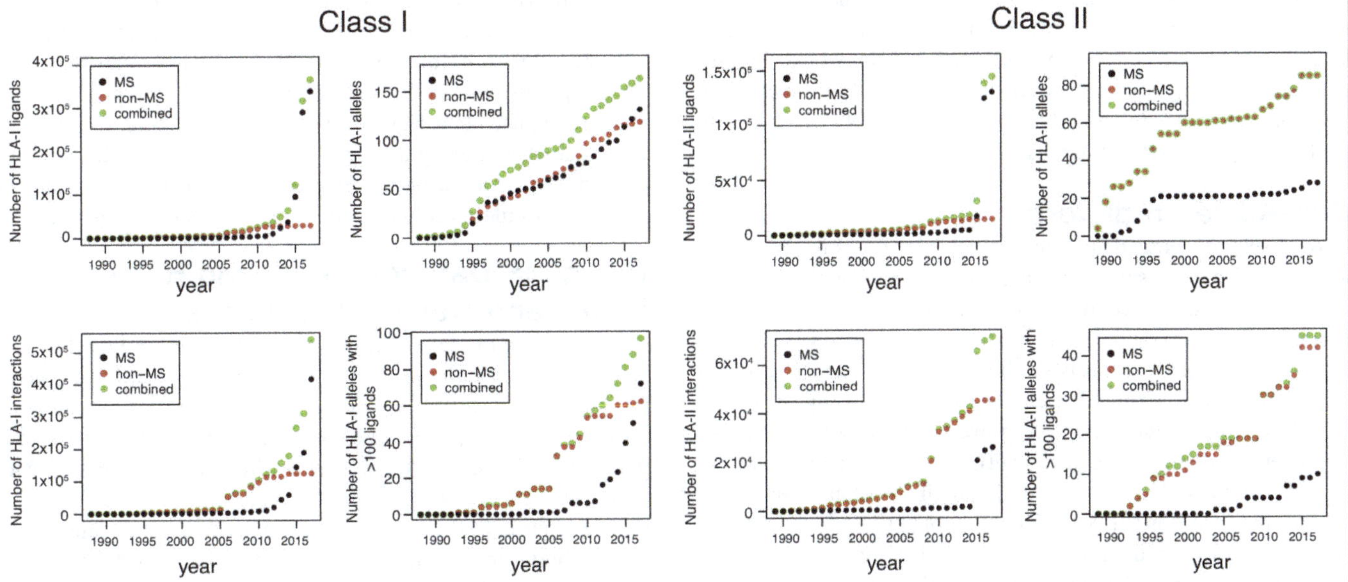


**FIGURE 1** | Analysis of HLA-I and HLA-II ligands obtained from human leukocyte antigen (HLA) peptidomics studies and *in vitro* assays. The number of unique HLA-I ligands, the number of unique interactions, the number of HLA alleles with at least one ligand, and the number of HLA alleles with at least 100 ligands are displayed for both class I and class II, as a function of years (cumulative distributions).

backgrounds for neoantigen discovery (15). Similar observations hold for HLA-II ligands, where the number of unique peptides identified by MS largely exceeds the number of peptides identified in *in vitro* assays. However, the number of HLA-II alleles with documented ligands is still larger for *in vitro* binding data. This likely reflects the fact that HLA-II ligands are easier to screen in a high-throughput way using peptide microarrays, and that allele restriction in HLA-II peptidomics data is still more difficult to determine with motif deconvolution or peptide clustering than for HLA-I peptidomics data.

## MODELING HLA-I BINDING SPECIFICITY

### Allele-Specific Predictors

Modeling HLA-I-binding specificity has been carried out for almost 30 years since the first evidence of HLA-I motifs. Early studies used simple sequence motifs [e.g., xLxxxxxx(L/V) for HLA-A02:01]. However, as more data started to accumulate, it became clear that simple motifs were too restrictive and not quantitative enough. To overcome these limitations, position weight matrices (PWM) (equally referred to as Position Specific Scoring Matrices or simply scoring matrices) were introduced (104–107). The basic idea is to compute the frequency of each amino acid at each position in a set of (pre-aligned) peptides. The score of a new peptide can then be computed by multiplying the PWM entries corresponding to the sequence of the new peptide (see Supplementary Material). Although the idea of computing amino acid frequencies is relatively simple to understand, several steps are important when building a predictor based on PWMs. First, one has to consider the amino acid background distribution and use this distribution to renormalize the scores (see Supplementary Material). In most existing approaches, amino acid frequencies of the human proteome have been used. However, this approach may not be fully justified when using viral epitopes to train predictors. Similarly, eluted HLA-I ligands do not show the same amino acid distribution as human proteins and much lower frequency of cysteine has been reported by ourselves and others (70, 72). As such, the optimal choice of background distribution may depend on the origin (both biological and technical) of the data. Second, in most cases, estimating the frequency of amino acids occurring only a few times (or never) at a given position is highly susceptible to statistical noise. To address this issue, pseudo-counts are often used. A widely used approach is based on the BLOSUM62 matrix (see Supplementary Material) (105, 108, 109). Third, biases due to the design of specific experiments can be found in many *in vitro* datasets. For instance, if a mutagenesis was carried out at a fairly non-specific position in a given epitope, many sequences will have identical amino acids at all positions except the one used in the mutagenesis. One way to correct for such biases is to add a weight to all peptides that is inversely proportional to the number of highly similar sequences in the dataset (see Supplementary Material).

Since the last decade, most allele-specific HLA-I ligand predictors use machine learning frameworks such as neural networks, hidden Markov Models, support vector machines, or convolutional neural networks (110–114). One attractive aspect of these models is the ability to consider potential correlations between different positions within HLA-I ligands. For instance, we recently observed in HLA-B07:02 ligands that arginine is preferred at P3 or at P6, but not at both positions at the same time (101). This type of correlation is not captured by simple PWMs. However, it is still unclear how frequent these correlations are for HLA-I ligands. In particular, although many studies reported improved predictions of HLA-I ligands using machine learning algorithms (112, 115), one has to be careful before concluding that correlation patterns are prevalent, since improvement in prediction accuracy may also result from more robust regularization frameworks. Finally, machine learning approaches are also susceptible to overfitting and correcting for potential biases in training sets can be more challenging than with simple PWMs.

## Pan-Allele Predictors

Enough experimental ligands are available for roughly 100 HLA-I alleles, which represents only a small fraction of the >12,000 HLA-I alleles observed in the human population. To address this issue, pan-allele predictors have been introduced, where the input of the algorithm consists of both the sequence of the ligand and the sequence of the HLA-I allele (or of its binding site) (107, 116–118). These algorithms are powerful at capturing correlations between amino acids in the HLA-I-binding site and in the ligand. The most widely used and likely the most elaborate pan-specific algorithm is the NetMHCpan tool (117), which includes several features specific for HLA-I molecules, such as combining peptides of different lengths in the training and incorporating peptide length preferences.

**Table 1** summarizes some of the most common predictors, together with information about the algorithm that is used, the type of training data and the output.

## Choosing the Right Training Set

While extensive work has been performed to optimize the algorithms used in HLA-I predictors, less attention has been devoted to the choice of the training set. Prior to 2016, most approaches aimed at predicting binding affinity values (i.e., IC50) and, therefore, were trained on *in vitro* data mainly obtained from IEDB (25). Although high accuracy could be reached for many common alleles, several potential biases suggest that such data can be suboptimal for training predictors. In particular, it is important to remember that most HLA-I ligands tested *in vitro* for binding were first predicted with older versions of HLA-I ligand predictors [some exceptions that used random peptide libraries include Ref. (58)]. Unfortunately, this can induce circularity when using these data to retrain predictors, and such biases are difficult to detect and correct for. Of note, the same circularity issue can also affect several published MS datasets when HLA-I ligand predictors or motifs were used to assign allele restriction and filter noise. Here, we argue that high-quality MS data not filtered with existing predictors provide a powerful solution toward overcoming the potential circularity inherent to many *in vitro* binding data.

## Using MS Data for Identifying HLA-I Motifs and Training Predictors

Mono-allelic samples or transfected soluble HLA-I alleles have been used since many years to study the binding motifs of specific HLA-I molecules (91, 92). However, due the experimental work implied by such approaches, they were never applied to a large panel of HLA-I alleles [the largest studies consist of 16 alleles for mono-allelic cell lines (70) and 17 alleles for transfected soluble HLA-I alleles (75)]. For pooled HLA peptidomics dataset, the impossibility to experimentally assign allelic restriction was often considered as an important hurdle to use such data toward studying HLA-I-binding motifs.

However, in the last few years, it became clear that pooled HLA peptidomics data can be used to study HLA-I motifs and improve predictions, thereby overcoming the need of genetically modifying cell lines or transfecting soluble HLA-I alleles. The first attempt to determine HLA-I-binding motifs from pooled HLA peptidomics data was published in 2015 (18). A year later, we published the first evidence that such data can be used to improve predictions of HLA-I ligands (101). Since then, many studies have confirmed these results both for the identification of new motifs (72, 81, 102, 103, 119) and for improving predictions of HLA-I ligands by integrating MS data in the training of predictors (70, 72, 117, 120).

As of today, two algorithms have been used for motif deconvolution and peptide clustering of pooled HLA peptidomics data. One of them (MixMHCp) is based on mixture models and was initially developed for multiple specificity analysis in large PDZ

**TABLE 1** | Summary of some of the most recent or most widely used human leukocyte antigen (HLA)-I predictors with available web interface or code repository.

| Name | Training data | Output | Algorithm | Allele coverage | Access | Reference |
|---|---|---|---|---|---|---|
| NetMHC4.0 | BA | BA | NN | S | http://www.cbs.dtu.dk/services/NetMHC/ | (110) |
| NetMHCpan4.0 | BA + MS | R (BA) | NN | Pan | http://www.cbs.dtu.dk/services/NetMHCpan-4.0/ | (117) |
| MixMHCpred | MS | R | PWM | S | https://github.com/GfellerLab/MixMHCpred | (72, 120) |
| MHCflurry | BA | BA | NN | S | https://github.com/openvax/mhcflurry | (113) |
| PickPocket | BA | BA | PWM | Pan | http://www.cbs.dtu.dk/services/PickPocket/ | (107) |
| NetMHCstabpan | BS | BS | NN | Pan | http://www.cbs.dtu.dk/services/NetMHCstabpan/ | (118) |
| NetMHCstab | BS | BS | NN | S | http://www.cbs.dtu.dk/services/NetMHCstab/ | (111) |
| NetMHCcons | BA | BA | C | S | http://www.cbs.dtu.dk/services/NetMHCcons/ | (181) |
| IEDB consensus | BA | R | C | S | http://tools.iedb.org/mhci/ | (182) |
| SMMPMBEC | BA | R | PWM | S | https://github.com/ykimbiology/smmpmbec | (104) |
| MHCnuggets | BA | BA | NN | S | https://github.com/KarchinLab/mhcnuggets-2.0 | (183) |
| ConvMHC | BA | R | NN | Pan | http://jumong.kaist.ac.kr:8080/convmhc | (116) |
| HLA-CNN | BA | R | NN | S | https://github.com/uci-cbcl/HLA-bind | (114) |
| SYFPEITHI | BA + MS | R | PWM | S | http://syfpeithi.de/0-Home.htm | (106) |
| PSSMHCpan | BA | BA | PWM | Pan | https://github.com/BGI2016/PSSMHCpan | (184) |

*Column 2, BA, binding affinity; BS, binding stability; MS, HLA peptidomics data; column 3, BA, binding affinity; R, ranking; column 4, NN, Neural network (including deep networks); PWM, position weight matrices; C, consensus; column 5, S, allele specific; Pan, pan-class I.*

or SH3 ligand datasets obtained by phage display (121–123). In this framework, the idea is to let the algorithm infer K distinct PWMs that optimally model the eluted peptides (101). Since peptides identified by MS come from K different HLA-I alleles ($K \leq 6$), it is not surprising that the motifs that optimally describe the data correspond precisely to the specificity of these alleles. The other algorithm (GibbsCluster) is based on simulated annealing to group the peptides into different clusters optimizing a global cost function that models how well each peptide fits into its respective cluster (103, 124). Somehow unexpectedly, both algorithms were initially developed for other purposes (i.e., multiple specificity analysis for MixMHCp and simultaneous clustering and alignments of short peptides for GibbsCluster) and their use for motif identification in HLA peptidomics data was realized only later (18, 101, 102). The two approaches have many conceptual similarities since the likelihood function optimized in MixMHCp differs only slightly from the cost function optimized in GibbsCluster. In practice, the two algorithms lead most of the time to very similar results for HLA-I peptidomics data (101) and nearly identical motifs as those obtained from mono-allelic samples or transfected soluble alleles (72) (see also examples in Figure S1 in Supplementary Material). In some cases, as we have reported, the mixture model tends to be slightly more sensitive to identify motifs supported by few peptides, such as those describing HLA-C alleles (101). Conversely, the GibbsCluster has several advantages, such as the ability to combine peptides of different lengths and the simultaneous clustering and alignment of the peptides (which is critical for HLA-II ligands) (102, 103). Both methods can be used as command line or through webservers (see http://www.mixmhcp.org and http://www.cbs.dtu.dk/services/GibbsCluster-2.0/). The availability of these algorithms strongly supports the notion that allele assignment in MS data should not be done based on HLA-I ligand predictors, since this may remove all peptides that are not well modeled with existing predictors, and hence bias determination of motifs and prevent improving the predictors. It is also important to emphasize that accurate motif deconvolution requires a large number of peptides, and ideally, many samples to test the robustness of the motifs (72). For this reason, it is likely the combination of higher accuracy and throughput of MS instruments (18) together with these novel algorithms that enabled accurate HLA-I motifs identification in pooled HLA peptidomics data.

Annotation of the motifs deconvolved from pooled HLA peptidomics data can be done in different ways. For alleles for which a reasonable description of the motifs is known, one can simply compare the motifs found in MS data to the known references (18). Using Euclidean distance to quantify the similarity between the PWMs appears to provide stable results and most of the time the mapping is quite obvious (72, 101). If the motifs are not known, two approaches have been developed. One fully unsupervised approach was proposed by ourselves based on cooccurrence of HLA-I alleles across different samples (72). In this way, we could identify and annotate HLA-I motifs for more than 40 alleles, including 7 alleles that had no experimental ligands at the time of this study. Another semi-supervised approach that works well in most cases consists of comparing with motifs predicted from pan-allele predictors such as NetMHCpan (119).

An important limitation of motif deconvolution approaches comes from the fact that motifs for some alleles (especially HLA-C alleles) are more difficult to detect in many samples. Also, in the presence of highly similar motifs (e.g., HLA-A23:01 and HLA-A24:02, or HLA-C07:01 and HLA-C07:02), the two motifs often cannot be split (72). Because of this, not all HLA peptidomics datasets are appropriate for training predictors for each allele expressed in the corresponding sample. This limitation can be alleviated by considering large collections of HLA peptidomics studies and focusing on cases where the motifs are clearly visible and can be unambiguously annotated (72). Finally, it is sometimes useful to consider more motifs than the number of alleles in order to identify motifs for each allele (Figure S2 in Supplementary Material).

**Figures 2–4** summarize the HLA-A, HLA-B, and HLA-C motifs currently available by combining motifs deconvolved from recent MS studies together with IEDB data (see Supplementary Material). As expected, the clustering based on the similarity between the motifs (see Supplementary Material) broadly recapitulates the supertype assignment for HLA-A and HLA-B alleles and helps highlighting differences among alleles classified within the same supertypes.

## Biases in MS Data

While MS data are not suffering from the potential circularity present in many *in vitro* binding data, they are not free from any biases. First, as already mentioned, only peptides that are part of the database used for spectral searches can be detected in HLA peptidomics data, or else, the less accurate *de novo* method may be applied. This has direct implication for cysteine-containing peptides. Since this amino acid can be chemically modified by oxidation and as such modifications are typically not included in standard MS searches, cysteine occurs at very low frequency in HLA peptidomics datasets. Attempts to correct for this bias when training predictors tried to renormalize PWMs based on observed amino acid frequencies at non-anchor positions (72) or expand the MS spectral search to include modified cysteines (70). Second, peptides that are too hydrophobic or too hydrophilic might be missed applying the common purification methods that rely on retaining peptides through hydrophobic interactions with the solid phase. Furthermore, some peptides have features that make them incompatible with ionization or lead to poor fragmentation. Combining fragmentation methods, such as higher-energy collision-induced dissociation and electron-transfer dissociation, have been shown to improve spectra annotation of HLA peptides (73). Despite these limitations, inspection of HLA peptidomics data and comparison with motifs obtained from *in vitro* data did not reveal major differences, except for the low frequency of cysteine [slightly higher frequency of charged amino acids at some positions has been reported in some studies (101, 102)]. Third, immuno-purification based MS data cannot distinguish between HLA-I ligands presented on the cell surface from those resident in the ER. This can be achieved by purifying HLA-I peptides from the cell surface by mild acid elution (125, 126). However, in a head-to-head comparison, the IP method outperformed the mild acid elution in terms of peptide recovery (127). Last, when considering MS

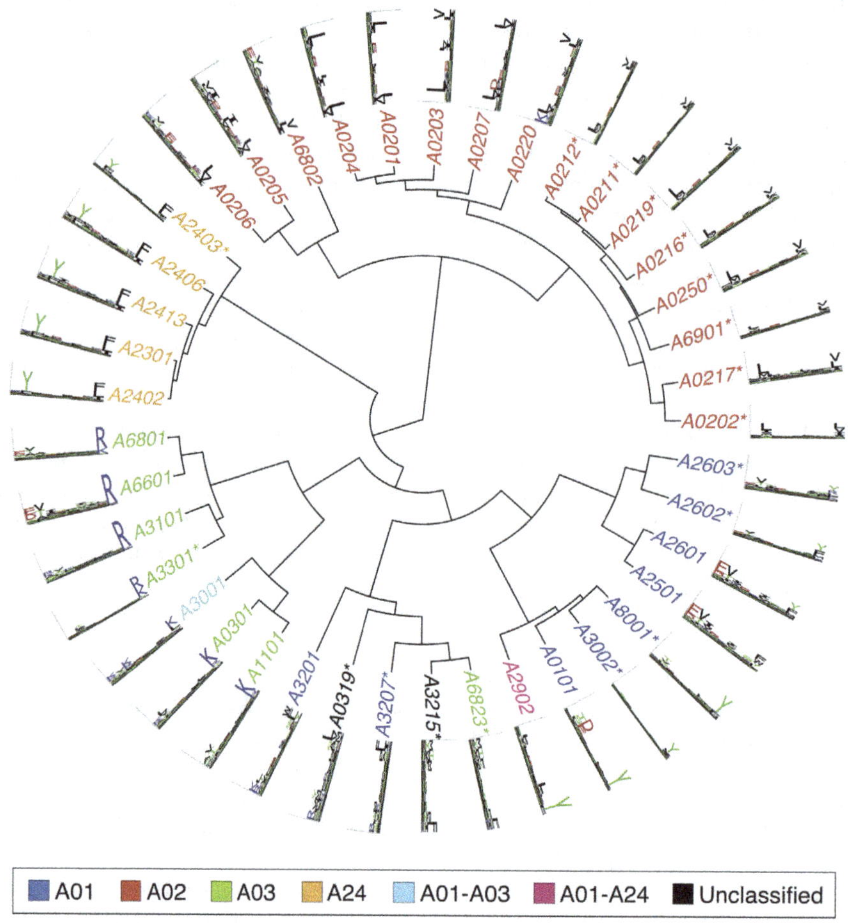


**FIGURE 2** | Hierarchical clustering of HLA-A alleles based on their binding specificity. Stars indicate cases where only *in vitro* binding data were available to generate the motifs. In all other cases, only mass spectrometry data were used. Name colors and their descriptions in the legend indicate supertypes as defined in Ref. (185).

data, it is important to remember that these peptides come from human proteins and that proteins or domains within proteins can display significant homology (especially for class II ligands where in addition many peptides can originate from the same core region). This can artificially enhance the frequency of some amino acids. This issue is especially important when building random models of MS data to infer whether amino acid frequencies (either within a motif or at flanking regions) differ from what is expected by chance.

## MODELING HLA-II-BINDING SPECIFICITY

Predictions of HLA-I ligands, especially with the recent incorporation of high-quality MS data in the training of predictors, have reached a high level of accuracy (70, 72, 117, 120). The situation is unfortunately not the same for HLA-II ligands, which are still much more difficult to predict despite the large amount of experimental data acquired over the years (**Figure 1**). Several challenges arise when modeling the binding specificity of HLA-II alleles. First, HLA-II alleles tend to have more degenerate and less specific motifs. Second, all current approaches rely on first aligning peptides with tools such as NN-align (128). Although these tools have been optimized to handle HLA-II ligands, automated alignment of small peptides is known to be a difficult computational problem. Finally, the fact that HLA-II molecules form dimers further increases the diversity for HLA-DP and HLA-DQ alleles where both members of the dimers are polymorphic. Allele-specific HLA-II ligand predictors include NetMHCII (129), ProPred Singh (130), MHCPred (131), TEPITOPE (132), and consensus methods (133). Pan-specific class II predictors mainly consist of NetMHCIIpan (129). While all these predictors show better than random performances, their accuracy is lower than for HLA-I ligand predictors. This may be due to the challenges of determining class II motifs, as well as to the complex machinery of class II presentation, whose specificity is still poorly understood from a quantitative and predictive point of view [see Ref. (7–10) for a detailed discussion of the more biological aspects of this process and the importance of HLA-DM and other enzymes]. In particular, it appears that properties such as conformational flexibility play a role in loading onto HLA-II molecules (134), and these properties are difficult to predict directly from peptide sequences.

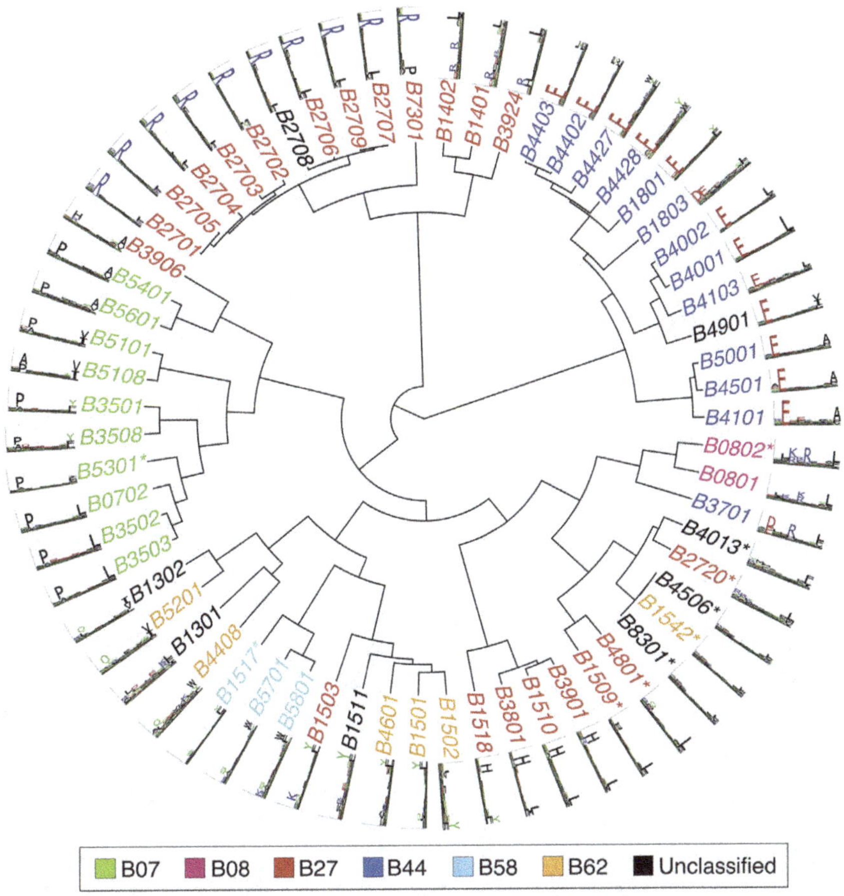


**FIGURE 3** | Hierarchical clustering of HLA-B alleles based on their binding specificity. Stars indicate cases where only *in vitro* binding data were available to generate the motifs. In all other cases, only mass spectrometry data were used. Name colors and their description in the legend indicate supertypes as defined in Ref. (185).

Whether similar improvement for class II predictions as for class I will be reached by incorporating class II peptidome data in the training of algorithms has not been investigated at a large scale. Nevertheless, it has been recognized already long ago that eluted ligands could provide important information about HLA-II-binding motifs (135). More recently, HLA-II peptidomics was performed in BALB/c and C57BL/6 mice and demonstrated that clear motifs for H-2 I-Ad and H-2 I-Ab could be obtained (136). A subsequent study suggested that predictors trained on these data perform better than NetMHCIIpan when repredicting the MS data (137). A similar strategy was carried out in transgenic DR1+ and DR15+ mice to identify the motifs of these two alleles (138). Recent studies also indicate that motif deconvolution with the GibbsCluster algorithm may work in pooled HLA-II peptidome datasets (21, 139), which could lead to refinement of HLA-II motifs and improved predictions in the coming years, as suggested in a recent preprint (140). However, the results are still more challenging to interpret and some motifs predicted by GibbsCluster are difficult to annotate, while the motifs for some alleles are sometimes not detected (21, 139, 141).

## INVESTIGATING OTHER PROPERTIES OF HLA–PEPTIDE INTERACTIONS

Many other important properties of HLA-I molecules beyond the 9-mer-binding motifs themselves can be studied through the analysis of HLA peptidomics data.

### Peptide Length Distribution

Arguably, the most important information beyond the binding motifs that can be extracted from MS data is the characterization of peptide length distributions. Many studies have demonstrated high heterogeneity of peptide length distributions between different alleles, with alleles such as HLA-B51:01 displaying high frequency of 8-mers (only slightly smaller than 9-mers) and very few longer peptide, while others such as HLA-A01:01 show high frequency of longer (≥12 amino acids) peptides, which can still be recognized by T cells (15, 70, 97, 103, 142). Structurally, most longer peptides are known to form bulges, with anchor residues conserved at the second and last positions of the peptides. Some patterns emerged from analysis of peptide length distributions. For instance, HLA-I alleles with anchor residues at middle

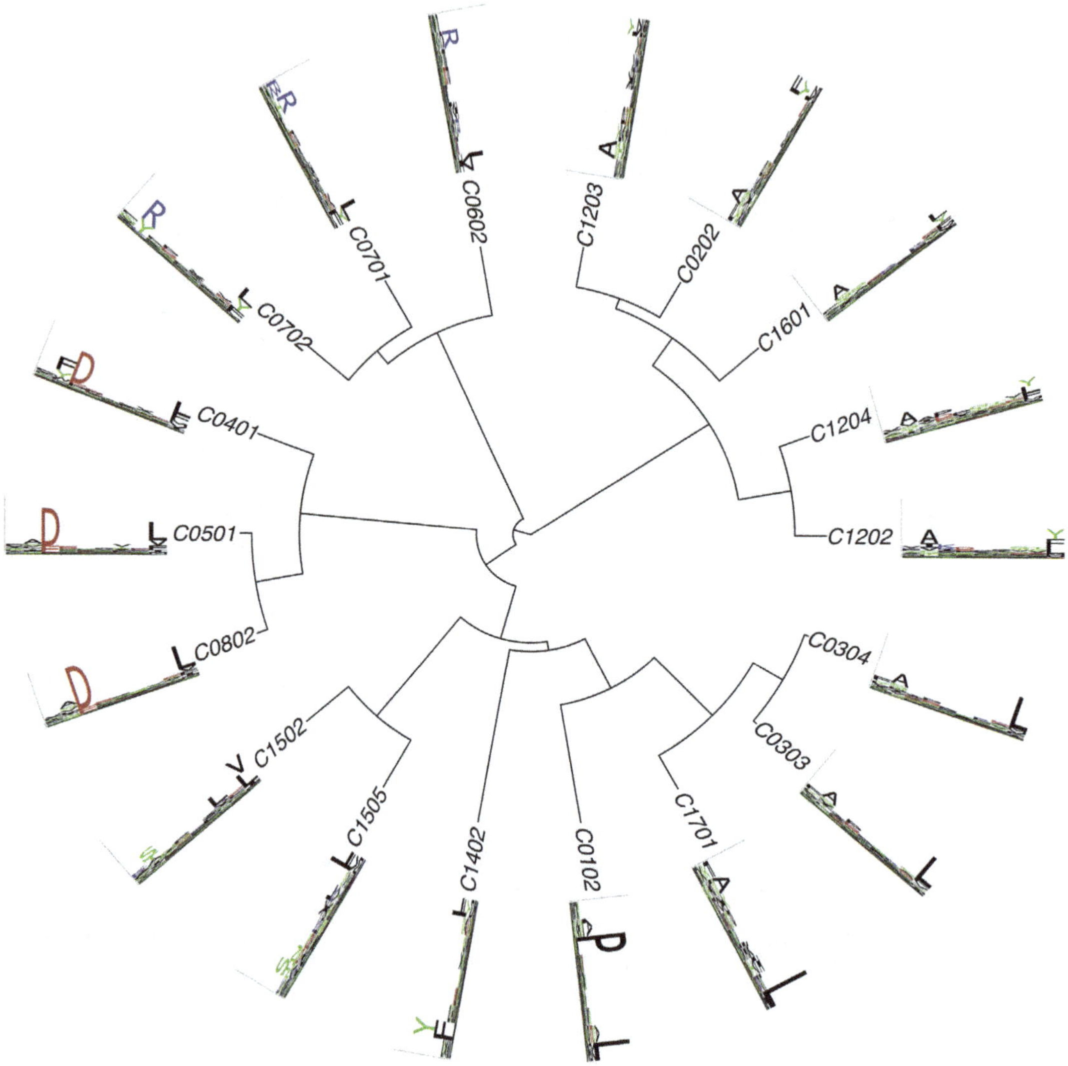


**FIGURE 4** | Hierarchical clustering of HLA-C alleles based on their binding specificity. Only mass spectrometry data were used. Peptides from both single allele and deconvolved pooled HLA peptidomics samples were used (see Supplementary Material).

positions (e.g., HLA-B08:01, HLA-B14:01, HLA-B14:02, HLA-B37:01) displayed peptide length distributions peaked at 9-mers, which is consistent with the fact that the middle anchor residue needs to be structurally conserved in the presence of an anchor at such positions (101). The study by Trolle and co-authors (97) demonstrated that peptide length distributions observed in MS data for five alleles could not be simply explained by differences in binding affinity, suggesting that the pool of peptides available for loading in the ER is skewed toward 9-mers. This likely implies that predictors trained on MS data will differ from those predicting binding affinity when comparing peptides of different lengths. In a recent preprint (143), we performed a large-scale analysis of peptide length distributions across 85 HLA-I alleles and could identify clusters of HLA-I molecules based on the similarity of their peptide length distributions. Peptide length distribution has been incorporated into the latest versions of NetMHC and NetMHCpan, by adding one additional input node encoding for peptide length in the neural networks (110, 117), and into MixMHCpred by directly fitting distributions observed in MS data (143).

As observed in our recent paper (21), peptide length distribution can also be affected by different treatments such as INFγ likely due to modulating the activity of catalytic subunits of the proteasome, and these aspects are not captured by existing predictors.

## C- And N-Terminal Extensions

Human leukocyte antigen peptidomics data have been instrumental in exploring non-canonical binding modes in HLA-I ligands. In particular, several recent studies have used MS data to study C- and N-terminal extensions in HLA-I ligands. Although such extensions had been identified long ago [first crystal structure in 1994 (144), PDB:2CLR, followed by another structure in 2009 (145), PDB:3GIV], their prevalence had remained unclear.

In 2016, HLA peptidomics profiling and X-ray crystallography were combined to explore C-terminal extensions in HLA-A02:01 and demonstrated that such extensions were especially common among peptides originating from pathogens (146). This was followed by additional work that better described the structural mechanisms and cellular origin of such extensions (147). N-terminal extensions have been identified in HLA-B57:01 (148) and HLA-B58:01 (149). More recently, we have demonstrated that C-terminal extension occur in a substantial fraction of HLA-I molecules and can be recognized by CD8 T cells (120). Our work further enabled us to identify both sequence and structural features predictive of such extensions. In particular, it appeared that C-terminal extensions are especially frequent in alleles displaying specificity for positively charged residues at the last anchor position (e.g., HLA-A03:01, HLA-A31:01, HLA-A68:01). While MS data potentially provide a rich source of information about C- and N-terminal extensions, identifying these extensions by looking at the sequence of the peptides can be challenging, especially when the residue at the extension has similar specificity as the anchor residue (i.e., same residues at P9 and P10 for putative C-terminal extensions, same residues a P2 and P3 for putative N-terminal extensions). Our work suggests that many ambiguous cases may actually follow the bulging conformation (120).

### Posttranslationally Modified HLA-I Ligands

Posttranslationally modified peptides have been identified by MS analysis of eluted ligands (15, 150–152). These include mainly phosphorylated peptides, which can be recognized by T cells (153–155). Phosphorylation was observed to occur mainly at position 4 (15), suggesting that it does not impact too much the binding to the HLA-I molecules. Existing HLA-I ligand predictors do not include phosphorylated peptides, although the increasingly larger MS datasets of phosphorylated HLA-I ligands suggest that predictions of phosphorylated HLAI ligands may soon become feasible. As for now, one approach is to treat the phosphorylated residue as its unmodified counterpart and use available predictors to predict such ligands.

### HLA-II Molecules

Fewer studies used MS data to investigate properties of HLA-II molecules other than the actual-binding motifs. Studies reported broad peptide length distributions peaked around 15-mers (15, 21, 139, 156, 157), but it is still unclear to what extent distinct alleles show distinct peptide length distributions. Other properties of HLA-II molecules that could be studied based on MS data include the cellular origin of class II peptides (156, 158, 159) and the impact of different biological processes such as autophagy (160). MS studies also indicated preference for proline at the second and second to last position of peptides degraded in the endolysosomal pathway (156, 161), and preference for lysine at the C-terminus and for aspartate at the N-terminally flanking residue of class II epitopes degraded in the cytosolic pathway (156). Along these lines, many studies support the idea that presentation of class II peptides is not only driven by the binding specificity to the HLA-II molecules but also involves some (still uncharacterized) specificity in the processing machinery, flanking regions (162), or presentation hotspots in the human proteome (159).

Considering the increasingly higher quality and throughput of class II HLA peptidomics data (15, 21, 86, 138, 139), we anticipate that analysis of HLA-II peptidomes will further enable researchers to investigate new properties of HLA-II molecules. For instance, it will be interesting to see whether the presence of bulging class II ligands, as recently reported from an analysis of *in vitro* binding data (163), can be confirmed in large-scale unbiased MS data.

## ANTIGEN PRESENTATION—BEYOND BINDING TO HLA

### Integrating Cleavage Site and TAP Transport Predictions, Signals from Flanking Regions and Other Proteomic Information

Mass spectrometry-based HLA peptidomics analysis can reveal crucial information about the rules underlying the biogenesis of the HLA peptidome, including signatures of cleavage site specificity, influence of source protein expression or other patterns characterizing naturally presented HLA ligands. Predictions of cleavage sites have been available since many years and have been used to narrow-down the list of predicted HLA-I ligands (164). Although some improvement has been observed, cleavage site predictions have only a limited effect on prediction accuracy of naturally presented HLA ligands. For this reason, it is not widely used in many existing pipelines for neoantigen predictions from exome sequencing data, for instance. Predictions of TAP transport has also been integrated with affinity and cleavage site predictions to model antigen presentation (165–167). Interrogation of properties of thousands of HLA-I ligands source-proteins has revealed that the proteome is not randomly sampled. Several biological determinants correlate with presentation, such as level of translation (71), expression, and turnover rate (18) and selective regions of the human proteome (71). Specific amino acid signals in flanking regions of naturally presented HLA-I ligands, like lower frequency of proline, have also been demonstrated (70). While binding to HLA still appears to be the most selective step of class I antigen presentation, integrating these additional features into a single predictor further improves the accuracy of predictions of naturally presented peptides (70, 71).

### Presentation Hotspots

After deep interrogation of HLA peptidomics large scale data, we and others have recently suggested that HLA ligands are not randomly distributed along the protein sequences but are located within "hotspots" (15, 71), which fit proteasomal cleavage, peptide processing, and HLA-binding rules (168). Recently, we envisioned that these hotspots reflect regions of proteins with enhanced proteasomal or endosomal peptide production prior to HLA loading and may, therefore, provide complementary information to HLA-binding predictions (159). To this end, we collected a large dataset of MS detected HLA class I and class

II ligands from different cancer and healthy tissues and variety of cell lines. We used this dataset to score potential neoantigens based on how well their un-mutated source proteins are naturally presented. In a proof of concept study, we tested this hypothesis with published data (33) and could show that MS-based features improved the prioritization of confirmed neoepitopes (159). Large scale databases of HLA peptidomics data capture the global nature of the *in vivo* peptidome averaged over many HLA alleles and, therefore, reflect the propensity of peptides to be presented, which can complement binding-affinity predictions.

## FUTURE PERSPECTIVES

### Expanding the Description of HLA Motifs

Accurate and unbiased binding motifs are available for a bit more than 100 HLA-I alleles (**Figures 1–4**). This is only a tiny fraction of the >12,000 HLA-I alleles listed in IMGT/HLA database (4). For this reason, much has still to be learned about the specificity of HLA-I molecules. We anticipate that the ability to deconvolve HLA-I motifs from pooled HLA peptidomics data will play an important role to expand our understanding of HLA-I-binding specificities. This is especially promising in light of the current interest in using MS to identify neoantigens in cancer patients. However, even with the current efforts in HLA peptidomics, extrapolation of the curves in **Figure 1** suggests that experimentally determined HLA-I ligands will remain available for only a small fractions of HLA-I alleles in the coming years. For this reason, development of pan-specific HLA-I ligand predictors leveraging high-quality MS data available for a few (~100) alleles to model the binding specificity of other alleles are expected to play an important role in broadening the scope of HLA-I ligand predictions to rarer alleles without document ligands (117). Accurate and in-depth HLA peptidomics data will also likely play an important role in improving our understanding and description of HLA-II motifs. Use of HLA-II gene-specific antibodies (i.e., pan-DR, pan-DP, or pan-DQ) may facilitate accurate motif deconvolution in such datasets.

### Better Understanding of Antigen Presentation

While binding to HLA molecules is the most specific and best quantitatively characterized step of the antigen presentation process, it is likely that some additional filtering comes from cleavage in the proteasome, transport with TAP, and loading in the ER. As mentioned earlier, several recent studies suggest that including these additional parameters further improves prediction accuracy (70, 71, 159, 166). One of the challenges there is to disentangle real biological signals from potential technical biases in MS data. Despite this caveat, it is likely that accumulating very large datasets of naturally presented HLA-I ligands is the only way to improve the accuracy of models of antigen presentation that go beyond the binding to HLA molecules. In addition, it could provide new information about how the HLA peptidome can be remodeled in response to extracellular signals, such as IFNγ stimulation (19, 21). We, therefore, envision that screening how inhibition or activation of components of the antigen processing and presentation affect the nature of naturally presented HLA ligands on a large scale may reveal their role in shaping the HLA peptidome.

### Non-Canonical HLA-I Ligands

Increasing evidences also suggest that non-canonical and cryptic peptides contribute to the HLA peptidome and expand the range of putative T cell epitopes. Laumont et al. have constructed a reference database of stop-to-stop translation products of six open reading frames of expressed RNAs and revealed that about 10% of the peptidome derive from presumably noncoding genomic sequences or exonic out-of-frame translation (87). Liepe et al. have reported that around 30% of the peptidome is derived from non-contiguous peptides spliced by the proteasome (169). Unexpectedly, spliced peptides displayed significantly lower predicted affinity than the normal peptides identified in the same samples (169) and did not show the expected HLA-I motifs. A very large database that is about two orders of magnitude larger than the typical protein-coding database was used to incorporate theoretical spliced products (169). Searching such large databases, especially in order to identify HLA peptides that have no enzymatic restrictions, may lead to improper control of false positives (170). In a recent preprint (171), we proposed an alternative, more conservative, approach to identify spliced peptides among HLA-I ligands based on *de novo* interpretation of high-quality spectra, suggesting that the number of such peptides may have been overestimated in the original study. The exact amount of spliced HLA-I ligands is still a matter of debate, and further studies will be needed to precisely estimate the fraction of spliced peptides actually displayed on HLA-I molecules. However, these potential issues suggest that putative spliced peptides may not all be appropriate for training HLA-I ligand predictors. Exploring non-canonical HLA ligands derived from translation of non-conventional regions in our genome or posttranslation events such as splicing is like finding a needle in a haystack. *In silico* predictions of such potential HLA ligands with existing tools may, therefore, lead to in-controlled numbers of false-positives, since the non-canonical space is theoretically orders of magnitude larger than the current canonical protein space. Hence, intensive proteogenomics based investigation of acquired HLA peptidomics data will likely play a central role in this endeavor and will require advanced computational tools and statistics to properly control for false positives.

### Toward Predictions of Immunogenicity

Recent years have witnessed an unprecedented growth of in-depth and accurate MS data (**Figure 1**) that significantly enhanced our ability to predict antigen presentation. Unfortunately, these data cannot inform us about the most critical step in immune recognition, namely, the recognition of presented antigens by T cells. Much less is known there, and it is for instance, a disappointing fact that most predicted neoantigens from mutations found by exome sequencing of tumors are not recognized by T cells, although many resulting peptides do bind to HLA-I molecules. While direct identification of mutated peptides presented on the surface of cancer cells will likely improve the fraction of truly immunogenic epitopes (101), it is likely that many mutated peptides seen by MS will still not be immunogenic. Moreover, although binding affinity has been demonstrated to be useful for enriching pools of peptide in immunogenic epitopes (especially for class I), many known immunogenic epitopes display low-binding affinity, suggesting that they would be missed by approaches based on affinity predictions only. This is especially true for class II epitopes, where clear evidences indicate that different enzymes, peptide exchange mediates by HLA-DM or HLA-DO, pH gradients and peptide conformational flexibility play a role in selecting immunodominant epitopes (8–10, 134). Unfortunately, currently, very little of this biological knowledge about class II antigen presentation could be used to improve predictions of class II epitopes.

Work by Calis et al. (172) suggested that some amino acids at non-anchor positions confer increased immunogenicity to HLA-I ligands. More recently, it has been observed that dissimilarity to self among mutated peptides predicted to have similar binding affinity as their wild-type counterpart can further help predicting immunogenic epitopes (173). Differences between the affinity of the wild-type and the mutated peptide, as well as stability of the MHC-I peptide interaction were also suggested to narrow down the list of immunogenic epitopes (174). Unfortunately, datasets of true immunogenic peptides from cancer or infectious diseases are still restricted to a few 100 peptides, limiting the power of machine learning approaches to infer properties of immunogenic epitopes (175, 176). This is likely the main bottleneck toward our understanding of the determinants of immunogenicity. Therefore, recent high-throughput methods for screening T cells using for instance DNA barcoded multimers have the potential to provide critical information about the differences between immunogenic and non-immunogenic peptides (46). Importantly, most of these approaches require to select *a priori* the HLA ligands to be screened [with the exception of a recent phage display system (177)]. Therefore, improved prediction of HLA ligands and antigen presentation will likely play an important role in optimizing the set of ligands currently tested for immunogenicity.

## CONCLUSION

The first HLA-I motifs were described almost 30 years ago by looking at sequences obtained from MS analysis of eluted MHC-I ligands (89, 90). Since then, much has been learned about HLA-I and HLA-II molecules through the analysis of their ligands. In human, this has resulted in a detailed description of HLA-I alleles binding specificities for the most common alleles and culminated with the development of pan-allele predictors. Recent years have witnessed an explosion of new high-quality data generated by MS about HLA-I ligands. Combined with advances in algorithms to analyze such data, this has led to refinement of known HLA-I motifs, discovery of new HLA-I motifs, characterization of peptide length distributions, analysis of N- and C-terminal extensions, characterization of antigen processing signals in flanking regions, analysis of the interplay between gene/protein expression, protein localization and peptide presentation, and evidences for presentation hotspots in the human proteome. For HLA-II ligands, MS studies have been recently used to study HLA-II motifs, suggesting that similar improvements may be observed there as well (21, 138–140). Moreover, the current interest in neoantigen discovery will likely result in many more HLA peptidomics datasets from donors with diverse HLA backgrounds and different pathogeneses. This will provide unique opportunities to further improve our understanding of the rules of antigen presentation. To this end, it will be crucial that raw MS data are made publicly available, and that the reporting of HLA peptidomics data will comply with the recent minimal information about an Immuno-Peptidomics Experiment (MIAIPE) guidelines (178). Databases such as IEDB (25), PRIDE (179), or the SysteMHC Atlas (180) play a key role in this process, and it is our hope that soon all journals publishing HLA peptidomics studies will require deposition of the raw MS data in PRIDE and unfiltered lists of peptides in appropriate databases, or at least accessible in supplementary datasets.

## AUTHOR CONTRIBUTIONS

DG and MB-S designed the review and wrote the manuscript. DG analyzed the data and prepared the figures.

## ACKNOWLEDGMENTS

We thank Julien Racle for insightful comments about the manuscript. DG is supported by the Swiss Cancer League (KFS-4104-02-2017-R).

## REFERENCES

1. Neefjes J, Jongsma MLM, Paul P, Bakke O. Towards a systems understanding of MHC class I and MHC class II antigen presentation. *Nat Rev Immunol* (2011) 11:823–36. doi:10.1038/nri3084
2. Blum JS, Wearsch PA, Cresswell P. Pathways of antigen processing. *Annu Rev Immunol* (2013) 31:443–73. doi:10.1146/annurev-immunol-032712-095910
3. Vyas JM, Van der Veen AG, Ploegh HL. The known unknowns of antigen processing and presentation. *Nat Rev Immunol* (2008) 8:607–18. doi:10.1038/nri2368
4. Robinson J, Halliwell JA, Hayhurst JD, Flicek P, Parham P, Marsh SGE. The IPD and IMGT/HLA database: allele variant databases. *Nucleic Acids Res* (2015) 43:D423–31. doi:10.1093/nar/gku1161
5. Roche PA, Furuta K. The ins and outs of MHC class II-mediated antigen processing and presentation. *Nat Rev Immunol* (2015) 15:203–16. doi:10.1038/nri3818
6. Crotzer VL, Blum JS. Autophagy and its role in MHC-mediated antigen presentation. *J Immunol* (2009) 182:3335–41. doi:10.4049/jimmunol.0803458
7. Yin L, Maben ZJ, Becerra A, Stern LJ. Evaluating the role of HLA-DM in MHC class II-peptide association reactions. *J Immunol* (2015) 195:706–16. doi:10.4049/jimmunol.1403190
8. Kim A, Sadegh-Nasseri S. Determinants of immunodominance for CD4 T cells. *Curr Opin Immunol* (2015) 34:9–15. doi:10.1016/j.coi.2014.12.005
9. Sadegh-Nasseri S, Kim A. MHC class II auto-antigen presentation is unconventional. *Front Immunol* (2015) 6:372. doi:10.3389/fimmu.2015.00372

10. Sadegh-Nasseri S. A step-by-step overview of the dynamic process of epitope selection by major histocompatibility complex class II for presentation to helper T cells. *F1000Res* (2016) 5:1305. doi:10.12688/f1000research.7664.1
11. Johnson DB, Estrada MV, Salgado R, Sanchez V, Doxie DB, Opalenik SR, et al. Melanoma-specific MHC-II expression represents a tumour-autonomous phenotype and predicts response to anti-PD-1/PD-L1 therapy. *Nat Commun* (2016) 7:10582. doi:10.1038/ncomms10582
12. West MA, Wallin RPA, Matthews SP, Svensson HG, Zaru R, Ljunggren H-G, et al. Enhanced dendritic cell antigen capture via toll-like receptor-induced actin remodeling. *Science* (2004) 305:1153–7. doi:10.1126/science.1099153
13. Ackerman AL, Cresswell P. Cellular mechanisms governing cross-presentation of exogenous antigens. *Nat Immunol* (2004) 5:678–84. doi:10.1038/ni1082
14. Cruz FM, Colbert JD, Merino E, Kriegsman BA, Rock KL. The Biology and underlying mechanisms of cross-presentation of exogenous antigens on MHC-I molecules. *Annu Rev Immunol* (2017) 35:149–76. doi:10.1146/annurev-immunol-041015-055254
15. Bassani-Sternberg M, Bräunlein E, Klar R, Engleitner T, Sinitcyn P, Audehm S, et al. Direct identification of clinically relevant neoepitopes presented on native human melanoma tissue by mass spectrometry. *Nat Commun* (2016) 7:13404. doi:10.1038/ncomms13404
16. Caron E, Kowalewski DJ, Chiek Koh C, Sturm T, Schuster H, Aebersold R. Analysis of major histocompatibility complex (MHC) immunopeptidomes using mass spectrometry. *Mol Cell Proteomics* (2015) 14:3105–17. doi:10.1074/mcp.M115.052431
17. Vaughan K, Xu X, Caron E, Peters B, Sette A. Deciphering the MHC-associated peptidome: a review of naturally processed ligand data. *Expert Rev Proteomics* (2017) 14:729–36. doi:10.1080/14789450.2017.1361825
18. Bassani-Sternberg M, Pletscher-Frankild S, Jensen LJ, Mann M. Mass spectrometry of human leukocyte antigen class I peptidomes reveals strong effects of protein abundance and turnover on antigen presentation. *Mol Cell Proteomics* (2015) 14:658–73. doi:10.1074/mcp.M114.042812
19. Caron E, Vincent K, Fortier M-H, Laverdure J-P, Bramoullé A, Hardy M-P, et al. The MHC I immunopeptidome conveys to the cell surface an integrative view of cellular regulation. *Mol Syst Biol* (2011) 7:533. doi:10.1038/msb.2011.68
20. Fortier M-H, Caron E, Hardy M-P, Voisin G, Lemieux S, Perreault C, et al. The MHC class I peptide repertoire is molded by the transcriptome. *J Exp Med* (2008) 205:595–610. doi:10.1084/jem.20071985
21. Chong C, Marino F, Pak H, Racle J, Daniel RT, Müller M, et al. High-throughput and sensitive immunopeptidomics platform reveals profound interferonγ-mediated remodeling of the human leukocyte antigen (HLA) ligandome. *Mol Cell Proteomics* (2018) 17:533–48. doi:10.1074/mcp.TIR117.000383
22. Ferrington DA, Gregerson DS. Immunoproteasomes: structure, function, and antigen presentation. *Prog Mol Biol Transl Sci* (2012) 109:75–112. doi:10.1016/B978-0-12-397863-9.00003-1
23. Kincaid EZ, Murata S, Tanaka K, Rock KL. Specialized proteasome subunits have an essential role in the thymic selection of CD8(+) T cells. *Nat Immunol* (2016) 17:938–45. doi:10.1038/ni.3480
24. Robek MD, Garcia ML, Boyd BS, Chisari FV. Role of immunoproteasome catalytic subunits in the immune response to hepatitis B virus. *J Virol* (2007) 81:483–91. doi:10.1128/JVI.01779-06
25. Vita R, Overton JA, Greenbaum JA, Ponomarenko J, Clark JD, Cantrell JR, et al. The immune epitope database (IEDB) 3.0. *Nucleic Acids Res* (2015) 43:D405–12. doi:10.1093/nar/gku938
26. Weiskopf D, Yauch LE, Angelo MA, John DV, Greenbaum JA, Sidney J, et al. Insights into HLA-restricted T cell responses in a novel mouse model of dengue virus infection point toward new implications for vaccine design. *J Immunol* (2011) 187:4268–79. doi:10.4049/jimmunol.1101970
27. van der Bruggen P, Traversari C, Chomez P, Lurquin C, De Plaen E, Van den Eynde B, et al. A gene encoding an antigen recognized by cytolytic T lymphocytes on a human melanoma. *Science* (1991) 254:1643–7. doi:10.1126/science.1840703
28. Reuschenbach M, von Knebel DM, Wentzensen N. A systematic review of humoral immune responses against tumor antigens. *Cancer Immunol Immunother* (2009) 58:1535–44. doi:10.1007/s00262-009-0733-4
29. Simpson AJG, Caballero OL, Jungbluth A, Chen Y-T, Old LJ. Cancer/testis antigens, gametogenesis and cancer. *Nat Rev Cancer* (2005) 5:615–25. doi:10.1038/nrc1669
30. Bobisse S, Genolet R, Roberti A, Tanyi JL, Racle J, Stevenson BJ, et al. Sensitive and frequent identification of high avidity neo-epitope specific CD8 + T cells in immunotherapy-naive ovarian cancer. *Nat Commun* (2018) 9:1092. doi:10.1038/s41467-018-03301-0
31. Carreno BM, Magrini V, Becker-Hapak M, Kaabinejadian S, Hundal J, Petti AA, et al. A dendritic cell vaccine increases the breadth and diversity of melanoma neoantigen-specific T cells. *Science* (2015) 348:803–8. doi:10.1126/science.aaa3828
32. Gros A, Parkhurst MR, Tran E, Pasetto A, Robbins PF, Ilyas S, et al. Prospective identification of neoantigen-specific lymphocytes in the peripheral blood of melanoma patients. *Nat Med* (2016) 22:433–8. doi:10.1038/nm.4051
33. Strønen E, Toebes M, Kelderman S, van Buuren MM, Yang W, van Rooij N, et al. Targeting of cancer neoantigens with donor-derived T cell receptor repertoires. *Science* (2016) 352:1337–41. doi:10.1126/science.aaf2288
34. Tran E, Turcotte S, Gros A, Robbins PF, Lu Y-C, Dudley ME, et al. Cancer immunotherapy based on mutation-specific CD4+ T cells in a patient with epithelial cancer. *Science* (2014) 344:641–5. doi:10.1126/science.1251102
35. Yadav M, Jhunjhunwala S, Phung QT, Lupardus P, Tanguay J, Bumbaca S, et al. Predicting immunogenic tumour mutations by combining mass spectrometry and exome sequencing. *Nature* (2014) 515:572–6. doi:10.1038/nature14001
36. Le DT, Uram JN, Wang H, Bartlett BR, Kemberling H, Eyring AD, et al. PD-1 blockade in tumors with mismatch-repair deficiency. *N Engl J Med* (2015) 372:2509–20. doi:10.1056/NEJMoa1500596
37. Rizvi NA, Hellmann MD, Snyder A, Kvistborg P, Makarov V, Havel JJ, et al. Cancer immunology. Mutational landscape determines sensitivity to PD-1 blockade in non-small cell lung cancer. *Science* (2015) 348:124–8. doi:10.1126/science.aaa1348
38. Snyder A, Makarov V, Merghoub T, Yuan J, Zaretsky JM, Desrichard A, et al. Genetic basis for clinical response to CTLA-4 blockade in melanoma. *N Engl J Med* (2014) 371:2189–99. doi:10.1056/NEJMoa1406498
39. Van Allen EM, Miao D, Schilling B, Shukla SA, Blank C, Zimmer L, et al. Genomic correlates of response to CTLA-4 blockade in metastatic melanoma. *Science* (2015) 350:207–11. doi:10.1126/science.aad0095
40. Tran E, Robbins PF, Lu Y-C, Prickett TD, Gartner JJ, Jia L, et al. T-cell transfer therapy targeting mutant KRAS in cancer. *N Engl J Med* (2016) 375:2255–62. doi:10.1056/NEJMoa1609279
41. Ott PA, Hu Z, Keskin DB, Shukla SA, Sun J, Bozym DJ, et al. An immunogenic personal neoantigen vaccine for patients with melanoma. *Nature* (2017) 547:217–21. doi:10.1038/nature22991
42. Sahin U, Derhovanessian E, Miller M, Kloke B-P, Simon P, Löwer M, et al. Personalized RNA mutanome vaccines mobilize poly-specific therapeutic immunity against cancer. *Nature* (2017) 547:222–6. doi:10.1038/nature23003
43. Gfeller D, Bassani-Sternberg M, Schmidt J, Luescher IF. Current tools for predicting cancer-specific T cell immunity. *Oncoimmunology* (2016) 5:e1177691. doi:10.1080/2162402X.2016.1177691
44. Andersen RS, Thrue CA, Junker N, Lyngaa R, Donia M, Ellebæk E, et al. Dissection of T-cell antigen specificity in human melanoma. *Cancer Res* (2012) 72:1642–50. doi:10.1158/0008-5472.CAN-11-2614
45. Bentzen AK, Hadrup SR. Evolution of MHC-based technologies used for detection of antigen-responsive T cells. *Cancer Immunol Immunother* (2017) 66:657–66. doi:10.1007/s00262-017-1971-5
46. Bentzen AK, Marquard AM, Lyngaa R, Saini SK, Ramskov S, Donia M, et al. Large-scale detection of antigen-specific T cells using peptide-MHC-I multimers labeled with DNA barcodes. *Nat Biotechnol* (2016) 34:1037–45. doi:10.1038/nbt.3662
47. Linnemann C, van Buuren MM, Bies L, Verdegaal EME, Schotte R, Calis JJA, et al. High-throughput epitope discovery reveals frequent recognition of neo-antigens by CD4+ T cells in human melanoma. *Nat Med* (2015) 21:81–5. doi:10.1038/nm.3773
48. Elvin J, Cerundolo V, Elliott T, Townsend A. A quantitative assay of peptide-dependent class I assembly. *Eur J Immunol* (1991) 21:2025–31. doi:10.1002/eji.1830210909
49. Harndahl M, Rasmussen M, Røder G, Dalgaard Pedersen I, Sørensen M, Nielsen M, et al. Peptide-MHC class I stability is a better predictor than

peptide affinity of CTL immunogenicity. *Eur J Immunol* (2012) 42:1405–16. doi:10.1002/eji.201141774

50. Sidney J, Assarsson E, Moore C, Ngo S, Pinilla C, Sette A, et al. Quantitative peptide binding motifs for 19 human and mouse MHC class I molecules derived using positional scanning combinatorial peptide libraries. *Immunome Res* (2008) 4:2. doi:10.1186/1745-7580-4-2
51. Townsend A, Elliott T, Cerundolo V, Foster L, Barber B, Tse A. Assembly of MHC class I molecules analyzed in vitro. *Cell* (1990) 62:285–95. doi:10.1016/0092-8674(90)90366-M
52. Wulf M, Hoehn P, Trinder P. Identification of human MHC class I binding peptides using the iTOPIA- epitope discovery system. *Methods Mol Biol* (2009) 524:361–7. doi:10.1007/978-1-59745-450-6_26
53. Bakker AH, Hoppes R, Linnemann C, Toebes M, Rodenko B, Berkers CR, et al. Conditional MHC class I ligands and peptide exchange technology for the human MHC gene products HLA-A1, -A3, -A11, and -B7. *Proc Natl Acad Sci U S A* (2008) 105:3825–30. doi:10.1073/pnas.0709717105
54. Hadrup SR, Toebes M, Rodenko B, Bakker AH, Egan DA, Ovaa H, et al. High-throughput T-cell epitope discovery through MHC peptide exchange. *Methods Mol Biol* (2009) 524:383–405. doi:10.1007/978-1-59745-450-6_28
55. Rodenko B, Toebes M, Hadrup SR, van Esch WJE, Molenaar AM, Schumacher TNM, et al. Generation of peptide-MHC class I complexes through UV-mediated ligand exchange. *Nat Protoc* (2006) 1:1120–32. doi:10.1038/nprot.2006.121
56. Sidney J, Southwood S, Moore C, Oseroff C, Pinilla C, Grey HM, et al. Measurement of MHC/peptide interactions by gel filtration or monoclonal antibody capture. *Curr Protoc Immunol.* (2013) 100:18.3.1–36. doi:10.1002/0471142735.im1803s100
57. Harndahl M, Rasmussen M, Røder G, Buus S. Real-time, high-throughput measurements of peptide-MHC-I dissociation using a scintillation proximity assay. *J Immunol Methods* (2011) 374:5–12. doi:10.1016/j.jim.2010.10.012
58. Rasmussen M, Harndahl M, Stryhn A, Boucherma R, Nielsen LL, Lemonnier FA, et al. Uncovering the peptide-binding specificities of HLA-C: a general strategy to determine the specificity of any MHC class I molecule. *J Immunol* (2014) 193:4790–802. doi:10.4049/jimmunol.1401689
59. Miles KM, Miles JJ, Madura F, Sewell AK, Cole DK. Real time detection of peptide-MHC dissociation reveals that improvement of primary MHC-binding residues can have a minimal, or no, effect on stability. *Mol Immunol* (2011) 48:728–32. doi:10.1016/j.molimm.2010.11.004
60. Justesen S, Harndahl M, Lamberth K, Nielsen L-LB, Buus S. Functional recombinant MHC class II molecules and high-throughput peptide-binding assays. *Immunome Res* (2009) 5:2. doi:10.1186/1745-7580-5-2
61. Salvat R, Moise L, Bailey-Kellogg C, Griswold KE. A high throughput MHC II binding assay for quantitative analysis of peptide epitopes. *J Vis Exp* (2014) (85):e51308. doi:10.3791/51308
62. Yin L, Stern LJ. Measurement of peptide binding to MHC class II molecules by fluorescence polarization. *Curr Protoc Immunol.* (2014) 106:5.10.1–12. doi:10.1002/0471142735.im0510s106
63. Gaseitsiwe S, Valentini D, Mahdavifar S, Reilly M, Ehrnst A, Maeurer M. Peptide microarray-based identification of *Mycobacterium tuberculosis* epitope binding to HLA-DRB1*0101, DRB1*1501, and DRB1*0401. *Clin Vaccine Immunol* (2010) 17:168–75. doi:10.1128/CVI.00208-09
64. Hammer J, Takacs B, Sinigaglia F. Identification of a motif for HLA-DR1 binding peptides using M13 display libraries. *J Exp Med* (1992) 176:1007–13. doi:10.1084/jem.176.4.1007
65. Jiang W, Boder ET. High-throughput engineering and analysis of peptide binding to class II MHC. *Proc Natl Acad Sci U S A* (2010) 107:13258–63. doi:10.1073/pnas.1006344107
66. Rajasagi M, Shukla SA, Fritsch EF, Keskin DB, DeLuca D, Carmona E, et al. Systematic identification of personal tumor-specific neoantigens in chronic lymphocytic leukemia. *Blood* (2014) 124:453–62. doi:10.1182/blood-2014-04-567933
67. Robbins PF, Lu Y-C, El-Gamil M, Li YF, Gross C, Gartner J, et al. Mining exomic sequencing data to identify mutated antigens recognized by adoptively transferred tumor-reactive T cells. *Nat Med* (2013) 19:747–52. doi:10.1038/nm.3161
68. Castle JC, Kreiter S, Diekmann J, Löwer M, van de Roemer N, de Graaf J, et al. Exploiting the mutanome for tumor vaccination. *Cancer Res* (2012) 72:1081–91. doi:10.1158/0008-5472.CAN-11-3722
69. Kreiter S, Castle JC, Türeci Ö, Sahin U. Targeting the tumor mutanome for personalized vaccination therapy. *Oncoimmunology* (2012) 1:768–9. doi:10.4161/onci.19727
70. Abelin JG, Keskin DB, Sarkizova S, Hartigan CR, Zhang W, Sidney J, et al. Mass spectrometry profiling of HLA-associated peptidomes in mono-allelic cells enables more accurate epitope prediction. *Immunity* (2017) 46:315–26. doi:10.1016/j.immuni.2017.02.007
71. Pearson H, Daouda T, Granados DP, Durette C, Bonneil E, Courcelles M, et al. MHC class I-associated peptides derive from selective regions of the human genome. *J Clin Invest* (2016) 126:4690–701. doi:10.1172/JCI88590
72. Bassani-Sternberg M, Chong C, Guillaume P, Solleder M, Pak H, Gannon PO, et al. Deciphering HLA-I motifs across HLA peptidomes improves neo-antigen predictions and identifies allostery regulating HLA specificity. *PLoS Comput Biol* (2017) 13:e1005725. doi:10.1371/journal.pcbi.1005725
73. Mommen GPM, Frese CK, Meiring HD, van Gaans-van den Brink J, de Jong APJM, van Els CACM, et al. Expanding the detectable HLA peptide repertoire using electron-transfer/higher-energy collision dissociation (EThcD). *Proc Natl Acad Sci U S A* (2014) 111:4507–12. doi:10.1073/pnas.1321458111
74. Dargel C, Bassani-Sternberg M, Hasreiter J, Zani F, Bockmann J-H, Thiele F, et al. T cells engineered to express a T-cell receptor specific for glypican-3 to recognize and kill hepatoma cells in vitro and in mice. *Gastroenterology* (2015) 149:1042–52. doi:10.1053/j.gastro.2015.05.055
75. Di Marco M, Schuster H, Backert L, Ghosh M, Rammensee H-G, Stevanović S. Unveiling the peptide motifs of HLA-C and HLA-G from naturally presented peptides and generation of binding prediction matrices. *J Immunol* (2017) 199:2639–51. doi:10.4049/jimmunol.1700938
76. Gloger A, Ritz D, Fugmann T, Neri D. Mass spectrometric analysis of the HLA class I peptidome of melanoma cell lines as a promising tool for the identification of putative tumor-associated HLA epitopes. *Cancer Immunol Immunother* (2016) 65:1377–93. doi:10.1007/s00262-016-1897-3
77. Guasp P, Alvarez-Navarro C, Gomez-Molina P, Martín-Esteban A, Marcilla M, Barnea E, et al. The peptidome of Behçet's disease-associated HLA-B*51:01 includes two subpeptidomes differentially shaped by endoplasmic reticulum aminopeptidase 1. *Arthritis Rheumatol* (2016) 68:505–15. doi:10.1002/art.39430
78. Hilton HG, McMurtrey CP, Han AS, Djaoud Z, Guethlein LA, Blokhuis JH, et al. The intergenic recombinant HLA-B*46:01 has a distinctive peptidome that includes KIR2DL3 ligands. *Cell Rep* (2017) 19:1394–405. doi:10.1016/j.celrep.2017.04.059
79. Jarmalavicius S, Welte Y, Walden P. High immunogenicity of the human leukocyte antigen peptidomes of melanoma tumor cells. *J Biol Chem* (2012) 287:33401–11. doi:10.1074/jbc.M112.358903
80. Kalaora S, Barnea E, Merhavi-Shoham E, Qutob N, Teer JK, Shimony N, et al. Use of HLA peptidomics and whole exome sequencing to identify human immunogenic neo-antigens. *Oncotarget* (2016) 7:5110–7. doi:10.18632/oncotarget.6960
81. Ritz D, Gloger A, Weide B, Garbe C, Neri D, Fugmann T. High-sensitivity HLA class I peptidome analysis enables a precise definition of peptide motifs and the identification of peptides from cell lines and patients' sera. *Proteomics* (2016) 16:1570–80. doi:10.1002/pmic.201500445
82. Shraibman B, Kadosh DM, Barnea E, Admon A. Human leukocyte antigen (HLA) peptides derived from tumor antigens induced by inhibition of DNA methylation for development of drug-facilitated immunotherapy. *Mol Cell Proteomics* (2016) 15:3058–70. doi:10.1074/mcp.M116.060350
83. Singh-Jasuja H, Emmerich NPN, Rammensee H-G. The Tübingen approach: identification, selection, and validation of tumor-associated HLA peptides for cancer therapy. *Cancer Immunol Immunother* (2004) 53:187–95. doi:10.1007/s00262-003-0480-x
84. Weinschenk T, Gouttefangeas C, Schirle M, Obermayr F, Walter S, Schoor O, et al. Integrated functional genomics approach for the design of patient-individual antitumor vaccines. *Cancer Res* (2002) 62:5818–27.
85. Gubin MM, Zhang X, Schuster H, Caron E, Ward JP, Noguchi T, et al. Checkpoint blockade cancer immunotherapy targets tumour-specific mutant antigens. *Nature* (2014) 515:577–81. doi:10.1038/nature13988
86. Khodadoust MS, Olsson N, Wagar LE, Haabeth OAW, Chen B, Swaminathan K, et al. Antigen presentation profiling reveals recognition of lymphoma immunoglobulin neoantigens. *Nature* (2017) 543:723–7. doi:10.1038/nature21433

87. Laumont CM, Daouda T, Laverdure J-P, Bonneil E, Caron-Lizotte O, Hardy M-P, et al. Global proteogenomic analysis of human MHC class I-associated peptides derived from non-canonical reading frames. *Nat Commun* (2016) 7:10238. doi:10.1038/ncomms10238

88. Erhard F, Halenius A, Zimmermann C, L'Hernault A, Kowalewski DJ, Weekes MP, et al. Improved Ribo-seq enables identification of cryptic translation events. *Nat Methods* (2018) 4:e08890. doi:10.1038/nmeth.4631

89. Falk K, Rötzschke O, Stevanović S, Jung G, Rammensee H-G. Allele-specific motifs revealed by sequencing of self-peptides eluted from MHC molecules. *Nature* (1991) 351:290–6. doi:10.1038/351290a0

90. Hunt DF, Henderson RA, Shabanowitz J, Sakaguchi K, Michel H, Sevilir N, et al. Characterization of peptides bound to the class I MHC molecule HLA-A2.1 by mass spectrometry. *Science* (1992) 255:1261–3. doi:10.1126/science.1546328

91. Barnea E, Beer I, Patoka R, Ziv T, Kessler O, Tzehoval E, et al. Analysis of endogenous peptides bound by soluble MHC class I molecules: a novel approach for identifying tumor-specific antigens. *Eur J Immunol* (2002) 32:213–22. doi:10.1002/1521-4141(200201)32:1<213::AID-IMMU213>3.0.CO;2-8

92. Prilliman K, Lindsey M, Zuo Y, Jackson KW, Zhang Y, Hildebrand W. Large-scale production of class I bound peptides: assigning a signature to HLA-B*1501. *Immunogenetics* (1997) 45:379–85. doi:10.1007/s002510050219

93. Scull KE, Dudek NL, Corbett AJ, Ramarathinam SH, Gorasia DG, Williamson NA, et al. Secreted HLA recapitulates the immunopeptidome and allows in-depth coverage of HLA A*02:01 ligands. *Mol Immunol* (2012) 51:136–42. doi:10.1016/j.molimm.2012.02.117

94. Bassani-Sternberg M, Barnea E, Beer I, Avivi I, Katz T, Admon A. Soluble plasma HLA peptidome as a potential source for cancer biomarkers. *Proc Natl Acad Sci U S A* (2010) 107:18769–76. doi:10.1073/pnas.1008501107

95. Mobbs JI, Illing PT, Dudek NL, Brooks AG, Baker DG, Purcell AW, et al. The molecular basis for peptide repertoire selection in the human leucocyte antigen (HLA) C*06:02 molecule. *J Biol Chem* (2017) 292:17203–15. doi:10.1074/jbc.M117.806976

96. Schittenhelm RB, Dudek NL, Croft NP, Ramarathinam SH, Purcell AW. A comprehensive analysis of constitutive naturally processed and presented HLA-C*04:01 (Cw4)-specific peptides. *Tissue Antigens* (2014) 83:174–9. doi:10.1111/tan.12282

97. Trolle T, McMurtrey CP, Sidney J, Bardet W, Osborn SC, Kaever T, et al. The length distribution of class I-restricted T cell epitopes is determined by both peptide supply and MHC allele-specific binding preference. *J Immunol* (2016) 196:1480–7. doi:10.4049/jimmunol.1501721

98. Giam K, Ayala-Perez R, Illing PT, Schittenhelm RB, Croft NP, Purcell AW, et al. A comprehensive analysis of peptides presented by HLA-A1. *Tissue Antigens* (2015) 85:492–6. doi:10.1111/tan.12565

99. Yair-Sabag S, Tedeschi V, Vitulano C, Barnea E, Glaser F, Melamed Kadosh D, et al. The peptide repertoire of HLA-B27 may include ligands with lysine at P2 anchor position. *Proteomics* (2018) 18:e1700249. doi:10.1002/pmic.201700249

100. Schittenhelm RB, Sian TCCLK, Wilmann PG, Dudek NL, Purcell AW. Revisiting the arthritogenic peptide theory: quantitative not qualitative changes in the peptide repertoire of HLA-B27 allotypes. *Arthritis Rheumatol* (2015) 67:702–13. doi:10.1002/art.38963

101. Bassani-Sternberg M, Gfeller D. Unsupervised HLA peptidome deconvolution improves ligand prediction accuracy and predicts cooperative effects in peptide-HLA interactions. *J Immunol* (2016) 197:2492–9. doi:10.4049/jimmunol.1600808

102. Alvarez B, Barra C, Nielsen M, Andreatta M. Computational tools for the identification and interpretation of sequence motifs in immunopeptidomes. *Proteomics* (2018) 14:1700252. doi:10.1002/pmic.201700252

103. Andreatta M, Alvarez B, Nielsen M. GibbsCluster: unsupervised clustering and alignment of peptide sequences. *Nucleic Acids Res* (2017) 45:W458–63. doi:10.1093/nar/gkx248

104. Kim Y, Sidney J, Pinilla C, Sette A, Peters B. Derivation of an amino acid similarity matrix for peptide: MHC binding and its application as a Bayesian prior. *BMC Bioinformatics* (2009) 10:394. doi:10.1186/1471-2105-10-394

105. Lund O, Nielsen M, Lundegaard C, Keşmir C, Brunak S. *Immunological Bioinformatics*. MIT Press (2005).

106. Rammensee H, Bachmann J, Emmerich NP, Bachor OA, Stevanović S. SYFPEITHI: database for MHC ligands and peptide motifs. *Immunogenetics* (1999) 50:213–9. doi:10.1007/s002510050595

107. Zhang H, Lund O, Nielsen M. The PickPocket method for predicting binding specificities for receptors based on receptor pocket similarities: application to MHC-peptide binding. *Bioinformatics* (2009) 25:1293–9. doi:10.1093/bioinformatics/btp137

108. Altschul SF, Madden TL, Schäffer AA, Zhang J, Zhang Z, Miller W, et al. Gapped BLAST and PSI-BLAST: a new generation of protein database search programs. *Nucleic Acids Res* (1997) 25:3389–402. doi:10.1093/nar/25.17.3389

109. Henikoff S, Henikoff JG. Amino acid substitution matrices from protein blocks. *Proc Natl Acad Sci U S A* (1992) 89:10915–9. doi:10.1073/pnas.89.22.10915

110. Andreatta M, Nielsen M. Gapped sequence alignment using artificial neural networks: application to the MHC class I system. *Bioinformatics* (2016) 32:511–7. doi:10.1093/bioinformatics/btv639

111. Jørgensen KW, Rasmussen M, Buus S, Nielsen M. NetMHCstab – predicting stability of peptide-MHC-I complexes; impacts for cytotoxic T lymphocyte epitope discovery. *Immunology* (2014) 141:18–26. doi:10.1111/imm.12160

112. Nielsen M, Lundegaard C, Worning P, Lauemøller SL, Lamberth K, Buus S, et al. Reliable prediction of T-cell epitopes using neural networks with novel sequence representations. *Protein Sci* (2003) 12:1007–17. doi:10.1110/ps.0239403

113. Rubinsteyn A, O'Donnell T, Damaraju N, Hammerbacher J. Predicting peptide-MHC binding affinities with imputed training data. *bioRxiv* (2016) 054775. doi:10.1101/054775

114. Vang YS, Xie X. HLA class I binding prediction via convolutional neural networks. *Bioinformatics* (2017) 33:2658–65. doi:10.1093/bioinformatics/btx264

115. Peters B, Tong W, Sidney J, Sette A, Weng Z. Examining the independent binding assumption for binding of peptide epitopes to MHC-I molecules. *Bioinformatics* (2003) 19:1765–72. doi:10.1093/bioinformatics/btg247

116. Han Y, Kim D. Deep convolutional neural networks for pan-specific peptide-MHC class I binding prediction. *BMC Bioinformatics* (2017) 18:585. doi:10.1186/s12859-017-1997-x

117. Jurtz V, Paul S, Andreatta M, Marcatili P, Peters B, Nielsen M. NetMHCpan-4.0: improved peptide-MHC class I interaction predictions integrating eluted ligand and peptide binding affinity data. *J Immunol* (2017) 199:3360–8. doi:10.4049/jimmunol.1700893

118. Rasmussen M, Fenoy E, Harndahl M, Kristensen AB, Nielsen IK, Nielsen M, et al. Pan-specific prediction of peptide-MHC class I complex stability, a correlate of T cell immunogenicity. *J Immunol* (2016) 197:1517–24. doi:10.4049/jimmunol.1600582

119. Nielsen M, Connelley T, Ternette N. Improved prediction of Bovine Leucocyte Antigens (BoLA) presented ligands by use of mass spectrometry-determined ligand- and in-vitro binding data. *J Proteome Res* (2017) 17(1):559–67. doi:10.1021/acs.jproteome.7b00675

120. Guillaume P, Picaud S, Baumgaertner P, Montandon N, Schmidt J, Speiser DE, et al. The C-terminal extension landscape of naturally presented HLA-I ligands. *Proc Natl Acad Sci U S A* (2018) 115:5083–8. doi:10.1073/pnas.1717277115

121. Gfeller D. Uncovering new aspects of protein interactions through analysis of specificity landscapes in peptide recognition domains. *FEBS Lett* (2012) 586:2764–72. doi:10.1016/j.febslet.2012.03.054

122. Gfeller D, Butty F, Wierzbicka M, Verschueren E, Vanhee P, Huang H, et al. The multiple-specificity landscape of modular peptide recognition domains. *Mol Syst Biol* (2011) 7:484. doi:10.1038/msb.2011.18

123. Kim T, Tyndel MS, Huang H, Sidhu SS, Bader GD, Gfeller D, et al. MUSI: an integrated system for identifying multiple specificity from very large peptide or nucleic acid data sets. *Nucleic Acids Res* (2012) 40:e47. doi:10.1093/nar/gkr1294

124. Andreatta M, Lund O, Nielsen M. Simultaneous alignment and clustering of peptide data using a Gibbs sampling approach. *Bioinformatics* (2013) 29:8–14. doi:10.1093/bioinformatics/bts621

125. Storkus WJ, Zeh HJ, Salter RD, Lotze MT. Identification of T-cell epitopes: rapid isolation of class I-presented peptides from viable cells by mild acid elution. *J Immunother Emphasis Tumor Immunol* (1993) 14:94–103. doi:10.1097/00002371-199308000-00003

126. Sugawara S, Abo T, Kumagai K. A simple method to eliminate the antigenicity of surface class I MHC molecules from the membrane of viable cells by acid treatment at pH 3. *J Immunol Methods* (1987) 100:83–90. doi:10.1016/0022-1759(87)90175-X

127. Lanoix J, Durette C, Courcelles M, Cossette É, Comtois-Marotte S, Hardy M-P, et al. Comparison of the MHC I immunopeptidome repertoire of B-cell lymphoblasts using two isolation methods. *Proteomics* (2018) 18(12): e1700251. doi:10.1002/pmic.201700251
128. Nielsen M, Lund O. NN-align. An artificial neural network-based alignment algorithm for MHC class II peptide binding prediction. *BMC Bioinformatics* (2009) 10:296. doi:10.1186/1471-2105-10-296
129. Jensen KK, Andreatta M, Marcatili P, Buus S, Greenbaum JA, Yan Z, et al. Improved methods for predicting peptide binding affinity to MHC class II molecules. *Immunology* (2018) 154:394–406. doi:10.1111/imm.12889
130. Singh H, Raghava GP. ProPred: prediction of HLA-DR binding sites. *Bioinformatics* (2001) 17:1236–7. doi:10.1093/bioinformatics/17.12.1236
131. Guan P, Doytchinova IA, Zygouri C, Flower DR. MHCPred: a server for quantitative prediction of peptide-MHC binding. *Nucleic Acids Res* (2003) 31:3621–4. doi:10.1093/nar/gkg510
132. Sturniolo T, Bono E, Ding J, Raddrizzani L, Tuereci O, Sahin U, et al. Generation of tissue-specific and promiscuous HLA ligand databases using DNA microarrays and virtual HLA class II matrices. *Nat Biotechnol* (1999) 17:555–61. doi:10.1038/9858
133. Wang P, Sidney J, Dow C, Mothé B, Sette A, Peters B. A systematic assessment of MHC class II peptide binding predictions and evaluation of a consensus approach. *PLoS Comput Biol* (2008) 4:e1000048. doi:10.1371/journal.pcbi.1000048
134. Yin L, Stern LJ. HLA-DM focuses on conformational flexibility around P1 pocket to catalyze peptide exchange. *Front Immunol* (2013) 4:336. doi:10.3389/fimmu.2013.00336
135. Vogt AB, Kropshofer H, Kalbacher H, Kalbus M, Rammensee H-G, Coligan JE, et al. Ligand motifs of HLA-DRB5*0101 and DRB1*1501 molecules delineated from self-peptides. *J Immunol* (1994) 153:1665–73.
136. Sofron A, Ritz D, Neri D, Fugmann T. High-resolution analysis of the murine MHC class II immunopeptidome. *Eur J Immunol* (2015) 46:319–28. doi:10.1002/eji.201545930
137. Fugmann T, Sofron A, Ritz D, Bootz F, Neri D. The MHC class II immunopeptidome of lymph nodes in health and in chemically induced colitis. *Journal Immunol* (2016) 198:1357–64. doi:10.4049/jimmunol.1601157
138. Ooi JD, Petersen J, Tan YH, Huynh M, Willett ZJ, Ramarathinam SH, et al. Dominant protection from HLA-linked autoimmunity by antigen-specific regulatory T cells. *Nature* (2017) 545:243–7. doi:10.1038/nature22329
139. Ritz D, Sani E, Debiec H, Ronco P, Neri D, Fugmann T. Membranal and blood-soluble HLA class II peptidome analyses using data-dependent and independent acquisition. *Proteomics* (2018) 34:1700246. doi:10.1002/pmic.201700246
140. Barra CM, Alvarez B, Andreatta M, Buus S, Nielsen M. Footprints of antigen processing boost MHC class II natural ligand binding predictions. *bioRxiv* (2018):285767. doi:10.1101/285767
141. Mommen GPM, Marino F, Meiring HD, Poelen MCM, van Gaans-van den Brink JAM, Mohammed S, et al. Sampling from the proteome to the human leukocyte antigen-DR (HLA-DR) ligandome proceeds via high specificity. *Mol Cell Proteomics* (2016) 15:1412–23. doi:10.1074/mcp.M115.055780
142. Hassan C, Chabrol E, Jahn L, Kester MGD, de Ru AH, Drijfhout JW, et al. Naturally processed non-canonical HLA-A*02:01 presented peptides. *J Biol Chem* (2015) 290:2593–603. doi:10.1074/jbc.M114.607028
143. Gfeller D, Guillaume P, Michaux J, Pak H-S, Daniel RT, Racle J, et al. Peptide length distribution and multiple specificity in naturally presented HLA-I ligands. *bioRxiv* (2018):335661. doi:10.1101/335661
144. Collins EJ, Garboczi DN, Wiley DC. Three-dimensional structure of a peptide extending from one end of a class I MHC binding site. *Nature* (1994) 371:626–9. doi:10.1038/371626a0
145. Tenzer S, Wee E, Burgevin A, Stewart-Jones G, Friis L, Lamberth K, et al. Antigen processing influences HIV-specific cytotoxic T lymphocyte immunodominance. *Nat Immunol* (2009) 10:636–46. doi:10.1038/ni.1728
146. McMurtrey C, Trolle T, Sansom T, Remesh SG, Kaever T, Bardet W, et al. Toxoplasma gondii peptide ligands open the gate of the HLA class I binding groove. *Elife* (2016) 5:246. doi:10.7554/eLife.12556
147. Remesh SG, Andreatta M, Ying G, Kaever T, Nielsen M, McMurtrey C, et al. Unconventional peptide presentation by major histocompatibility complex (MHC) class I Allele HLA-A*02:01: BREAKING CONFINEMENT. *J Biol Chem* (2017) 292:5262–70. doi:10.1074/jbc.M117.776542
148. Pymm P, Illing PT, Ramarathinam SH, O'Connor GM, Hughes VA, Hitchen C, et al. MHC-I peptides get out of the groove and enable a novel mechanism of HIV-1 escape. *Nat Struct Mol Biol* (2017) 219:277. doi:10.1038/nsmb.3381
149. Li X, Lamothe PA, Walker BD, Wang J-H. Crystal structure of HLA-B*5801 with a TW10 HIV Gag epitope reveals a novel mode of peptide presentation. *Cell Mol Immunol* (2017) 14:631–4. doi:10.1038/cmi.2017.24
150. Alpízar A, Marino F, Ramos-Fernández A, Lombardía M, Jeko A, Pazos F, et al. A molecular basis for the presentation of phosphorylated peptides by HLA-B antigens. *Mol Cell Proteomics* (2016) 16(2):181–93. doi:10.1074/mcp.M116.063800
151. Marino F, Bern M, Mommen GPM, Leney AC, van Gaans-van den Brink JAM, Bonvin AMJJ, et al. Extended O-GlcNAc on HLA class-I-bound peptides. *J Am Chem Soc* (2015) 137:10922–5. doi:10.1021/jacs.5b06586
152. Marino F, Mommen GPM, Jeko A, Meiring HD, van Gaans-van den Brink JAM, Scheltema RA, et al. Arginine (Di)methylated human leukocyte antigen class I peptides are favorably presented by HLA-B*07. *J Proteome Res* (2017) 16:34–44. doi:10.1021/acs.jproteome.6b00528
153. Andersen MH, Bonfill JE, Neisig A, Arsequell G, Sondergaard I, Valencia G, et al. Phosphorylated peptides can be transported by TAP molecules, presented by class I MHC molecules, and recognized by phosphopeptide-specific CTL. *J Immunol* (1999) 163:3812–8.
154. Petersen J, Wurzbacher SJ, Williamson NA, Ramarathinam SH, Reid HH, Nair AKN, et al. Phosphorylated self-peptides alter human leukocyte antigen class I-restricted antigen presentation and generate tumor-specific epitopes. *Proc Natl Acad Sci U S A* (2009) 106:2776–81. doi:10.1073/pnas.0812901106
155. Zarling AL, Polefrone JM, Evans AM, Mikesh LM, Shabanowitz J, Lewis ST, et al. Identification of class I MHC-associated phosphopeptides as targets for cancer immunotherapy. *Proc Natl Acad Sci U S A* (2006) 103:14889–94. doi:10.1073/pnas.0604045103
156. Ciudad MT, Sorvillo N, van Alphen FP, Catalán D, Meijer AB, Voorberg J, et al. Analysis of the HLA-DR peptidome from human dendritic cells reveals high affinity repertoires and nonconventional pathways of peptide generation. *J Leukoc Biol* (2017) 101:15–27. doi:10.1189/jlb.6HI0216-069R
157. Collado JA, Alvarez I, Ciudad MT, Espinosa G, Canals F, Pujol-Borrell R, et al. Composition of the HLA-DR-associated human thymus peptidome. *Eur J Immunol* (2013) 43:2273–82. doi:10.1002/eji.201243280
158. Clement CC, Becerra A, Yin L, Zolla V, Huang L, Merlin S, et al. The dendritic cell major histocompatibility complex II (MHC II) peptidome derives from a variety of processing pathways and includes peptides with a broad spectrum of HLA-DM sensitivity. *J Biol Chem* (2016) 291:5576–95. doi:10.1074/jbc.M115.655738
159. Müller M, Gfeller D, Coukos G, Bassani-Sternberg M. "Hotspots" of antigen presentation revealed by human leukocyte antigen ligandomics for neoantigen prioritization. *Front Immunol* (2017) 8:1367. doi:10.3389/fimmu.2017.01367
160. Dengjel J, Schoor O, Fischer R, Reich M, Kraus M, Müller M, et al. Autophagy promotes MHC class II presentation of peptides from intracellular source proteins. *Proc Natl Acad Sci U S A* (2005) 102:7922–7. doi:10.1073/pnas.0501190102
161. Kropshofer H, Max H, Halder T, Kalbus M, Muller CA, Kalbacher H. Self-peptides from four HLA-DR alleles share hydrophobic anchor residues near the NH2-terminal including proline as a stop signal for trimming. *J Immunol* (1993) 151:4732–42.
162. Godkin AJ, Smith KJ, Willis A, Tejada-Simon MV, Zhang J, Elliott T, et al. Naturally processed HLA class II peptides reveal highly conserved immunogenic flanking region sequence preferences that reflect antigen processing rather than peptide-MHC interactions. *J Immunol* (2001) 166:6720–7. doi:10.4049/jimmunol.166.11.6720
163. Andreatta M, Jurtz VI, Kaever T, Sette A, Peters B, Nielsen M. Machine learning reveals a non-canonical mode of peptide binding to MHC class II molecules. *Immunology* (2017) 152:255–64. doi:10.1111/imm.12763
164. Nielsen M, Lundegaard C, Lund O, Keşmir C. The role of the proteasome in generating cytotoxic T-cell epitopes: insights obtained from improved predictions of proteasomal cleavage. *Immunogenetics* (2005) 57:33–41. doi:10.1007/s00251-005-0781-7
165. Doytchinova IA, Guan P, Flower DR. EpiJen: a server for multistep T cell epitope prediction. *BMC Bioinformatics* (2006) 7:131. doi:10.1186/1471-2105-7-131

166. Tenzer S, Peters B, Bulik S, Schoor O, Lemmel C, Schatz MM, et al. Modeling the MHC class I pathway by combining predictions of proteasomal cleavage, TAP transport and MHC class I binding. *Cell Mol Life Sci* (2005) 62: 1025–37. doi:10.1007/s00018-005-4528-2
167. Zhang GL, Petrovsky N, Kwoh CK, August JT, Brusic V. PRED(TAP): a system for prediction of peptide binding to the human transporter associated with antigen processing. *Immunome Res* (2006) 2:3. doi:10.1186/1745-7580-2-3
168. Jappe EC, Kringelum J, Trolle T, Nielsen M. Predicted MHC peptide binding promiscuity explains MHC class I "hotspots" of antigen presentation defined by mass spectrometry eluted ligand data. *Immunology* (2018) 154:407–17. doi:10.1111/imm.12905
169. Liepe J, Marino F, Sidney J, Jeko A, Bunting DE, Sette A, et al. A large fraction of HLA class I ligands are proteasome-generated spliced peptides. *Science* (2016) 354:354–8. doi:10.1126/science.aaf4384
170. Nesvizhskii AI. Proteogenomics: concepts, applications and computational strategies. *Nat Methods* (2014) 11:1114–25. doi:10.1038/nmeth.3144
171. Mylonas R, Beer I, Iseli C, Chong C, Pak H, Gfeller D, et al. Estimating the contribution of proteasomal spliced peptides to the HLA-I ligandome. *bioRxiv* (2018):288209. doi:10.1101/288209
172. Calis JJA, Maybeno M, Greenbaum JA, Weiskopf D, De Silva AD, Sette A, et al. Properties of MHC class I presented peptides that enhance immunogenicity. *PLoS Comput Biol* (2013) 9:e1003266. doi:10.1371/journal.pcbi.1003266
173. Bjerregaard A-M, Nielsen M, Jurtz V, Barra CM, Hadrup SR, Szallasi Z, et al. An analysis of natural T cell responses to predicted tumor neoepitopes. *Front Immunol* (2017) 8:1566. doi:10.3389/fimmu.2017.01566
174. Duan F, Duitama J, Al Seesi S, Ayres CM, Corcelli SA, Pawashe AP, et al. Genomic and bioinformatic profiling of mutational neoepitopes reveals new rules to predict anticancer immunogenicity. *J Exp Med* (2014) 211:2231–48. doi:10.1084/jem.20141308
175. van Buuren MM, Calis JJ, Schumacher TN. High sensitivity of cancer exome-based CD8 T cell neo-antigen identification. *Oncoimmunology* (2014) 3:e28836. doi:10.4161/onci.28836
176. Fritsch EF, Rajasagi M, Ott PA, Brusic V, Hacohen N, Wu CJ. HLA-binding properties of tumor neoepitopes in humans. *Cancer Immunol Res* (2014) 2:522–9. doi:10.1158/2326-6066.CIR-13-0227
177. Gee MH, Han A, Lofgren SM, Beausang JF, Mendoza JL, Birnbaum ME, et al. Antigen identification for orphan t cell receptors expressed on tumor-infiltrating lymphocytes. *Cell* (2018) 172:549.e–63.e. doi:10.1016/j.cell.2017.11.043
178. Lill JR, van Veelen PA, Tenzer S, Admon A, Caron E, Elias J, et al. Minimal information about an immuno-peptidomics experiment (MIAIPE). *Proteomics* (2018) 18(12):e1800110. doi:10.1002/pmic.201800110
179. Vizcaíno JA, Csordas A, Del-Toro N, Dianes JA, Griss J, Lavidas I, et al. 2016 update of the PRIDE database and its related tools. *Nucleic Acids Res* (2016) 44:11033–11033. doi:10.1093/nar/gkv1145
180. Shao W, Pedrioli PGA, Wolski W, Scurtescu C, Schmid E, Vizcaíno JA, et al. The SysteMHC Atlas project. *Nucleic Acids Res* (2018) 46:D1237–47. doi:10.1093/nar/gkx664
181. Karosiene E, Lundegaard C, Lund O, Nielsen M. NetMHCcons: a consensus method for the major histocompatibility complex class I predictions. *Immunogenetics* (2012) 64:177–86. doi:10.1007/s00251-011-0579-8
182. Moutaftsi M, Peters B, Pasquetto V, Tscharke DC, Sidney J, Bui H-H, et al. A consensus epitope prediction approach identifies the breadth of murine T(CD8+)-cell responses to vaccinia virus. *Nat Biotechnol* (2006) 24:817–9. doi:10.1038/nbt1215
183. Bhattacharya R, Sivakumar A, Tokheim C, Guthrie VB, Anagnostou V, Velculescu VE, et al. Evaluation of machine learning methods to predict peptide binding to MHC Class I proteins. *bioRxiv* (2017) 154757. doi:10.1101/154757
184. Liu G, Li D, Li Z, Qiu S, Li W, Chao C-C, et al. PSSMHCpan: a novel PSSM-based software for predicting class I peptide-HLA binding affinity. *GigaScience* (2017) 6:1–11. doi:10.1093/gigascience/gix017
185. Sidney J, Peters B, Frahm N, Brander C, Sette A. HLA class I supertypes: a revised and updated classification. *BMC Immunol* (2008) 9:1. doi:10.1186/1471-2172-9-1

3

# ASAP - A Webserver for Immunoglobulin-Sequencing Analysis Pipeline

**_Oren Avram†, Anna Vaisman-Mentesh†, Dror Yehezkel, Haim Ashkenazy, Tal Pupko and Yariv Wine*_**

*George S. Wise Faculty of Life Sciences, School of Molecular Cell Biology and Biotechnology, Tel Aviv University, Ramat Aviv, Israel*

***Correspondence:**
*Yariv Wine*
*yarivwine@tauex.tau.ac.il*

*†These authors have contributed equally to this work.*

Reproducible and robust data on antibody repertoires are invaluable for basic and applied immunology. Next-generation sequencing (NGS) of antibody variable regions has emerged as a powerful tool in systems immunology, providing quantitative molecular information on antibody polyclonal composition. However, major computational challenges exist when analyzing antibody sequences, from error handling to hypermutation profiles and clonal expansion analyses. In this work, we developed the ASAP (A webserver for Immunoglobulin-Seq Analysis Pipeline) webserver (https://asap.tau.ac.il). The input to ASAP is a paired-end sequence dataset from one or more replicates, with or without unique molecular identifiers. These datasets can be derived from NGS of human or murine antibody variable regions. ASAP first filters and annotates the sequence reads using public or user-provided germline sequence information. The ASAP webserver next performs various calculations, including somatic hypermutation level, CDR3 lengths, V(D)J family assignments, and V(D)J combination distribution. These analyses are repeated for each replicate. ASAP provides additional information by analyzing the commonalities and differences between the repeats ("joint" analysis). For example, ASAP examines the shared variable regions and their frequency in each replicate to determine which sequences are less likely to be a result of a sample preparation derived and/or sequencing errors. Moreover, ASAP clusters the data to clones and reports the identity and prevalence of top ranking clones (clonal expansion analysis). ASAP further provides the distribution of synonymous and non-synonymous mutations within the V genes somatic hypermutations. Finally, ASAP provides means to process the data for proteomic analysis of serum/secreted antibodies by generating a variable region database for liquid chromatography high resolution tandem mass spectrometry (LC-MS/MS) interpretation. ASAP is user-friendly, free, and open to all users, with no login requirement. ASAP is applicable for researchers interested in basic questions related to B cell development and differentiation, as well as applied researchers who are interested in vaccine development and monoclonal antibody engineering. By virtue of its user-friendliness, ASAP opens the antibody analysis field to non-expert users who seek to boost their research with immune repertoire analysis.

**Keywords: high throughput sequencing, antibodies, B cell receptor, next generation sequencing, Ig-Seq, AIRR-Seq, antibody repertoire analysis, immune repertoire**

## INTRODUCTION

The power of the adaptive immune system relies on its ability to generate an exceptional diversity in the genes encoding the variable region of B cell receptors and their secreted form, the antibodies. This diversity of antibodies is achieved by several unique molecular mechanisms, including chromosomal V(D)J rearrangement during B cell maturation in the bone marrow, N-P addition/deletion in the ligated V(D)J genes and somatic hypermutations (SHM) following antigen stimuli in the peripheral lymph nodes (1) (**Figure 1A**).

Antibodies can reach an enormous theoretical diversity of $10^{13}$–$10^{18}$. However, the actual diversity is more restricted and was estimated to reach $10^{11}$–$10^{12}$ in humans (2). Due to labor and cost considerations, as well as the lack of suitable high-throughput technologies, analysis of such complex repertoires using traditional Sanger sequencing was impractical for many years, resulting in major knowledge gaps regarding antibodies molecular composition. This precluded the ability to address many fundamental immunological questions related to the development of the immune response in health, disease, and following vaccination.

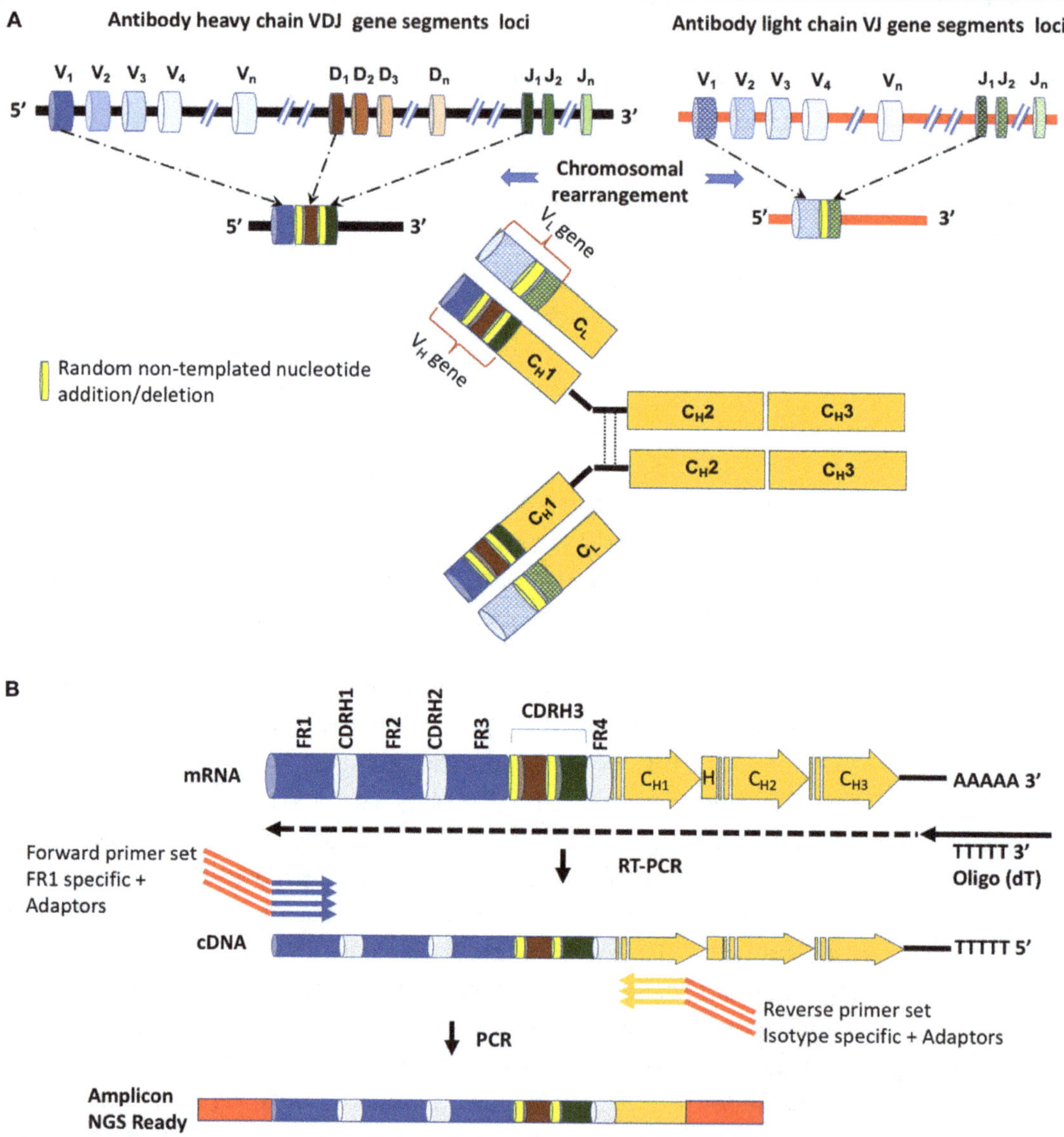


**FIGURE 1** | The diversity of antibody sequences and structures and molecular methodologies for next-generation sequencing. **(A)** Antibodies are comprised of two identical heavy chains and two identical light chains, each encoded on a different chromosome, both in human and in mouse. Diversity is achieved by chromosomal rearrangement, where different V, D, and J (V and J) genes are combined to construct the variable region of the heavy (light) chain of the antibody. In yellow are random nucleotides introduced during the chromosomal rearrangement process. **(B)** A detailed view of the variable region. Shown are the forward and reverse primers used for amplification. Several alternative primers, both forward and reverse, are used in order to capture the diversity of the variable region and its associated isotypes. The forward primers anneal to the framework 1 (FR1) region. Red regions within the primers represent adaptor sequences.

The introduction of next-generation sequencing (NGS) platforms has significantly advanced research in many scientific fields and opened new avenues in genomics and transcriptomics research. For immunoglobulin sequencing (Ig-Seq), which is also termed adaptive immune receptor repertoire sequencing (AIRR-Seq), NGS provided the means to underline quantitative measures of the immune response in an unprecedented throughput and since 2009 (3), the number of studies that applied NGS to analyze immune repertoires has increased substantially.

AIRR-Seq is based on targeted sequencing of genomic DNA or mRNA and in principle focuses on recording the diversity of the variable region (which includes the V(D)J genes) encoding the heavy ($V_H$) and/or light ($V_L$) chains of antibodies (**Figure 1B**). The variable region encodes the most diversified sites of the antibodies as they are the product of chromosomal rearrangements and SHMs and comprise three complementary determining regions (CDR1-3) in each antibody chain (**Figure 1B**). Due to the recombination and non-templated diversification mechanisms that generate the CDR3 of the heavy chain (CDR-H3), it is considered the most diverse determinant in terms of length and sequence of AIRR. CDR-H3 is thus pivotal for antibody specificity, although it was recently suggested that CDR-H3 is necessary, albeit insufficient, for specific antibody binding (4).

Accumulating AIRR-Seq data provide invaluable insights regarding the nature of the immune response in health and disease. These data were shown to be important for isolation and expression of antigen-specific monoclonal antibodies (5, 6), sequencing and cloning antibodies from single cells (7, 8), and proteomic analyses of secreted antibodies (9–11). These sequencing data can further facilitate the elucidation of the properties of antigen-specific antibodies that mediate protection against infectious diseases, are induced following vaccination, and generated in cancer and autoimmune diseases.

While AIRR-Seq is a powerful tool for immune repertoire analysis, errors accumulated during the experimental procedure (e.g., PCR and sequencing errors) make it extremely difficult to confidently/reliably determine the qualitative and quantitative measurements of the immune repertoire and establish an error-free antibody variable region sequence database. High confidence antibody variable region archives are particularly important when AIRR-Seq is combined with the utilization of serum antibodies proteomics (12–16), as these archives define the search space to interpret the proteomic spectra.

To overcome these challenges, experimental and computational strategies can be employed to reduce error-derived "noise" (17, 18). One such strategy utilizes replicate samples (either technical or biological) (19, 20). The main advantage of this approach is that it does not require complex experimental protocols that may prevent researchers from exploring the potential usage of AIRR-Seq in their research. Noteworthy, while great effort is invested in the development AIRR-Seq analysis tools, there is still no consensus on standard operating procedures for data processing and deposition. To address these issues, the AIRR Community was established in 2014 (http://airr.irmacs.sfu.ca/home) (21, 22).

Here, we report ASAP (A webserver for Ig-Seq Analysis Pipeline), a webserver for the analysis of AIRR-Seq data from several replicates, that is user-friendly, simple, free, and open to all users. ASAP is easily accessible to researchers who are interested to address basic questions related to B-cell development and differentiation in health and disease, as well as to researchers

**TABLE 1** | Summary of the analyses supported in ASAP compared to other related webservers.

| Feature | ASAP | BRepertoire | ARGalaxy | Vidjil | VDJviz | VDJServer |
|---|---|---|---|---|---|---|
| Paired-end alignment | + | − | + | + | − | + |
| VDJ annotation | + | − | + | + | − | + |
| Framework and CDR3 annotation | + | − | + | + | − | + |
| Filtering | + | − | + | + | − | + |
| Data trimming | + | − | + | + | − | + |
| Unique molecular identifier clustering | + | − | − | − | − | + |
| Inclusion of novel germline alleles | + | − | − | + | − | − |
| CDR3 length distribution | + | + | + | + | + | + |
| Somatic hypermutations level | + | − | + | − | − | + |
| Synonymous/non-synonymous mutations | + | + | + | − | − | + |
| Isotype distribution | + | − | + | − | − | − |
| Joint analysis for replicates | + | − | − | − | − | + |
| Clonal analysis | + | + | + | + | + | + |
| V(D)J usage | + | + | + | + | + | + |
| V-D-J combination analysis | + | + | + | + | + | + |
| Clone ranking detailed analysis | + | − | − | − | + | + |
| Integrative database of all unique variable region sequences including sequence metadata | + | − | − | − | − | − |
| MS ready database for proteomics analysis of secreted antibodies | + | − | − | − | − | − |
| Amino acid level sequences linked to nucleotide level | + | − | − | − | − | − |
| Single push-button for all analysis steps | + | − | + | − | − | − |

interested in applicable vaccine development and monoclonal antibody engineering. ASAP provides several unique features that are absent from other published webservers dedicated for AIRR-Seq data processing, analysis, and visulation (**Table 1**). ASAP and its associated source code are freely available at https://asap.tau.ac.il and https://github.com/orenavram/ASAP, respectively.

## RESULTS

The webserver ASAP allows analysis of the complete B cell receptor repertoire based on NGS replicates of antibody variable region sequencing experiments. Implemented in Python 3, ASAP is simple, user-friendly, and freely available for all users.

The simplicity of the webserver allows researchers of diversified expertise levels to submit up to six replicates, given that the replicates use different barcodes. ASAP consists of two major parts: the individual part, in which each replicate is analyzed separately, and a joint part, in which the commonalities and differences among the replicates are analyzed. A complete overview of the ASAP workflow and output information is shown in **Figure 2**. A detailed description of all types of analyses provided by ASAP can be found on the webserver's Gallery section.

To exemplify the advantages of ASAP, we present here a demonstration of the entire webserver workflow by analyzing previously published antibody sequence data (23). These data were obtained from murine pools of plasmablasts and plasma cells in technical triplicates, i.e., three samples prepared from the same starting cDNA pool. All samples were sequenced using Illumina MiSeq platform, 2 × 250 bp paired-end reads (European nucleotide archive study accession: PRJEB4643).

### Individual Processing

The input to ASAP is two FASTQ files for each replicate (paired end files). These files are initially processed by the ASAP webserver using the MiXCR software (24), which provides full V(D)J assignment, frameworks, and CDR3 annotations.

Alignment files that were generated by MiXCR are further processed. Aligned sequences are filtered out if at least one of the following conditions is met: (1) sequence contains a stop codon in the variable region ORF; (2) the two paired-end reads do not overlap; (3) the obtained sequences are shorter than a specified threshold (default set to be 300 nucleotides); (4) read quality is lower than a specified threshold (default set to be 20). A file describing the number of sequences filtered due to each criterion is provided. In case the reads are associated with a unique molecular identifier (UMI), reads with the same UMI are collapsed to a single sequence and errors are corrected based on the consensus sequence (25). For UMI analyses, the user has to provide the UMI pattern according to the IUPAC nucleotide code. Notably, UMI are handled in cases where the UMI is found only on the forward read, only on the reverse read, or both, as described in Ref. (19).

Each chain type has a different output section as follows. The first output of the processed data is an annotation file (e.g., "IGH_aa_sequence_annotations," for the IGH chain). In this file, each row contains the following information regarding unique amino acid sequences (identical sequences are grouped to a single line): [1] chain type ($V_H$, $V_\kappa$, or $V_\lambda$); [2] antibody isotype associated with the $V_H$ sequences (e.g., for human sequences: IgM, IgD, IgG, IgA1, IgA2, or IgE); [3] the trimmed nucleotide read (without the adapter sequence); [4] the corresponding amino acid sequence; [5] amino acid sequence of the CDR3 region; [6] V family subgroup; [7] D family subgroup; [8] J family subgroup; [9] the number of reads for this amino acid sequence (counts).

The isotype assignment is computed by string matching to peptides defining each isotype. These peptides correspond to the N terminus of the antibody $C_H1$ region (**Figure 1A**) and were derived from IMGT (26) (**Table 2**). Isotypes are assigned by

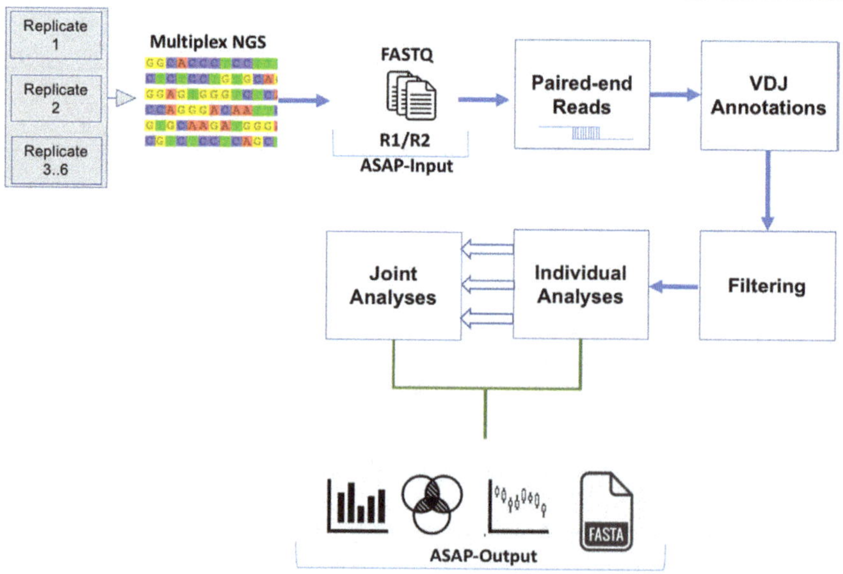


**FIGURE 2** | Schematic flowchart for the analysis of each next-generation sequencing replicate (individual) as well as the analyses of the entire set of replicates (joint).

searching for an exact match between a substring of the translated read and these peptides. Specifically, the peptides are searched against the C terminal region to the Framework-4. This region is defined by the string VTVSS in human and by the strings VTVSS, LTVSS, and VTVSA in mouse. In case no match is found, the server searches for the closest match. In case the difference between the closest match is more than a single amino acid mismatch, the isotype is classified as "unknown." In addition, for certain human samples, the server is unable to distinguish between the A1 and A2 isotypes, e.g., when the relevant peptide motif information used for this classification is ambiguous (the peptide motif ends with CSTQP for A1 and DSTPQ for A2; **Table 2**). In this case, the isotype is defined as "IgA." This isotype information is included in the annotation file described above. The frequencies of each isotype are graphically presented as a pie chart (**Figure 3**). Of note, the ability to detect the various isotypes depends on the primers used within the experimental setup.

**TABLE 2** | The sequence fingerprint characteristic of each isotype in human and mouse.

| Isotype | Human | Mouse |
|---|---|---|
| M | GSASAPT | ESQSFP |
| D | APTKAP | GDKKEP |
| G | ASTKGPS | AKTT[A/P]P |
| A | ASPTSP | ESARNP |
| A1 | ASPTSPKVFPLSLCSTQP | – |
| A2 | ASPTSPKVFPLSLDSTPQ | – |
| E | ASTQSP | ASIRNP |

Next, ASAP provides information regarding SHM. For each DNA read, the number of mutations with respect to the germline is recorded (**Figure 4A**). Mutations are stratified to silent and non-silent (synonymous and non-synonymous, respectively). These data are provided as a file and are also displayed as boxplots (**Figure 4B**). ASAP additionally allow conducting this step using germline sequences provided by a user.

CDR3 length distribution was shown to vary in response to specific challenges (27–30). ASAP hence provides the distribution of CDR3 length for each replicate, both as a file and as a histogram (**Figure 5**).

Each of the V, D, and J genes can be encoded by several distinct alleles termed subgroups (26). Thus, for each gene, the server provides the frequency of unique amino acid sequences included in each subgroup. These data are graphically shown as three histograms. An example of such a histogram is shown in (**Figure 6**). Data regarding the subgroup usage and combination were previously shown to be important for understanding the nature and dynamics of the immune response, facilitating the distinction between cell types (31, 32). ASAP thus also provides the frequencies of all possible subgroup combinations. An example of the histogram is shown in **Figure 7**.

A clone is defined as the collection of antibody sequences that likely originated from a single B cell lineage. Clonal analysis may provide insights into the evolution of the antigen-specific response of that lineage (11). In practice, clones are defined by clustering variable region sequences that comprise highly similar

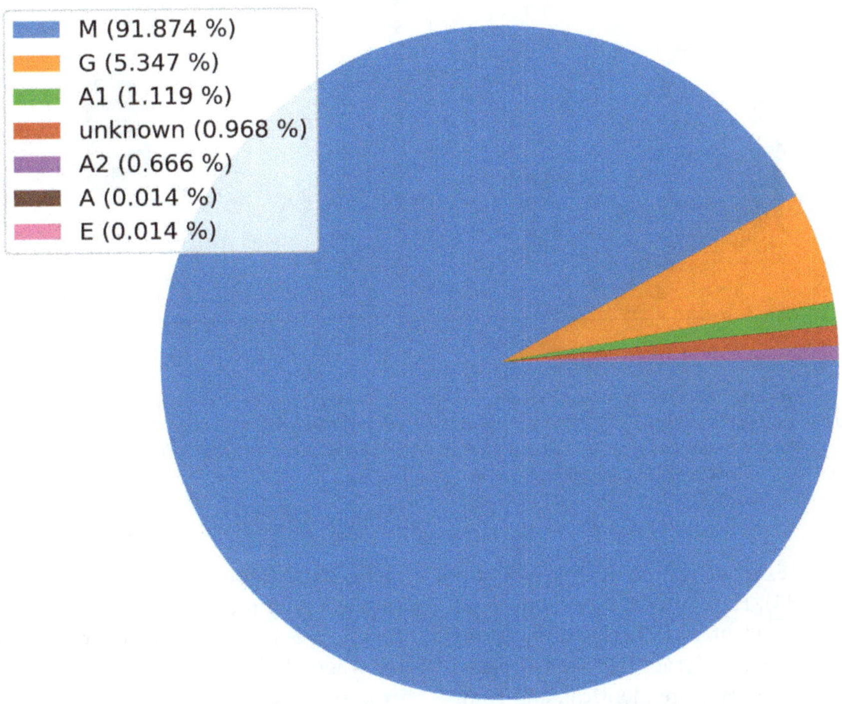


**FIGURE 3** | A pie chart showing the distribution of isotypes in a specific next-generation sequencing (NGS) replicate. Note, this chart was generated using unpublished human NGS data.

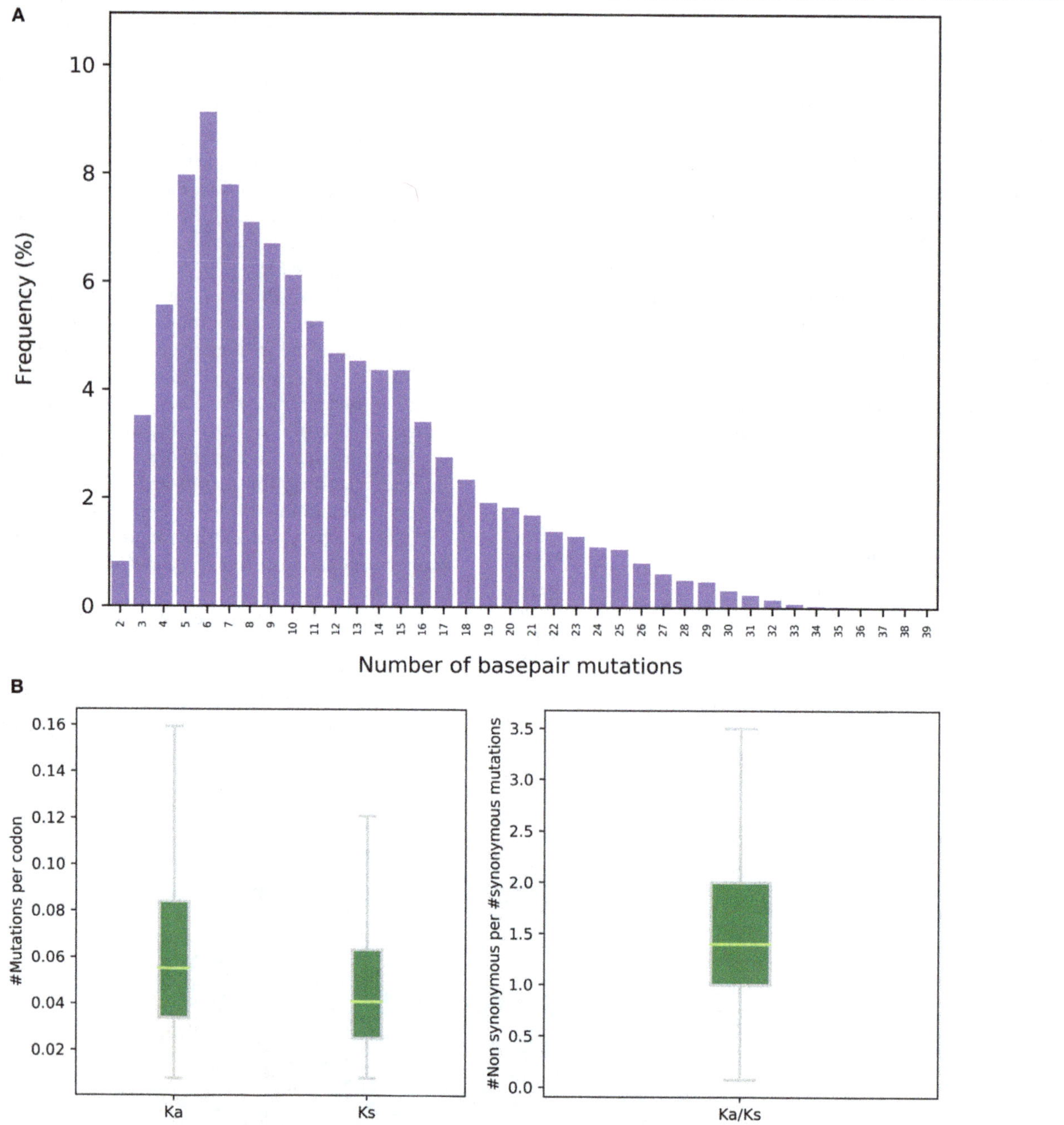


**FIGURE 4** | Somatic hypermutation analysis. **(A)** A histogram showing the frequency of the number of base pair mutations in a next-generation sequencing replicate. The *X* axis represents the number of mutations (both synonymous and non-synonymous) defined by comparison to the germline genes. **(B)** The number of non-synonymous (Ka) and synonymous (Ks) mutations and their ratios (Ka/Ks), based on comparison to the germline genes. The *Y* axis is the number of mutations per codon. Each dot represents a unique variable region nucleotide sequence.

CDRH3 regions, although the exact definition of this similarity varies among studies (10, 15, 33). Here, we define a clone as all variable region sequences with an identical CDRH3 region (at the amino acid level). Let $y$ be the number of reads that are associated with a specific clone. Some of the reads are identical, and some differ in their nucleotide sequence. Let $x$ be the number of unique amino acid sequences within a clone (these sequences differ in regions other than the CDRH3 region; $x \leq y$). Both $x$ and $y$ are biologically important: $y$ is indicative of the level of sequence variance within a clone, a phenomenon called clonal expansion (2) and $x$ is indicative of the proliferation tendency of the clone (or when cDNA is used, high values of $x$ may also indicate high expression levels). In ASAP, the data regarding these $x$ and $y$ values are provided for each clone, as well as a graph showing these values for the $K$ clones (the default is $K = 100$) with the highest $y$ values (**Figure 8**).

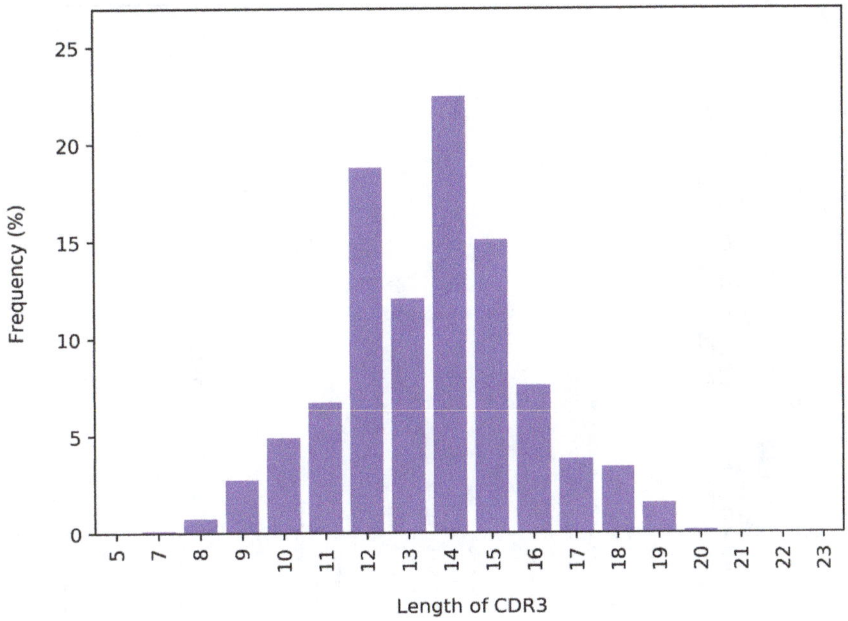


**FIGURE 5** | The distribution of CDR3 length (number of amino acids) in a next-generation sequencing replicate.

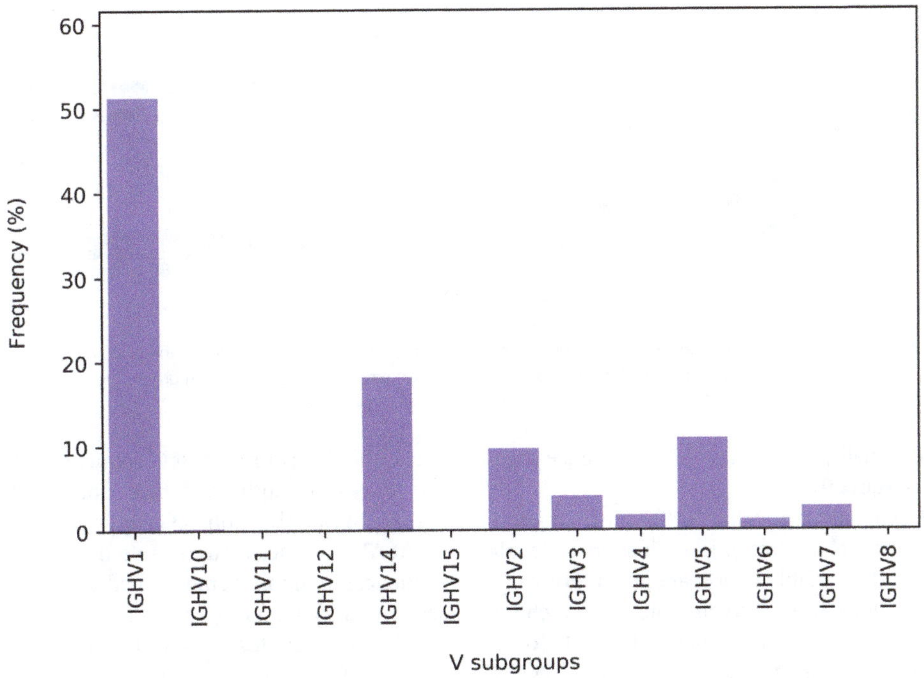


**FIGURE 6** | The distribution of V subgroups in a replicate. Shown is the distribution of the subgroup families for the heavy chain of IgG.

For each of the above *K* clones, ASAP also provides a file for the multiple sequence alignment between all clone members. These multiple sequence alignments are also visualized by Wasabi (34). An addition annotation file includes the following information for each clone: [1] CDRH3 amino acid sequence; [2] CDRH3 counts (the *y* parameter described above); [3] unique variable region amino acid sequence counts (the *x* parameter described above); [4] the consensus sequence; [5] the amino acid sequence of the clone member which is most similar to the consensus sequence; [6] the similarity score; [7] the DNA sequence of the

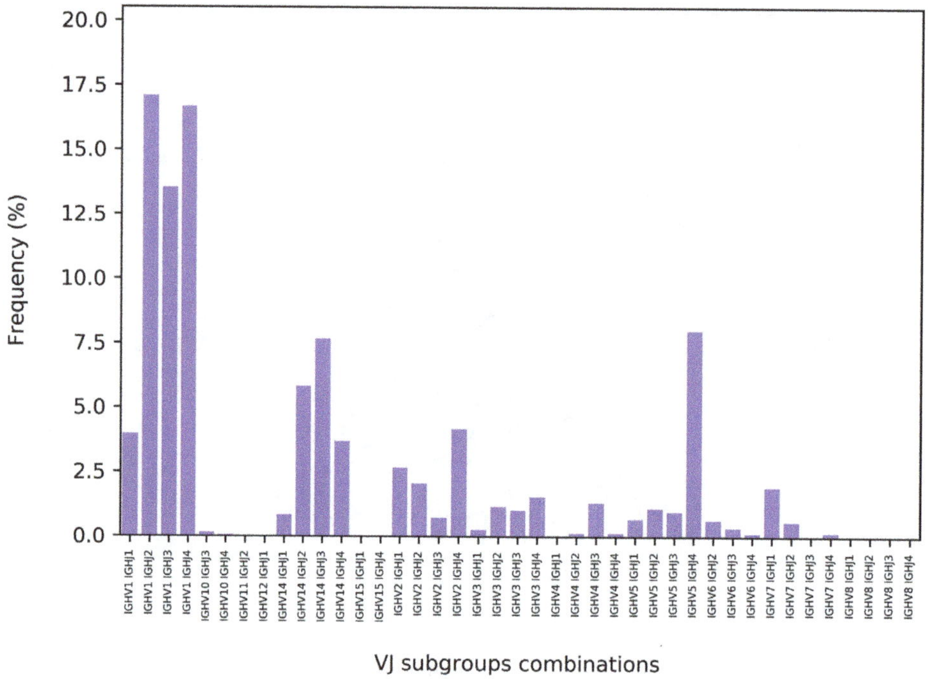


**FIGURE 7** | The distribution of the V(D)J combinations in a next-generation sequencing replicate. Shown are the frequencies of the various combinations between the V and J subgroups.

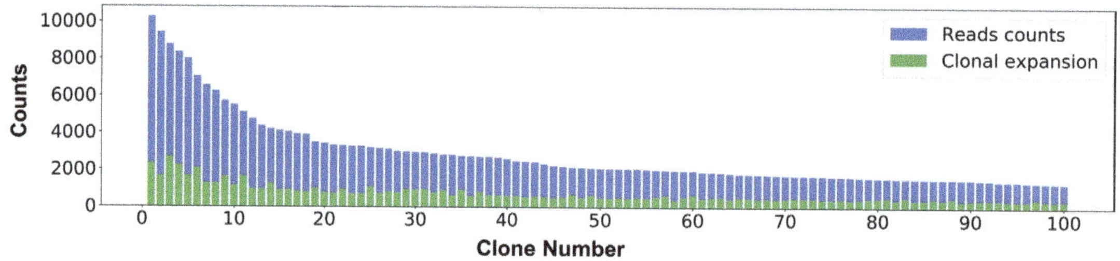


**FIGURE 8** | Clonal expansion. The *X* axis shows the most prevalent 100 clones. For each clone, the *Y* axis represents the number of variable region amino acid reads supporting each clone (in blue) and the number of contributing unique variable region amino acid sequences (in green).

most similar sequence. Finally, for each clone a sequence logo graph is also provided (**Figure 9**).

In addition, ASAP generates a specific FASTA file for each chain type (e.g., $V_H$ AA Sequences.fasta). In each such a file, all amino acid sequences of the variable region are given. For each sequence, the following information is given in its header: chain type and isotype, the CDR3 amino acid sequence, the V, D (only in $V_H$), and J subgroup families, and unique variable region occurrences (at the amino acid level). For proteomic analyses, and in particular, those aimed to analyze antibody repertoires, the C terminus of the variable region sequence (i.e., the N terminal of the $C_H1$ region) must include a proteolytic cleavage site (9). To this end, the server allows concatenating for each of the sequences in the above FASTA file a proteolytic cleavage site. By default, the "ASTK" and "AK" peptides are added after the FR4 motif (**Figure 1B**) of the heavy chain, for the human and mouse sequences, respectively. These suffixes introduce a trypsin cleavage site at the C terminus of IgG sequences. Alternatively, users can introduce other suffixes of their choice, including isotype-specific suffixes in case that non-IgG isotypes are proteomically analyzed.

ASAP provides a supportive file that maps each amino acid sequences in the abovementioned file to the associated nucleotide sequences. A file is provided for each chain type (e.g., $V_H$ AA TO DNA reads, fasta). Within each file, for each amino acid sequence the following information is given: the header includes the variable region amino acid sequence itself. For each header, the nucleotide sequences that are associated with the amino acid sequences are provided coupled with the original index from the FASTQ file.

## Joint Analysis

After each replicate is analyzed as outlined above, the server also reports statistics based on replicate integration (a "joint" analysis). Importantly, while valuable information can be obtained by

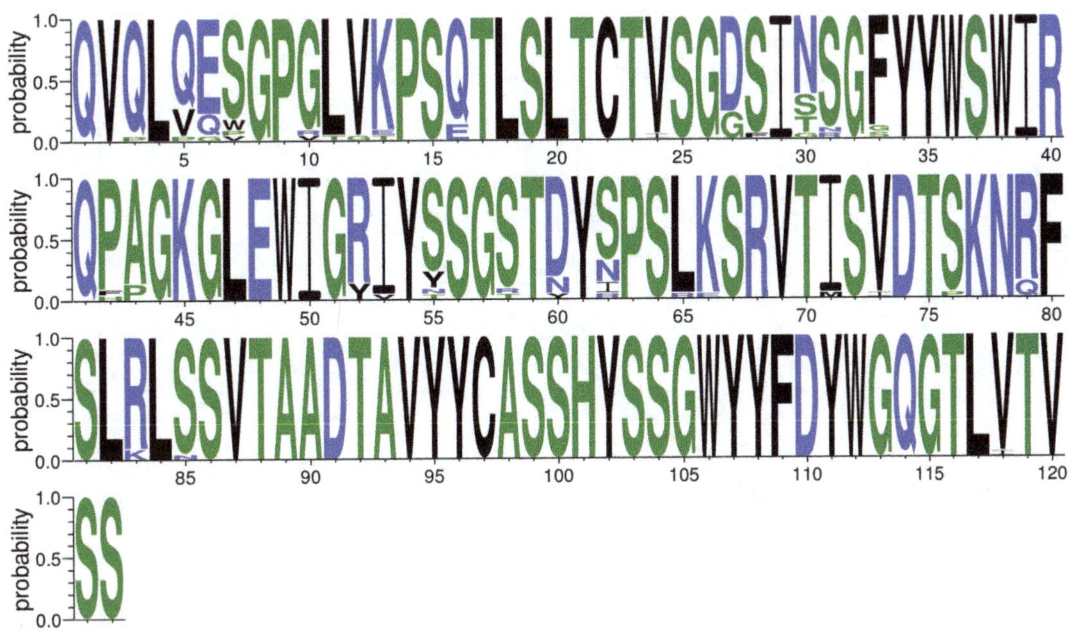

**FIGURE 9** | Sequence logo of one of the top clones.

analyzing individual runs, the benefit of the joint analysis is that a single graph for each attribute of the data is generated based on shared reads, e.g., the top K clones based on the ensemble of all repeats. Thus, the joint analysis is beneficial for filtering out dataset specific reads, which may be unreliable, for pointing out problematic repeats, and as a platform to get characteristics and statistical measurements from the entire data. Notably, establishing a single reliable data is of vast importance for downstream applications, such as mass spectrometry (see below).

The first step in this joint analysis is to construct a joint annotation file, in which the reads from all replicates are aggregated, and which is otherwise in the same format as the individual files for each replicate analysis (individual analysis). Based on this joint analysis, ASAP produces the entire set of statistics, as described above for the single replicates (see previous section). The differences and commonalities among the multiple runs are further characterized, as outline below.

The correlation between each pair of runs is reported in terms of the frequencies of each sequence. High correlation (**Figure 10A**) point to reproducible replicates while lower levels of correlations (**Figure 10B**) can point to biases that may be derived from experimental or sequencing problems.

Similar to the single individual processing, ASAP generates a FASTA file, which provides the entire list of amino acid sequences shared among all replicates. Unlike the individual processing file, information regarding the unique variable region occurrences summed over all replicates (at the amino acid level) and a comma separated list of these occurrences in each replicate is also provided. The server additionally provides a Venn diagram that depicts the intersections among the different replicates, presenting the number of unique variable region amino acid sequences shared between the replicates (**Figure 11**).

## DISCUSSION

The ASAP webserver described here provides bioinformatic support for AIRR-Seq analysis. It is simple, free, and does not require a login information. Several webservers for analyzing AIRR-Seq obtained *via* NGS have been recently reported (35–39). However, the ASAP server offers a number of unique advantages, including the analysis of multiple replicates, defining custom search space to include new germlines, preparation of the data for proteomic analyses, and single push button analysis of raw data directly obtained from the NGS platform, without requiring any pre-analyses. This latter feature allows non-expert users to readily use ASAP for analyzing their data. **Table 1** summarizes the analyses supported by ASAP compared to other related webservers.

Clonality is an important concept in antibody repertoire analysis. Yet, its exact definition varies among different studies and tools. For example, clonality may be defined based on either DNA or amino-acid sequences. Most commonly, computational clustering of variable region sequences into clones is based on the CDR-H3 region (2). Clearly, with the enormous increase in NGS data available for such studies, concepts such as clonality are rapidly evolving and choosing a specific criterion may result in too narrow or too wide clustering (under-clustering and over-clustering, respectively). Thus, clustering analysis such as the one provided in this webserver should be taken with a grain of salt when interpreting biological data.

We rely on the MiXCR software for the initial processing that uses germline information from IMGT. Novel germline alleles are inferred and discovered in an accelerated pace (40–42). Thus, it is clear that the set of germline sequences found in IMGT is restricted. This emphasizes the need to enable flexibility in defining the annotation search space to include new germlines. The inclusion of such

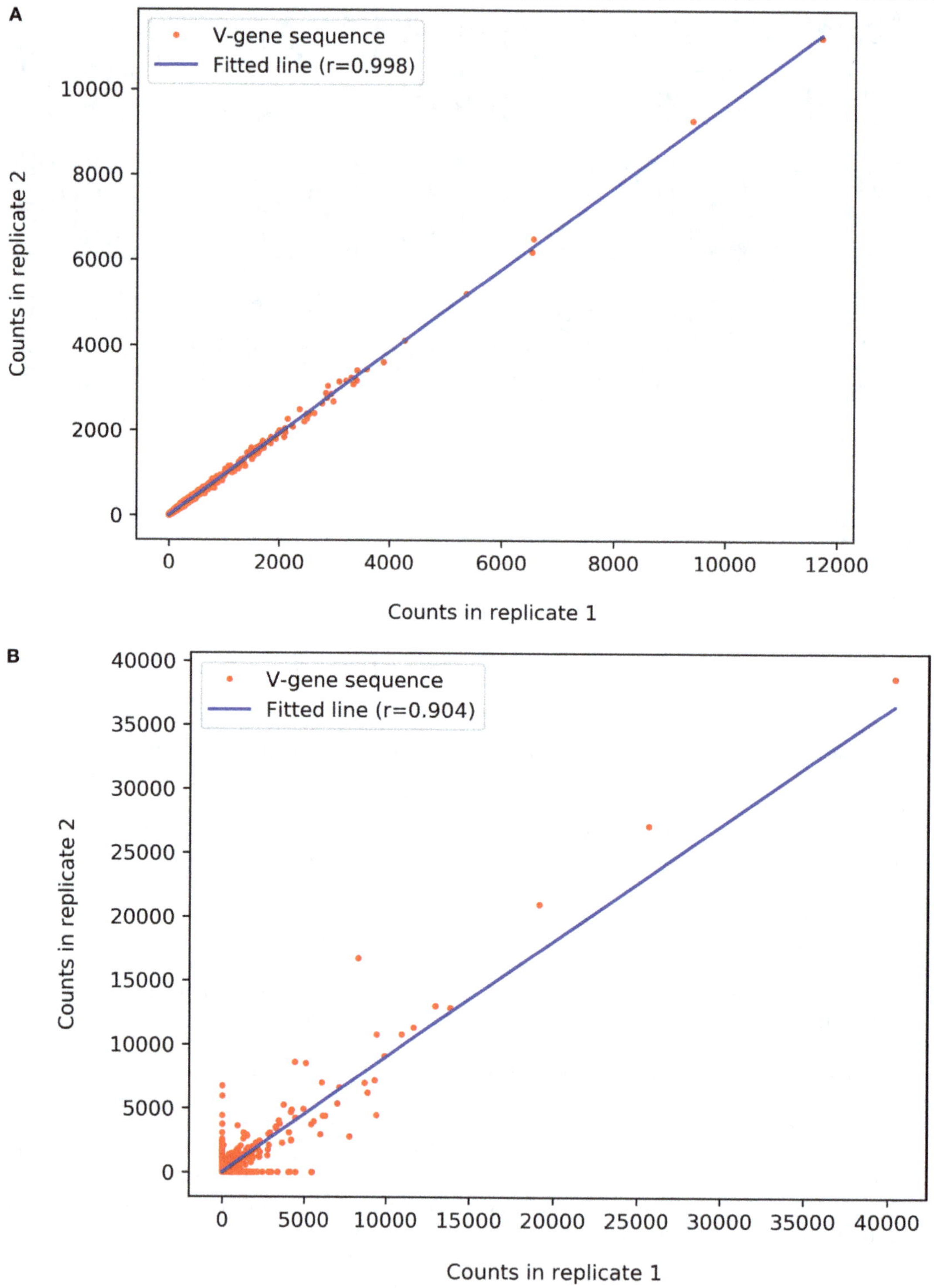


**FIGURE 10** | Pearson correlation between two next-generation sequencing replicates. Each dot represents a unique amino acid variable region. The *X* and *Y* axes indicate the number of times each such read appears in the first and the second replicate, respectively. **(A)** Replicates with high reproducibility and **(B)** with lower reproducibility between replicates.

alleles will directly affect the V(D)J usage profile, clonality, and level of SHM, thus eventually reflecting on the obtained biological insights. ASAP provides the option to append the germline space with provisional novel alleles. This option enables to annotate the AIRR-Seq data with these alleles and to inspect the impact of missing germline alleles on downstream analyses.

In various fields of biology, analyzing multiple repeats is a requirement, e.g., in expression analyses (43) or ChiP Seq data (44).

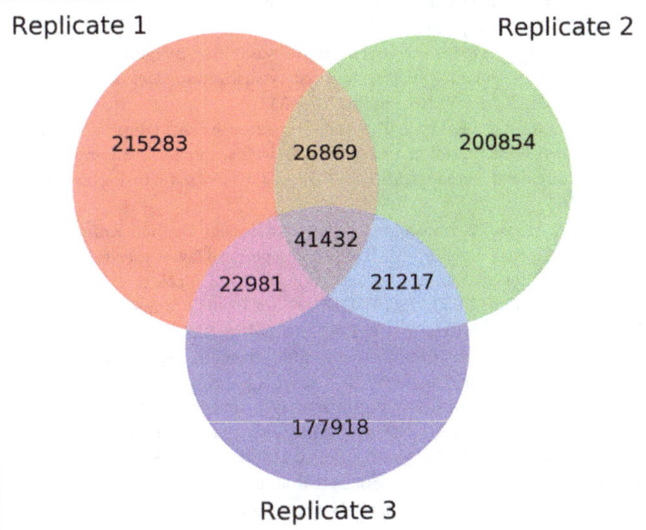


**FIGURE 11** | Venn diagram showing the number of variable region amino acid sequences that are shared among next-generation sequencing replicates.

The importance of repeats is critical in high-throughput analyses in order to remove random noise, thereby increasing the signal to noise ratio. While experimental and computational methodologies to increase this ratio do exist (19, 45, 46), these approaches often require sophisticated experimental setups, precluding their utilization by non-experts. Moreover, even when applying these experimental approaches, a further increase in signal to noise ratio can be achieved by experimental repeats. This motivated us to implement robust inference procedures for analyzing multiple repeats, e.g., the correlations between repeats, a Venn diagram showing the intersections among repeats, etc. Given the constant reduction in NGS costs, we expect repetitions in NGS experiments to become the standard procedure in the field of AIRR-Seq.

AIRR-Seq can also be used for proteomic identification of monoclonal antibodies within the polyclonal pool present in biological fluids. B cells effector function is the expression and secretion of antibodies into the blood or mucosal tissues. However, the composition of these antibodies remained elusive for many years. Proteomic identification of secreted antibodies requires the consolidation of a high confidence individual specific antibody archive in order to interpret the LC-MS/MS spectra. The utilization of proteomic analysis of antibodies from serum or secretion is emerging as a powerful tool to investigate their molecular composition, relative concentrations, temporal dynamics, and the relationship to well-studied B cells (6, 8–10, 12, 13, 15).

ASAP currently allows analyzing antibody sequences obtained from either human or mouse. While most studies involving AIRR-Seq focus on these two model organisms, in the future, antibody repertoire analyses from an extended taxonomical sampling should provide information about the differences among organisms, thereby providing insights into the evolution of the adaptive immune response.

## AUTHOR CONTRIBUTIONS

AV-M, DY, OA, TP, and YW designed the research; OA, DY, HA, TP, and YW implemented the webserver; OA, TP, and YW wrote the paper; OA and AV-M equally contributed.

## FUNDING

This study was supported in part by a fellowship from the Edmond J. Safra Center for Bioinformatics at Tel Aviv University and ISF Grant No. 1282/17.

## REFERENCES


1. Tonegawa S. Somatic generation of antibody diversity. *Nature* (1983) 302(5909):575–81. doi:10.1038/302575a0
2. Miho E, Yermanos A, Weber CR, Berger CT, Reddy ST, Greiff V. Computational strategies for dissecting the high-dimensional complexity of adaptive immune repertoires. *Front Immunol* (2018) 9:224. doi:10.3389/fimmu.2018.00224
3. Weinstein JA, Weinstein JA, Jiang N, Jiang N, White RA, White RA, et al. High-throughput sequencing of the zebrafish antibody repertoire. *Science* (2009) 324(5928):807–10. doi:10.1126/science.1170020
4. D'Angelo S, Ferrara F, Naranjo L, Erasmus MF, Hraber P, Bradbury ARM. Many routes to an antibody heavy-chain CDR3: necessary, yet insufficient, for specific binding. *Front Immunol* (2018) 9:395. doi:10.3389/fimmu.2018.00395
5. Reddy ST, Ge X, Miklos AE, Hughes RA, Kang SH, Hoi KH, et al. Monoclonal antibodies isolated without screening by analyzing the variable-gene repertoire of plasma cells. *Nat Biotechnol* (2010) 28(9):965–U20. doi:10.1038/nbt.1673
6. Cheung WC, Beausoleil SA, Zhang X, Sato S, Schieferl SM, Wieler JS, et al. A proteomics approach for the identification and cloning of monoclonal antibodies from serum. *Nat Biotechnol* (2012) 30(5):447–52. doi:10.1038/nbt.2167
7. DeKosky BJ, Kojima T, Rodin A, Charab W, Ippolito GC, Ellington AD, et al. In-depth determination and analysis of the human paired heavy- and light-chain antibody repertoire. *Nat Med* (2014) 21(1):86–91. doi:10.1038/nm.3743
8. DeKosky BJ, Ippolito GC, Deschner RP, Lavinder JJ, Wine Y, Rawlings BM, et al. High-throughput sequencing of the paired human immunoglobulin heavy and light chain repertoire. *Nat Biotechnol* (2013) 31(2):166–9. doi:10.1038/nbt.2492
9. Boutz DR, Horton AP, Wine Y, Lavinder JJ, Georgiou G, Marcotte EM. Proteomic identification of monoclonal antibodies from serum. *Anal Chem* (2014) 86(10):4758–66. doi:10.1021/ac4037679
10. Lavinder JJ, Wine Y, Giesecke C, Ippolito GC, Horton AP, Lungu OI, et al. Identification and characterization of the constituent human serum antibodies elicited by vaccination. *Proc Natl Acad Sci U S A* (2014) 111(6):2259–64. doi:10.1073/pnas.1317793111
11. Wine Y, Boutz DR, Lavinder JJ, Miklos AE, Hughes RA, Hoi KH, et al. Molecular deconvolution of the monoclonal antibodies that comprise the polyclonal serum response. *Proc Natl Acad Sci U S A* (2013) 110(8):2993–8. doi:10.1073/pnas.1213737110
12. Iversen R, Snir O, Stensland M, Kroll JE, Steinsbø Ø, Korponay-Szabó IR, et al. Strong clonal relatedness between serum and gut IgA despite different plasma cell origins. *Cell Rep* (2017) 20(10):2357–67. doi:10.1016/j.celrep.2017.08.036
13. Tipton CM, Fucile CF, Darce J, Chida A, Ichikawa T, Gregoretti I, et al. Diversity, cellular origin and autoreactivity of antibody-secreting cell population expansions in acute systemic lupus erythematosus. *Nat Immunol* (2015) 16(7):755. doi:10.1038/ni.3175
14. VanDuijn MM, Dekker LJ, van IJcken WFJ, Sillevis Smitt PAE, Luider TM. Immune repertoire after immunization as seen by next-generation sequencing and proteomics. *Front Immunol* (2017) 8:1286. doi:10.3389/fimmu.2017.01286
15. Lee J, Boutz DR, Chromikova V, Joyce MG, Vollmers C, Leung K, et al. Molecular-level analysis of the serum antibody repertoire in young adults

before and after seasonal influenza vaccination. *Nat Med* (2016) 22(12):1456. doi:10.1038/nm.4224
16. Chen J, Zheng Q, Hammers CM, Ellebrecht CT, Mukherjee EM, Tang H-Y, et al. Proteomic analysis of pemphigus autoantibodies indicates a larger, more diverse, and more dynamic repertoire than determined by B cell genetics. *Cell Rep* (2017) 18(1):237–47. doi:10.1016/j.celrep.2016.12.013
17. Greiff V, Miho E, Menzel U, Reddy ST. Bioinformatic and statistical analysis of adaptive immune repertoires. *Trends Immunol* (2015) 36(11):738–49. doi:10.1016/j.it.2015.09.006
18. Yaari G, Kleinstein SH. Practical guidelines for B-cell receptor repertoire sequencing analysis. *Genome Med* (2015) 7(1):121. doi:10.1186/s13073-015-0243-2
19. Khan TA, Friedensohn S, de Vries ARG, Straszewski J, Ruscheweyh H-J, Reddy ST. Accurate and predictive antibody repertoire profiling by molecular amplification fingerprinting. *Sci Adv* (2016) 2(3):e1501371. doi:10.1126/sciadv.1501371
20. Wang C, Liu Y, Cavanagh MM, Le Saux S, Qi Q, Roskin KM, et al. B-cell repertoire responses to varicella-zoster vaccination in human identical twins. *Proc Natl Acad Sci U S A* (2015) 112(2):500–5. doi:10.1073/pnas.1415875112
21. Breden F, Luning Prak ET, Peters B, Rubelt F, Schramm CA, Busse CE, et al. Reproducibility and reuse of adaptive immune receptor repertoire data. *Front Immunol* (2017) 8:1817. doi:10.3389/fimmu.2017.01418
22. Rubelt F, Busse CE, Bukhari SAC, Burckert JP, Mariotti-Ferrandiz E, Cowell LG, et al. Adaptive immune receptor repertoire community recommendations for sharing immune-repertoire sequencing data. *Nat Immunol* (2017) 18(12): 1274–8. doi:10.1038/ni.3873
23. Greiff V, Menzel U, Haessler U, Cook SC, Friedensohn S, Khan TA, et al. Quantitative assessment of the robustness of next-generation sequencing of antibody variable gene repertoires from immunized mice. *BMC Immunol* (2014) 15:40. doi:10.1186/s12865-014-0040-5
24. Bolotin DA, Poslavsky S, Mitrophanov I, Shugay M, Mamedov IZ, Putintseva EV, et al. MiXCR: software for comprehensive adaptive immunity profiling. *Nat Methods* (2015) 12(5):380–1. doi:10.1038/nmeth.3364
25. Smith T, Heger A, Sudbery I. UMI-tools: modeling sequencing errors in Unique Molecular Identifiers to improve quantification accuracy. *Genome Res* (2017) 27(3):491–9. doi:10.1101/gr.209601.116
26. Lefranc MP, Giudicelli V, Ginestoux C, Bodmer J, Müller W, Bontrop R, et al. IMGT, the international ImMunoGeneTics database. *Nucleic Acids Res* (1999) 27(1):209–12. doi:10.1093/nar/27.1.209
27. Galson JD, Trück J, Fowler A, Clutterbuck EA, Münz M, Cerundolo V, et al. Analysis of B cell repertoire dynamics following hepatitis B vaccination in humans, and enrichment of vaccine-specific antibody sequences. *EBioMedicine* (2015) 2(12):2070–9. doi:10.1016/j.ebiom.2015.11.034
28. Douthwaite JA, Sridharan S, Huntington C, Hammersley J, Marwood R, Hakulinen JK, et al. Affinity maturation of a novel antagonistic human monoclonal antibody with a long VH CDR3 targeting the class A GPCR formyl-peptide receptor 1. *MAbs* (2015) 7(1):152–66. doi:10.4161/19420862.2014.985158
29. Wu Y-C, Kipling D, Leong HS, Martin V, Ademokun AA, Dunn-Walters DK. High-throughput immunoglobulin repertoire analysis distinguishes between human IgM memory and switched memory B-cell populations. *Blood* (2010) 116(7):1070–8. doi:10.1182/blood-2010-03-275859
30. Wu Y-C, Kipling D, Dunn-Walters DK. The relationship between CD27 negative and positive B cell populations in human peripheral blood. *Front Immunol* (2011) 2:81. doi:10.3389/fimmu.2011.00081
31. Wu GC, Cheung N-KV, Georgiou G, Marcotte EM, Ippolito GC. Temporal stability and molecular persistence of the bone marrow plasma cell antibody repertoire. *Nat Commun* (2016) 7:13838. doi:10.1038/ncomms13838
32. Martin VG, Wu Y-CB, Townsend CL, Lu GHC, O'Hare JS, Mozeika A, et al. Transitional B cells in early human B cell development – time to revisit the paradigm? *Front Immunol* (2016) 7:546. doi:10.3389/fimmu.2016.00546
33. Greiff V, Menzel U, Miho E, Weber C, Riedel R, Cook S, et al. Systems analysis reveals high genetic and antigen-driven predetermination of antibody repertoires throughout B cell development. *Cell Rep* (2017) 19(7):1467–78. doi:10.1016/j.celrep.2017.04.054
34. Veidenberg A, Medlar A, Löytynoja A. Wasabi: an integrated platform for evolutionary sequence analysis and data visualization. *Mol Biol Evol* (2016) 33(4):1126–30. doi:10.1093/molbev/msv333
35. Margreitter C, Lu H-C, Townsend C, Stewart A, Dunn-Walters DK, Fraternali F. BRepertoire: a user-friendly web server for analysing antibody repertoire data. *Nucleic Acids Res* (2018) 46(W1):W264–70. doi:10.1093/nar/gky276
36. IJspeert H, van Schouwenburg PA, van Zessen D, Pico-Knijnenburg I, Stubbs AP, van der Burg M. Antigen receptor galaxy: a user-friendly, web-based tool for analysis and visualization of T and B cell receptor repertoire data. *J Immunol* (2017) 198(10):4156–65. doi:10.4049/jimmunol.1601921
37. Duez M, Giraud M, Herbert R, Rocher T, Salson M, Thonier F. Vidjil: a web platform for analysis of high-throughput repertoire sequencing. *PLoS One* (2016) 11(11):e0166126. doi:10.1371/journal.pone.0166126
38. Bagaev DV, Zvyagin IV, Putintseva EV, Izraelson M, Britanova OV, Chudakov DM, et al. VDJviz: a versatile browser for immunogenomics data. *BMC Genomics* (2016) 17(1):453. doi:10.1186/s12864-016-2799-7
39. Christley S, Scarborough W, Salinas E, Rounds WH, Toby IT, Fonner JM, et al. VDJServer: a cloud-based analysis portal and data commons for immune repertoire sequences and rearrangements. *Front Immunol* (2018) 9:976. doi:10.3389/fimmu.2018.00976
40. Gadala-Maria D, Yaari G, Uduman M, Kleinstein SH. Automated analysis of high-throughput B-cell sequencing data reveals a high frequency of novel immunoglobulin V gene segment alleles. *Proc Natl Acad Sci U S A* (2015) 112(8):E862–70. doi:10.1073/pnas.1417683112
41. Corcoran MM, Phad GE, Bernat NV, Stahl-Hennig C, Sumida N, Persson MAA, et al. Production of individualized V gene databases reveals high levels of immunoglobulin genetic diversity. *Nat Commun* (2016) 7:13642. doi:10.1038/ncomms13642
42. Ma K-Y, He C, Wendel BS, Williams CM, Xiao J, Yang H, et al. Immune repertoire sequencing using molecular identifiers enables accurate clonality discovery and clone size quantification. *Front Immunol* (2018) 9:33. doi:10.3389/fimmu.2018.00033
43. Mortazavi A, Williams BA, McCue K, Schaeffer L, Wold B. Mapping and quantifying mammalian transcriptomes by RNA-Seq. *Nat Methods* (2008) 5(7):621–8. doi:10.1038/nmeth.1226
44. Tang X, Srivastava A, Liu H, Machiraju R, Huang K, Leone G. annoPeak: a web application to annotate and visualize peaks from ChIP-seq/ChIP-exo-seq. *Bioinformatics* (2017) 33(10):1570–1. doi:10.1093/bioinformatics/btx016
45. Vollmers C, Sit RV, Weinstein JA, Dekker CL, Quake SR. Genetic measurement of memory B-cell recall using antibody repertoire sequencing. *Proc Natl Acad Sci U S A* (2013) 110(33):13463–8. doi:10.1073/pnas.1312146110
46. Vander Heiden JA, Yaari G, Uduman M, Stern JNH, O'Connor KC, Hafler DA, et al. pRESTO: a toolkit for processing high-throughput sequencing raw reads of lymphocyte receptor repertoires. *Bioinformatics* (2014) 30(13):1930–2. doi:10.1093/bioinformatics/btu138

# 4

# Immune Repertoire Sequencing Using Molecular Identifiers Enables Accurate Clonality Discovery and Clone Size Quantification

*Ke-Yue Ma[1†], Chenfeng He[2†], Ben S. Wendel[3], Chad M. Williams[2], Jun Xiao[4], Hui Yang[5,6] and Ning Jiang[1,2*]*

*[1] Institute for Cellular and Molecular Biology, The University of Texas at Austin, Austin, TX, United States, [2] Department of Biomedical Engineering, Cockrell School of Engineering, The University of Texas at Austin, Austin, TX, United States, [3] McKetta Department of Chemical Engineering, Cockrell School of Engineering, The University of Texas at Austin, Austin, TX, United States, [4] ImmuDX, LLC, Austin, TX, United States, [5] School of Life Sciences, Northwestern Polytechnical University, Xi'an, Shaanxi, China, [6] Research Center of Special Environmental Biomechanics & Medical Engineering, Xi'an, Shaanxi, China*

***Correspondence:**
*Ning Jiang*
*jiang@austin.utexas.edu*

*†These authors have contributed equally to this work.*

Unique molecular identifiers (MIDs) have been demonstrated to effectively improve immune repertoire sequencing (IR-seq) accuracy, especially to identify somatic hypermutations in antibody repertoire sequencing. However, evaluating the sensitivity to detect rare T cells and the degree of clonal expansion in IR-seq has been difficult due to the lack of knowledge of T cell receptor (TCR) RNA molecule copy number and a generalized approach to estimate T cell clone size from TCR RNA molecule quantification. This limited the application of TCR repertoire sequencing (TCR-seq) in clinical settings, such as detecting minimal residual disease in lymphoid malignancies after treatment, evaluating effectiveness of vaccination and assessing degree of infection. Here, we describe using an MID Clustering-based IR-Seq (MIDCIRS) method to quantitatively study TCR RNA molecule copy number and clonality in T cells. First, we demonstrated the necessity of performing MID sub-clustering to eliminate erroneous sequences. Further, we showed that MIDCIRS enables a sensitive detection of a single cell in as many as one million naïve T cells and an accurate estimation of the degree of T cell clonal expression. The demonstrated accuracy, sensitivity, and wide dynamic range of MIDCIRS TCR-seq provide foundations for future applications in both basic research and clinical settings.

**Keywords: MID clustering-based IR-Seq TCR repertoire sequencing, molecular identifiers, sub-clustering, naïve T cells, CMV-specific T cells**

## INTRODUCTION

Immune repertoire sequencing (IR-seq) has become a useful tool to quantify the composition of B or T cell antigen receptor repertoires in basic research, such as vaccination (1–3), immune repertoire development (4–9), and lymphocyte lineage tracking (2, 9), as well as in various clinical settings, such as minimal residual disease (MRD) monitoring (10), hematopoietic stem cell transplant recovery monitoring (11), and cancer patient prognosis (12, 13). However, early IR-seq experiments suffered from high PCR and sequencing errors that limited their ability to perform accurate repertoire diversity and abundance quantification. This bottleneck also limits the sensitivity of many IR-seq-based assays, such as MRD monitoring. Recently, we and others introduced molecular identifiers (MIDs) to IR-seq and DNA/RNA sequencing to reduce errors by tracking each RNA molecule through PCR and sequencing. This approach has significantly improved the accuracy of repertoire profiling (9, 14–19), especially to distinguish antibody somatic hypermutations from PCR and sequencing errors. However, several challenges remain regarding how to use MIDs correctly and how to use MIDs for cell clone size estimate. First, erroneous MIDs resulting from PCR or sequencing errors make accurate MID counting difficult. Second, there is a lack of general guidelines of required sequencing depth to saturate MID counts. Third, how to use RNA molecular counting to estimate T cell clone size has yet to be established.

These challenges become roadblocks to accurately quantify T cell receptor (TCR) or BCR RNA molecule copy number, which is important in estimating clonal expansion and identifying rare clones. Robins et al. developed QuanTILfy to attempt to address this problem by counting TILs and assessing T cell clonality in tissue samples through droplet digital PCR (dPCR) of rearranged TCRβ loci (20). However, by partitioning TCR Vβ into eight non-overlapping subgroups, this method lacks the sensitivity to identify unique CDR3 of each clonality, not to mention rare clones. Therefore, a more comprehensive method to quantify TCR or antibody transcripts with high sensitivity while retaining accurate clonal diversity is needed for both standardizing basic IR-seq studies and applying it in clinical decision-making, such as detecting MRD in lymphoid malignancies after treatment, evaluating effectiveness of vaccination, and assessing degree of infection.

We recently developed a more generalized approach with reduced MID length to identify each individual RNA molecule using a sequence-similarity-based clustering method to separate sequencing reads into sub-clusters within a group of sequencing reads that have the same MID. We applied this MID Clustering-based IR-Seq (MIDCIRS) to study age-related antibody repertoire development and diversification during acute malaria (9). In this study, we applied MIDCIRS to TCR [MIDCIRS TCR repertoire sequencing (TCR-seq)] and used CD8$^+$ T cells as a test bed to build a model to count TCR RNA molecule copy number based on input cell numbers, percentage of RNA input, and sequencing depth. We also demonstrated a significant improvement in detection sensitivity. A previous study using a different repertoire sequencing methodology reported the capacity to resolve one in 10,000 cells (21). With MIDCIRS TCR-seq, we were able to detect one unique T cell clone in 1,000,000 T cells. In addition, we applied MIDCIRS TCR-seq to examine T cell clonal expansion in CMV infection and showed that sensitive and accurate quantification of the TCR RNA molecule copy number is essential to quantify a single-cell's worth of TCR transcripts and to assess the degree of clonal expansion. In summary, we showed the significance of the sub-clustering step of MIDCIRS in preventing false MID group generation, which enabled highly accurate clonal type discovery. This study provides a framework for leveraging the sensitivity and accuracy of molecular barcoded IR-seq in MRD detection and assessing clonal expansion in infection and vaccination.

## MATERIALS AND METHODS

### Naïve CD8$^+$ T Cell Sorting

Human leukocyte reduction system chambers were obtained from de-identified donors at We Are Blood (Austin, TX, USA) with strict adherence to guidelines from the Institutional Review Board of the University of Texas at Austin. CD8$^+$ T cell enrichment was done following the protocol described previously (22) using RosetteSep CD8$^+$ T Cell Enrichment Cocktail (STEMCELL) together with Ficoll-Paque (GE Healthcare). Then, RBCs were lysed using ACK Lysing Buffer (Lonza). After washing in phosphate-buffered saline with fetal bovine serum, the cell mixture was passed through a cell strainer (Corning) and ready for use. Naïve CD8$^+$ T cells were FACS-sorted into RLT Plus buffer (Qiagen) supplemented with 1% β-mercaptoethanol (Sigma) based on the phenotype of CD8$^+$CD4$^-$CCR7$^+$CD45RA$^+$ using BD FACSAria II cell sorter.

### CMV CD8$^+$ T Cell Enrichment and Sorting

CMVpp65:482-490 (NLVPMVATV) was used to prepare streptamers as previously described (23). Miltenyi anti-phycoerythrin microbeads and magnetic column were used to bind and enrich CMVpp65-specific T cells (22). The flow-through was collected for background staining. The enriched fraction was eluted off the column and washed into cell buffer. The following antibody panel was used to stain both the enriched and flow-through fractions: CD4, CD14, CD16, CD19, CD32, and CD56 (BioLegend) as a dump channel to stain residual non-CD8 T cells, and CD45RA, CCR7, CD27, and IL7R (BioLegend). 7-aminoactinomycin D was used as a viability marker. Dump$^-$Streptmer$^+$CD45RA$^+$CCR7$^-$CD27$^-$IL7R$^{lo}$ live T cells were sorted into RLT Plus buffer supplemented with 1% β-mercaptoethanol using BD FACSAria II cell sorter.

### Bulk TCR Library Generation and Sequencing

Total RNA was purified using All Prep DNA/RNA kit (Qiagen) following the manufacturer's protocol. Library preparation and QC were similar to protocols described previously (9) using TCR primers (Table S5 in Supplementary Material). Reads of the same library from all runs were combined and analyzed.

### dPCR of TCR

Total RNA purified from sorted CD8$^+$ T cells and cultured CMV-specific CD8$^+$ T cell lines were reverse transcribed with polyT primers (Table S5 in Supplementary Material) using Superscript III in 20 μl reaction following the manufacturer's protocol. 2 μl of cDNA was subsequently used on QuantStudio 3D dPCR system following manufacturer's protocol.

### Preliminary Read Processing

We followed the similar procedure as described previously to generate consensus sequences (9). First, only reads that have exact TCR constant sequences were kept for further analysis. These reads were then cut to 150 nt starting from constant region to eliminate high error-prone region at the end of reads. These preprocessed reads were split into MID groups according to 12-nt barcodes.

## MID Sub-Cluster Generating and Filtering

For each MID group, a quality threshold clustering was used to group reads derived from a common ancestor RNA molecule and separate reads derived from distinct RNAs as previously described (9). Briefly, a Levenshtein distance of 15% of the read length was used as the threshold (9). For each subgroup, a consensus sequence was built based on the average nucleotide at each position, weighted by the quality score. In the case that there were only two reads in an MID subgroup, we only considered them useful reads if both were identical. Each MID subgroup is equivalent to an RNA molecule. Next, we merged all of the identical consensus to form unique consensus sequences. Further, we applied filtering of unique consensus sequences after sub-cluster generation by (a) removing non-functional TCR sequences and (b) removing sequences with lower MID counts that are one Levenshtein distance away from the other. Then, for each unique consensus sequence, we removed MID sub-clusters if their reads are less than 20% of maximum read count based on the fitting of two negative binomial distribution (Figure S5 in Supplementary Material). Scripts for this section can be downloaded at https://github.com/utjianglab/MIDCIRS.

## Theoretical Percentage of MIDs That Need Sub-Clustering

We modeled the process of MID labeling as a Poisson distribution. Given the total number of MIDs being $M$ and the number of target molecules being $N$, the probability that a unique MID will occur $k$ time(s) is:

$$P_k = \frac{(\frac{N}{M})^k}{k!} \times e^{-\frac{N}{M}}. \quad (1)$$

Thus, $P_0$ and $P_1$ are the probability that a MID will be tagged 0 and 1 time, respectively, and the percentage of MIDs that need sub-clustering, $F(k > 1)$, is given by:

$$F(k>1) = \frac{\left[1 - e^{-\frac{N}{M}} - \frac{N}{M} \times e^{-\frac{N}{M}}\right]}{1 - e^{-\frac{N}{M}}}. \quad (2)$$

With over 16 million MID combinations from 12 random nucleotides, when the number of target molecules, $N$ is less than 5,000,000, Eq. 2 is an approximate linear function (**Figure 1B**).

## Diversity Coverage and RNA Copy Number Simulation

The estimation of diversity will be affected by the initial RNA input (percentage of initial RNA used to construct the sequencing library). We used a statistical model to estimate the diversity coverage for the naïve T cells we sorted based on RNA sampling depth.

For $N$ observed RNA molecules, there are $K$ different RNA clones. The RNA molecule copy number of each clone is $m_i$ ($i \in (1,K)$), whose sum equals $N$. After fitting the data, $m_i$ follows a power law distribution (Figure S9 in Supplementary Material):

$$m_i = m \times x_i \quad (3)$$

$$f(x_i) = (\alpha - 1) x_i^{-\alpha}, (\alpha > 1) \quad (4)$$

where, $m$ is the RNA molecule copy number per cell, which is a constant across all T cells (see **Figure 3C**). $x_i$ represents the cell numbers of each clone, which follows a power law distribution (24), and the parameter $\alpha$ was fitted with an algorithm combining maximum-likelihood fitting and goodness-of-fit test based on Kolmogorov–Smirnov statistic (25) "fit_power_law" function in R package igraph was applied (26).

Specifically, we fitted the RNA molecule distribution (Figure S9 in Supplementary Material) with Eq. 5:

$$f(m_i) = \left(\frac{\alpha - 1}{m_{\min}}\right)\left(\frac{m_i}{m_{\min}}\right)^{-\alpha}, (\alpha > 1). \quad (5)$$

Since "$m$" is a constant (see **Figure 3C**), the alpha in Eqs 4 and 5 should be equal. We fitted across all libraries on log–log scale, and the average slope was taken as $\alpha$ in the above model.

When we sample $n$ RNA molecules from this population, the expected detected diversity, $E(\mathrm{D})$, can be calculated as the following:

$$E(D \mid m, x_i) = K - \frac{\sum_{i=1}^{K} \binom{N - m \times x_i}{n}}{\binom{N}{n}}, x_i = (x_1, x_2, \ldots, x_K). \quad (6)$$

And $x_i$ can be sampled from the fitted power law distribution. Then, the percentage of the RNA diversity coverage, $P(\mathrm{D})$, can be estimated as:

$$P(D \mid m, x_i) = \frac{E(D \mid m, x_i)}{K}. \quad (7)$$

We scaled the diversity coverage of unique CDR3s to the estimated diversity coverage with 90% RNA input, $D_{\mathrm{obs}}$. We then used Eq. 8 to get estimated $m$:

$$\min_{m} \sum_{i} \left(P(D_i \mid m, x_i) - D_{\mathrm{obs}}\right)^2, m \in \{1, 2, \ldots\}. \quad (8)$$

## Statistical Analysis

Mann–Whitney $U$ test was used to calculate the significance of copy number difference between pairs in naïve, effector, effector memory, and central memory CD8+ T cells and $p$ values was adjusted with Benjamini–Hochberg procedure. Adjusted $p$-value that was less than 0.05 was considered significant.

# RESULTS

## MIDCIRS Sub-Clustering Improves Repertoire Diversity Estimation Accuracy

Molecular identifiers have been adopted in IR-seq and DNA/RNA sequencing to reduce error rate. However, during reverse

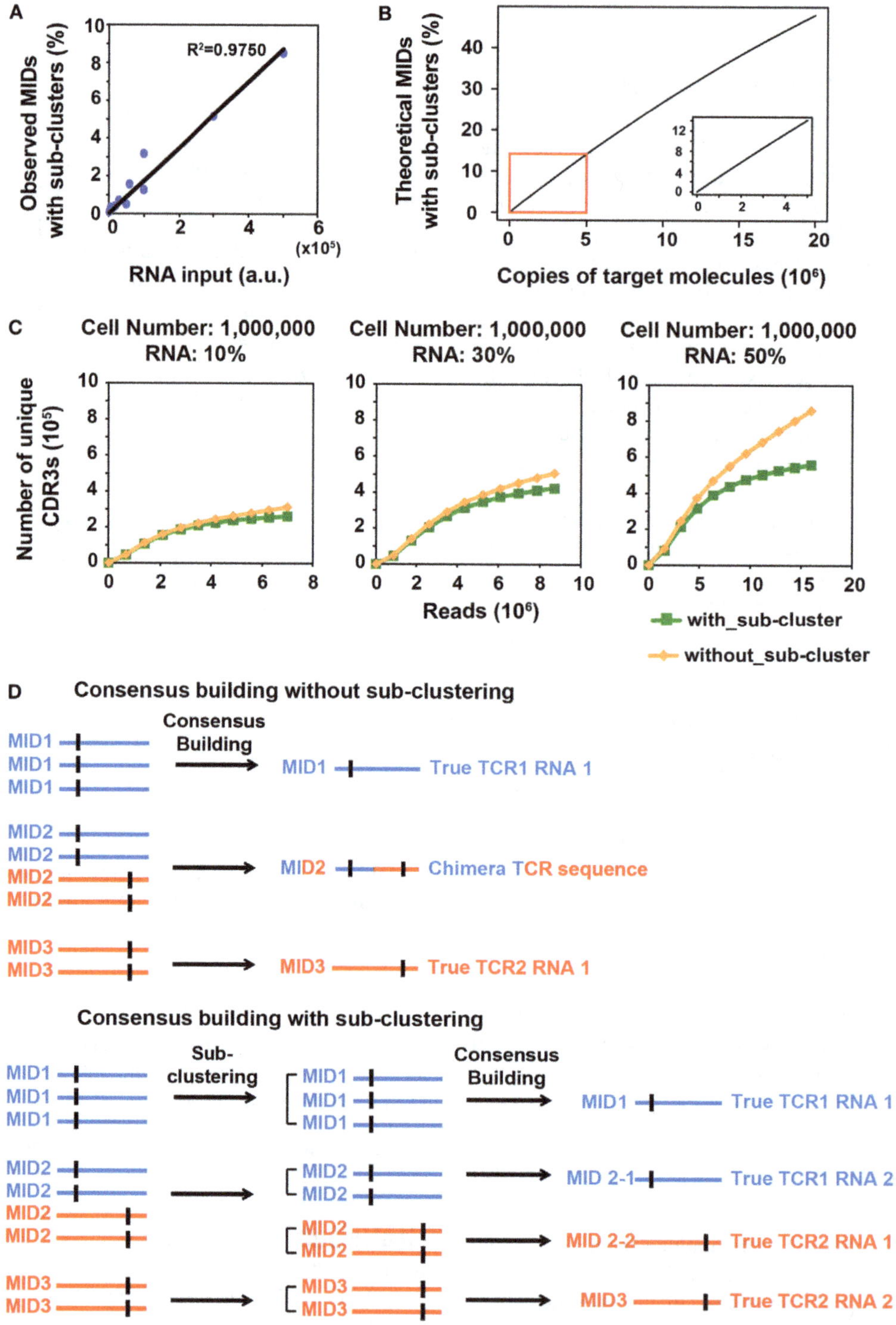


**FIGURE 1** | MID Clustering-based IR-Seq improves accuracy of T cell receptor (TCR) diversity estimation with sub-clustering. **(A)** The percentage of observed molecular identifiers (MIDs) containing sub-clusters is linearly dependent on RNA input, which is defined as cell number multiplied by percentage of RNA (e.g., 20,000 cells with 10%RNA is equivalent to 2,000 RNA input). Line represents linear regression fit, *F*-test on the slope, $p < 10^{-9}$. **(B)** The theoretical percentage of MIDs with sub-clusters is approximately linearly dependent on copies of target molecules when copies of target molecules are less than 5,000,000 (bottom right insert). The theoretical percentage of MIDs with sub-clusters was calculated by Eq. 2 in Section "Materials and Methods." **(C)** Rarefaction curve of unique complementarity-determining regions 3 (CDR3s) with or without sub-clustering. Number of unique CDR3s in three libraries made with three different RNA inputs from sorted one million naïve $CD8^+$ T cells are shown here. Data from other cell inputs are in Figure S2 in Supplementary Material. **(D)** Illustration of consensus TCR sequence building without (top) and with (bottom) sub-clustering. Top: without sub-clustering, chimera sequences are generated when different TCR RNA molecules are tagged with the same MID; bottom: TCR RNA molecules that are tagged with same MID are sub-clustered to reveal truly represented TCR sequences. Short vertical black lines indicate nucleotide differences between two TCR sequences.

transcription, multiple transcripts could stochastically be tagged with same MID. Previous strategies relied on increasing the length of MID to reduce the probability of non-unique MID tagging when the total RNA molecule copy number was either unknown or very large (27). However, longer MID length could reduce the efficiency of reverse transcription (28, 29). Thus, we developed a more generalized approach (MIDCIRS) with reduced MID length. A sequence-similarity-based clustering method was implemented in MIDCIRS to separate sequencing reads into sub-clusters within a group of sequencing reads that have the same MID (9). Here, we developed metrics to validate the accuracy of this sub-clustering method. In addition, we demonstrated the robust ability of MIDCIRS to faithfully represent the diversity and abundance of the TCR repertoire using a large range of RNA inputs.

We reasoned that in order to comprehensively quantify the overall diversity, a large portion of its RNA must be sampled. However, this will inevitably increase the number of TCR transcripts that need to be tagged with MIDs, which increases the portion of MIDs tagging multiple TCR transcripts. We sought to closely examine the relationship between RNA input and multiple TCR RNA tagging by the same MID. The process of MID labeling can be modeled as a Poisson distribution (see Materials and Methods). The percentage of MIDs with sub-clusters follows an approximate linear trend when the copies of target RNA molecules are less than 5,000,000 (**Figure 1B**). To experimentally validate this, we applied MIDCIRS TCR-seq on a range of sorted naïve CD8$^+$ T cells (from 20,000 to 1 million) with three different RNA inputs (10, 30, and 50%) (Table S1 in Supplementary Material). We have previously used control template sequences and evaluated the clustering threshold that would separate TCR RNA molecules accidentally tagged with the same MID, which is 15% of the sequence length (9). As expected, we found that the observed percentage of MIDs that need sub-clustering is approximately linear with respect to copies of target RNA molecules used in this study (**Figure 1A**). With the highest amount of RNA molecules used in this study, approximately 8.5% of MIDs require further clustering, while previous method treated these sequences as ambiguous (17). Thus, MIDCIRS sub-clustering significantly improves repertoire diversity coverage.

To evaluate the accuracy of the sub-clustering step by an alternative means, we examined the TCR sequence lengths within MIDs that contain sub-clusters. We reasoned that if indeed each TCR RNA molecule was tagged with a unique MID, then the lengths of CDR3 for all reads would be identical under each MID. However, we showed that of the 8.5% of MIDs that contain sub-clusters, about 87% of MIDs contain TCR sequencing reads of different CDR3 lengths while only 13% have the same length for one million naïve CD8$^+$ T cells (50% RNA input). After performing sub-clustering, over 97% of sub-clusters have a uniform length (Figure S1 in Supplementary Material), demonstrating the accuracy of sub-clustering step in MIDCIRS.

More importantly, to our surprise, we found that, without performing sub-clustering, the number of unique consensus sequences (unique CDR3 sequences) was overestimated, especially in samples with one million cells (**Figure 1C**; Figure S2 in Supplementary Material). This is because chimera sequences were generated in the consensus building step for two scenarios. In one scenario, multiple true TCR sequences could be tagged with the same MID and quality score weighted consensus building will generate chimera sequences (**Figure 1D**; Figure S3A in Supplementary Material). In the second scenario, PCR or sequencing errors on MIDs group multiple singletons (MIDs that contain only one read) under the new MID. If sub-clustering is applied, then these singletons will be separated and discarded under the singleton category. However, without sub-clustering, these singletons will be forced to generate a chimera sequence (Figure S3B in Supplementary Material). Taking together, these chimera sequences cause overestimation of the total TCR diversity. The percentage of chimera sequences can be as high as 47% (Table S1 in Supplementary Material). Thus, compared with previous IR-seq with MID method (17), MIDCIRS not only can increase diversity coverage of CDR3 but improve the accuracy of diversity estimation.

## MID Read-Distribution-Based Barcode Correction Improves Accuracy and Sensitivity of Counting TCR Transcripts

Besides correcting PCR and sequencing errors, MIDs have also been used for absolute quantification of RNA molecule copy number in single-cell studies to improve precision (30–33). Here, we demonstrated how to use MIDCIRS TCR-seq to digitally count TCR transcripts. The absolute quantification of TCR transcripts is fundamental for accurate clonal size estimation. We noticed that PCR and sequencing errors also affected MIDs, as seen in single-cell RNA sequencing studies (29, 34), leading to an inflated number of RNA molecules when libraries were sequenced exhaustively with respective to the total TCR transcripts in the sample (**Figure 2A**; Figure S4 in Supplementary Material). To correct MID errors, we first removed singleton reads, which cannot be confidently used in generating MID groups due to sequencing errors. Then, we adopted a similar approach applied in single-cell RNA-seq by fitting the distribution of reads under each MID subgroup into two negative binomial distributions (Figure S5 in Supplementary Material) (34). Erroneous MIDs generated due to PCR errors generally have distinctively lower read counts compared with true MIDs. These two negative binomial distributions distinctly separated true MIDs from erroneous MIDs. MIDs with low read counts were removed accordingly (see Materials and Methods). After MID correction, number of RNA molecules saturated across libraries (**Figure 2A**; Figure S4 in Supplementary Material).

We found that a shallower sequencing depth is required to saturate unique CDR3s than RNA molecules (**Figure 2B**). In addition, the amount of diversity covered increased with increasing RNA input. Thus, to exhaustively measure the TCR repertoire diversity, with 30–50% of RNA input, a sequencing depth equivalent to 10 times the cell number covers most of the CDR3 diversity (**Figure 1C**; Figure S2 in Supplementary Material), while a sequencing depth equivalent to about 100 times the relative RNA input (defined as cell number multiplied by percentage of RNA input) is required to saturate the RNA molecules (**Figure 2A**; Figure S4 in Supplementary Material). For example, 30% RNA of

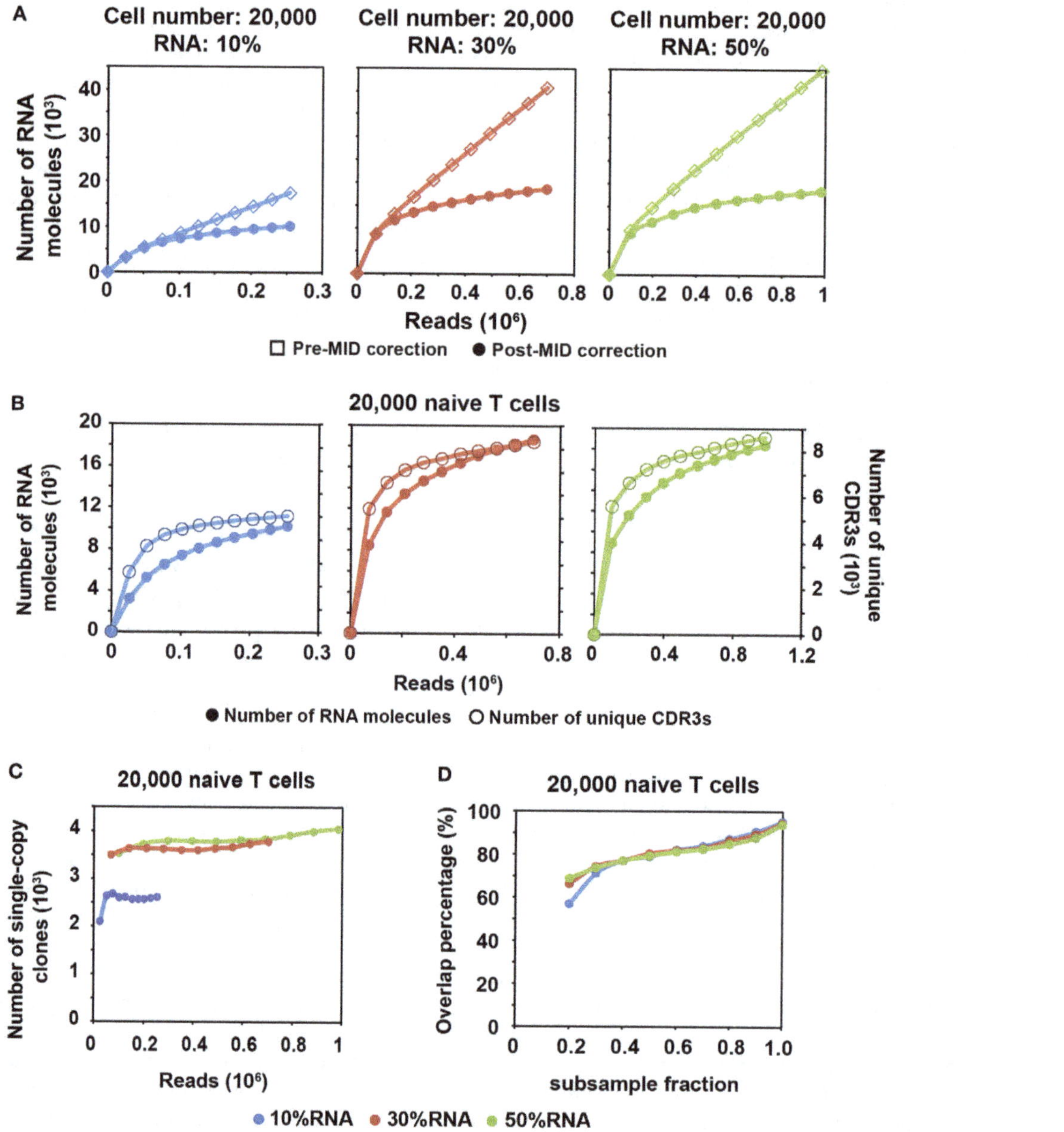


**FIGURE 2** | MID Clustering-based IR-Seq is capable of accurate digital counting of T cell receptor (TCR) RNA molecules. **(A)** Rarefaction curve of detected TCR RNA molecules before and after error correction on molecular identifiers (MIDs) in 20,000 naïve CD8+ T cells for three RNA input amounts. Data from other cell inputs are in Figure S4 in Supplementary Material. **(B)** Comparison of rarefaction curve of detected RNA molecules and unique complementarity-determining regions 3 (CDR3s) in 20,000 naïve CD8+ T cells for three RNA input amounts. **(C)** Rarefaction curve of number of unique CDR3s with single RNA copy in 20,000 naïve CD8+ T cells for three RNA input amounts. Sequencing reads were subsampled to different depth and unique CDR3s were tallied. Data from other cell inputs are in Figure S6A in Supplementary Material. **(D)** The percentage of overlapping clones with single RNA copy at different sequencing depths by sub-sampling in 20,000 naïve CD8+ T cells for three RNA input amounts. The overlapping clones were compared between two adjacent sub-samplings and overlap percentage was calculated by dividing the number of overlapping clones by the total number of clones observed in the deeper sub-sampling. Data from other cell input are in Figure S6B in Supplementary Material.

20,000 cells is equivalent to 6,000 RNA input. Then, it takes about 600,000 reads to saturate the RNA molecules but only 200,000 reads to saturate the unique CDR3s (**Figure 2A**, middle panel).

After MID correction, with optimal sequencing depth, we stably detected TCR clones with a single TCR RNA molecule (single-copy clones with at least two identical sequencing reads). The number of single-copy clones saturates with adequate sequencing depth (**Figure 2C**; Figure S6A in Supplementary Material). Meanwhile, we compared the degree of overlapping clones within these single-copy clones at different sequencing depths. To do this, we subsampled each library to different fractions of the total reads. The overlapping clones were compared between two adjacent subsamples, and the overlap percentage was calculated by dividing the number of overlapping clones by the total number of clones observed in the deeper subsample. Thus, for total of 10 subsamples, 9 clonal overlap percentages were calculated and plotted with respect to sequencing depth (**Figure 2D**; Figure S6B in Supplementary Material). More than 90% of single-copy clones were repeatedly detected between the full sequencing reads and the 0.9 subsample fraction. The overlap percentage was above 80% for the latter part of curve (**Figure 2D**; Figure S6B in Supplementary Material), which suggested that we have reached optimal sequencing depth to detect single-copy TCR clones.

## Estimating TCR RNA Molecule Copy Number and Validation with dPCR

From early analysis, we know that the diversity coverage of unique CDR3s increased as RNA input increased. Here, we performed an in depth analysis on the relationship between these two parameters and found that the diversity coverage of unique CDR3s increased significantly as the RNA input increased initially, then reached a plateau, which resulted in a nonlinear increasing of the diversity coverage of unique CDR3s (**Figures 3A,B**). We assumed that total diversity for a sample is the diversity discovered when combining all sequencing reads from 10, 30, and 50% RNA input libraries into a pseudo-90% RNA input. With 50% RNA, we could recover about 60% of total diversity (**Figure 3B**).

Since the observed diversity is dependent on total TCR RNA molecules in a sample, which is a function of TCR RNA molecule copy number per cell and RNA input percentage, we next sought to use a probability model to predict TCR RNA molecule copy number per cell using the observed diversity coverage of unique CDR3s as a function of RNA input percentage (see Materials and Methods). We used the estimated diversity coverage of different RNA inputs, including 10, 30, and 50% RNA, as well as the computationally combined pseudo-40% (10 + 30%) and pseudo-90% RNA inputs as data points to fit the probability model. The best fit resulted in three copies of TCR RNA molecule per cell (**Figure 3B**). In another independent experiment, RNA from 20,000 and 100,000 naïve $CD8^+$ T cells were evenly separated into five aliquots, respectively. Four of five aliquots were sequenced (Table S2 in Supplementary Material). Results showed that CDR3 diversity detected by MIDCIRS is very reproducible among the four aliquots and is also proportional to the cell input numbers. In addition, we bioinformatically combined the aliquots into pseudo-40, -60, and -80% of RNA inputs and fitted the diversity coverage using the probability model described in the Section "Materials and Methods." As with previously, the best fit resulted in three copies of TCR RNA molecule per cell (Figure S7 in Supplementary Material).

However, in order to apply this TCR RNA molecule copy number in estimating T cell clone size, we need to validate it using a different method and also test to see if different phenotypes of T cells might have different TCR RNA molecule copy numbers, which would be similar to the differences seeing in naïve B cells and plasmablasts (35). Next, we validated TCR RNA molecule copy number using dPCR and found that various types of T cells have similar TCR RNA copies (8–12 copies per cell) (**Figure 3C**). Thus, with MIDCIRS TCR-seq, we could achieve about 30% efficiency in recovering the target TCR RNA molecules, which is expected given dPCR in a nanoliter volume is more efficient than bulk PCR in tubes (36). This ratio also establishes a reference point for rare T cell clone frequency estimate using MIDCIRS method.

## Detecting Single-Cell Worth of TCR RNA Using MIDCIRS

The lack of accurate and absolute quantitation of TCR clones limited the evaluation of the sensitivity of various IR-seq methods

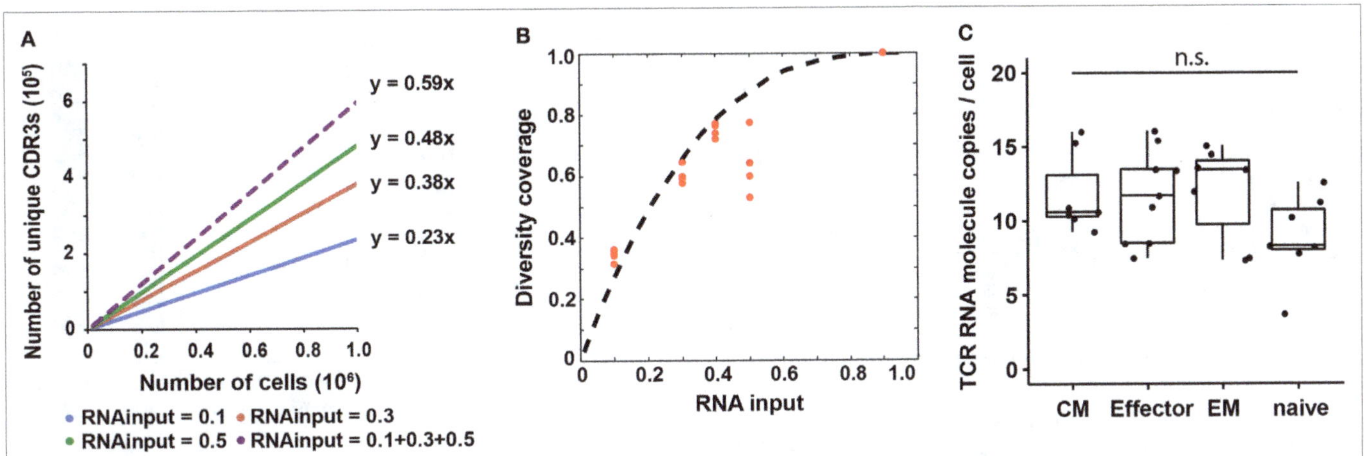


**FIGURE 3** | T cell receptor (TCR) RNA copy number per cell estimation and experimental validation. **(A)** Diversity coverage of unique productive complementarity-determining regions 3 with different RNA inputs and cell numbers (Line represents linear regression fit, *F*-test on the slope, $R^2 > 0.99$ and $p < 10^{-3}$ for all different RNA inputs). **(B)** Diversity coverages with different RNA inputs using 3 as a predicted TCR RNA molecule copy number per cell. Dashed line is the theoretical prediction (see Materials and Methods); red dots are diversity coverages observed in libraries with different RNA inputs as illustrated in panel **(A)**, assuming diversity coverage at 90% RNA input is 1. **(C)** Digital PCR results of TCR RNA molecule copies per cell in different $CD8^+$ T cell subset (N, naïve; CM, central memory; EM, effector memory; E, effector; NTC, no template control; n.s: *p*-value > 0.05 by Mann–Whitney *U* test).

(37), which slowed the application of detecting rare TCR clones in both basic research and clinical practice. To address the detection sensitivity using MIDCIRS, we spiked-in control TCR RNA with varying copy numbers into naïve T cells and validated the robustness of detecting spiked-in TCRs. 5, 20, and 5 copies of three spike-in cell lines with known TCR sequences were added into 20,000 and 100,000 naïve CD8$^+$ T cells. 3, 13, and 3 copies of three spike-ins were reliably detected, respectively (**Figure 4A**).

We also analyzed the ability to detect a single T cell's worth of control RNA in a larger number of other T cells. We digitally counted the concentration of TCR RNA molecule from the Jurkat cell line and spiked-in 10 copies of TCR RNA into 20,000–1,000,000 naïve CD8$^+$ T cells (Table S1 in Supplementary Material). In all 1,000,000 cells we sequenced, we were capable of detecting Jurkat TCR sequences (**Table 1**). This sensitivity was a significant improvement compared with previous method, which was demonstrated to be 1 in 10,000 (21). These results demonstrated that MIDCIRS is highly sensitive, capable of detecting a single-cell's amount of TCR transcripts, and rare clones could be readily and robustly detected. Those single-copy clones (minimum two identical reads) we discovered are thus likely to come from single cells (**Figure 2C**; Figure S6A in Supplementary Material).

Meanwhile, we compared the sensitivity of MIDCIRS and 5′RACE protocol using the diversity coverage as the parameter. Briefly, the 5′RACE protocol that was used in Smart-seq2 protocol was used for TCR-seq, which has been demonstrated to significantly improve RNA capture efficiency (38). Equal amount of RNA (20%) from same purification was used for both MIDCIRS and 5′RACE protocol. We then processed sequencing results with MIDCIRS-TCR pipeline and found that 5′RACE protocol only recovered about 44% of diversity compared to what MIDCIRS protocol obtained (Table S3 in Supplementary Material). With improved accuracy and sensitivity to detect rare clones, MIDCIRS is promising in being applied to detect MRD after treatment.

## Quantifying T Cell Clonal Expansion in Infection Using MIDCIRS

It has been shown that the clonality and quantity of T cells are strongly correlated with efficacy of therapies, such as cancer chemotherapy and antiviral therapy (20, 39). Accurate quantification of diversity and abundance of T cell clones is important for application of TCR-seq in clinical settings, ranging from prognosis to treatment decision-making. However, there lacks an accurate approach to evaluate the degree of T cell clonal expansion in humans. Therefore, we applied MIDCIRS TCR-seq to examine T cell clonal expansion in infection. We sorted 20,000 and 200,000 CMVpp65-specific effector CD8$^+$ T cells from CMV-infected patients and used 30% of RNA input to perform TCR-seq (Table S4 in Supplementary Material). CMV pp65 peptide has been shown to be the immunodominant target of CD8$^+$ T cell response (40). TCR RNA molecules were digitally counted through MIDCIRS pipeline. We defined TCR sequences with over 20 copies of RNA molecules as expanded clones according to TCR abundance distribution comparing between naïve CD8$^+$ T cells and CMV tetramer positive effector CD8$^+$ T cells (**Figure 4B**). Over 99% unique RNA molecules were from these expanded clones in CMVpp65-specific effector CD8$^+$ T cells. On the other hand, although we observed uneven clonal distribution in naïve CD8$^+$ T cells, these expanded clones only account for less than 1% unique RNA molecules (**Figure 4C**). Our data showed that in CMV infection, single CMV-specific TCR clone can have about 70,000 T cell progenies in 200,000 polyclonal CMV-specific effector CD8$^+$ T cells (Table S4 in Supplementary Material). These polyclonal CMV-specific effector CD8$^+$ T cells represent about 2.6% of total CD8$^+$ T cells. In addition, our previous study showed that tetramer positive polyclonal CMV precursor cells existed at

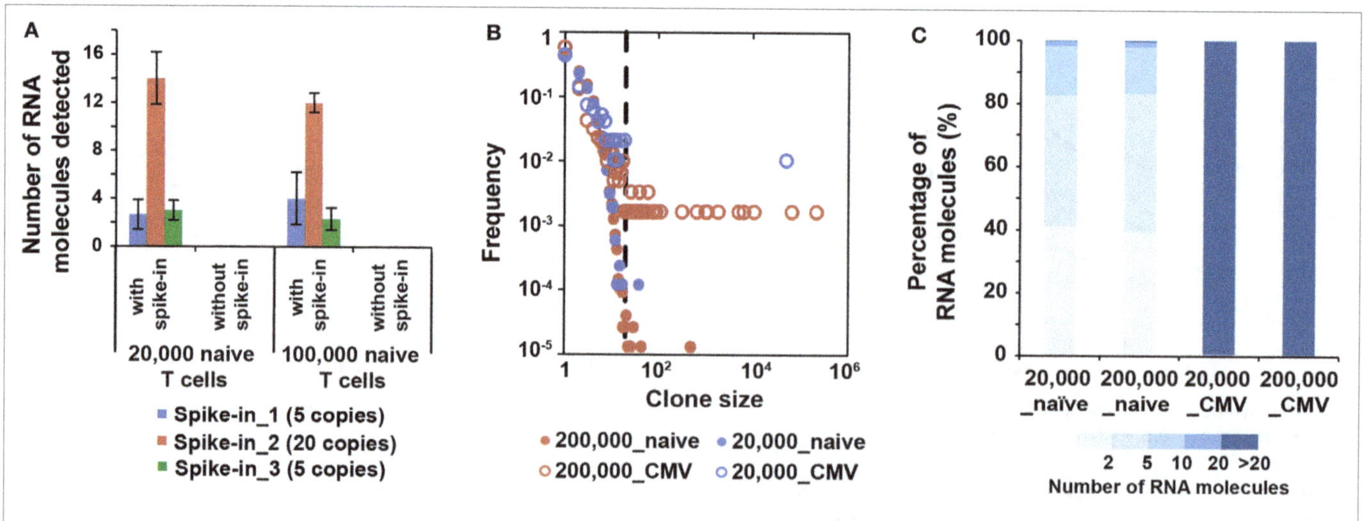


**FIGURE 4** | MID Clustering-based IR-Seq is sensitive to detect both low copy and highly clonal expanded T cell receptors (TCRs). **(A)** Number of RNA molecules detected by sequencing for each spike-in TCR control sequences (the numbers in the legend denote copies of each TCR spike-in control sequence added). **(B)** Comparison of clone size distribution in naïve CD8$^+$ T cells and CMVpp65-specific effector CD8$^+$ T cells (dashed line indicates TCR sequences with 20 copies of RNA molecules). **(C)** The percentage of RNA molecules that varying degree of clonally expanded complementarity-determining region 3 account for.

**TABLE 1** | Spike-in Jurkat T cell receptor (TCR) RNA detection in naïve CD8+ T cells.

| Sample | Jurkat TCR copies detected |
|---|---|
| 20,000Tn_10%RNA | 7 |
| 20,000Tn_30%RNA | 0 |
| 20,000Tn_50%RNA | 1 |
| 100,000Tn_10%RNA | 5 |
| 100,000Tn_30%RNA | 4 |
| 100,000Tn_50%RNA | 1 |
| 200,000Tn_10%RNA | 7 |
| 200,000Tn_30%RNA | 3 |
| 200,000Tn_50%RNA | 3 |
| 1,000,000Tn_10%RNA | 4 |
| 1,000,000Tn_30%RNA | 8 |
| 1,000,000Tn_50%RNA | 17 |

*10 TCR-copy worth of Jurkat RNA was added to each sample during the reverse transcription step. Number of molecular identifiers for RNA molecules that are tagged with jurkat TCR sequences were counted.*

a frequency of 1 in 100,000 CD8+ T cells in CMV seronegative individuals (22). Taking together, these results suggest that single T cell clone can have about 900-fold proliferation in infection in humans. Thus, MIDCIRS can be applied to evaluate clone size and degree of clonal expansion in viral infection.

## DISCUSSION

In this study, we applied the MIDCIRS, recently developed by our group (9), in T cells to demonstrate (1) the necessity of MID sub-clustering to improve accuracy of repertoire diversity estimation; (2) the accuracy of counting TCR RNA molecules *via* MID read-distribution based barcode correction; (3) the sensitivity of detecting a single cell in as many as one million naïve T cells; and (4) the ability to quantify T cell clonal expansion due to infection in CMV-seropositive patients.

Previous MID-based IR-seq methods, such as MIGEC, build TCR consensus sequences by grouping MIDs (17, 41). However, the number of target molecules could vary significantly with different sample inputs, which could be challenging for choosing the appropriate MID length to ensure that each target RNA molecule is uniquely tagged by MID. Longer MIDs are likely to decrease the reverse transcription efficiency (28, 29). Thus, the MIDCIRS method offers a flexible strategy for MID-barcoded IR-seq. In addition, MIGEC triages MIDs with high diversity as ambiguous. We compared TCR diversity discovered using MIDCIRS with that of MIGEC, using MID with at least two reads as the threshold for both approaches (see Materials and Methods) and found that MIGEC led to an underestimated TCR diversity (Figure S8 in Supplementary Material, $p < 0.001$, effect size $r = 0.62$). We demonstrated that using MID-based sub-clustering approach, MIDCIRS could identify new diversities, prevent chimera sequences from being built, and digitally count RNA molecules (**Figure 1**; Figures S2 and S3 in Supplementary Material). This corrected diversity is highly consistent with cell input numbers.

While MIDs are useful to correct for sequencing errors and PCR errors that occur on TCR sequences, such errors are also likely to show up on MID sequences. Although these errors do not affect TCR diversity estimation, they lead to an overestimation of transcript copies, thus misestimating TCR clone size (**Figure 2**; Figure S4 in Supplementary Material). We corrected MID errors based on the distribution of MID read counts under MID subgroups. With MID correction, we were able to accurately count TCR RNA molecule copy number, estimate MIDCIRS detection limit as well as detect T cell clonal expansion.

Noteworthy, we found uneven CDR3 clone size distribution in naïve CD8+ T cells (**Figure 4B**). The most expanded clone was enriched about 0.27% (Table S1 in Supplementary Material). This could be due to convergent recombination as has been previously noted (42, 43) or uneven clonal expansion during thymocyte maturation and selection in thymus (44, 45).

Furthermore, there is a lack of standard guidelines of how much RNA input to use for library preparation and sequencing. Also, the capacity to evaluate immune repertoire and gene expression profile simultaneously will facilitate clinical practice, such as cancer immunotherapies. Efforts have been made to reconstruct antibody and TCR repertoire from RNA-seq data. This, however, requires very deep sequencing to recover highly expanded T cell clones in the sample, and the exact degree of repertoire coverage is difficult to assess (46–48). Here, we demonstrated that 50% RNA is enough to cover about 60% of CDR3 diversity (**Figure 3B**), making it beneficial to take advantage of the rest of the RNA from the same sample for other applications, e.g., RNA-seq.

Based on the TCR diversity estimation and its dependency on RNA input, we built a probability model to estimate TCR RNA molecule copies, which resulted in three copies per cell (**Figure 3B**). We would like to point out that this does not mean that on average there are three copies of TCR RNA in a T cell. Because of the efficiency of RNA purification and reverse transcription, we expect our observed RNA molecule per cell to be lower than the true value. In Fact, dPCR results showed an average of 10 copies of TCR RNA molecule per cell (**Figure 3C**), suggesting the efficiency of MIDCIRS in TCR RNA molecule digital counting is about 30%, which is consistent with previous finding that nanoliter reaction volume significantly improved PCR efficiency. Thus, quantifying TCR RNA molecule per cell enables us to estimate the extent of T cell clonal expansion that was not possible until now.

We also used spike-in TCR RNA to validate the sensitivity of MIDCIRS. We showed that spiked-in TCR RNA at as few as five copies can be reliably detected across multiple libraries (**Figure 4A**). More importantly, we were also able to detect a single-cell worth of RNA in as many as one million cells (**Table 1**). With this demonstrated sensitivity, this method could be extremely useful in MRD detection.

Last, we applied MIDCIRS to evaluate T cell clonal expansion in CMV-infected patients. Through accurate digital counting of TCR RNA molecules and in combination of precursor T cell frequency, we showed that CMV-specific effector CD8+ T cells can expand at least 900 times, and there could be more than 70,000 effector CD8+ T cells derived from the same CMV-specific T cell clone in total of 7,700,000 of CD8+ T cell in infection. We also noticed that there is a potential of same TCR sequences tagged with same MID, which would under estimate the clonal size, especially in highly expanded clones. We calculated the expected number of collisions where same MIDs tag same RNA molecules (Supplementary Methods in Supplementary Material). With MID length being 12, when there are 200,000 identical RNA molecules, the percentage of identical RNA molecules tagged with same MID is only 1%. While long MID decreases the percentage of identical RNA molecules tagged with same MID, it also decreases efficiency of reverse transcription. Our analysis revealed that MID with 12 nucleotides is appropriate. Therefore, MIDCIRS provides the foundation of accurate assessment of clone size and clonal expansion in infection and vaccination, which would be a useful technology to provide a comprehensive quantification of the T cell repertoire in various basic studies and clinical settings.

## AUTHOR CONTRIBUTIONS

K-YM performed all library preparation, data analysis, and wrote the manuscript; CH developed MIDCIRS-TCR analysis pipeline and RNA copy number simulation model; BW helped with naïve T cell sorting and manuscript editing; CW helped with CMV-specific T cell sorting and CMV-specific T cell line culture; JX helped to optimize MIDCIRS pipeline. HY helped with sequencing. NJ conceived the idea, designed the study, directed data analysis, and revised the manuscript with contributions from all coauthors.

## ACKNOWLEDGMENTS

The authors would like to thank We Are Blood (Austin, TX, USA), for providing the blood samples, Jessica Podnar, and Dr. Michael Wilson at the Genomic Sequencing and Analysis Facility at UT Austin for helping with the sequencing runs.

## FUNDING

This work was supported by NIH grants R00AG040149 (NJ) and S10OD020072 (NJ), NSF CAREER Award 1653866 (NJ), the Welch Foundation grant F1785 (NJ), and National Natural Science Foundation of China grants 1147222 and 11672246 (HY). NJ is a Cancer Prevention and Research Institute of Texas (CPRIT) Scholar and a Damon Runyon-Rachleff Innovator. BW is a recipient of the Thrust 2000—George Sawyer Endowed Graduate Fellowship in Engineering.

## REFERENCES

1. Ellebedy AH, Jackson KJ, Kissick HT, Nakaya HI, Davis CW, Roskin KM, et al. Defining antigen-specific plasmablast and memory B cell subsets in human blood after viral infection or vaccination. *Nat Immunol* (2016) 17(10):1226–34. doi:10.1038/ni.3533
2. Jiang N, He J, Weinstein JA, Penland L, Sasaki S, He XS, et al. Lineage structure of the human antibody repertoire in response to influenza vaccination. *Sci Transl Med* (2013) 5(171):171ra19. doi:10.1126/scitranslmed.3004794
3. Lee J, Boutz DR, Chromikova V, Joyce MG, Vollmers C, Leung K, et al. Molecular-level analysis of the serum antibody repertoire in young adults before and after seasonal influenza vaccination. *Nat Med* (2016) 22(12):1456–64. doi:10.1038/nm.4224
4. IJspeert H, van Schouwenburg PA, van Zessen D, Pico-Knijnenburg I, Driessen GJ, Stubbs AP, et al. Evaluation of the antigen-experienced B-cell receptor repertoire in healthy children and adults. *Front Immunol* (2016) 7:410. doi:10.3389/fimmu.2016.00410
5. Jiang N, Weinstein JA, Penland L, White RA III, Fisher DS, Quake SR. Determinism and stochasticity during maturation of the zebrafish antibody repertoire. *Proc Natl Acad Sci U S A* (2011) 108(13):5348–53. doi:10.1073/pnas.1014277108
6. Prabakaran P, Chen W, Singarayan MG, Stewart CC, Streaker E, Feng Y, et al. Expressed antibody repertoires in human cord blood cells: 454 sequencing and IMGT/HighV-QUEST analysis of germline gene usage, junctional diversity, and somatic mutations. *Immunogenetics* (2012) 64(5):337–50. doi:10.1007/s00251-011-0595-8
7. Rechavi E, Lev A, Lee YN, Simon AJ, Yinon Y, Lipitz S, et al. Timely and spatially regulated maturation of B and T cell repertoire during human fetal development. *Sci Transl Med* (2015) 7(276):276ra25. doi:10.1126/scitranslmed.aaa0072
8. Weinstein JA, Jiang N, White RA III, Fisher DS, Quake SR. High-throughput sequencing of the zebrafish antibody repertoire. *Science* (2009) 324(5928):807–10. doi:10.1126/science.1170020
9. Wendel BS, He C, Qu M, Wu D, Hernandez SM, Ma KY, et al. Accurate immune repertoire sequencing reveals malaria infection driven antibody lineage diversification in young children. *Nat Commun* (2017) 8(1):531. doi:10.1038/s41467-017-00645-x
10. Faham M, Zheng J, Moorhead M, Carlton VE, Stow P, Coustan-Smith E, et al. Deep-sequencing approach for minimal residual disease detection in acute lymphoblastic leukemia. *Blood* (2012) 120(26):5173–80. doi:10.1182/blood-2012-07-444042
11. Logan AC, Gao H, Wang C, Sahaf B, Jones CD, Marshall EL, et al. High-throughput VDJ sequencing for quantification of minimal residual disease in chronic lymphocytic leukemia and immune reconstitution assessment. *Proc Natl Acad Sci U S A* (2011) 108(52):21194–9. doi:10.1073/pnas.1118357109
12. Huang AC, Postow MA, Orlowski RJ, Mick R, Bengsch B, Manne S, et al. T-cell invigoration to tumour burden ratio associated with anti-PD-1 response. *Nature* (2017) 545(7652):60–5. doi:10.1038/nature22079
13. Jia Q, Zhou J, Chen G, Shi Y, Yu H, Guan P, et al. Diversity index of mucosal resident T lymphocyte repertoire predicts clinical prognosis in gastric cancer. *Oncoimmunology* (2015) 4(4):e1001230. doi:10.1080/2162402X.2014.1001230
14. Khan TA, Friedensohn S, Gorter de Vries AR, Straszewski J, Ruscheweyh HJ, Reddy ST. Accurate and predictive antibody repertoire profiling by molecular amplification fingerprinting. *Sci Adv* (2016) 2(3):e1501371. doi:10.1126/sciadv.1501371
15. Kinde I, Wu J, Papadopoulos N, Kinzler KW, Vogelstein B. Detection and quantification of rare mutations with massively parallel sequencing. *Proc Natl Acad Sci U S A* (2011) 108(23):9530–5. doi:10.1073/pnas.1105422108
16. Shugay M, Bagaev DV, Turchaninova MA, Bolotin DA, Britanova OV, Putintseva EV, et al. VDJtools: unifying post-analysis of T cell receptor

repertoires. *PLoS Comput Biol* (2015) 11(11):e1004503. doi:10.1371/journal.pcbi.1004503

17. Shugay M, Britanova OV, Merzlyak EM, Turchaninova MA, Mamedov IZ, Tuganbaev TR, et al. Towards error-free profiling of immune repertoires. *Nat Methods* (2014) 11(6):653–5. doi:10.1038/nmeth.2960
18. Vander Heiden JA, Yaari G, Uduman M, Stern JN, O'Connor KC, Hafler DA, et al. pRESTO: a toolkit for processing high-throughput sequencing raw reads of lymphocyte receptor repertoires. *Bioinformatics* (2014) 30(13):1930–2. doi:10.1093/bioinformatics/btu138
19. Vollmers C, Sit RV, Weinstein JA, Dekker CL, Quake SR. Genetic measurement of memory B-cell recall using antibody repertoire sequencing. *Proc Natl Acad Sci U S A* (2013) 110(33):13463–8. doi:10.1073/pnas.1312146110
20. Robins HS, Ericson NG, Guenthoer J, O'Briant KC, Tewari M, Drescher CW, et al. Digital genomic quantification of tumor-infiltrating lymphocytes. *Sci Transl Med* (2013) 5(214):214ra169. doi:10.1126/scitranslmed.3007247
21. Ruggiero E, Nicolay JP, Fronza R, Arens A, Paruzynski A, Nowrouzi A, et al. High-resolution analysis of the human T-cell receptor repertoire. *Nat Commun* (2015) 6:8081. doi:10.1038/ncomms9081
22. Yu W, Jiang N, Ebert PJ, Kidd BA, Muller S, Lund PJ, et al. Clonal deletion prunes but does not eliminate self-specific alphabeta CD8(+) T lymphocytes. *Immunity* (2015) 42(5):929–41. doi:10.1016/j.immuni.2015.05.001
23. Zhang SQ, Parker P, Ma KY, He C, Shi Q, Cui Z, et al. Direct measurement of T cell receptor affinity and sequence from naive antiviral T cells. *Sci Transl Med* (2016) 8(341):341ra77. doi:10.1126/scitranslmed.aaf1278
24. Mora T, Walczak A. Quantifying lymphocyte receptor diversity. *ArXiv e-prints* (2016) 1604. Available from: http://adsabs.harvard.edu/abs/2016arXiv160400487M
25. Clauset A, Shalizi CR, Newman MEJ. Power-law distributions in empirical data. *SIAM Rev* (2009) 51(4):661–703. doi:10.1137/070710111
26. Csardi G, Nepusz T. The igraph software package for complex network research. *Int J Complex Syst* (2006) 1695(5):1–9.
27. Briney B, Le K, Zhu J, Burton DR. Clonify: unseeded antibody lineage assignment from next-generation sequencing data. *Sci Rep* (2016) 6:23901. doi:10.1038/srep23901
28. Shiao YH. A new reverse transcription-polymerase chain reaction method for accurate quantification. *BMC Biotechnol* (2003) 3:22. doi:10.1186/1472-6750-3-22
29. Zajac P, Islam S, Hochgerner H, Lonnerberg P, Linnarsson S. Base preferences in non-templated nucleotide incorporation by MMLV-derived reverse transcriptases. *PLoS One* (2013) 8(12):e85270. doi:10.1371/journal.pone.0085270
30. Fan HC, Fu GK, Fodor SP. Combinatorial labeling of single cells for gene expression cytometry. *Science* (2015) 347(6222):1258367. doi:10.1126/science.1258367
31. Fu GK, Hu J, Wang PH, Fodor SP. Counting individual DNA molecules by the stochastic attachment of diverse labels. *Proc Natl Acad Sci U S A* (2011) 108(22):9026–31. doi:10.1073/pnas.1017621108
32. Islam S, Zeisel A, Joost S, La Manno G, Zajac P, Kasper M, et al. Quantitative single-cell RNA-seq with unique molecular identifiers. *Nat Methods* (2014) 11(2):163–6. doi:10.1038/nmeth.2772
33. Shiroguchi K, Jia TZ, Sims PA, Xie XS. Digital RNA sequencing minimizes sequence-dependent bias and amplification noise with optimized single-molecule barcodes. *Proc Natl Acad Sci U S A* (2012) 109(4):1347–52. doi:10.1073/pnas.1118018109
34. Fu GK, Wilhelmy J, Stern D, Fan HC, Fodor SP. Digital encoding of cellular mRNAs enabling precise and absolute gene expression measurement by single-molecule counting. *Anal Chem* (2014) 86(6):2867–70. doi:10.1021/ac500459p
35. Shi W, Liao Y, Willis SN, Taubenheim N, Inouye M, Tarlinton DM, et al. Transcriptional profiling of mouse B cell terminal differentiation defines a signature for antibody-secreting plasma cells. *Nat Immunol* (2015) 16(6):663–73. doi:10.1038/ni.3154
36. Warren L, Bryder D, Weissman IL, Quake SR. Transcription factor profiling in individual hematopoietic progenitors by digital RT-PCR. *Proc Natl Acad Sci U S A* (2006) 103(47):17807–12. doi:10.1073/pnas.0608512103
37. Warren RL, Freeman JD, Zeng T, Choe G, Munro S, Moore R, et al. Exhaustive T-cell repertoire sequencing of human peripheral blood samples reveals signatures of antigen selection and a directly measured repertoire size of at least 1 million clonotypes. *Genome Res* (2011) 21(5):790–7. doi:10.1101/gr.115428.110
38. Picelli S, Bjorklund AK, Faridani OR, Sagasser S, Winberg G, Sandberg R. Smart-seq2 for sensitive full-length transcriptome profiling in single cells. *Nat Methods* (2013) 10(11):1096–8. doi:10.1038/nmeth.2639
39. Heather JM, Best K, Oakes T, Gray ER, Roe JK, Thomas N, et al. Dynamic perturbations of the T-cell receptor repertoire in chronic HIV infection and following antiretroviral therapy. *Front Immunol* (2015) 6:644. doi:10.3389/fimmu.2015.00644
40. Wills MR, Carmichael AJ, Mynard K, Jin X, Weekes MP, Plachter B, et al. The human cytotoxic T-lymphocyte (CTL) response to cytomegalovirus is dominated by structural protein pp65: frequency, specificity, and T-cell receptor usage of pp65-specific CTL. *J Virol* (1996) 70(11):7569–79.
41. Egorov ES, Merzlyak EM, Shelenkov AA, Britanova OV, Sharonov GV, Staroverov DB, et al. Quantitative profiling of immune repertoires for minor lymphocyte counts using unique molecular identifiers. *J Immunol* (2015) 194(12):6155–63. doi:10.4049/jimmunol.1500215
42. Quigley MF, Greenaway HY, Venturi V, Lindsay R, Quinn KM, Seder RA, et al. Convergent recombination shapes the clonotypic landscape of the naive T-cell repertoire. *Proc Natl Acad Sci U S A* (2010) 107(45):19414–9. doi:10.1073/pnas.1010586107
43. Venturi V, Price DA, Douek DC, Davenport MP. The molecular basis for public T-cell responses? *Nat Rev Immunol* (2008) 8(3):231–8. doi:10.1038/nri2260
44. Qi Q, Liu Y, Cheng Y, Glanville J, Zhang D, Lee JY, et al. Diversity and clonal selection in the human T-cell repertoire. *Proc Natl Acad Sci U S A* (2014) 111(36):13139–44. doi:10.1073/pnas.1409155111
45. Surh CD, Sprent J. Homeostatic T cell proliferation: how far can T cells be activated to self-ligands? *J Exp Med* (2000) 192(4):F9–14. doi:10.1084/jem.192.4.F9
46. Blachly JS, Ruppert AS, Zhao W, Long S, Flynn J, Flinn I, et al. Immunoglobulin transcript sequence and somatic hypermutation computation from unselected RNA-seq reads in chronic lymphocytic leukemia. *Proc Natl Acad Sci U S A* (2015) 112(14):4322–7. doi:10.1073/pnas.1503587112
47. Brown SD, Raeburn LA, Holt RA. Profiling tissue-resident T cell repertoires by RNA sequencing. *Genome Med* (2015) 7:125. doi:10.1186/s13073-015-0248-x
48. Li B, Li T, Pignon JC, Wang B, Wang J, Shukla SA, et al. Landscape of tumor-infiltrating T cell repertoire of human cancers. *Nat Genet* (2016) 48(7):725–32. doi:10.1038/ng.3581

5

# The CAIRR Pipeline for Submitting Standards-Compliant B and T Cell Receptor Repertoire Sequencing Studies to the National Center for Biotechnology Information Repositories

*Syed Ahmad Chan Bukhari[1], Martin J. O'Connor[2], Marcos Martínez-Romero[2], Attila L. Egyedi[2], Debra Willrett[2], John Graybeal[2], Mark A. Musen[2], Florian Rubelt[3], Kei-Hoi Cheung[4,5,6†] and Steven H. Kleinstein[1,6*†]*

*[1] Department of Pathology, Yale School of Medicine, Yale University, New Haven, CT, United States, [2] Stanford Center for Biomedical Informatics Research, Stanford University, Stanford, CA, United States, [3] Department of Microbiology and Immunology, Institute for Immunity, Transplantation and Infection, Stanford University School of Medicine, Stanford, CA, United States, [4] Department of Emergency Medicine, Yale School of Medicine, Yale University, New Haven, CT, United States, [5] Yale Center for Medical Informatics, Yale School of Medicine, Yale University, New Haven, CT, United States, [6] Interdepartmental Program in Computational Biology and Bioinformatics, Yale University, New Haven, CT, United States*

***Correspondence:**
Steven H. Kleinstein
steven.kleinstein@yale.edu*

*†Co-senior authors.*

The adaptation of high-throughput sequencing to the B cell receptor and T cell receptor has made it possible to characterize the adaptive immune receptor repertoire (AIRR) at unprecedented depth. These AIRR sequencing (AIRR-seq) studies offer tremendous potential to increase the understanding of adaptive immune responses in vaccinology, infectious disease, autoimmunity, and cancer. The increasingly wide application of AIRR-seq is leading to a critical mass of studies being deposited in the public domain, offering the possibility of novel scientific insights through secondary analyses and meta-analyses. However, effective sharing of these large-scale data remains a challenge. The AIRR community has proposed minimal information about adaptive immune receptor repertoire (MiAIRR), a standard for reporting AIRR-seq studies. The MiAIRR standard has been operationalized using the National Center for Biotechnology Information (NCBI) repositories. Submissions of AIRR-seq data to the NCBI repositories typically use a combination of web-based and flat-file templates and include only a minimal amount of terminology validation. As a result, AIRR-seq studies at the NCBI are often described using inconsistent terminologies, limiting scientists' ability to access, find, interoperate, and reuse the data sets. In order to improve metadata quality and ease submission of AIRR-seq studies to the NCBI, we have leveraged the software framework developed by the Center for Expanded Data Annotation and Retrieval (CEDAR), which develops technologies involving the use of data standards and ontologies to improve metadata quality. The resulting CEDAR-AIRR (CAIRR) pipeline enables data submitters to: (i) create web-based templates whose entries are controlled by ontology terms, (ii) generate and validate metadata, and (iii) submit the ontology-linked metadata and sequence files (FASTQ) to the NCBI BioProject, BioSample, and Sequence Read Archive databases. Overall, CAIRR provides a web-based metadata submission interface that supports compliance with the MiAIRR standard. This pipeline is available at http://cairr.miairr.org, and will facilitate the NCBI submission process and improve the metadata quality of AIRR-seq studies.

**Keywords: immune-repertoire sequencing, Rep-seq, antibody, B cell receptor, T cell receptor, National Center for Biotechnology Information, ontology**

## INTRODUCTION

Recent advances in next-generation sequencing technology have made it possible to profile the adaptive immune receptor repertoire (AIRR) in exquisite detail. AIRR sequencing (AIRR-seq) (1) studies can generate tens- to hundreds-of-millions of B and T cell receptor gene rearrangements per experiment. Categorization of receptor diversity and gene segment usage, along with identification of clonal lineages and shared hypervariable region motifs provide a rich and detailed view of the adaptive immune landscape (1). Since first developed in 2009 (2, 3), AIRR-seq has been broadly applied in basic and clinical research settings. For example, it has been used to monitor immune responses to vaccines and natural infections, cancer therapies, and to track autoimmune and malignant clones over time (2, 4). Secondary analyses and meta-analyses, which combine independent AIRR-seq studies, could enhance reproducibility and facilitate new scientific discoveries provided that the AIRR-seq data adhere to the findable, accessible, interoperable, and reusable (FAIR) data principles (5).

Effective sharing of large-scale experimental data is a significant challenge. Minimal information about an adaptive immune receptor repertoire (MiAIRR) sequencing experiment (6) was proposed by the AIRR Community (7) as a standard for making AIRR-seq studies sharable. Community-accepted data standards, such as MiAIRR, lower the barriers to data sharing, as experimental results can easily be transferred without the need for lengthy and error-prone descriptions of experimental conditions. In addition, analysis software can be written once to work on all data, and the standards specify the availability of key information in a machine readable format. More broadly, the availability of common standards for AIRR-Seq studies benefits the wider immunology community, with implications for both basic research and clinical medicine.

We used Center for Expanded Data Annotation and Retrieval (CEDAR) technology (8) to develop a submission pipeline for AIRR-seq studies into National Center for Biotechnology Information (NCBI) repositories. Four NCBI repositories are needed to cover the full set of required MiAIRR data elements (6): BioProject, BioSample (9), the Sequence Read Archive (SRA) (10), and GenBank (11). Study, subject, and sample information is submitted to BioProject and BioSample, while the sequencing information and linked raw sequencing data are submitted to SRA. Processed sequencing data are submitted to GenBank. Submissions of AIRR-seq data to the NCBI repositories typically use a combination of web-based and flat-file templates and include only a minimal amount of terms validation. As a result, metadata at these NCBI repositories are often described using inconsistent terminologies, limiting scientists' ability to access, find, interpret, and reuse the data sets, and to understand how the experiments were performed. Ontologies help to contextually interpret the heterogeneous metadata by associating the metadata concepts with ontology classes (12, 13). CEDAR develops technology that takes advantage of data standards and ontologies to improve metadata consistency and interoperability (8, 14, 15). We have leveraged CEDAR technology to improve metadata quality and ease the AIRR-seq study submission process by developing an AIRR-seq data submission pipeline named CEDAR-AIRR (CAIRR) (**Figure 1**).

CAIRR uses CEDAR technology to: (i) create web-based data submission templates whose values are mapped to ontology terms, (ii) generate and validate metadata, and (iii) submit the ontology-linked metadata and sequence files (FASTQ) (16) to the NCBI BioProject, BioSample, and SRA databases. Overall, CAIRR provides a web-based metadata submission interface that supports compliance with MiAIRR standard, with the exception of GenBank data submission (which is still in progress). The interface enables ontology-based validation for several data fields, including: organism, disease, cell type and subtype, and tissue (17). This pipeline (**Figure 1**) will facilitate the NCBI submission process and improve the metadata quality of AIRR-seq studies.

## MIAIRR-COMPLIANT TEMPLATE DEVELOPMENT LEVERAGING CEDAR TEMPLATE EDITOR

The CEDAR Workbench provides the CEDAR Template Designer, a module to create metadata templates or web forms for metadata editing. These templates consist of fields each of which contains one or more atomic pieces of information, such as a text or date field, or may be recursively composed from other template fields (**Figure 2**, right panel) (18). Fields can be restricted to accept certain data types (e.g., number and text) and can be configured to make them mandatory or to accept multiple values. To enrich the template fields with controlled vocabularies or ontologies, the CEDAR Template Designer provides a utility for searching and linking the ontology-controlled vocabularies from the NCBO (National Center for Biomedical Ontology) BioPortal. BioPortal is a repository for biomedical ontologies (**Figure 2**, organism panel view) (18, 19). Linking ontologies with template fields makes the resulting metadata interoperable, which helps to accelerate the meta-analysis process and enhances study reproducibility.

We used the CEDAR Template Designer to design metadata submission templates implementing the MiAIRR standard. To effectively share AIRR-seq studies, MiAIRR specifies a list of 82 fields (**Figure 2** left panel) which are categorized into six sets: (i) study, subject, and diagnosis, (ii) sample collection, (iii) sample processing and sequencing, (iv) raw sequences, (v) data processing, and (vi) processed sequences with annotations (6). The CEDAR-based MiAIRR template currently includes the first four MiAIRR sets with 66 fields because the CAIRR pipeline is not covering the submission to GenBank yet. In addition, we have included four SRA database specific fields (library_startegy, library_source, library_layout), which are not part of MiAIRR, but are mandatory elements for the repositories (e.g., isolate, geolocation, and library information in SRA, etc.) (20). The MiAIRR elements are mapped to BioProject, BioSample, and the SRA repositories in the NCBI. Overall, we have created three templates for the BioProject, BioSample, and the SRA and then grouped them into a single template called "MiAIRR Template."

To make an AIRR study findable, we devised a scheme to link the components (e.g., BioSample and the SRA records of

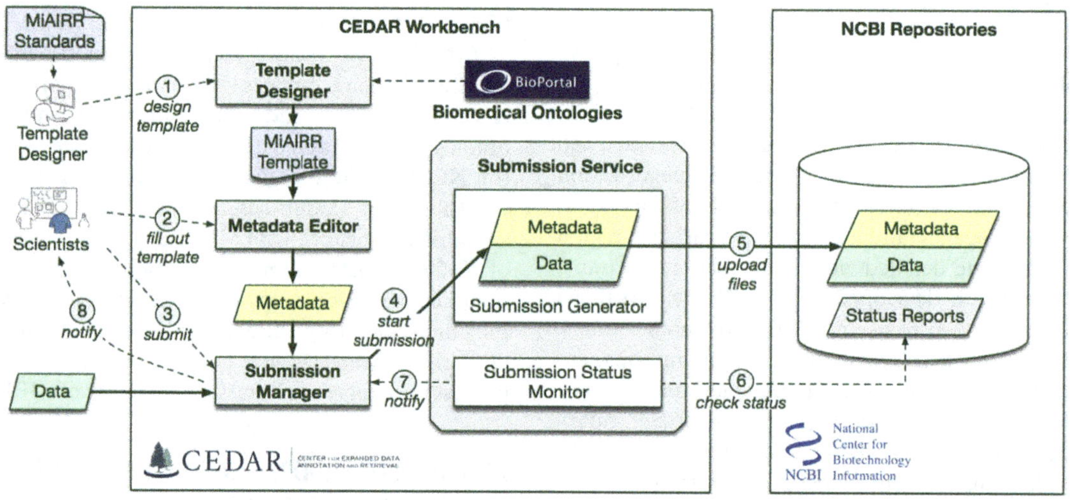


**FIGURE 1** | CAIRR Submission Pipeline Workflow. (1) The CEDAR Template Designer is employed to create a set of templates according to the Minimal Information about an Adaptive Immune Receptor Repertoire (MiAIRR) standard. (2) Scientists can log into the CEDAR Workbench and use these templates to edit ontology-controlled metadata associated with their AIRR-sequencing study. The edited metadata is pre-validated through the National Center for Biotechnology Information (NCBI) validation service. (3) Scientists can start the submission process by accessing the Submission Manager within their CEDAR Workbench workspace. (4) The Submission Manager connects the CEDAR Workbench to the NCBI. (5) The Submission Manager facilitates uploading the metadata and data (FASTQ files) to the NCBI. (6) The CAIRR pipeline periodically checks the submission status at the NCBI. (7) Alert messages from NCBI are received by the Submission Manager. (8) These alert messages provide step-by-step processing detail to the scientists.

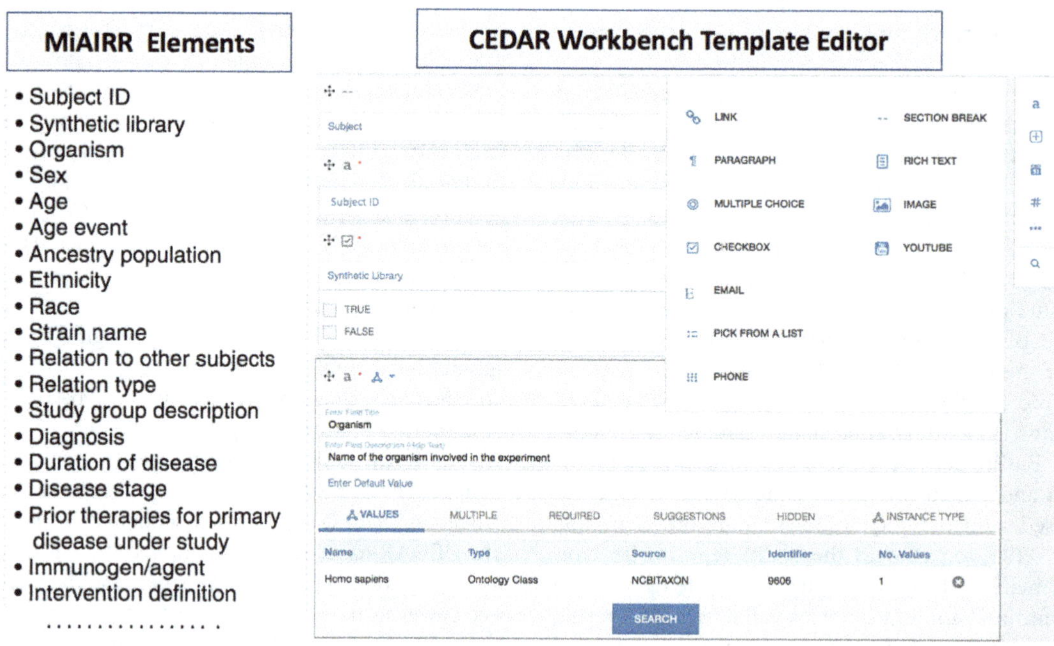


**FIGURE 2** | The Minimal Information about an Adaptive Immune Receptor Repertoire (MiAIRR) fields are transformed into a CEDAR template using the CEDAR Template Designer. Fields specified by MiAIRR (left panel) are transformed into a CEDAR template (right panel).

an AIRR study) to each other through unique identifiers in the MiAIRR template. For example, a typical AIRR study consists of multiple BioSample and SRA records and these records should be anchored to each other in a way that a human or machine can navigate from a particular BioSample record to the related SRA record. Since each BioSample is represented with a unique identifier, we used BioSample identifier as a *prime identifier* and linked BioSample records to the related SRA records with unique BioSample identifiers. This functionality helps to reduce an AIRR study metadata creation and submission time, since users can

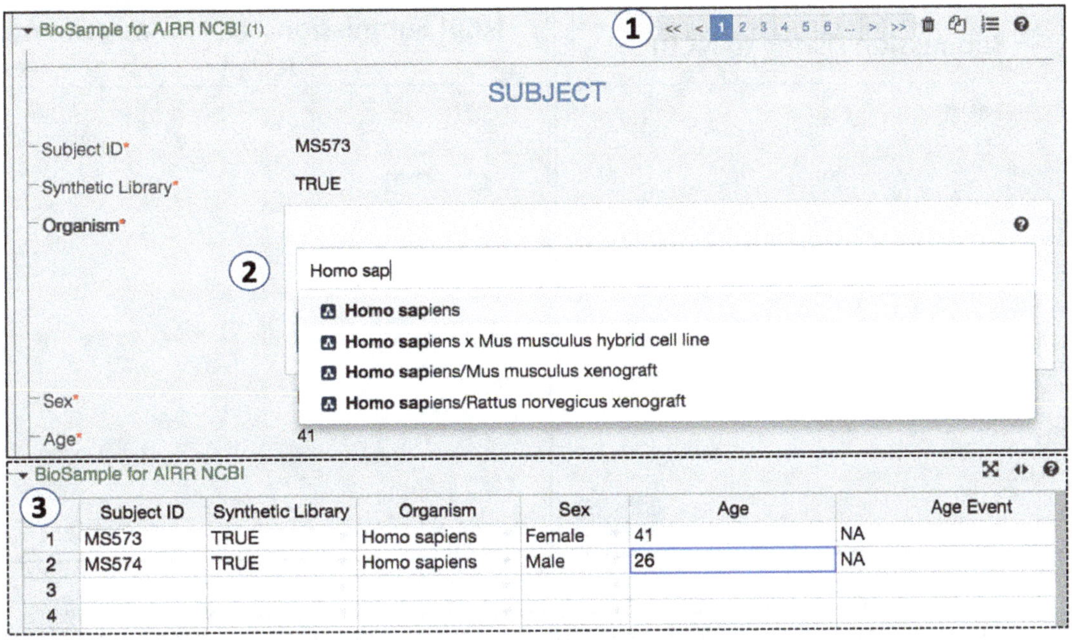


**FIGURE 3** | An ontology-controlled adaptive immune receptor repertoire study metadata editing process. (1) CEDAR's Metadata Editor presents this web form based on the MiAIRR template produced by the Template Designer. The paging option allows a data submitter to add or delete BioSample and sequence read archive (SRA) records. (2) Some of BioSample and the SRA metadata are controlled through ontologies, which allow for auto-completion during data entry. (3) The toggle spreadsheet option allows data submitters to edit metadata using a traditional spreadsheet view.

instantiate multiple BioSample and the SRA submission without worrying how the NCBI translates the resulting AIRR study data.

Linking ontologies with template fields can help make the entered metadata interoperable. In the MiAIRR template, we have constrained the field values to ontology terms. For instance, we restricted the organism, cell type, cell subtype, disease, and tissue fields to terms from AIRR community recommended ontologies such as: National Center for Biotechnology Information Taxonomy Ontology (NCBITAXON) (21), cell ontology (CL) (22), Brenda Tissue Ontology (23), and Human Disease Ontology (DOID) (24) (note that CL covers both the cell type and cell subtype). By employing the CEDAR Template Designer module, we created a MiAIRR template to fulfill the AIRR data submission needs.

## ONTOLOGY-CONTROLLED METADATA EDITING

In the CAIRR pipeline, fields are associated with available ontologies. These associations allow CEDAR to provide autocomplete functionality using the controlled vocabularies from the linked ontologies. Moreover, CEDAR ensures that all ontology-linked field values come only from ontologies and prevents free text from being used. For instance, when a user starts typing "*Homo sapiens*" in the *organism* field, controlled metadata from the NCBITAXON ontology shows up (**Figure 2**) (21). This ontology-based auto-completion reduces typographical errors and promotes consistent metadata entry practices. Moreover, filling a template with ontology-linked metadata enhances the ability to carry out semantic search of the submitted studies. NCBI does not make pervasive use of controlled terms as NCBI does employ the NCBI taxonomy for the organism field but features are not still implemented for the semantic search. If semantic search interface is implemented at the NCBI, a study could be searched based on its related metadata. For example, since *Homo sapiens* is a subclass of mammalia in the ontology hierarchy of NCBITAXON, it would be possible to expand the query search scope based on parent class or to narrow down the scope of a query based on the subclasses of "*Homo sapiens*" only.

The CAIRR pipeline provides a user-friendly interface for metadata creation. Features such as spreadsheet mode make the metadata editing process easy and efficient (**Figure 3**). For example, an AIRR study may hold multiple BioSample and SRA records, and the CAIRR pipeline allows users to add multiple records. Entering metadata into web-based templates is not always the preferred option for scientists who already have metadata available in spreadsheets (**Figure 3**). Therefore, we introduced a toggle spreadsheet view which works like any other traditional spreadsheet. Scientists can import existing spreadsheet hosted data into CAIRR pipeline by copying and pasting through the CAIRR spreadsheet toggle feature. Importantly, metadata validation based on ontologies and other template level constraints still works in spreadsheet view, which otherwise is not possible without writing special macros in programs like Microsoft Excel (25) or by using third-party spreadsheet ontology utilities such as RightField (26). Thus, CAIRR helps scientists to edit ontology-controlled metadata with ease and efficiency.

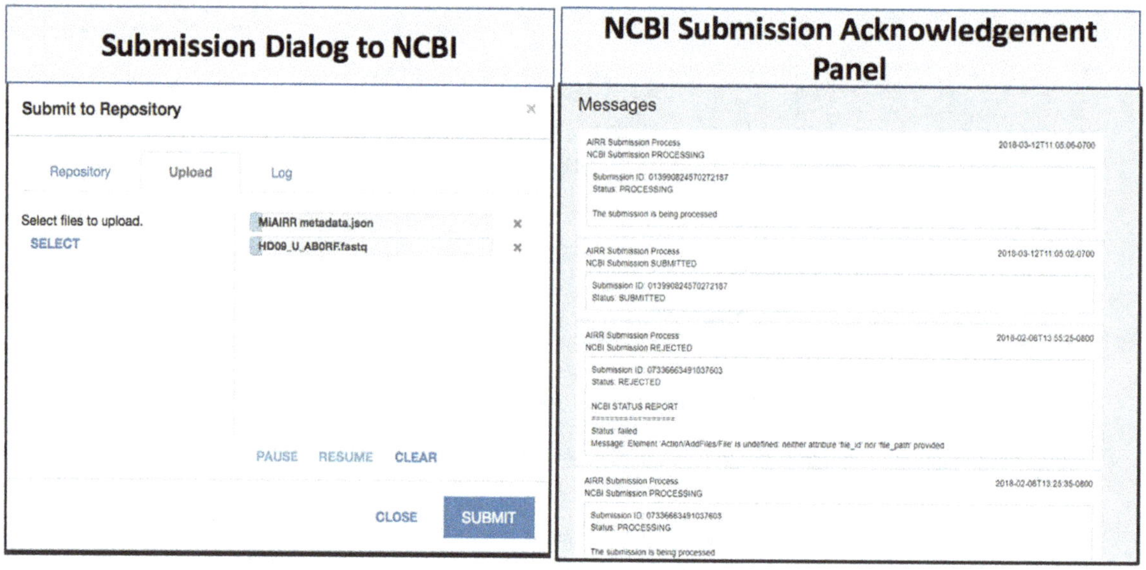


**FIGURE 4** | CAIRR data submission. (1) Data submitters choose National Center for Biotechnology Information (NCBI) Sequence Read Archive (SRA) as the target repository, and then upload the related datasets to submit. (2) CAIRR provides submission acknowledgment and data-processing-level messages generated by the NCBI system.

## AIRR STUDY METADATA VALIDATION AND SUBMISSION

The CAIRR pipeline provides ontology-controlled suggestions at entry-time along with data type checks for the entered values (e.g., date, string, and number). To ensure the quality of the submitted metadata to the NCBI, we have designed a metadata validation module by employing the NCBI validation service which provides an additional layer of quality control (**Figure 4**). The NCBI validation service is publicly available for any external user or application. It detects missing mandatory BioSample fields, such as BioSample Identifier, age, isolate, and sex, and generates alerts with error messages. To use the validation service inside the CAIRR pipeline, a user fills in an AIRR study's metadata in the MiAIRR template and invokes the validation service through the Validate Metadata option within the Metadata Editor. The validation service fetches the entered metadata and reports any non-compliant metadata. This validation service could be invoked multiple times by a data submitter during the AIRR study metadata authoring process. Thus, the CAIRR pipeline includes multi-layered validation mechanism to ensure that the submitted metadata is of a high quality and compliant with the NCBI repositories.

An AIRR study consists of AIRR metadata along with raw and processed sequence reads which are stored in FASTQ format (16). The available options for data and metadata submission using the NCBI submission interface are depositing through email or submitting through the file transfer protocol (FTP) using command line or third-party FTP utilities. In order to make the submission process easier, the CAIRR pipeline provides a user-friendly data submission interface. This data uploading facility can be accessed through the CEDAR Workspace—the first CEDAR interface users see after logging in—where users can select the generated metadata file and submit it to the NCBI repositories (**Figure 4**, submission dialog to the NCBI).

The CAIRR pipeline provides post-submission processing information to the submitters. Data submitters are informed within the CAIRR pipeline if any error is automatically detected after an AIRR study submission to the NCBI. The post-processing at the NCBI involves both computer-based validation and a human curator check. The computer automatically checks for the sequence reads length and its format details while a human curator looks for data relevancy and submitted metadata anomalies. Each computerized stage generates processing logs which are stored as a report. The logs capture the submitter detail, IP address, number of submitted files, and time zone information, along with the NCBI approval and rejection status information. The CAIRR pipeline parses this log file and displays the messages in the submitter's workspace (**Figure 4**, NCBI submission acknowledgment panel).

## DISCUSSION

The CAIRR pipeline was designed in compliance with the MiAIRR standard to facilitate AIRR study metadata generation and submission (see Figure S1 in Supplementary Material). In order to help users improve their metadata quality through ontology-constrained AIRR metadata selections, the CAIRR pipeline employs CEDAR technology in conjunction with NCBO BioPortal ontologies to develop the MiAIRR template. CAIRR makes AIRR study submission to the NCBI straightforward by providing a Submission Manager which handles data uploading and notifies users about post-submission processing at the NCBI.

CAIRR also generates its output in JSON-LD and RDF (Resource Description Framework) formats which could be deposited into other AIRR-specific repositories such as VDJServer (27) and iReceptor (28), or into general repositories such as Zenodo.[1]

The possibility of re-analysis and meta-analysis of datasets made available through the NCBI offers the potential for important insights. However, such analyses largely depend on the effective sharing of large-scale experimental data such as that generated by AIRR sequencing studies. As next-generation sequencing technologies continue to improve, scientists are adopting these technologies to get insights into the adaptive immune response in healthy individuals and in individuals with a wide range of diseases (29, 30). The number of published and publicly available AIRR-seq datasets is also steadily increasing in repositories such as NCBI. Because metadata production is not a straightforward process, we observe some existing metadata at the NCBI with several metadata anomalies (31). The CAIRR pipeline simplifies AIRR study metadata editing and submission, thus improving the production and sharing of AIRR-seq data for further analysis.

The CAIRR pipeline can be extended in several ways. The current production version of the CAIRR pipeline supports the generation of metadata and deposition into three repositories at the NCBI (BioProject, BioSample, and the SRA). MiAIRR standard also mandates the deposition of processed data, which is not covered by these repositories. To address this, CAIRR will be extended to support submission to the NCBI GenBank. Another future extension will involve the development of an AIRR ontology, which will address the fact that not all the MiAIRR template fields are linked to ontology classes because of the unavailability of the appropriate ontology classes (e.g., forward and reverse PCR primer target locations, physical linkage of different loci). Finally, a community-level evaluation will be carried out to supplement the more limited evaluation described here.

## CONCLUSION

To improve AIRR study metadata quality and to facilitate the metadata creation and submission process we have developed the CAIRR pipeline[2] using the CEDAR Workbench. By linking MiAIRR template fields with ontologies, and providing validation checks, CAIRR minimizes metadata anomalies, such as metadata inconsistency, incomplete metadata, and incorrect metadata. Through CAIRR, users can submit MiAIRR-compliant data to the NCBI BioProject, BioSample, and the SRA repositories. To promote the maximum use of CAIRR, we have created a mailing list, online documentation with step-by-step instructions[3] along with a video tutorial. More generally, CAIRR demonstrates how the CEDAR Workbench can be tailored for metadata editing and submission according to the needs of a particular scientific community.

[1]http://zenodo.org (Accessed: August 6, 2017).
[2]http://cairr.miairr.org (Accessed: August 6, 2017).

## AUTHOR CONTRIBUTIONS

Study conception and design: SACB, K-HC, SHK, MC, JG, and MM. Code implementation: SACB, MC, MM-R, DW, and AE. Validated and interpreted the results: SACB, JG, FR, MC, and DW. Drafting of manuscript: SACB, SHK, and K-HC. Critical revision: MAM, MM-R, and FR. All authors read and approved the final manuscript.

## ACKNOWLEDGMENTS

We acknowledge Susanna Marquez and Hailong Meng from Yale University for their participation in the evaluation of CAIRR and for providing valuable suggestions.

## FUNDING

This work was supported by grant U54 AI117925 awarded by the National Institute of Allergy and Infectious Diseases through funds provided by the trans-NIH Big Data to Knowledge (BD2K) initiative (www.bd2k.nih.gov), as well as by grant R01 AI104739 awarded by the National Institute of Allergy and Infectious Diseases. FR was supported by NIH grant U19 AI57229.

[3]http://cairr-docs.miairr.org/ (Accessed: August 6, 2017).

## REFERENCES

1. Hou D, Chen C, Seely EJ, Chen S, Song Y. High-throughput sequencing-based immune repertoire study during infectious disease. *Front Immunol* (2016) 7:336. doi:10.3389/fimmu.2016.00336
2. Weinstein JA, Jiang N, White RA III, Fisher DS, Quake SR. High-throughput sequencing of the zebrafish antibody repertoire. *Science* (2009) 324:807–10. doi:10.1126/science.1170020
3. Freeman JD, Warren RL, Webb JR, Nelson BH, Holt RA. Profiling the T-cell receptor beta-chain repertoire by massively parallel sequencing. *Genome Res* (2009) 19:1817–24. doi:10.1101/gr.092924.109
4. Robinson WH. Sequencing the functional antibody repertoire – diagnostic and therapeutic discovery. *Nat Rev Rheumatol* (2015) 11:171–82. doi:10.1038/nrrheum.2014.220
5. Wilkinson MD, Dumontier M, Aalbersberg IJJ, Appleton G, Axton M, Baak A, et al. The FAIR guiding principles for scientific data management and stewardship. *Sci Data* (2016) 3:160018. doi:10.1038/sdata.2016.18
6. Rubelt F, Busse CE, Bukhari SAC, Bürckert J-P, Mariotti-Ferrandiz E, Cowell LG, et al. Adaptive immune receptor repertoire community recommendations for sharing immune-repertoire sequencing data. *Nat Immunol* (2017) 18:1274–8. doi:10.1038/ni.3873
7. Breden F, Luning Prak ET, Peters B, Rubelt F, Schramm CA, Busse C, et al. Reproducibility and reuse of adaptive immune receptor repertoire data. *Front Immunol* (2017) 8:1418. doi:10.3389/fimmu.2017.01418
8. Musen MA, Bean CA, Cheung K-H, Dumontier M, Durante KA, Gevaert O, et al. The center for expanded data annotation and retrieval. *J Am Med Inform Assoc* (2015) 22:1148–52. doi:10.1093/jamia/ocv048

9. Barrett T, Clark K, Gevorgyan R, Gorelenkov V, Gribov E, Karsch-Mizrachi I, et al. BioProject and BioSample databases at NCBI: facilitating capture and organization of metadata. *Nucleic Acids Res* (2012) 40:D57–63. doi:10.1093/nar/gkr1163
10. Leinonen R, Sugawara H, Shumway M. International nucleotide sequence database collaboration. The sequence read archive. *Nucleic Acids Res* (2011) 39:D19–21. doi:10.1093/nar/gkq1019
11. Benson DA, Clark K, Karsch-Mizrachi I, Lipman DJ, Ostell J, Sayers EW. GenBank. *Nucleic Acids Res* (2015) 43:D30–5. doi:10.1093/nar/gku1216
12. Bukhari SAC, Cheung KH. *Towards Ontological Mapping of Immunological Data Standards*. Orlando: Bio-Ontologies SIG at the ISMB (2016).
13. Bukhari SAC, Bashir AK, Malik KM. Semantic web in the age of big data: a perspective. (2018). doi:10.31219/osf.io/mwjtq
14. Bukhari SAC, O'Connor MJ, Graybeal J, Musen MA, Cheung KH, Kleinstein SH. *Leveraging the CEDAR Workbench for Ontology-Linked Submission of Adaptive Immune Receptor Repertoire Data to the Sequence Read Archive (SRA)*. Bethesda: Zenodo (2016).
15. Bukhari SAC, Martínez-Romero M, O'Connor MJ, Egyedi AL, Willrett D, Graybeal J, et al. CEDAR OnDemand: a browser extension to generate ontology-based scientific metadata. *BMC Bioinformatics* (2018) 19(1):268. doi:10.1186/s12859-018-2247-6
16. Cock PJA, Fields CJ, Goto N, Heuer ML, Rice PM. The Sanger FASTQ file format for sequences with quality scores, and the Solexa/Illumina FASTQ variants. *Nucleic Acids Res* (2010) 38:1767–71. doi:10.1093/nar/gkp1137
17. Wache H, Voegele T, Visser U, Stuckenschmidt H, Schuster G, Neumann H, et al. Ontology-based integration of information-a survey of existing approaches. *IJCAI-01 Workshop: Ontologies and Information Sharing* (2001). p. 108–17.
18. Mattingly CJ, McKone TE, Callahan MA, Blake JA, Cohen Hubal EA. Providing the missing link: the exposure science ontology ExO. *Environ Sci Technol* (2012) 46(6):3046–53. doi:10.1021/es2033857
19. NCBO BioPortal. *Exposure Ontology*. Available from: https://bioportal.bioontology.org/ontologies/EXO (Accessed: September 6, 2017).
20. Authority SR. *SRA Handbook*. Bethesda: Law Society (2015).
21. Federhen S. The NCBI Taxonomy database. *Nucleic Acids Res* (2012) 40:D136–43. doi:10.1093/nar/gkr1178
22. Meehan TF, Masci AM, Abdulla A, Cowell LG, Blake JA, Mungall CJ, et al. Logical development of the cell ontology. *BMC Bioinformatics* (2011) 12:6. doi:10.1186/1471-2105-12-6
23. Gremse M, Chang A, Schomburg I, Grote A, Scheer M, Ebeling C, et al. The BRENDA tissue ontology (BTO): the first all-integrating ontology of all organisms for enzyme sources. *Nucleic Acids Res* (2011) 39:D507–13. doi:10.1093/nar/gkq968
24. Schriml LM, Arze C, Nadendla S, Chang Y-WW, Mazaitis M, Felix V, et al. Disease ontology: a backbone for disease semantic integration. *Nucleic Acids Res* (2012) 40:D940–6. doi:10.1093/nar/gkr972
25. Dory RA. Macros in a spreadsheet. *Comput Phys Commun* (1990) 4:558. doi:10.1063/1.4822947
26. Wolstencroft K, Owen S, Horridge M, Krebs O, Mueller W, Snoep JL, et al. RightField: embedding ontology annotation in spreadsheets. *Bioinformatics* (2011) 27:2021–2. doi:10.1093/bioinformatics/btr312
27. Christley S, Scarborough W, Salinas E, Rounds WH, Toby IT, Fonner JM, et al. VDJServer: a cloud-based analysis portal and data commons for immune repertoire sequences and rearrangements. *Front Immunol* (2018) 9:976. doi:10.3389/fimmu.2018.00976
28. iReceptor. *What is iReceptor?* Available from: http://ireceptor.irmacs.sfu.ca/ (Accessed: August 6, 2017).
29. Goodwin S, McPherson JD, McCombie WR. Coming of age: ten years of next-generation sequencing technologies. *Nat Rev Genet* (2016) 17:333–51. doi:10.1038/nrg.2016.49
30. Georgiou G, Ippolito GC, Beausang J, Busse CE, Wardemann H, Quake SR. The promise and challenge of high-throughput sequencing of the antibody repertoire. *Nat Biotechnol* (2014) 32:158–68. doi:10.1038/nbt.2782
31. Gonçalves RS, O'Connor MJ, Martínez-Romero M, Graybeal J, Musen MA. *Metadata in the BioSample Online Repository are Impaired by Numerous Anomalies. 1st International Workshop SemSci 2017 (Enabling Open Semantic Science), co-located with ISWC 2017*. Vienna (2017). Available from: http://ceur-ws.org/Vol-1931/paper-06.pdf (Accessed: August 6, 2017).

# 6

# Optimized Threshold Inference for Partitioning of Clones From High-Throughput B Cell Repertoire Sequencing Data

*Nima Nouri[1] and Steven H. Kleinstein[1,2]**

[1] *Department of Pathology, Yale School of Medicine, New Haven, CT, United States,* [2] *Interdepartmental Program in Computational Biology and Bioinformatics, Yale University, New Haven, CT, United States*

***Correspondence:***
*Steven H. Kleinstein*
*steven.kleinstein@yale.edu*

During adaptive immune responses, activated B cells expand and undergo somatic hypermutation of their B cell receptor (BCR), forming a clone of diversified cells that can be related back to a common ancestor. Identification of B cell clones from high-throughput Adaptive Immune Receptor Repertoire sequencing (AIRR-seq) data relies on computational analysis. Recently, we proposed an automated method to partition sequences into clonal groups based on single-linkage hierarchical clustering of the BCR junction region with length-normalized Hamming distance metric. This method could identify clonal sequences with high confidence on several benchmark experimental and simulated data sets. However, determining the threshold to cut the hierarchy, a key step in the method, is computationally expensive for large-scale repertoire sequencing data sets. Moreover, the methodology was unable to provide estimates of accuracy for new data. Here, a new method is presented that addresses this computational bottleneck and also provides a study-specific estimation of performance, including sensitivity and specificity. The method uses a finite mixture model fitting procedure for learning the parameters of two univariate curves which fit the bimodal distribution of the distance vector between pairs of sequences. These distributions are used to estimate the performance of different threshold choices for partitioning sequences into clones. These performance estimates are validated using simulated and experimental data sets. With this method, clones can be identified from AIRR-seq data with sensitivity and specificity profiles that are user-defined based on the overall goals of the study.

**Keywords: AIRR-seq data, B-cell clonal partitioning, hierarchical clustering, optimized distance threshold, immcantation portal**

## 1. INTRODUCTION

Next-generation sequencing technologies are increasingly being applied to carry out detailed profiling of B cell receptors (BCRs, also referred to as the immunoglobulin (Ig) receptors). Identification of B cell clones (sequences that are related through descent from a single naive B cell) from these high-throughput AIRR-seq data relies on computational analysis. Accurate identification of clonal members is important, as these clonal groups form the basis for a wide range of repertoire analysis, including diversity analysis, lineage reconstruction, and detection of antigen-specific sequences (1).

Hierarchical clustering is a widely used approach for partitioning sequences into clones (1) and several associated software tools have been developed (2–4). Identifying clonally related BCRs is typically accomplished in two steps. First, sequences are split into groups that share the same V-gene annotation, J-gene annotation, and number of nucleotides in their junction region (5–9). Here, the junction region is defined as the CDR3 plus the conserved flanking amino acid residues. Next, these groups are hierarchically clustered based on the nucleotide similarity of their junction region, and partitioned by cutting the dendrogram at a fixed distance threshold. We previously developed an automated approach for determining this threshold, and demonstrated that using this threshold with single-linkage clustering based on the length-normalized Hamming distance (i.e., the absolute count of differences between two sequences divided by the length of the sequence) detects clones with high confidence on several benchmark data sets (4). However, the actual sensitivity and specificity may differ on any particular data set, and existing methods do not provide a mechanism to estimate or tune study-specific performance. Here, we propose and validate a computationally efficient threshold inference algorithm for partitioning BCR sequences into clones that also allows for study-specific performance estimation.

## 2. METHOD

The proposed method extends the approach developed by Gupta et al. (4), where identifying clonally related BCRs is accomplished in two steps. First, sequences are split into groups that share the same V-gene annotation, J-gene annotation, and number of nucleotides in their junction region. Next, these groups are hierarchically clustered based on the nucleotide similarity of their junction quantified by Hamming distance, and partitioned by cutting the dendrogram at a fixed distance threshold. In this paper, we specifically develop a new model-based method for determining the fixed distance threshold for partitioning sequences, which allows for estimation of sensitivity and specificity. First, the "distance-to-nearest" distribution is determined using length-normalized nucleotide Hamming distance (i.e., the distribution of minimum distances from each sequence to every other non-identical sequence). This is typically a bimodal distribution (8, 9), with the first mode representing sequences with clonal relatives and the second mode representing those without clonal relatives (i.e., singletons) in the data set. Next, the bimodal distance-to-nearest distribution is explicitly modeled as a mixture of two univariate distribution functions (e.g., a mixture of Gaussian or Gamma distribution) of the form:

$$f(x) = \lambda_1 f_1(x \mid \phi_1) + \lambda_2 f_2(x \mid \phi_2), \tag{1}$$

where $\lambda_1$ and $\lambda_2$ represent the mixing weights (summing to one), $x$ represents the nearest neighbor distances, and $\phi$ represents the vector of each component parameters. Here, we investigate all combinations of $f_1$ and $f_2$ as Gaussian and Gamma distributions so $\phi$ is either the mean and SD ($\mu$, $\sigma$) of a Gaussian distribution, or the shape and scale ($k$, $\theta$) of a Gamma distribution. A maximum-likelihood fitting procedure (function `fitdistr` from MASS R package) is used to estimate the parameters of the model as follows: (1) parameters of the model are initialized using a standard Gaussian mixture model (GMM). The GMM estimates mixing weight $\lambda_i$, mean $\mu_i$, and SD $\sigma_i$ where $i \in \{1,2\}$ refers to the first and second distributions. (2) These parameters are then used as initial values to begin the maximum-likelihood fitting procedure (if Gamma distribution is chosen, the initial values are translated accordingly).

After fitting, the two distributions are used to estimate sensitivity (SEN) and specificity (SPC) by the fractions TP/(TP + FN) and TN/(TN + FP), respectively. The statistical rates [true positive (TP), false negative (FN), false positive (FP), and true negative (TN)] are then given by the area under the curves:

$$\mathrm{TP} = \int_{t_1}^{t} \lambda_1 f_1(x \mid \phi_1)dx, \quad \mathrm{FN} = \int_{t}^{t_2} \lambda_1 f_1(x \mid \phi_1)dx,$$
$$\mathrm{FP} = \int_{t_1}^{t} \lambda_2 f_2(x \mid \phi_2)dx, \quad \mathrm{TN} = \int_{t}^{t_2} \lambda_2 f_2(x \mid \phi_2)dx, \tag{2}$$

where $t_1$ and $t_2$ are the minimum and maximum values of the distance-to-nearest distribution, respectively. Finally, the optimized threshold $t$ is chosen in the distance interval ($t_1$, $t_2$) to maximize the average of sensitivity and specificity:

$$\max_{t_1 < t < t_2} \left( \frac{SEN(t) + SPC(t)}{2} \right). \tag{3}$$

## 3. RESULTS

### 3.1. Mixture of Gamma Distributions Is Used to Fit the Bimodal Distribution

To determine the optimal distributions to use for the mixture model, we tested the method using simulated and experimental data sets. Specifically, we used the simulated data sets from Gupta et al. (4). These simulations start with a set of observed lineage tree topologies from lymph node samples from each of four individuals (M2, M3, M4, and M5 from Ref. (6)), and generate a simulated data set for each individual (R1, R2, R3, and R4, respectively) by randomly selecting a new germline sequence for every lineage and then stochastically re-introducing mutations along the lineage branches. This process was repeated 10 times for each individual to create a collection of 40 simulated data sets. We also invoked experimental data from BCR sequencing of PBMCs from 58 individuals with acute dengue virus infection (note that two individuals with total reads <1k sequences were excluded) (10). These samples each contained ~1–13k total reads.

We evaluated all four combinations of Gaussian and Gamma distributions for $f_1$ and $f_2$ on both simulated and experimental data sets. For each combination, the log likelihood was determined once for 40 simulated and 58 experimental data sets. We found that in 80% of trials the choice of Gamma distribution for both $f_1$ and $f_2$ yielded the highest likelihood. Furthermore, in each trial, visual inspection suggested that this choice placed the threshold approximately equidistant between the two distributions. Therefore, Gamma distributions were selected as the default choices and used in all of the analyses below (**Figures 1A–C**). We note that the Gamma distribution is known to be skewed positively (i.e., an asymmetric distribution with longer right-tail). However, the Gamma distribution becomes more symmetric as its shape parameter $k \to \infty$. This intrinsic feature of the Gamma distribution makes it a strong tool which behaves flexibly according to the notion of how symmetric/asymmetric the observed distributions are. By contrast, the Gaussian distribution is always symmetric, and thus unable to adapt itself to an asymmetric distribution of observed data points.

## 3.2. High Correlation Between Actual and Estimated Performance Is Achieved in Simulated Data

The ability of the proposed method to estimate sensitivity and specificity for clonal relatedness was evaluated on simulated data. First, sensitivity and specificity were evaluated using ten simulated data sets (set R1 generated by Gupta et al. (4)). On each data set, a wide range of potential thresholds for partitioning sequences into clones was considered. At each threshold value, we calculated the actual performance based on the known clonal relationships from the simulation (actual), as well as the estimated performance based on the mixture modeling and equation set 2 using the area under the fitted distribution curves (estimated). We found a high correlation between the actual and estimated sensitivity ($R^2 = 92\%$) and specificity ($R^2 = 98\%$) on average over all ten simulated data sets (**Figures 2A,B**). We believe that the correlation is useful, as we see that method provides a lower bound on actual performance. On the other hand, sensitivity shows some lack of proportionality. Specifically, at high values for the threshold (between 0.12 and 0.15), the sensitivity estimated from the mixture model becomes saturated (i.e., the area under fitted left distribution reaches one). Although, using the positively skewed-shape Gamma distribution is better than using a Gaussian distribution, the right-tail of the first Gamma distribution still falls off too fast relative to the actual intra-clonal distance distribution in some cases.

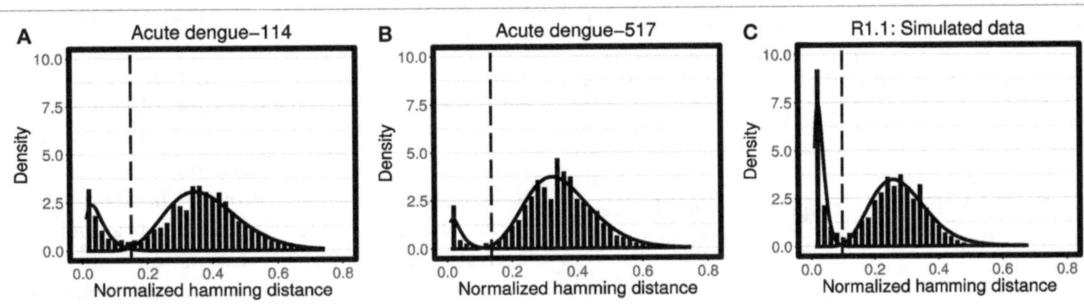


**FIGURE 1** | Analysis of the distance-to-nearest neighbor plot to define the distance threshold for partitioning clones. For each sequence, the length-normalized nucleotide Hamming distance to every other sequence was calculated, and the nearest (non-identical) neighbor was identified. The histogram of nearest neighbor distances is fitted using Gamma distribution for both modes (solid line) for **(A,B)** representative peripheral blood B cell samples from patients with acute dengue virus infection (10), and **(C)** representative simulated data from Gupta et al. (4). For each data set the optimum threshold, where the average of sensitivity and specificity reaches its maximum, was calculated by the `findThreshold` function (dashed vertical line). Note that the choice of bin size impacts the shape of plotted histograms, while the fitting procedure is independent of this bin size.

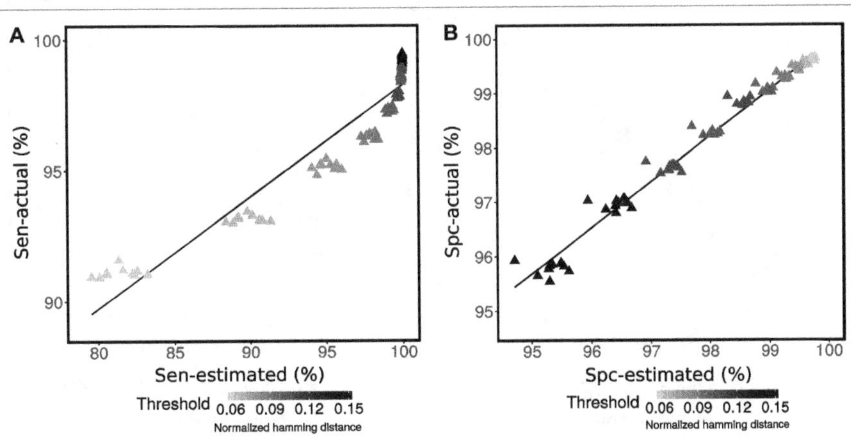


**FIGURE 2** | Performance assessment of **(A)** sensitivity (Sen) and **(B)** specificity (Spc) for determining membership in a multi-sequence clone. Mixture modeling of the distance-to-nearest distribution was used to estimate sensitivity and specificity for each specified value of the threshold (points) according to equation set 2. The estimated performance (Sen-estimated and Spc-estimated) was compared with actual performance (Sen-actual and Spc-actual) for simulated R1.1–R1.10 data from Gupta et al. (4) across a wide range of thresholds (shades of gray for each point).

## 3.3. High Correlation Between Actual and Estimated Specificity Is Achieved in Experimental Data

The underlying clonal relationships among sequences in experimental data sets are not known with certainty. However, we reasoned that two sequences are unrelated when they are derived from two separate individuals since, by definition, a B cell clone cannot span two individuals. Therefore, false positives are defined as sequences from different individuals being grouped together in a clone, whereas true negatives are defined as sequences from different individuals that are grouped into separate clones. Specificity is then calculated by dividing the number of true negative classifications by the sum over the number of true negative and false positive classifications. We used this approach to further evaluate the ability of the method to estimate specificity on experimental BCR sequencing data from 58 individuals with acute dengue infection (10). First, one of the individuals was chosen as the "base." Next, a single sequence was chosen randomly from each of the remaining individuals and added to the sequencing data from the base individual. Specificity was then defined by how often the sequences from non-base individuals were correctly determined to be singletons. Any grouping of these sequences into larger clones must be a false positive. Like the simulated data, specificity was calculated both using the known source of the sequences (actual) and for the mixture model (estimated). This procedure was then repeated 50 times for each of 58 different base individuals. The results indicated a high correlation between the actual and estimated specificity ($R^2 = 95\%$) across all 58 base individuals (**Figure 3A**).

## 3.4. High Correlation Between Actual and Estimated Specificity Is Achieved Across Experimental Data Sets

Within a single study, spurious sharing of BCRs may occur by cross clustering within the same flow cell, by contamination or by chance with low frequency. To address the possibility that these occurrences impacted our estimation of specificity, we repeated the same specificity analysis described in the previous section, but using individuals from two independent experimental data sets. First, subject M2 (with ~100k total reads from lymph node samples collected by Stern et al. (6)) was chosen as the "base." Next, a single sequence was chosen randomly from each of the 58 individuals with acute dengue infection (10) and added to the sequencing data from the base. Like the previous analysis, specificity was then defined by how often the sequences from non-base individuals were correctly determined to be singletons, and was calculated both using the known source of the sequences (actual) and for the mixture model (estimated). This procedure was then repeated 50 times. High correlation between the actual and estimated specificity ($R^2 = 97\%$) was obtained (**Figure 3B**). These results show that the proposed approach provides a reliable estimate of specificity on experimental data.

## 3.5. The Mixture Method Is Computationally Efficient

The threshold inference algorithm developed in this work (`gmm`) is computationally more efficient than its density-based predecessor by Gupta et al. (4) (**Figure 4**). The improvement does not arise from the nearest neighbor identification, which is identical for both methods. Rather, the improvement comes in how to identify the fixed threshold to cut the hierarchy in order to identify discrete clonal groups. The density-based approach is computationally demanding since it is associated with a fourth derivative kernel density estimation with a sequential time complexity of $O(n^3)$, where $n$ denotes the number of sequences. The `gmm` exhibits faster performance by replacing this computationally expensive step with an optimization algorithm with a sequential time complexity of $O(n)$, where $n$ denotes the number of sequences. We compared the run times of both approaches using the implementations under the `findThreshold` function as part of the **SHazaM** R package (version 0.1.9) in the

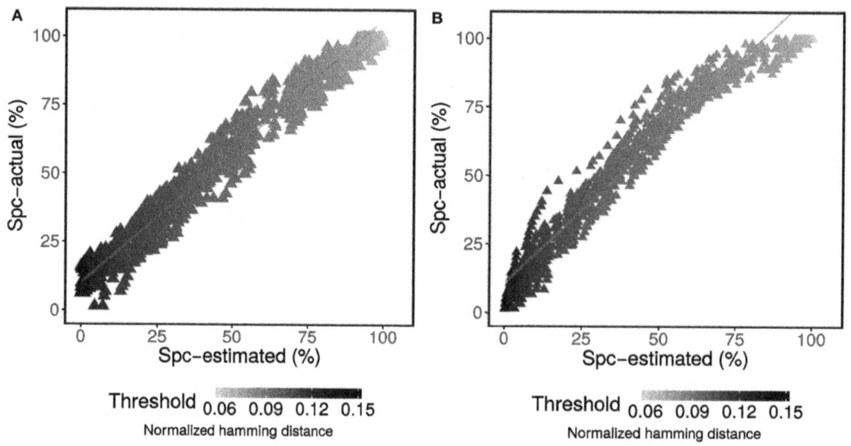


**FIGURE 3** | Performance assessment of specificity (Spc) for determining membership in a multi-sequence clone. Mixture modeling of the distance-to-nearest distribution was used to estimate specificity for each specified value of the threshold (points) according to equation set 2. **(A)** The estimated performance was compared with actual performance for experimental data from patients with acute dengue infection (10) across a wide range of thresholds (shades of gray for each point). **(B)** The estimated performance (Spc-estimated) was compared with actual performance (Spc-actual) across two independent experimental studies (6, 10) across a wide range of thresholds (shades of gray for each point).

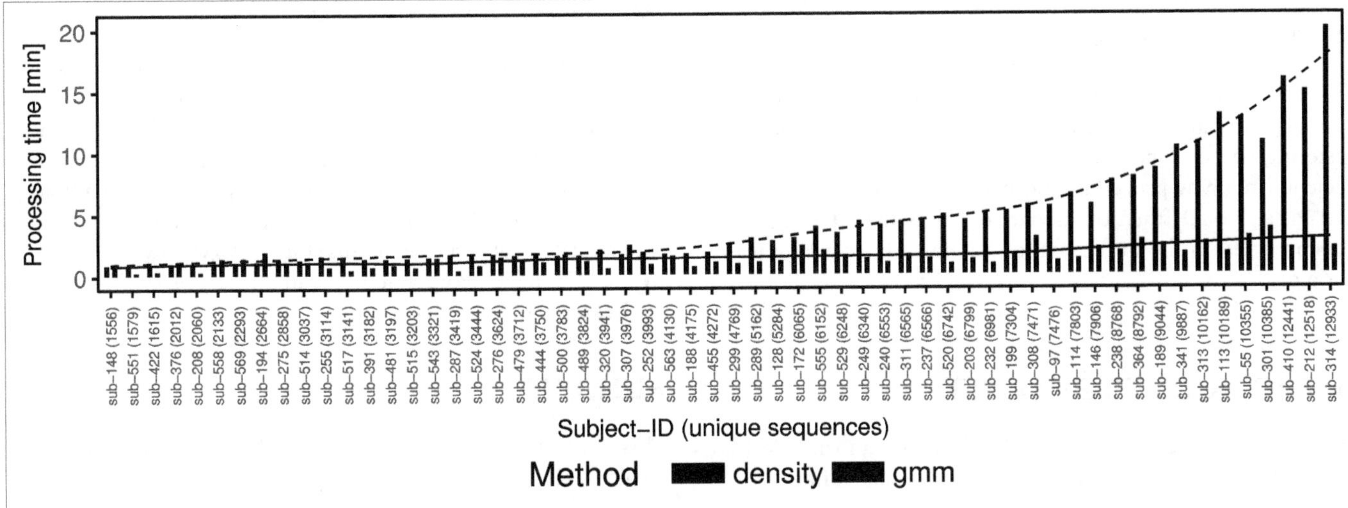


**FIGURE 4** | The gmm approach is computationally efficient while the `density` approach run time scales exponentially. Comparison of running times (*y*-axis) between `density` (dashed line and gray bars) and gmm (solid line and black bars) approaches performed over 58 individuals from a study of acute dengue infection (10) (*x*-axis). The *x*-axis is ordered ascending by the number of sequences in the individual sample.

Immcantation framework (www.immcantation.org). The density-based method by Gupta et al. (4) and the model-based method described here are implemented as methods `density` and gmm, respectively. On a Linux computer with a 2.20 GHz Intel processor and 32 GB RAM, we found, for example, that using the gmm approach it took <5 min to find the threshold in a data set of ~10k sequences, while the `density` approach completed in ~15 min (**Figure 4**).

## 4. CONCLUSION

We have proposed and validated a computationally efficient threshold inference algorithm that can be used to automatically partition BCR sequences into clonally related groups. The method gmm is based on a mixture model fit to the bimodal distance-to-nearest distribution, and allows for direct estimation of the sensitivity and specificity for membership in a multi-sequence clone. This is an important advantage over previous methods, such as the density-based method by Gupta et al. (4), which are unable to provide estimates of accuracy for new data. The ability to estimate sensitivity and specificity directly from a BCR sequencing data set allows researchers to identify B cell clones with performance characteristics that optimize study-specific goals. For instance, a threshold with high-sensitivity may be ideal for identifying sequences that are part of a clone expansion including a known antigen-specific sequence, while a threshold with high-specificity may be ideal for determining biological connections between tissue compartments or B cell subsets. In the evaluations presented in this study, we have chosen to maximize the average of sensitivity and specificity.

BCR sequencing data contain errors, although methods such as the inclusion of UMIs (11) can dramatically reduce their frequency. Thus, the distance-to-nearest distributions being fit by the mixture model contain a combination of true somatic hypermutation and errors (e.g., PCR and sequencing errors). Rather than being a problem, this is an important feature of the method. It is critical to take both sources of diversity into account when determining the threshold for partitioning sequences into clones. If members of a clone were truly <10% different, but experimental errors increased their difference to <11%, then the proper choice is to use the 11% as the threshold.

The choice of distributions (e.g., Gaussian or Gamma) that accurately describe the observed distance-to-nearest distribution for clonally related sequences in one data set may not be ideal for other sequencing data sets. The shape of the distance-to-nearest distribution depends on various experimental and physiological factors such as initial B-cell population, sampling depth, sequencing error, polarized or flat repertoire, and unusual BCR junction length distribution. These factors may influence the quality of mixture model fits. Therefore, we recommend users visually inspect the resulting fit from each data set. If a mixture of Gamma distributions results in a poor fit, then other combinations of mixture models should be tried. The `density` method provides a robust backup to these model-based methods, although it would be at the cost of losing the estimation of cloning performance. Our empirical observations of peripheral blood B cell repertoires suggest the bimodality of the distance-to-nearest distribution is detectable for a repertoire of minimum 1k total reads. From statistical point of view, increasing number of sequences will improve the fitting procedure, although it would be at the potential expense of higher demand in computational time complexity.

The method used in this study has been developed for partitioning BCR heavy (H) chain sequences. More specifically, the method leverages the high diversity of the H chain junction region as the main "fingerprint" to infer clonal relatedness. Emerging techniques, including single-cell sequencing, can provide paired H and L chain data (12–14). The methods presented here can be applied to such data by extending the criteria for the initial grouping of sequences to include the same $V_H$ gene, $J_H$ gene, $CDR3_H$ length, $V_L$ gene, $J_L$ gene, and $CDR3_L$ length. Clustering of the H chain junction region can then be carried out as before on these more refined groups. The low diversity of the L chain junction region (12) makes it unlikely that including this region in the clustering will provide a significant performance improvement.

Overall, the results on the simulated and experimental data sets indicate that the mixture modeling method provides an accurate estimate of sensitivity and specificity for hierarchical clustering-based clonal partitioning of BCRs, and is also time-efficient. This new procedure has been implemented under the `findThreshold` function as part of the **SHazaM** R package (version 0.1.9) in the Immcantation framework (www.immcantation.org).

## AUTHOR CONTRIBUTIONS

NN and SHK have made a substantial, direct, and intellectual contribution to the work and approved it for publication.

## ACKNOWLEDGMENTS

The authors thank Dr. Namita T. Gupta for providing the simulated data set and S. Marquez for useful comments on code. We are also grateful to Dr. Jason Vander Heiden, Department of Neurology at Yale School of Medicine, for his useful comments on the manuscript, and Dr. Hailong Meng, Department of Pathology at Yale School of Medicine, for development of a website to share the simulated data set used in this study. This work was supported by the HPC facilities operated by, and the staff of, the Yale Center for Research Computing.

## FUNDING

This work was supported in part by the National Institutes of Health (NIH) under award number R01AI104739.

## REFERENCES


1. Yaari G, Kleinstein SH. Practical guidelines for B-cell receptor repertoire sequencing analysis. *Genome Med* (2015) 7:121. doi:10.1186/s13073-015-0243-2
2. Chen Z, Collins AM, Wang Y, Gaëta BA. Clustering-based identification of clonally-related immunoglobulin gene sequence sets. *Immunome Res* (2010) 6:S4. doi:10.1186/1745-7580-6-S1-S4
3. Gupta NT, Vander Heiden JA, Uduman M, Gadala-Maria D, Yaari G, Kleinstein SH. Change-o: a toolkit for analyzing large-scale B cell immunoglobulin repertoire sequencing data. *Bioinformatics* (2015) 31:3356–8. doi:10.1093/bioinformatics/btv359
4. Gupta NT, Adams KD, Briggs AW, Timberlake SC, Vigneault F, Kleinstein SH. Hierarchical clustering can identify B cell clones with high confidence in ig repertoire sequencing data. *J Immunol* (2017) 198:2489–99. doi:10.4049/jimmunol.1601850
5. Boyd SD, Marshall EL, Merker JD, Maniar JM, Zhang LN, Sahaf B, et al. Measurement and clinical monitoring of human lymphocyte clonality by massively parallel VDJ pyrosequencing. *Sci Transl Med* (2009) 1:12ra23. doi:10.1126/scitranslmed.3000540
6. Stern JN, Yaari G, Vander Heiden JA, Church G, Donahue WF, Hintzen RQ, et al. B cells populating the multiple sclerosis brain mature in the draining cervical lymph nodes. *Sci Transl Med* (2014) 6:248ra107. doi:10.1126/scitranslmed.3008879
7. Tsioris K, Gupta NT, Ogunniyi AO, Zimnisky RM, Qian F, Yao Y, et al. Neutralizing antibodies against West Nile virus identified directly from human B cells by single-cell analysis and next generation sequencing. *Integr Biol (Camb)* (2015) 7:1587–97. doi:10.1039/c5ib00169b
8. Jiang N, He J, Weinstein JA, Penland L, Sasaki S, He X-S, et al. Lineage structure of the human antibody repertoire in response to influenza vaccination. *Sci Transl Med* (2013) 5:171ra19. doi:10.1126/scitranslmed.3004794
9. Glanville J, Kuo TC, von Büdingen H-C, Guey L, Berka J, Sundar PD, et al. Naive antibody gene-segment frequencies are heritable and unaltered by chronic lymphocyte ablation. *Proc Natl Acad Sci U S A* (2011) 108:20066–71. doi:10.1073/pnas.1107498108
10. Parameswaran P, Liu Y, Roskin KM, Jackson KK, Dixit VP, Lee J-Y, et al. Convergent antibody signatures in human dengue. *Cell Host Microbe* (2013) 13:691–700. doi:10.1016/j.chom.2013.05.008
11. Vollmers C, Sit RV, Weinstein JA, Dekker CL, Quake SR. Genetic measurement of memory b-cell recall using antibody repertoire sequencing. *Proc Natl Acad Sci U S A* (2013) 110:13463–8. doi:10.1073/pnas.1312146110
12. DeKosky BJ, Kojima T, Rodin A, Charab W, Ippolito GC, Ellington AD, et al. In-depth determination and analysis of the human paired heavy- and light-chain antibody repertoire. *Nat Med* (2015) 21:86. doi:10.1038/nm.3743
13. Macosko EZ, Basu A, Satija R, Nemesh J, Shekhar K, Goldman M, et al. Highly parallel genome-wide expression profiling of individual cells using nanoliter droplets. *Cell* (2015) 161:1202–14. doi:10.1016/j.cell.2015.05.002
14. Briggs AW, Goldfless SJ, Timberlake S, Belmont BJ, Clouser CR, Koppstein D, et al. Tumor-infiltrating immune repertoires captured by single-cell barcoding in emulsion. *bioRxiv* (2017) 134841. doi:10.1101/134841

# 7

# Stochastically Timed Competition Between Division and Differentiation Fates Regulates the Transition From B Lymphoblast to Plasma Cell

*Jie H. S. Zhou* [1,2], *John F. Markham* [1,3†], *Ken R. Duffy* [4‡] *and Philip D. Hodgkin* [1,2*‡]

[1] *Immunology Division, The Walter and Eliza Hall Institute of Medical Research, Parkville, VIC, Australia,* [2] *Department of Medical Biology, The University of Melbourne, Parkville, VIC, Australia,* [3] *Victoria Research Laboratory, National ICT Australia, The University of Melbourne, Parkville, VIC, Australia,* [4] *Hamilton Institute, Maynooth University, Maynooth, Ireland*

***Correspondence:**
*Philip D. Hodgkin*
*hodgkin@wehi.edu.au*

**†Present Address:**
*John F. Markham,*
*Peter MacCallum Cancer Centre,*
*Parkville, VIC, Australia*

*‡These authors have contributed equally to this work*

In response to external stimuli, naïve B cells proliferate and take on a range of fates important for immunity. How their fate is determined is a topic of much recent research, with candidates including asymmetric cell division, lineage priming, stochastic assignment, and microenvironment instruction. Here we manipulate the generation of plasmablasts from B lymphocytes *in vitro* by varying CD40 stimulation strength to determine its influence on potential sources of fate control. Using long-term live cell imaging, we directly measure times to differentiate, divide, and die of hundreds of pairs of sibling cells. These data reveal that while the allocation of fates is significantly altered by signal strength, the proportion of siblings identified with asymmetric fates is unchanged. In contrast, we find that plasmablast generation is enhanced by slowing times to divide, which is consistent with a hypothesis of competing timed stochastic fate outcomes. We conclude that this mechanistically simple source of alternative fate regulation is important, and that useful quantitative models of signal integration can be developed based on its principles.

**Keywords: B cells, anti-CD40 stimulation titration, fate regulation, lineage priming, competing stochastic timers**

## INTRODUCTION

Increased understanding of the regulation of cell differentiation, division and death is crucial in many fields of biology (1–5). While population-level consistency in the proportion of cells taking on distinct fates has long-since been observed, advancing technologies that enable direct observations of individual cells and their lineages reveal significant heterogeneity (6–14). In order to manipulate population-level fate allocation, determining the primary drivers of this cell-level heterogeneity is an essential precursor to designing interventions, and so the search for the sources of heterogeneity has been a topic of much recent research.

B lymphocytes are an essential component of the immune response and provide a useful model for assessing methods of fate control. During activation, they integrate signals from multiple sources that modify the resulting cell response by altering lifespan, the type of antibody made, the speed of cell proliferation, and the rate of development into antibody secreting plasma cells (15).

T cells provide one important source of signals that influence the B cell (16, 17). During an immune response, antigen captured by the B cell is presented to reactive T cells that are, in turn, induced to express CD40L on their surface. This ligand engages the constitutively expressed receptor CD40 found on the B cell surface. CD40 stimulation alone can activate and promote B cell proliferation, but its impact is amplified by T cell derived cytokines, such as IL-4 and IL-5, that further shape fate changes including isotype switching and the rate of development into Antibody Secreting Cells (ASCs) (18). Importantly for quantitative studies, a CD40 agonist and cytokines can replace the T cell, making it an excellent model system for studying the impact of variations in signals on fate outcomes *in vitro*.

Activated lymphocytes vary in the times they take to divide and, in culture, are usually found spread across multiple generations. Notwithstanding that, numerous studies report that the greater the number of divisions cells have experienced, the more likely they are to have undergone a change, regardless of time from stimulation. For example, isotype switching is linked to division, and is influenced by the concentration of switch-inducing cytokines (19–21). Similarly, the development into ASC also has been reported to be promoted by progressive passage through division cycles, and this likelihood, in turn, is modulated by the concentration of cytokine delivered signals (18, 22). These studies proposed that alternative division-linked cell changes, such as switching and development to ASC, could arise as the combination of a series of independent fate decisions underway in each cell (18, 20, 23–25).

This hypothesis of independent fate competition was evaluated and extended upon by Duffy et al. (26), by assessing data taken from experiments where individual B cells that had undergone given numbers of divisions, as determined by CTV staining, were sorted by flow cytometry and subsequently followed with long-term imaging. Once these cells were observed to divide, their sibling offspring were examined with times to divide, to die, to differentiate to ASC, and to antibody isotype-switch from last mitosis recorded. Probabilistic analysis established that the complex array of heterogeneous fate outcomes and times to fates were consistent with a simple hypothesis where, within each single cell, times to each fate (isotype switching, differentiation, death, and division) were selected independently from a probability distribution and behaved in competition with each other, such that short times to fate censor later fate outcomes (26). Sibling fates, however, had significantly greater commonality than unrelated cells of the same generation, indicating a substantial element of familial lineage priming.

As external regulators are known to influence the proportions of cells assuming fates at a population level, we reasoned that investigation of their impact at the single cell level would provide additional discriminating insight. Here we examine the cell-level impact of changing CD40 stimulation strength on ASC development. This analysis suggests that CD40 has no direct impact on differentiation rate or asymmetric fate changes, but exerts its influence by altering the time to divide distribution, thereby regulating the proportion of cells that differentiate as the result of alterations to the inherent cellular competition.

# MATERIALS AND METHODS

## Mice

Blimp-1-GFP reporter mice on a C57BL/6 background (22) were bred and maintained in specific pathogen free conditions at the Walter and Eliza Hall Institute (WEHI) animal facility according to institutional guidelines. All experiments were approved by the WEHI Animal Ethics Committee. Ten-week-old female reporter (Blimp-$1^{+/GFP}$) and wild type (Blimp-$1^{+/+}$) mice were used for the flow cytometry and filming experiments.

## Cell Isolation and Labeling

Naïve, resting B cells were isolated from murine spleens using a discrete Percoll (GE Healthcare, cat#17089101) density gradient (50/65/80%, cells collected from 65/80% interface), followed by purification using magnetic beads (negative selection, mouse B cell isolation kit, Miltenyi Biotech cat#130-090-862). Enriched cells were verified to be >98% B220$^+$ and CD19$^+$ by flow cytometry. Cells were labeled with CellTrace Violet (Invitrogen, cat#C34557) at 7.5 μM final concentration, with $10^7$ cells/mL in phosphate buffered saline containing 0.1% bovine serum albumin (PBS/0.1%BSA), and incubated in a 37°C water bath for 20 min. Cells were washed twice with cold culture medium prior to culture.

## Cell Culture

For flow cytometry and for bulk cultures, cells were cultured in "B cell medium," made from Advanced RPMI 1640 (Gibco cat#12633-012) supplemented with 5% fetal calf serum (Gibco, cat#10099-141, Australian origin), 10 mM HEPES (Gibco, cat#15630-130), 2 mM GlutaMAX (Gibco, cat#35050-061), 10 U/mL penicillin, 100 μg/mL streptomycin (Penicillin/Streptomycin, Gibco, cat#15140-148), and 50 μM 2-mercaptoethanol (2-ME, Sigma-Aldrich, cat#M7522). For filming, cells were cultured in phenol red-free Advanced RPMI 1640 (Gibco custom order) with the same supplements. Imaged cells were stimulated with 1,000 U/mL IL-4 (WEHI), and 10, 2.5, or 0.625 μg/mL anti-CD40 antibody (1C10, WEHI Antibody Facility), and incubated at 37°C with 5% $CO_2$. Differentiation promoting effects of IL-4 were saturating at concentrations above 316 U/ml [(18) and data not shown].

## Flow Cytometry

For flow cytometry experiments, 200 μL wells containing $10^4$ cells were cultured in triplicates across 96 well flat-bottomed plates. Blimp-$1^{+/GFP}$ and wild type cells stimulated with IL-4 and 10, 2.5, or 0.625 μg/mL of anti-CD40 antibody, or IL-4 alone were harvested periodically for flow cytometry analyses (BD FACSCantoII). Propidium iodide (PI, 0.5 μg/mL final, Sigma cat#287075) for dead cell exclusion and 5,000 beads (Sphero Rainbow Calibration particles [6 peaks] 6.0-6.4 μm, BD Biosciences, cat#556288) for cell counting were added just prior to sample acquisition.

## Cell Sorting and Long-Term Live Cell Imaging

For filming, 5 mL cultures ($2 \times 10^5$ cells/mL) of cells stimulated with IL-4 and 10, 2.5, or 0.625 μg/mL of anti-CD40 antibody were harvested 85 h after stimulation. Cells were labeled for expression of IgG1 (clone X56, BD Pharmingen cat#550874), and sorted (BD FACSAriaIIu), for generation four cells that were undifferentiated (Blimp-1-GFP$^-$) and unswitched (IgG1-APC$^-$), to ensure that cells with a similar starting phenotype were tracked and compared in each CD40 stimulation condition.

Sorted cells were re-cultured in phenol red-free B cell medium with the same stimuli concentrations as prior to the sort, at $5 \times 10^4$ cells/mL. For each of the three anti-CD40 conditions, 250 μL of cell suspension was placed into a separate well of a pre-prepared chamber slide (Ibidi, cat#80826) where each well was lined with a polymer imprinted with a microgrid array of cell "paddocks" (Microsurfaces, cat#MGA-050-02) (27). Microgrids were prepared aseptically, rinsed with 100% ethanol for sterilization, then left to dry completely to ensure adherence; before wetting again with ethanol such that B cell medium could be introduced to the hydrophobic grids. Chambers were rinsed 10 times with B cell medium, prior to resting overnight in an incubator to aid the dissolution of any air bubbles. Chambers and polydimethylsiloxane (PDMS) microgrids were exposed to 470 nm LEDs (custom made) for at least 30 min prior to the addition of cells, to photobleach the grids and reduce autofluorescence during imaging. The seeding cell density was determined to yield not more than an average of one cell per paddock for filming.

Microscopy images were acquired using a Zeiss Axiovert 200M widefield inverted microscope, equipped with an incubation chamber (37°C, 5% $CO_2$, humidifier), plan-apochromat 20x objective (0.8 n.a.), 0.63x c-mount, and a Zeiss AxioCam MRm (1.4 MP) camera. Fluorescence (GFP) and bright field images were acquired for 141 positions, at 15-min intervals, encompassing 7,896 paddocks for the three culture conditions, across 360 time points over the following 89.75 h. The remainder of the sorted cells were placed into triplicate or duplicate cultures in 96-well plates for a concurrent flow-cytometry time course of events, and were run twice-daily for the duration of the filming experiment as a parallel control.

## Single Cell Fates Were Manually Tracked With Visual Cues and Fluorescence Thresholding

For consistent tracking of imaged cells, fluorescence images were first processed using the pipeline reported by Duffy et al. (26). All images from the GFP channel were corrected for uneven illumination of the microscopy stage, thresholded for fluorescence, and binarized to produce an objective indicator of GFP positivity. The image processing method is automatic, and threshold values were computed relative to background illumination using intensity histograms for each image. Resultant images were cropped into individual paddocks, and the processed GFP, unthresholded GFP, and bright field images with GFP overlay for each paddock were concatenated for ease of viewing and stacked into time-lapse films.

Paddocks with individual, undifferentiated cells were identified, and those observed to divide were followed to record the fates of paired offspring. Bright field images were used to manually track cells using their location, size, shape, granularity and trajectory. These properties allowed for the reliable identification of division, as well as death. Shortly before division, cells appeared to lose adhesion and formed large spheres, before cleaving into two smaller cells that do not immediately produce pseudopodia. For death, cells sharply increased in granularity and the circumference of the membrane appeared ruffled, likely due to blebbing, several frames before cell fragmentation was observed, or the membrane perforated and the cell swelled from osmotic intake. This first change in texture was recorded as the cell death time.

For identifying differentiation to ASC, thresholded and binarized images in the GFP channel were followed as a reporter for Blimp-1 expression. Dim light settings are required for extended imaging to avoid phototoxicity, hence chosen voltage and exposure settings also allowed some noise to be detected above the low threshold, from the autofluorescence of the cells and grids. Consequently, differentiation times were only recorded when the cell's fluorescence remained above threshold for three or more consecutive frames (45 min), and then did not disappear for more than one frame at a time; GFP expression would later brighten and cover a larger area. Unthresholded images from the GFP channel were referenced for noise exclusion, and also used for cell identification and tracking based on differentiation status and level of fluorescence.

Sister cells fates were tracked until they either divided again or died. Some cells survived until the end of filming, or were lost due to falling out of focus, migration away from their paddock, or failure to maintain cell ID—these times were also recorded. Homotypic adhesion prevented the tracking of four or more cells using this experimental design.

## Statistical Analysis

Data was processed in Matlab 2017b by custom software utilizing in-built functionality. Pearson's correlation coefficient was evaluated using `corr`, and the reported confidence intervals (CIs) were determined by Fisher's Transformation. We used Yule's Q, a traditional measure of association between pairs of variables, to quantify association between division and death or differentiation and no differentiation. Its asymmetric CIs were determined from a normal approximation to errors in the logarithm of the Odds Ratio. Non-parametric survival function (i.e., Kaplan-Meier) estimates were made using the censoring option of the in-built function `ecdf`.

## Parametric Model Fitting Procedure

Custom software utilizing the Optimization Toolbox in Matlab 2017b was used for model fitting. The uncensored distributions were assumed to lie in the class of log-normal distributions. For all stimulation conditions, there was a single log-normal time to death $T_{death}$ parameterized by a mean $\mu_{death}$ and covariance $\sigma^2_{death}$. For all stimulation conditions, there was a probability, $p_{diff}$, that the differentiation process is active in the cell whereupon it occurs at a log-normally distributed time with parameters $\mu_{diff}$ and $\sigma^2_{diff}$. If the process was not on, then the differentiation time was set to be $+\infty$. For each of the three concentrations of 1C10 (0.625, 2.5 and 10 μg/mL), labeled j in (1, 2, 3), it was assumed there was a distinct probability, $p^j_{div}$, that the division process is active in the cell whereupon it occurs at a concentration-dependent log-normally distributed time with parameters $\mu^j_{div}$ and $\sigma^{2,j}_{div}$. If division was not active, the time was set to be $+\infty$.

For $\theta = (\mu_{death}, \sigma^2_{death}, p_{diff}, \mu_{diff}, \sigma^2_{diff}, p^1_{div}, \mu^1_{div}, \sigma^{2,1}_{div}, p^2_{div}, \mu^2_{div}, \sigma^{2,2}_{div}, p^3_{div}, \mu^3_{div}, \sigma^{2,3}_{div})$, a function was written that numerically calculates the likelihood of generating a data point $d \in D$ given that parameterization. For example, if a time-lapse frame is taken every h units of time, for a data point $d \in D$ in which a cell in stimulation condition j is observed to differentiate in the frame number $f_{diff}$ and undergo death in the frame number $f_{death}$, the likelihood of generating that data point d given the model parameterization $\theta$ is

$$L(d|\theta) = P(f_{diff} \leq T_{diff}/h < f_{diff} + 1)P(f_{death} \leq T_{death}/h < f_{death} + 1)P(T^j_{div.}/h > f_{death.}),$$

where the cumulative distribution functions were evaluated using Matlab's `logncdf`. For a set D composed of the fates of stochastically independent cells, the likelihood of generating the set is the product of the likelihoods of generating each point in the data

$$L(D|\theta) := \Pi_{d \in D} L(d|\theta).$$

We used Matlab 2017b's Optimization Toolbox function `fmincon` to identify the maximum likelihood model parameters $\theta$ that would generate the data:

$$\theta_{MAP} := \text{argsup}_\theta L(D|\theta).$$

As sibling cells have correlated times to fate, they are not independent and so the function given above does not describe their likelihoods. Despite that, assuming symmetry in the joint underlying distribution of times to each fate of siblings, the maximum likelihood marginal parameters are obtained by optimizing over the same objective function given above computed on all data, including siblings.

## Reshaped Distributions

Competition and censorship alters the underlying distributions of times to differentiation, division and death into those that are observed. For example, the observed marginal probability density function for division under stimulation condition j is related to the uncensored distributions for division and death through the following equation:

$$dP(T^{obs,j}_{div} \leq t)/dt = dP(T^j_{div} \leq t)/dtP(T_{death} > t) \Big/ \int dP(T^j_{div} \leq s)P(T_{death} > s),$$

which differs from the uncensored density of $T^j_{div}$. Similar expressions hold for $T^{obs,j}_{diff}$ and $T^{obs,j}_{death}$. Rather than perform numerical integrals to evaluate these, a Monte Carlo approach was taken where $10^6$ samples were drawn from the uncensored distributions parameterized by $\theta_{MAP}$, censoring rules were applied to the sampled values, and the resulting empirical distribution functions and densities of the observed variables were determined.

# RESULTS

## Population-Level Generation-Based Rate of Differentiation Is Increased by Weak CD40 Stimulation

To determine the effect of modulating CD40 signal strength, we utilized B cells from Blimp-1-GFP reporter mice to indicate expression of the ASC differentiation program within plasmablasts. In this system, cells expressing GFP secrete Ig at high efficiency (22). Purified resting naïve B cells from reporter mice were labeled with CellTrace Violet (CTV), and equal numbers of cells were placed in culture with varying concentrations of anti-CD40 agonist antibody (clone 1C10) (28) and saturating IL-4 (500 U/mL), and harvested over time (**Figures S1, 1**). As expected, increasing concentrations of CD40 led to greater cell numbers and increased progression through consecutive generations (**Figures S1A,B**). Furthermore, division-linked effects on ASC development were apparent as a greater proportion of cells produced Blimp-1-GFP in the advanced generations (**Figures 1C,D**), consistent with published findings (18). These data also confirmed the observation of Hawkins et al. (29) that lower CD40 stimulation levels resulted in a greater proportion of ASC per generation when compared to equivalent generations in cultures with high CD40 stimulation (**Figures 1C,D**). An increased rate of differentiation was also measurable in the population as a whole (**Figure 1C**). Thus, modulating CD40 stimulation strength has two distinct effects on the B cell response: high concentrations promote increased proliferation, whilst low concentrations increase the rate of observed differentiation events per generation. To identify the mechanism that alters cell differentiation by changes in stimulation strength, we undertook direct observation by live imaging.

## Long-Term Imaging Allocates Fate Assignments for Single Cells

B lymphoblasts stimulated by CpG can be tracked individually through multiple cell generations (30, 31). In contrast, observing differentiation by live imaging following CD40 stimulation is challenging due to homotypic adhesion. The development of cell aggregates restricts tracking of individual progenitor cells for more than one or two generations (30). A new method was introduced in Duffy et al. (32) to circumvent this problem. By harvesting and disaggregating CTV labeled, proliferating B cells after a few days in culture, then seeding sorted, individual cells into microgrids to maintain segregation,

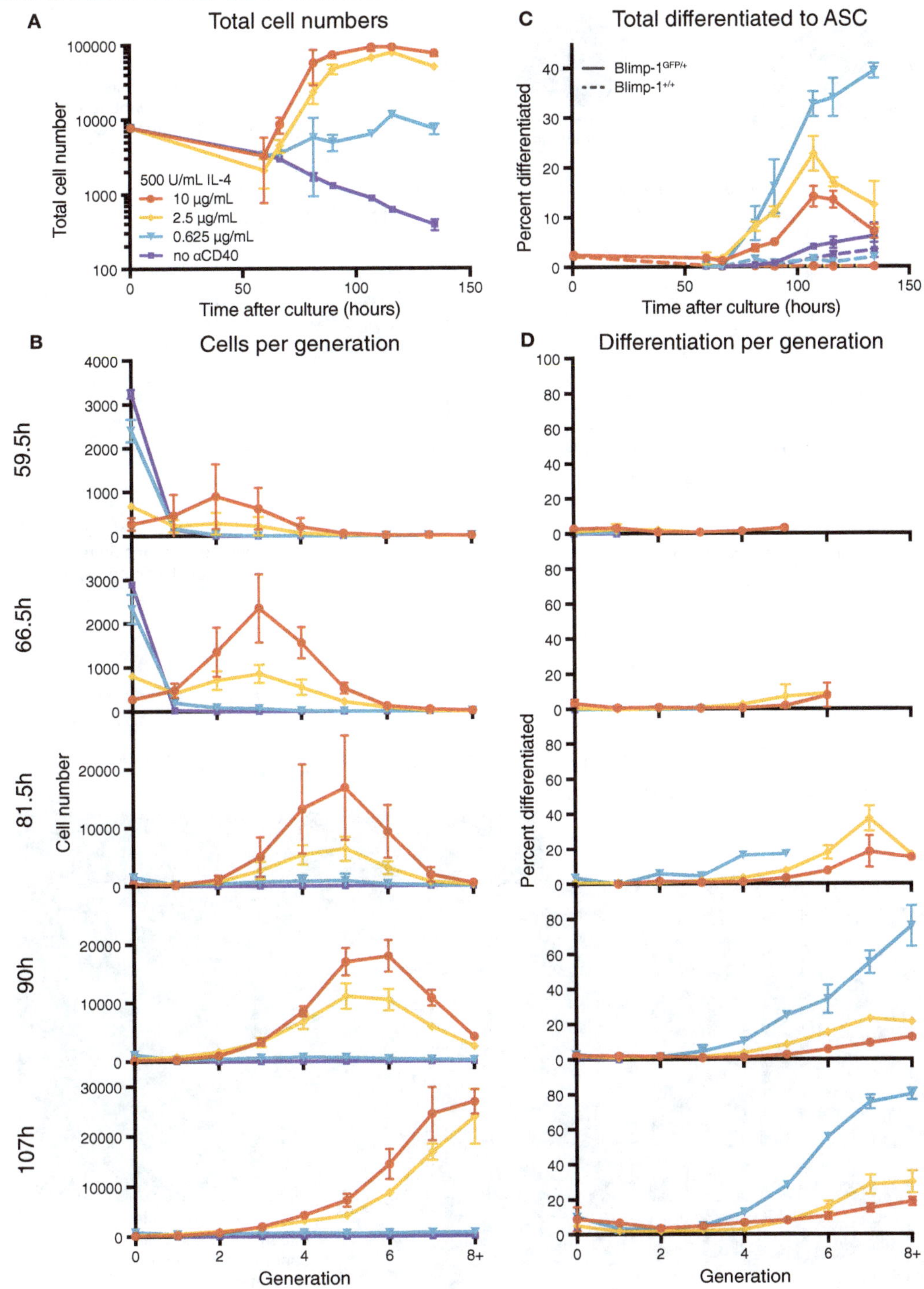


**FIGURE 1 |** Anti-CD40 concentration alters division and differentiation rates. CTV labeled resting Blimp-1$^{gfp/+}$ B cells were cultured in 500 U/mL IL-4 and 10, 2.5, 0.625, or 0 µg/mL anti-CD40 and harvested over time for flow cytometry analysis. **(A)** Total cell numbers over time. **(B)** Total cells found in each generation. **(C)** The proportion of total viable cells also GFP$^+$ (ASC). Dashed lines are from equivalent wild-type control cells used to set GFP gates. **(D)** The proportion of cells in each generation that were GFP$^+$. Data points are mean of triplicate cultures ± SEM, and representative of several repeated titration experiments.

(27) cells from different generations were observed to divide and their progeny followed until their next fate (32). Here we adapted this protocol, illustrated in **Figure 2**, to observe the effect of CD40 stimulation strength changes on differentiation and division times, as well as concordance in sibling fates.

In initial bulk cultures CTV labeled Blimp-1-GFP reporter B cells were incubated with IL-4 and varying concentrations of

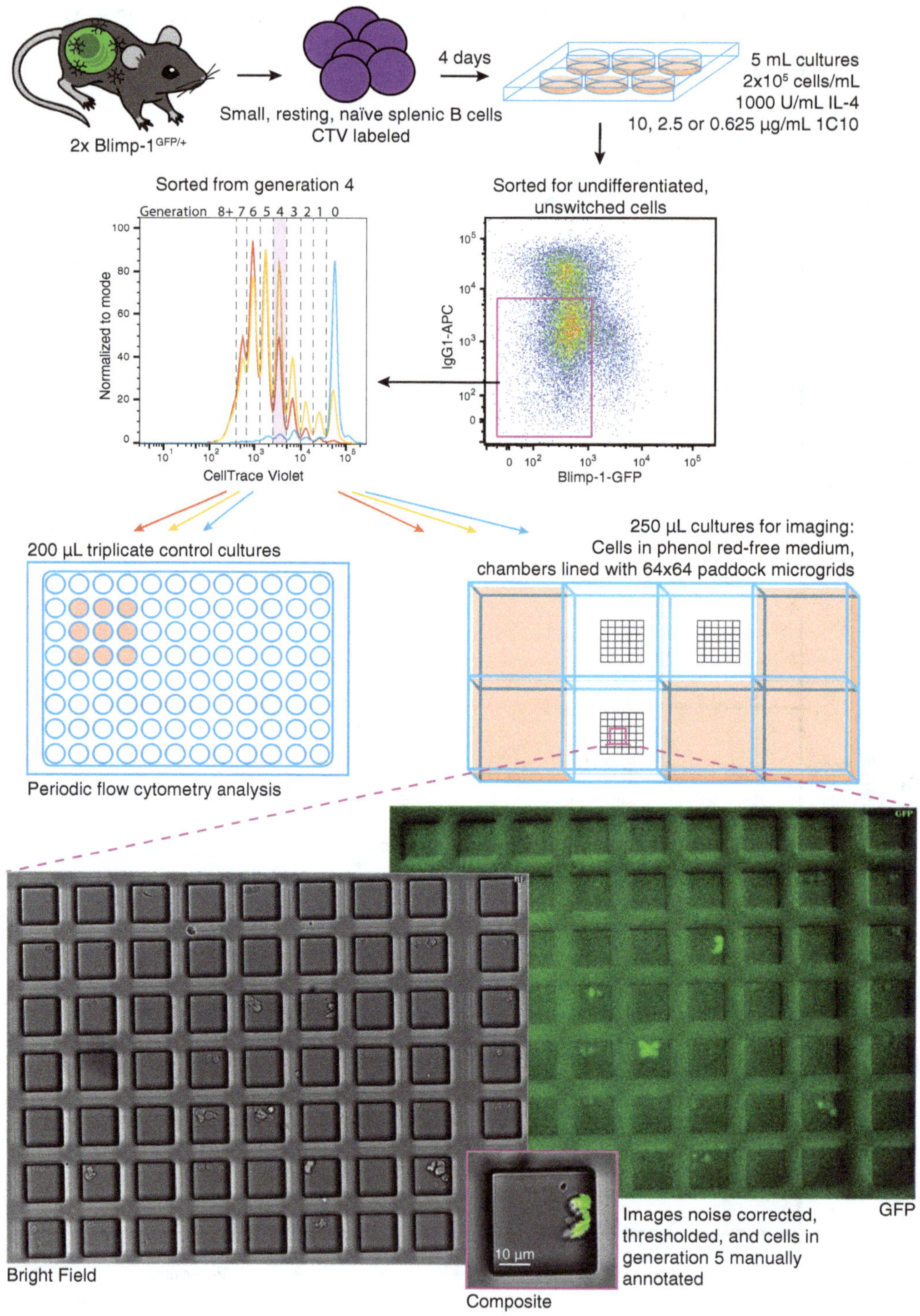


**FIGURE 2 |** Schematic of live cell imaging experiment. CTV labeled Blimp-1$^{gfp/+}$ B cells were incubated in two stages. Upper panels indicate the initial bulk culture at multiple anti-CD40 concentrations. After 85 h, cells were harvested, labeled with anti-IgG1, and unswitched, GFP$^{-}$ cells identified and sorted from generation 4. Cells were returned to stimulation conditions identical to that prior to sorting, and a portion plated into control cultures for flow cytometry. For microscopy, phenol red-free media was used, and cells from each culture condition were placed into a separate chamber of an imaging slide, each lined with a microgrid of 50 µM cell paddocks. Once settled, the cell density was such that, on average one cell would randomly deposit within one paddock. Media containing pH indicator was placed in surrounding wells to buffer for evaporation and monitor CO$^{2}$ availability. Micrograds were tiled and imaged at 15 min intervals for 89.75 h. Acquired bright field and fluorescence images were processed and manually annotated to record cell fate.

anti-CD40 (10, 2.5, 0.625, and 0 μg/ml) for 4 days, resulting in the expected variation in division and differentiation rates (**Figure S1A**). To compare the subsequent fate of undifferentiated cells from the same generation, cells from each culture were sorted by flow cytometry for those in generation 4, and seeded into 250 μL chambers containing microgrids for a further 90 h of live cell imaging (see Materials and Methods). Control cell cultures were prepared in parallel at the same density in 96 well plates, and triplicate 200 μL cultures were analyzed periodically to ensure the overall population response of the sorted cells was consistent (**Figure S2**). Control analyses indicated that sorted cells were $GFP^-$ and in generation 4 at the time they were re-cultured (**Figure S2B**). These cultures also confirmed that cells stimulated with higher concentrations of anti-CD40 divided faster, resulting in greater CTV dye dilution (**Figure S2B**), and higher total cell numbers (**Figure S2C**). Despite the variation in progression through generations, a greater proportion of cells in 2.5 μg/mL anti-CD40 were $GFP^+$ than in 10 μg/mL (**Figure S2D**). As these proliferation and differentiation features were consistent with earlier studies, manual tracking and analysis of the parallel single cell imaged cultures were undertaken.

## Single Cell Data Recapitulated Fate Changes Seen at Population Level

Acquired images were processed and thresholded to facilitate GFP scoring, as described in Methods and illustrated in **Figure 3A**. After initial visual inspection, "paddocks" identified with single cells that undertook their first division as $GFP^-$ cells were selected, and the resulting two siblings followed manually, to record their times to changes in fates (**Figure 3**). For the data presented here, the time of the cell's first division (therefore from generation 4 to 5) is set as time 0, the initiating event time, and the siblings being tracked are in generation 5. The complete annotated data set was converted to such times by calculating the times between the first observed division and subsequent fates (differentiation to ASC, division or death). Histograms of these times are plotted in **Figure 3B**, illustrating the heterogeneity in each outcome.

To visualize differences between culture conditions, observed proportions to undergo each fate are shown in **Figure 4A**, and mean times to reach each fate in **Figure 4B**. These data suggest that cells stimulated with high concentrations of anti-CD40 were more likely to divide and less likely to die (**Figure 4A**), and when they did divide they completed mitosis more quickly (**Figure 4B**) The proportion of cells observed to differentiate is also consistent with flow cytometry time courses, in that a higher proportion of cells differentiated to ASC with lower CD40 stimulation (**Figure 4A**). Thus, despite segregation into cell paddocks by the microgrids, the filmed cells recapitulated the fate outcomes measured by flow cytometry at the population level.

## Stimulation Strength Does Not Affect Sibling Correlations or Concordance

Whether stimulation strength affected differentiation by influencing asymmetry in fate was first assessed. For each of the three concentrations (0.625, 2.5, and 10 μg/mL, respectively) 78, 68 and 75% (±8, 9, 8% as 95% CIs) of siblings take the same differentiation or no differentiation and death or division fates. **Figure 4C** plots Yule's Q, a measure of concordance for opposing fates (division vs. death, and differentiation vs. no differentiation) relative to their frequency of occurrence in the population. The consistent, high values of Q indicate the significant concordance found for both division-death and differentiation-no differentiation fates of siblings was not affected by CD40 stimulation strength. Thus, strong sibling concordances and correlations were found in this experiment, in line with earlier findings. Interestingly, these sibling similarities did not appear to be controlled by altered CD40 stimulation strengths, despite the marked changes in division times, and differentiation rates.

## Uncensoring Cell Fate Time Distributions

Having eliminated modulation of asymmetric fates as a control feature regulated by anti-CD40 concentration, we turned to the theory of competing fates as a potential driver of heterogeneity. Under this hypothesis, autonomous processes leading to each fate are underway within the cell. The order in which they complete determines the fate that the cell is observed to take. As observed times to fate are heterogeneous, the mathematical framework of probability is necessary to describe them. It encapsulates the heterogeneity irrespective of whether its source is truly stochastic processes within each single cell, or arises as a result of unidentified heterogeneous lineage properties. The hypothesis suggests that the apparently complex correlation structures observed in cell fate data are a consequence of observed times to fate being the product of competition and censorship, and leads one to query the role of external regulation on each of the autonomous processes (26, 32).

**Figures 4D,E** shows the result of applying the standard non-parametric survival function estimator, the Kaplan-Meier estimator (33), to the raw cumulative frequency data for each fate (**Figure 4D**) to reveal the pre-competition, uncensored time-to-fate distributions (**Figure 4E**), assuming probabilistic independence of these underlying timed mechanisms. For these plots division is assumed to censor death, death censor division, and both division and death censor differentiation. In some instances, the remaining proportion is >0 (i.e., plot does not reach a height of 1), indicating the observation time was too short to capture all possible events in this category; or alternatively that the remaining proportion of cells were incapable of undergoing that fate.

Within this competing timers model, these results are consistent with the hypothesis that CD40 stimulation strength had a significant impact on cell division times with little direct effect on the underlying distributions of times to death or differentiation. Higher levels of anti-CD40 reduces division times, positively impacting the proportion of cells in the population that progress to the next generation, while reducing the proportion of cells that differentiate. Together, these results are consistent with the hypothesis that CD40 stimulation controls the time to divide, but not the times to differentiate or die.

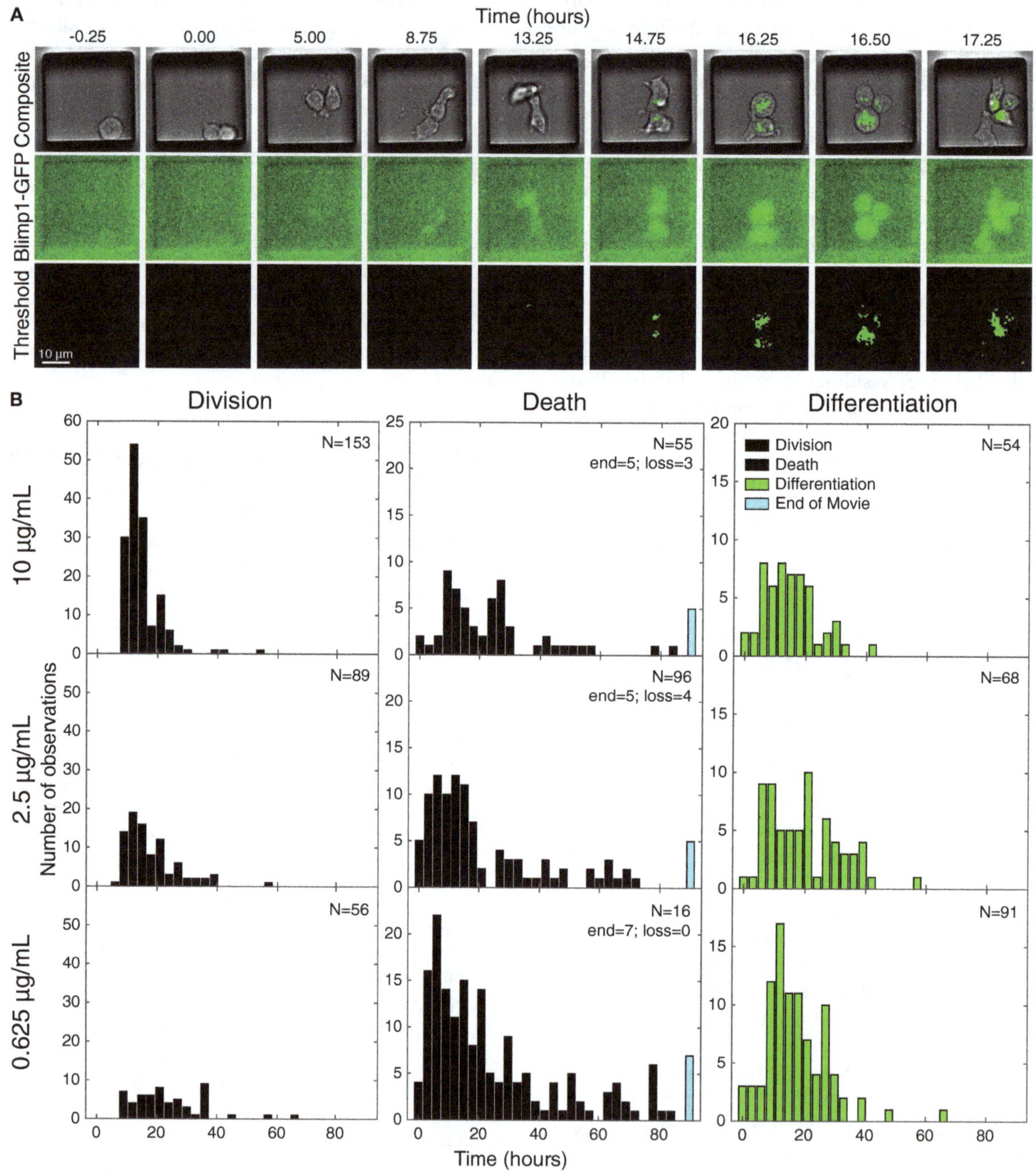


**FIGURE 3 |** Tracking individual cell fates over time. **(A)** Example microscopy images from one cell paddock, with selected frames from the bright field and GFP channels over time. Sorted cells (generation 4) observed to divide (generation 5) and, if still GFP$^{-}$, were tracked further to record subsequent division, death, and differentiation times. The initial mitotic event was assigned time = 0 in subsequent analyses. Division and death were visually discernible in the bright field channel (top row). Fluorescence images in the GFP channel (middle row) were corrected for uneven illumination, thresholded, and binarized for annotating differentiation to ASC (bottom row). **(B)** Histograms of the total data for each fate recorded, timed from first observed cell division and allocated to 3 h bins. Number of recorded cells indicated in panels (*N*). Cells that reached the end of the imaging period and had neither divided nor died were recorded as "end" and appear in the blue bar. Number of lost cells also indicated.

## Parametric Model Based on Competition and Changes in Division Time Only

Under the stochastic competition hypothesis, not all processes need to be in operation in every cell. In particular, there is a possibility that neither differentiation nor division partake in the competition. To extract these propensities to differentiate and divide (i.e., likelihood that the underlying division or differentiation machinery is active within a cell), we created a

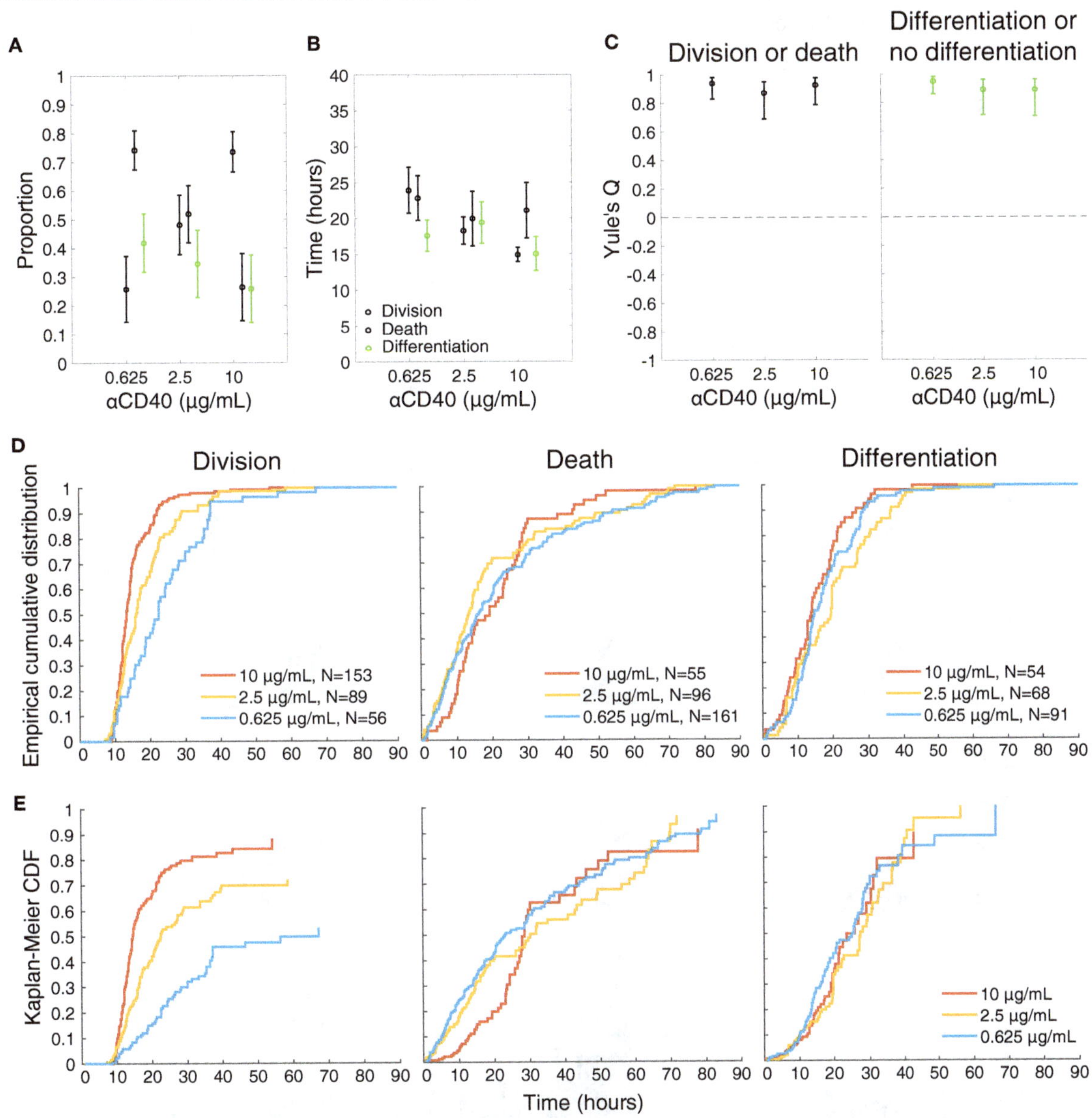


**FIGURE 4 |** Features of single cell imaged data. **(A)** The proportion of tracked single cells that underwent each fate. Fisher's exact test was performed to compare proportions of cells to undergo fates between 0.625 vs. 2.5, 0.625 vs. 10, 2.5 vs. 10 μg/mL anti-CD40. Division vs. death: $p = 4.18 \times 10^{-6}$, $1.77 \times 10^{-23}$, and $3.01 \times 10^{-7}$, respectively. Differentiation vs. no-differentiation: $p = 0.15$, 0.0007, and 0.078, respectively. **(B)** For cells reaching each fate the average time is shown with 95% CIs. Kruskal-Wallis test was performed to compare the times to fates between different anti-CD40 concentrations. Division: $p = 3.8741 \times 10^{-8}$, death: $p = 0.2386$ and differentiation: $p = 0.1354$. **(C)** Yule's Q, a measure of concordance in fate, shows that sibling fate selection (death or division, differentiation or no differentiation) is highly symmetric at all anti-CD40 stimulation levels with 95% CIs indicated by bars. **(D)** Cumulative frequency distributions of raw data for time to each fate. **(E)** Uncensored times to fate as determined by Kaplan-Meier survival function estimates overlaid for each anti-CD40 concentration. Division was uncensored from the influence of death, death was uncensored from division, and differentiation was uncensored from both division and death. Data from all tracked cells are included.

parametric statistical model by assuming that underlying time-to-fate distributions are log-normal given fate is in operation, but with a possibility that differentiation and division are inactive (discussed in Materials and Methods). Based on the observations from application of the Kaplan-Meier estimator, we assumed that the uncensored differentiation and death distributions were unchanging with stimulus and that only the division distribution and the propensity to divide were altered. This resulted in a single three-parameter description for differentiation (mean, variance, propensity to differentiate) and a two-parameter description for death (mean, variance) across all three stimulation conditions, along with a three-parameter description for division (mean, variance, propensity) per stimulation condition.

The uncensored lognormal curves with the highest likelihood of fitting to the data are shown in **Figure 5A** for comparison with the per-condition non-parametric uncensoring. The parametric

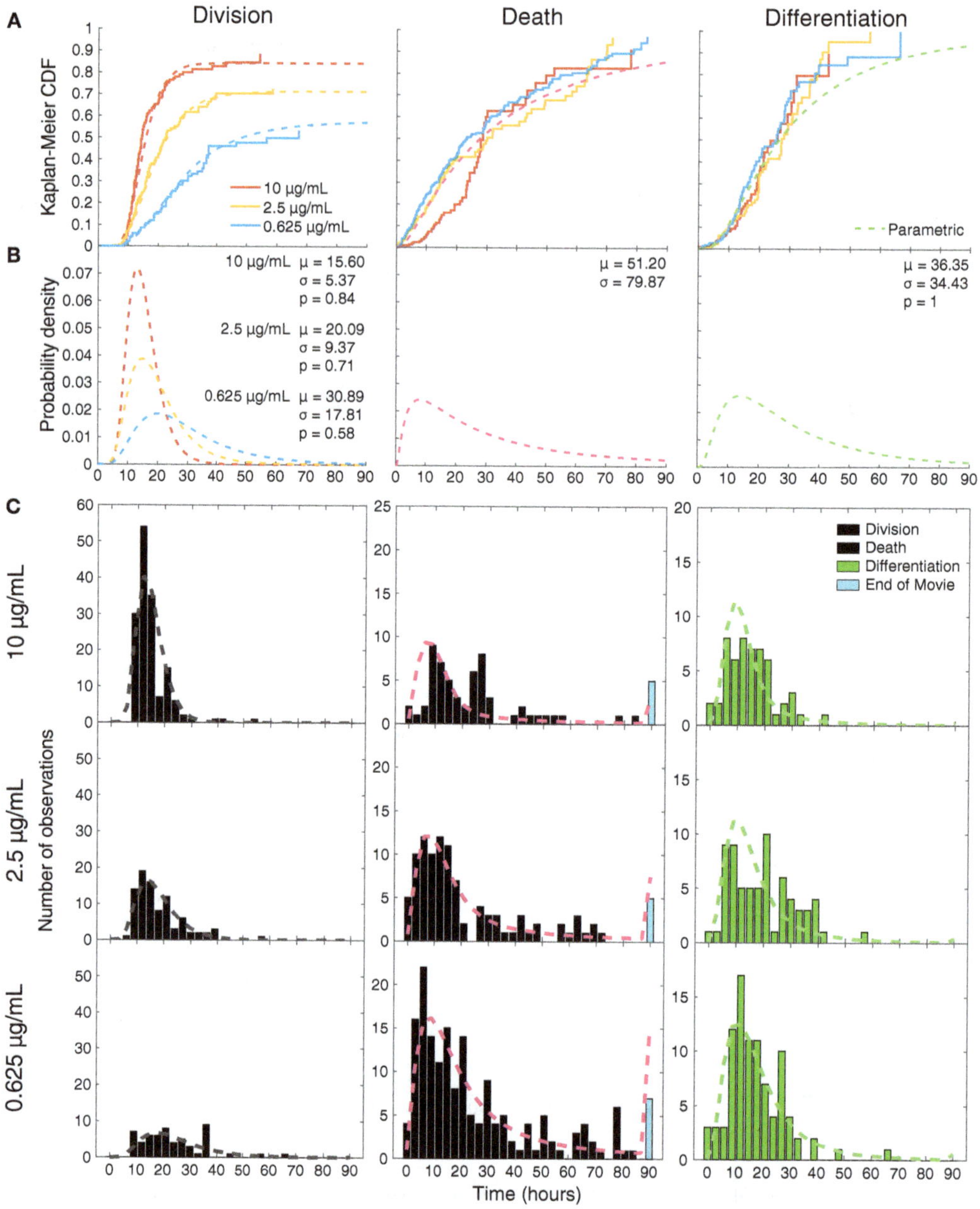


**FIGURE 5 |** Parametric model fitting with constrained parameters to censored data. **(A)** Maximum likelihood parametric model-fits to the data, under the constraints that death and differentiation time distributions were the same for all conditions, while the division time distribution and propensity for division could change with CD40 stimulation; overlaid with Kaplan-Meier analyses. **(B)** Uncensored parametric plots drawn as probability density functions; mean division times (μ) get longer with less CD40 stimulation, as variance (σ) increases and propensity (p) to divide decreases. **(C)** Predicted outcomes calculated from these constrained parametric distributions overlaid onto the observed data.

and non-parametric estimates are in good agreement, further supporting the hypotheses of the parametric model. Having ascribed lognormal curves to the probability distributions of times to fate, fitted parameters from different conditions could be compared for deviations in means, variations, and probabilities (**Figure 5B**). For decreasing anti-CD40 concentrations (10, 2.5, 0.625 μg/mL), the model fit division time distributions to the data with increasing mean (15.60, 20.09, 30.89 h) and variance (5.37, 9.37, 17.81 h), while the propensity for division being "on" in the cell decreased (0.84, 0.71, and 0.58, respectively). Death times (mean 51.20 h, variance 79.87 h) and differentiation times (mean 36.35 h, variance 34.43 h, propensity 1) were fitted with one distribution each for all of the CD40 stimulation concentrations, with the assumption that the probability of death is always ultimately 1. The best-fit propensity for differentiation was 1, suggesting that differentiation is always "on" in a

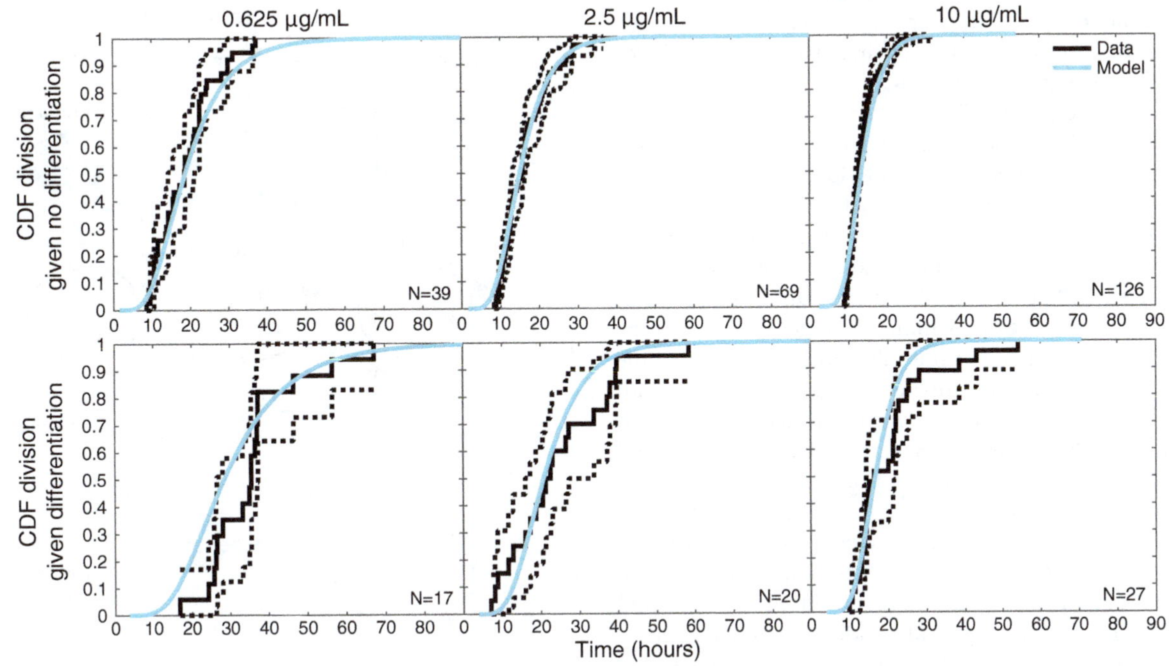


**FIGURE 6 |** Times to divide given differentiation or not. For each stimulation condition, upper panels display the empirical distribution of times to divide for cells that did not differentiate (solid black lines) with 95% confidence intervals (dotted black lines) computed with Greenwood's Formula. The lower panels display the same information for cells that were observed to differentiate before dividing. Also shown on both are the model-predicted distributions (cyan) of times to divide conditional on a cell differentiating or not, which differ as a consequence of the reshaping by competition.

stimulated cell and so is the default action that occurs when either division or death does not censor it. Overlaying the raw data, **Figure 5C** provides the extrapolation from these best-fit uncensored probability distribution functions to what they predict would be observed as a consequence of competition and censorship. The model predicts that a small proportion of cells will take their fate, typically death, after cessation of filming. A small number of cells are, indeed, observed to have neither died nor divided by the end of the microscopy session, and these are plotted at the end of the death-time histograms, according well with the out-of-sample model prediction.

## Further Features of the Data Consistent With Competition

**Figure 6** plots an additional interesting feature of the data that might appear to require an involved explanation. The upper panels display the empirical cumulative distribution of the times to divide of cells that did not differentiate for each stimulation condition, while the corresponding lower panels display the times to divide for cells that were observed to differentiate. For each condition, these two distributions are distinct, with division times being—on average—longer for cells that differentiated. The equivalent plots for times to death can be found in **Figure S3**, where the same phenomenon is exhibited.

Outside of the competition model, this seems to suggest distinct distributions for times to division or death fates dependent on whether a cell differentiates or not. Within the competition hypothesis, however, it is instead an intrinsic consequence of the model structure. Also displayed in the upper panel of **Figure 6** is the conditional distribution of the time to divide given that the cell did not differentiate as determined by the model, while the lower panel displays the model's conditional distribution of the time to divide given a cell did differentiate. Within the competition model, these two observed distributions are expected to be distinct as a consequence of censoring: knowing that a cell differentiates ensures a lower bound on the time to divide, conditioning it to be larger. Thus, the competition model inherently anticipates and accounts for these apparently involved features of the data within one mechanistically simple hypothesis that would otherwise require a model with significantly more parameters to explain.

# DISCUSSION

The B lymphocyte is an ideal model system for studying cell fate control, being highly tractable to *in vitro* manipulation and sensitive to many alternative receptor driven signals that alter its behavior. Here we adopted this system and sought an answer to how varying the strength of one significant signal, transmitted through CD40 on the B cell surface, could affect the rate of development to ASC. This question is of particular interest as earlier studies noted the effect to be "paradoxical": weaker stimulation leads to a greater rate of differentiation with each generation (29). Building on previous filming experiments (26, 30), chamber slides were used to sustain and image cells in varying levels of anti-CD40 stimulation. Miniature paddocks segregated the individual cells and reduced interference from homotypic adhesion (27). These data consisted of the recorded times to fates of hundreds of sibling pairs, making it suitable for quantitatively challenging hypotheses.

Analyzing these data allowed the elimination of the hypothesis that the paradoxical differentiation effect was due to changes in asymmetric cell division, as siblings had a high concordance in fate that was unaffected by stimulation strength. Our attention turned to ask whether the theory of competing fates (26, 32) could explain the phenomena. We hypothesized that increased differentiation could arise by cells transitioning faster within each generation, or by division times slowing, and thus allowing cells more time to differentiate before they divided again. Consistent with the latter hypothesis, the data, when uncensored, revealed that CD40 stimulation level regulated division times and division proportions, but had no effect on either differentiation or death times. Parametric fitting to differentiation times only required one set of parameters (mean, variance, propensity), whereas constraining division times to a single set of parameters would have produced poorly fitted outcomes. Hence, assuming independently timed control of fates, we were able to reject the hypothesis that CD40 stimulation was controlling either the proportions of cells capable of differentiating to ASC, or the time required for cells to differentiate. Instead, changes in division times were sufficient to re-create the differentiation patterns seen with flow cytometry.

This analysis supported the hypothesis that low CD40 stimulation slows division times, and consequently allows more time for cells to differentiate. Thus, regulation of division time by stimulation strength is identified as a controlling feature of fate decisions by the stimulated B cell. An influence of cell cycle length on differentiation has been noted in other cell systems suggesting this may be a biologically widespread regulatory mechanism (34, 35). We also assume the likelihood of differentiation is dependent on, and in turn altered by, the concentration of cytokines in culture. Further experiments will be required to assess this possibility.

These studies raise the question of how signals and internal molecular processes alter the time to different fates. One mechanism reported to date posits accumulation of transcriptional regulators. Kueh et al. (36) imaged hematopoietic progenitor cells and noted the choice between becoming a macrophage-lineage cell or a B cell was dependent upon the timed accumulation of transcriptional regulator PU.1. The longer cells took to divide, the more likely they were to accumulate the higher levels of PU.1 needed for macrophage commitment. A variant of this mechanism requiring both timed production and loss was noted by Heinzel et al. (37) for expression of Myc as a controller of division progression. Myc accumulated in proportion to signal strength and decayed at a constant rate, independently of division, eventually leading to a timed cessation of mitosis. As transcriptional regulators are important drivers for many fate changes, equivalent timed changes in expression level based on accumulation are likely

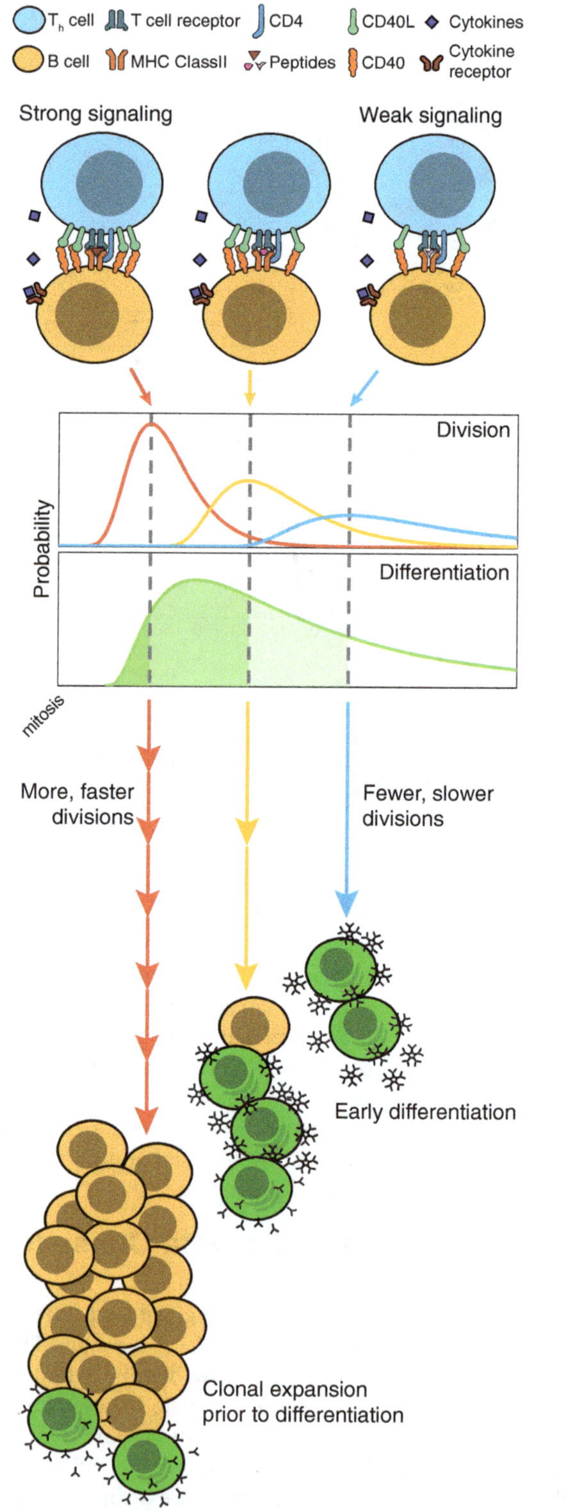


**FIGURE 7 |** Model of division-based control of B cell fate. Quantitative differences in CD40 signaling leads to proportional differences in division times, as well as the number of divisions completed. Even without modifications to underlying differentiation times, cell populations can differentiate as a result of competing cell fates. With slow divisions, the multitude of weakly stimulated

*(Continued)*

**FIGURE 7 |** cells automatically differentiate, and rapidly form large numbers of unswitched, low affinity antibody secreting cells. Meanwhile, those cells that receive strong stimulation divide rapidly, and hold back their differentiation mechanism until the clone has undergone expansion and isotype modifications, thus leading to an increased net number of higher affinity plasmablasts.

to be in operation in mature B cells. Further experiments measuring levels of transcriptional regulators and correlating levels with fate outcomes in individual cells will be informative to identify this and other putative molecular mechanisms (15).

These findings also offer insights into the controlling systems for antibody generation during a T-dependent immune response. T and B cell cooperation is an active process that occurs in two distinct sites during an immune response. Initial engagement occurs in the extrafollicular zones of lymphoid tissue and leads to the heterogeneous production of antibody secreting plasmablasts, that are typically short-lived and of weak to moderate affinity (38). Effective T and B cell collaboration requires an unbroken sequence of graded quantitative events that begins with antigen capture by the B cell receptor (BCR) and upregulation of T cell costimulatory surface molecules such as CD28, class II MHC and CD40 (39, 40). For effective stimulation by T cells, antigen must also be internalized by the B cell and presented on the cell surface, providing further opportunities for quantitative titration of the outcome (41). These variables in turn determine the level of stimulation received by an engaged T cell and subsequently the level of CD40L expression, and the rate of cytokine production provided to the B cell during the collaborative event (42). While the combinatorial possibilities are large, given the results here, we can identify a key principle in operation: even if holding all other variables constant, quantitative differences in CD40L, as the result of the chain of early events, will lead to proportional variations in average division times as well as the number of divisions completed (43). By slowing division, the weaker cells automatically assume a greater likelihood of differentiating and of dying. The more strongly stimulated cells will divide rapidly, automatically holding back their differentiation to ASC and leading to greater selection and expansion. Based on these findings we suggest that, as stimulated cells lose access to T cells, B cells slow division and automatically transition to secreting plasmablasts, provided cytokines are also present. Thus, the more avid and competent B cells are naturally selected for expansion while their differentiation is suppressed, leading, ultimately, to an increased net number of higher affinity plasmablasts overall (illustrated in **Figure 7**). This model is consistent with the studies of Paus et al. showing greater proliferation and overall generation of plasmablasts by higher affinity B cells (44). As antibody isotype switching is also strongly linked to progressive division and unaffected by the strength of CD40 stimulation (18, 19), this selection mechanism will, without additional cellular machinery, result in higher affinity clones that transition, automatically, to produce specialized antibody subtypes. It seems likely that the quantitative relation between all of these processes has evolved to provide an optimal balance for generating protective antibody over time.

An important second site of T-B cell collaboration is the germinal center. A subset of activated T and B cells migrate to primary follicles to initiate and sustain this reaction (45–47). At this site B cells undertake successive rounds of somatic hypermutation and selection that generates fully differentiated plasma cells and long-lived high affinity, memory B cells. Selection of B cell clones in the germinal center is critically dependent upon T cells and CD40-CD40L interactions (17, 48, 49). B lineage cells in the germinal center are distinct from those generated *in vitro*, and seen in extrafollicular sites (50). However, labeling studies *in vivo* have determined that the division rate is affected by the strength of stimulation provided by T cell help (51, 52). These observations taken together with the *in vitro* findings of the present paper, imply a general mechanism where the rate of proliferation is linked to, and tempers, the fate of competent, highly stimulated cells to achieve an optimal dynamic outcome with minimal direct control over differentiation.

## AUTHOR CONTRIBUTIONS

JZ, PH, and KD designed all experiments and analyzed and interpreted experiments and wrote manuscript. JZ performed experiments and undertook all data annotation. JM developed the data pipeline, conducted the image processing, and oversaw microscopy setup.

## ACKNOWLEDGMENTS

This work was supported by the National Health and Medical Research Council via Project Grants 1010654 and 1057831, and Program Grant 1054925, and fellowships to PH and Science Foundation Ireland grant No. 12IP1263 to KD. This work was made possible through Victorian State Government Operational Infrastructure Support and Australian Government NHMRC Independent Research Institutes Infrastructure Support Scheme Grant 361646. JZ was supported by an Australian Postgraduate Award. JM was supported by National ICT Australia (NICTA), which was funded by the Australian Research Council and the Australian Department of Broadband, Communications and the Digital Economy. We thank S. Nutt and A. Kallies for Blimp-1-GFP reporter mice.

## REFERENCES


1. Sun J, Ramos A, Chapman B, Johnnidis JB, Le L, Ho YJ, et al. Camargo: clonal dynamics of native haematopoiesis. *Nature* (2014) 514:322–7. doi: 10.1038/nature13824
2. Carulli AJ, Samuelson LCS. Schnell: unraveling intestinal stem cell behavior with models of crypt dynamics. *Integr Biol (Camb).* (2014) 6:243–57. doi: 10.1039/c3ib40163d
3. Livesey FJ, Cepko CL. Vertebrate neural cell-fate determination: lessons from the retina. *Nat Rev Neurosci.* (2001) 2:109–18. doi: 10.1038/35053522
4. Homem CC, Knoblich JA. Drosophila neuroblasts: a model for stem cell biology. *Development* (2012) 139:4297–310. doi: 10.1242/dev.080515
5. Tyson JJ, Novak B. Control of cell growth, division and death: information processing in living cells. *Interface Focus* (2014) 4:20130070. doi: 10.1098/rsfs.2013.0070
6. Naik SH, Perie L, Swart E, Gerlach C, van Rooij N, de Boer RJ, et al. Diverse and heritable lineage imprinting of early haematopoietic progenitors. *Nature* (2013) 496:229–32. doi: 10.1038/nature12013
7. Papalexi E, Satija R. Single-cell RNA sequencing to explore immune cell heterogeneity. *Nat Rev Immunol.* (2018) 18:35–45. doi: 10.1038/nri.2017.76
8. Altschuler SJ, Wu LF. Cellular heterogeneity: do differences make a difference? *Cell* (2010) 141:559–63. doi: 10.1016/j.cell.2010.04.033
9. Rodriguez-Fraticelli AE, Wolock SL, Weinreb CS, Panero R, Patel SH, Jankovic M, et al. Camargo: clonal analysis of lineage fate in native haematopoiesis. *Nature* (2018) 553:212–216. doi: 10.1038/nature25168
10. Pei W, Feyerabend TB, Rossler J, Wang X, Postrach D, Busch K, et al. Polylox barcoding reveals haematopoietic stem cell fates realized *in vivo*. *Nature* (2017) 548:456–460. doi: 10.1038/nature23653
11. Paul F, Arkin Y, Giladi A, Jaitin DA, Kenigsberg E, Keren-Shaul H, et al. Transcriptional heterogeneity and lineage commitment in myeloid progenitors. (2016) *Cell* 164:325. doi: 10.1016/j.cell.2015.12.046
12. Perie L, Duffy KR, Kok L, de Boer RJ, Schumacher TN. The branching point in erythro-myeloid differentiation. *Cell* (2015) 163:1655–62. doi: 10.1016/j.cell.2015.11.059
13. Gerlach C, Rohr JC, Perie L, van Rooij N, van Heijst JW, Velds A, et al. Heterogeneous differentiation patterns of individual CD8$^+$ T cells. *Science* (2013) 340:635–9. doi: 10.1126/science.1235487
14. Buchholz VR, Flossdorf M, Hensel I, Kretschmer L, Weissbrich B, Graf P, et al. Disparate individual fates compose robust CD8$^+$ T cell immunity. *Science* (2013) 340:630–5. doi: 10.1126/science.1235454
15. Nutt SL, Hodgkin PD, Tarlinton DM, Corcoran LM. The generation of antibody-secreting plasma cells. *Nat Rev Immunol.* (2015) 15:160–71. doi: 10.1038/nri3795
16. Crotty S. A brief history of T cell help to B cells. *Nat Rev Immunol.* (2015) 15:185–9. doi: 10.1038/nri3803
17. Vinuesa CG, Linterman MA, Yu D, MacLennan IC. Follicular helper T cells. *Annu Rev Immunol.* (2016) 34:335–68. doi: 10.1146/annurev-immunol-041015-055605
18. Hasbold J, Corcoran LM, Tarlinton DM, Tangye SG, Hodgkin PD. Evidence from the generation of immunoglobulin G-secreting cells that stochastic mechanisms regulate lymphocyte differentiation. *Nat Immunol.* (2004) 5:55–63. doi: 10.1038/ni1016
19. Hodgkin PD, Lee JH, Lyons AB. B cell differentiation and isotype switching is related to division cycle number. *J Exp Med.* (1996) 184:277–81.
20. Deenick EK, Hasbold J, Hodgkin PD. Switching to IgG3, IgG2b, and IgA is division linked and independent, revealing a stochastic framework for describing differentiation. *J Immunol.* (1999) 163:4707–14.
21. Hasbold J, Lyons AB, Kehry MR, Hodgkin PD. Cell division number regulates IgG1 and IgE switching of B cells following stimulation by CD40 ligand and IL-4. *Eur J Immunol.* (1998) 28:1040–51. doi: 10.1002/(SICI)1521-4141(199803)28:03<1040::AID-IMMU1040>3.0.CO;2-9
22. Kallies A, Hasbold J, Tarlinton DM, Dietrich W, Corcoran LM, Hodgkin PD, et al. Plasma cell ontogeny defined by quantitative changes in blimp-1 expression. *J Exp Med.* (2004) 200:967–77. doi: 10.1084/jem.20040973
23. Hawkins ED, Turner ML, Dowling MR, van Gend C, Hodgkin PD. A model of immune regulation as a consequence of randomized lymphocyte division and death times. *Proc Natl Acad Sci USA.* (2007) 104:5032–7. doi: 10.1073/pnas.0700026104
24. Duffy KR, Subramanian VG. On the impact of correlation between collaterally consanguineous cells on lymphocyte population dynamics. *J Math Biol.* (2009) 59:255–85. doi: 10.1007/s00285-008-0231-x
25. Subramanian VG, Duffy KR, Turner ML, Hodgkin PD. Determining the expected variability of immune responses using the cyton model. *J Math Biol.* (2008) 56:861–92. doi: 10.1007/s00285-007-0142-2
26. Duffy KR, Wellard CJ, Markham JF, Zhou JH, Holmberg R, Hawkins ED, et al. Activation-induced B cell fates are selected by intracellular stochastic competition. *Science* (2012) 335:338–41. doi: 10.1126/science.1213230
27. Day D, Pham K, Ludford-Menting MJ, Oliaro J, Izon D, Russell SM, et al. A method for prolonged imaging of motile lymphocytes. *Immunol Cell Biol.* (2009) 87:154–8. doi: 10.1038/icb.2008.79
28. Heath AW, Wu WW, Howard MC. Monoclonal antibodies to murine CD40 define two distinct functional epitopes. *Eur J Immunol.* (1994) 24:1828–34. doi: 10.1002/eji.1830240816
29. Hawkins ED, Turner ML, Wellard CJ, Zhou JH, Dowling MR, Hodgkin PD. Quantal and graded stimulation of B lymphocytes as alternative strategies for regulating adaptive immune responses. *Nat Commun.* (2013) 4:2406. doi: 10.1038/ncomms3406
30. Hawkins ED, Markham JF, McGuinness LP, Hodgkin PD. A single-cell pedigree analysis of alternative stochastic lymphocyte fates. *Proc Natl Acad Sci USA.* (2009) 106:13457–62. doi: 10.1073/pnas.0905629106
31. Mitchell S, Roy K, Zangle TA, Hoffmann A. Nongenetic origins of cell-to-cell variability in B lymphocyte proliferation. *Proc Natl Acad Sci USA.* (2018) 115:E2888–97. doi: 10.1073/pnas.1715639115
32. Duffy KR, Hodgkin PD. Intracellular competition for fates in the immune system. *Trends Cell Biol.* (2012) 22:457–64. doi: 10.1016/j.tcb.2012.05.004
33. Cox DR, Oakes, D. *Analysis of Survival Data.* London; New York, NY: Chapman and Hall (1984).
34. Calegari F, Huttner WB. An inhibition of cyclin-dependent kinases that lengthens, but does not arrest, neuroepithelial cell cycle induces premature neurogenesis. *J Cell Sci.* (2003) 116(Pt 24):4947–55. doi: 10.1242/jcs.00825
35. Coronado D, Godet M, Bourillot PY, Tapponnier Y, Bernat A, Petit M, et al. A short G1 phase is an intrinsic determinant of naive embryonic stem cell pluripotency. *Stem Cell Res.* (2013) 10:118–31. doi: 10.1016/j.scr.2012.10.004
36. Kueh HY, Champhekar A, Nutt SL, Elowitz MB, Rothenberg EV. Positive feedback between PU.1 and the cell cycle controls myeloid differentiation. *Science* (2013) 341:670–3. doi: 10.1126/science.1240831
37. Heinzel S, Binh Giang T, Kan A, Marchingo JM, Lye BK, Corcoran LM, et al. Myc-dependent division timer complements a cell-death timer to regulate T cell and B cell responses. *Nat Immunol.* (2017) 18:96–103. doi: 10.1038/ni.3598
38. MacLennan IC, Toellner KM, Cunningham AF, Serre K, Sze DM, Zuniga E, et al. Extrafollicular antibody responses. *Immunol Rev.* (2003) 194:8–18. doi: 10.1034/j.1600-065X.2003.00058.x
39. Harwood NE, Batista FD. Early events in B cell activation. *Annu Rev Immunol.* (2010) 28:185–210. doi: 10.1146/annurev-immunol-030409-101216
40. Linterman MA, Vinuesa CG. Signals that influence T follicular helper cell differentiation and function. *Semin Immunopathol.* (2010) 32:183–96. doi: 10.1007/s00281-009-0194-z
41. Batista FD, Neuberger MS. Affinity dependence of the B cell response to antigen: a threshold, a ceiling, and the importance of off-rate. *Immunity* (1998) 8:751–9.
42. Crotty S. Follicular helper CD4 T cells (TFH). *Annu Rev Immunol.* (2011) 29:621–63. doi: 10.1146/annurev-immunol-031210-101400
43. Rush JS, Hodgkin PD. B cells activated via CD40 and IL-4 undergo a division burst but require continued stimulation to maintain division, survival and differentiation. *Eur J Immunol.* (2001) 31:1150–9. doi: 10.1002/1521-4141(200104)31:4<1150::AID-IMMU1150>3.0.CO;2-V
44. Paus D, Phan TG, Chan TD, Gardam S, Basten A, Brink, R. Antigen recognition strength regulates the choice between extrafollicular plasma cell and germinal center B cell differentiation. *J Exp Med.* (2006) 203:1081–91. doi: 10.1084/jem.20060087
45. Phan TG, Paus D, Chan TD, Turner ML, Nutt SL, Basten A, et al. High affinity germinal center B cells are actively selected into the plasma cell compartment. *J Exp Med.* (2006) 203:2419–24. doi: 10.1084/jem.20061254
46. Shlomchik MJ, Weisel, F. Germinal centers. *Immunol Rev.* (2012) 247:5–10. doi: 10.1111/j.1600-065X.2012.01125.x

47. Victora GD, Nussenzweig MC. Germinal centers. *Annu Rev Immunol.* (2012) 30:429–57. doi: 10.1146/annurev-immunol-020711-075032
48. Liu YJ, Joshua DE, Williams GT, Smith CA, Gordon J, MacLennan IC. Mechanism of antigen-driven selection in germinal centres. *Nature* (1989) 342:929–31. doi: 10.1038/342929a0
49. Foy TM, Laman JD, Ledbetter JA, Aruffo A, Claassen E, Noelle RJ. gp39-CD40 interactions are essential for germinal center formation and the development of B cell memory. *J Exp Med.* (1994) 180:157–63.
50. Victora GD, Dominguez-Sola D, Holmes AB, Deroubaix S, Dalla-Favera R, Nussenzweig MC. Identification of human germinal center light and dark zone cells and their relationship to human B-cell lymphomas. *Blood* (2012) 120:2240–8. doi: 10.1182/blood-2012-03-415380
51. Victora GD, Schwickert TA, Fooksman DR, Kamphorst AO, Meyer-Hermann M, Dustin ML, et al. Germinal center dynamics revealed by multiphoton microscopy with a photoactivatable fluorescent reporter. *Cell* (2010) 143:592–605. doi: 10.1016/j.cell.2010.10.032
52. Gitlin AD, Mayer CT, Oliveira TY, Shulman Z, Jones MJ, Koren A, et al. Humoral Immunity. T cell help controls the speed of the cell cycle in germinal center B cells. *Science* (2015) 349:643–6. doi: 10.1126/science.aac4919

# 8

# iBCE-EL: A New Ensemble Learning Framework for Improved Linear B-Cell Epitope Prediction

*Balachandran Manavalan[1], Rajiv Gandhi Govindaraj[2], Tae Hwan Shin[1,3], Myeong Ok Kim[4] and Gwang Lee[1,3]**

*[1] Department of Physiology, Ajou University School of Medicine, Suwon, South Korea, [2] Department of Biological Sciences, Louisiana State University, Baton Rouge, LA, United States, [3] Institute of Molecular Science and Technology, Ajou University, Suwon, South Korea, [4] Division of Life Science and Applied Life Science (BK21 Plus), College of Natural Sciences, Gyeongsang National University, Jinju, South Korea*

***Correspondence:** Gwang Lee glee@ajou.ac.kr*

Identification of B-cell epitopes (BCEs) is a fundamental step for epitope-based vaccine development, antibody production, and disease prevention and diagnosis. Due to the avalanche of protein sequence data discovered in postgenomic age, it is essential to develop an automated computational method to enable fast and accurate identification of novel BCEs within vast number of candidate proteins and peptides. Although several computational methods have been developed, their accuracy is unreliable. Thus, developing a reliable model with significant prediction improvements is highly desirable. In this study, we first constructed a non-redundant data set of 5,550 experimentally validated BCEs and 6,893 non-BCEs from the Immune Epitope Database. We then developed a novel ensemble learning framework for improved linear BCE predictor called iBCE-EL, a fusion of two independent predictors, namely, extremely randomized tree (ERT) and gradient boosting (GB) classifiers, which, respectively, uses a combination of physicochemical properties (PCP) and amino acid composition and a combination of dipeptide and PCP as input features. Cross-validation analysis on a benchmarking data set showed that iBCE-EL performed better than individual classifiers (ERT and GB), with a Matthews correlation coefficient (MCC) of 0.454. Furthermore, we evaluated the performance of iBCE-EL on the independent data set. Results show that iBCE-EL significantly outperformed the state-of-the-art method with an MCC of 0.463. To the best of our knowledge, iBCE-EL is the first ensemble method for linear BCEs prediction. iBCE-EL was implemented in a web-based platform, which is available at http://thegleelab.org/iBCE-EL. iBCE-EL contains two prediction modes. The first one identifying peptide sequences as BCEs or non-BCEs, while later one is aimed at providing users with the option of mining potential BCEs from protein sequences.

**Keywords: B-cell epitope, ensemble learning, extremely randomized tree, gradient boosting, immunotherapy**

## INTRODUCTION

The humoral immune system is a complex network of cells that work together to protect the body against foreign substances or antigens such as bacteria, viruses, fungi, parasites, and cancerous cells. Generally, antigens are larger in size, however, only certain parts of antigenic determinants, called B-cell epitopes (BCEs), are recognized by specific receptors on the B-cell surface, generating soluble forms of antigen-specific antibodies (1). These antibodies play an important role in neutralization, cell-mediated cytotoxicity, and phagocytosis for the adaptive arm of immunity (2, 3). Thus, the identification and characterization of BCEs is a fundamental step in the development of vaccines, therapeutic antibodies, and other immunodiagnostic tools (4–7). Today, interest in epitope-based antibodies in biopharmaceutical research and development is rising due to their selectivity, biosafety, tolerability, and high efficacy.

B-cell epitopes are broadly classified into two categories: continuous/linear and discontinuous/conformational. Continuous/linear BCEs comprise linear stretches of residues in the antigen protein sequence, while the discontinuous/conformational BCEs comprise residues placed far apart in the antigen protein sequence, which are brought together in three-dimensional space through folding (8, 9). Experimental methods to identify BCEs include X-ray crystallography, cryo-EM, nuclear magnetic resonance, hydrogen–deuterium exchange coupled to mass spectroscopy, peptide-based approaches, mutagenesis, and antigen fragmentation (5, 10). However, these methods could be expensive and time-consuming. Therefore, new sequence-based computational methods need to be developed for rapid identification of potential BCEs. To this end, several computational methods based on machine learning (ML) algorithms have been developed to predict linear BCEs. These methods can be classified into local and global methods. Local methods such as Bcepred (11), BepiPred (12), and COBEpro (13) classify each residue as a BCE or non-BCE in a given protein sequence; global methods such as ABCpred (14), SVMTriP (15), IgPred (16), and LBtope (17) predict whether a given peptide is a BCE or non-BCE. Among global methods, LBtope is the most recently developed one and is also publicly available.

Although global prediction methods for linear BCEs have contributed to some development in this field, further studies are needed for the following reasons. (i) With the rapidly increasing number of BCEs in the Immune Epitope Database (IEDB) (18, 19), developing more accurate prediction methods using non-redundant (nr) benchmark data sets remain an important and urgent task. (ii) Most of the existing methods use random peptides as negative data sets. Experimentally determined negative data sets are necessary for developing efficient methods. Thus, better methods that use ML algorithms based on high-quality benchmarking data sets are necessary to accurately predict BCEs.

In this study, we constructed an nr data set of experimentally validated BCEs and non-BCEs from the IEDB and excluded sequences that showed more than 70% sequence similarity to avoid performance bias. We investigated six different ML algorithms [support vector machine (SVM), random forest (RF), extremely randomized tree (ERT), AdaBoost (AB), gradient boosting (GB), and $k$-nearest neighbors ($k$-NN)], five compositions [amino acid composition (AAC), amino acid index (AAI), dipeptide composition (DPC), chain-transition-distribution (CTD), and physicochemical properties (PCP)], 23 hybrid features (different combinations of the five compositions), and six binary profiles (BPF). We propose a novel ensemble approach, called iBCE-EL for predicting BCEs. The ensemble approach combines two different ML classifiers (ERT and GB) and uses the average predicted probabilities to make a final prediction. Furthermore, iBCE-EL achieved a significantly better overall performance on benchmarking and independent data sets and was capable of more accurate prediction than state-of-the-art predictor.

# MATERIALS AND METHODS

## Construction of Benchmarking and Independent Data Sets

To build an ML model, an experimentally well-characterized data set is required. Therefore, we extracted a set of linear peptides from IEDB that tested positive for immune recognition (BCEs) and another set that tested negative (non-BCEs) (18, 19). Less than 1% of the peptides had lower than 5 or greater than 25 amino acid residues. We excluded these peptides from our data set because including them may result in outliers during prediction model development.

As mentioned in IEDB, one of the following seven different B-cell experimental assays (Qualitative binding, decreased disease, neutralization, disassociation constant KD, antibody-dependent cellular cytotoxicity, off rate, and on rate) are used to determine whether a peptide belongs to a positive or negative set of epitopes. Indeed, all this assay information is clearly specified for each peptide in IEDB (sixth column of the following link: http://www.iedb.org/bcelldetails_v3.php). It is worth mentioning that the criteria for categorizing positive and negative data set are the same as the one used in the recent study (12). To generate high confidence in our data set, we carefully examined each peptide assay information and considered as positive only when it has been confirmed as positive in two or more separate B-cell experiments. Similarly, peptides shown as negative in two or more separate experiment and never observed as positive in any of the above assays were considered as negative ones. To avoid potential bias and over-fitting in the prediction model development, sequence clustering and homology reduction using CD-HIT were performed, thus removing sequence redundancy from the retrieved data set. Based on the design of previous studies (20, 21), pairs of sequences that showed a sequence identity greater than 70% were excluded, thus obtaining an nr data set of 5,550 BCEs and 6,893 non-BCEs. Furthermore, each peptide present in our nr data set was mapped onto the original protein sequence, thus confirming the nature of linear epitopes. From this nr data set, 80% of the data was randomly selected as the benchmarking data set (4,440 BCEs and 5,485 non-BCEs) for development of a prediction model and the remaining 20% was used as the independent data set (1,110 BCEs and 1,408 non-BCEs).

## Feature Representation of Peptides

A peptide sequence (P) can be represented as:

$$P = p_1 p_2 p_3 \ldots p_N \quad (1)$$

where $p_1$, $p_2$, and $p_3$, respectively, denotes the first, second, and third residues in the peptide $P$, and so forth. $N$ denotes the peptide length. It should be noted that the residue $p_i$ is an element of the standard amino acid {A, C, D, E, F, G, H, I, K, L, M, N, P, Q, R, S, T, V, W, Y}. To train a ML model, we formulated diverse-length peptides as fixed-length feature vectors. We exploited five different compositions and BPF that cover different aspects of sequence information as described below:

(i) AAC

Amino acid composition is the percentage of standard amino acids; it has a fixed length of 20 features. AAC can be formulated as follows:

$$AAC(P) = (f_1, f_2, f_3, \ldots\ldots, f_{20}) \quad (2)$$

where $f_1 = \frac{R_i}{N}(i = 1,2,\ldots,20)$ is the percentage of composition of amino acid type $i$, $R_i$ is the number of type I appearing in the peptide, while $N$ is the peptide length.

(ii) DPC

Dipeptide composition is the rate of dipeptides normalized by all possible dipeptide combinations; it has a fixed length of 400 features. DPC can be formulated as follows:

$$DPC(P) = (f_1, f_2, f_3, \ldots\ldots, f_{400}) \quad (3)$$

where $f_1 = \frac{R_i}{N}(i = 1,2,\ldots,400)$ is the percentage of composition of dipeptide type $i$, $R_i$ is the number of type $i$ appearing in the peptide, while $N$ is the peptide length.

(iii) CTD

Chain-transition-distribution was introduced by Dubchak et al. (22) for predicting protein-folding classes. It has been widely applied in various classification problems. A detailed description of computing CTD features was presented in our previous study (23). Briefly, standard amino acids (20) are classified into three different groups: polar, neutral, and hydrophobic. Composition (C) consists of percentage composition values from these three groups for a target peptide. Transition (T) consists of percentage frequency of a polar followed by a neutral residue, or that of a neutral followed by a polar residue. This group may also contain a polar followed by a hydrophobic residue or a hydrophobic followed by a polar residue. Distribution (D) consists of five values for each of the three groups. It measures the percentage of the length of the target sequence within which 25, 50, 75, and 100% of the amino acids of a specific property are located. CTD generates 21 features for each PCP; hence, seven different PCPs (hydrophobicity, polarizability, normalized van der Waals volume, secondary structure, polarity, charge, and solvent accessibility) yields a total of 147 features.

(iv) AAI

The AAindex database has a variety of physiochemical and biochemical properties of amino acids (24). However, utilizing all this information as input features for the ML algorithm may affect the model performance due to redundancy. Therefore, Saha et al. (25) classified these amino acid indices into eight clusters by fuzzy clustering method, and the central indices of each cluster were considered as high-quality amino acid indices. The accession numbers of the eight amino acid indices in the AAindex database are BLAM930101, BIOV880101, MAXF760101, TSAJ990101, NAKH920108, CEDJ970104, LIFS790101, and MIYS990104. These high-quality indices encode as 160-dimensional vectors from the target peptide sequence. Furthermore, the average of eight high-quality amino acid indices (i.e., a 20-dimensional vector) was used as an additional input feature. As our preliminary analysis indicated that both feature sets (160 and 20) produced similar results, we employed the 20-dimensional vector to save computational time.

(v) PCP

Amino acids can be grouped based on their PCP, and this has been used to study protein sequence profiles, folding, and functions (26). The PCP computed from the target peptide sequence included (i) hydrophobic residues (i.e., F, I, W, L, V, M, Y, C, A), (ii) hydrophilic residues (i.e., S, Q, T, R, K, N, D, E), (iii) neutral residues (i.e., H,G, P); (iv) positively charged residues (i.e., K, H, R); (v) negatively charged residues (i.e., D, E), (vi) fraction of turn-forming residues [i.e., (N + G + P + S)/n, where $n$ = sequence length], (vii) absolute charge per residue (i.e., $\left|\frac{R+K-D-E}{n} - 0.03\right|$), (viii) molecular weight, and (ix) aliphatic index [i.e., (A + 2.9V + 3.9I + 3.9L)/$n$].

(vi) BPF

Each amino acid type of 20 different standard amino acids is encoded with the following feature vector 0/1. For instance, the first amino acid type A is encoded as b(A) = (1, 0, 0, …., 0), the second amino acid type C is encoded as b(C) = (0, 1, 0,…., 0), and so on. Subsequently, for a given peptide sequence P, its N or C-terminus with length of $k$ amino acids was encoded as:

$$BPF(k) = [b(p_1), b(p_2), \ldots, b(p_k)] \quad (4)$$

The dimension of BPF($k$) is 20 × $k$. Here, we considered $k$ = 5 and 10 both at N-terminus and C-terminus, which resulted BPFN5, BPFN10, BPFC5, and BPFC10. In addition to this, we also generated BPFN5-BPFC5 and BPFN10-BPFC10.

## Performance Assessment

A brief description of ML method employed in this study is given in the supplementary information, whose performances were evaluated using the receiver operating characteristic (ROC) analysis and the corresponding area under the ROC curve (AUC). An AUC value of 0.5 is equivalent to random prediction and an AUC value of 1 represents perfection. ROC analysis is based on the true positive rate and false positive rate at various thresholds. Furthermore, we used sensitivity, specificity, accuracy, and Matthews correlation coefficient (MCC) to assess prediction quality, which were defined as:

$$\begin{aligned}
\text{Sensitivity} &= \frac{\text{TP}}{\text{TP}+\text{FN}} \\
\text{Specificity} &= \frac{\text{TN}}{\text{TN}+\text{FP}} \\
\text{Accuracy} &= \frac{\text{TP}+\text{TN}}{\text{TP}+\text{TN}+\text{FP}+\text{FN}} \\
\text{MCC} &= \frac{\text{TP}\times\text{TN-FP}\times\text{FN}}{\sqrt{(\text{TP}+\text{FP})(\text{TP}+\text{FN})(\text{TN}+\text{FP})(\text{TN}+\text{FN})}}
\end{aligned} \quad (5)$$

where TP is the number of true positives, i.e., BCEs classified correctly as BCEs, and TN is the number of true negatives, i.e., non-BCEs classified correctly as non-BCEs. FP is the number of false positives, i.e., BCEs classified incorrectly as non-BCEs, and FN is the number of false negatives, i.e., non-BCEs classified incorrectly as BCEs.

## Cross-Validation

In this study, we adopted the 5-fold cross-validation method, where benchmarking data set is randomly divided into five parts, from which four parts were used for training, and the fifth part was used for testing. This process was repeated until all the parts were used at least once as a test set, and the overall performance with all five parts was evaluated.

# RESULTS

## Methodology Overview

**Figure 1** shows a flowchart illustrating the methodology of iBCE-EL, which comprises four stages: (1) construction of an nr benchmarking data set of 9,925 peptides (4,440 BCEs and 5,485 non-BCEs) and an independent data set of 2,518 peptides (1,110 BCEs and 1,408 non-BCEs) from IEDB; (2) extraction of various features from peptide sequences, including AAC, AAI, CTD, DPC, and PCP, and generation of hybrid features (various combinations of individual compositions); (3) exploration of six different ML algorithms and selection of the appropriate ones and their corresponding features; and (4) construction of an ensemble model.

## Compositional and Positional Information Analysis

Prior to the development of the ML-based prediction model, we performed compositional analysis using combined data set (i.e., benchmarking and independent) to understand the nature of the preference of amino acid residues in BCEs and non-BCEs. AAC analysis showed that Asn (N), Asp (D), Pro (P), and Tyr (Y) were predominant in BCEs (**Figure 2A**). However, Ala (A), Glu (E), Leu (L), Val (V), and Met (M) were predominant in non-BCEs (Welch's *t*-test; $P \leq 0.05$). DPC analysis showed that 32.25% of dipeptides differed significantly between BCEs and non-BCEs (Welch's *t*-test; $P \leq 0.05$). Of these, the 10 most abundant dipeptides in BCEs and non-BCEs were PP, SP, NK, NN, PN, NP, KY, QP, PY, and DP and LA, LT, KE, LL, VL, LQ, GL, AL, LE, and LS, respectively (**Figure 2B**). These results suggested that the most abundant dipeptides in BCEs were mostly pairs of aromatic–aromatic residues or a positively or negatively charged residue paired with proline. The most abundant dipeptides in non-BCEs were aliphatic-aliphatic residues with hydroxyl group and aliphatic–aromatic amino acids. Overall, the differences observed in compositional analyses (AAC and DPC) can be used as an input feature for ML algorithms, where it can capture hidden relationships between features allowing a better classification. Therefore, we considered them as input features.

To better understand the positional information of each residue, sequence logos of the first 10 residues from the N- and C-terminals of BCEs and non-BCEs were generated using two

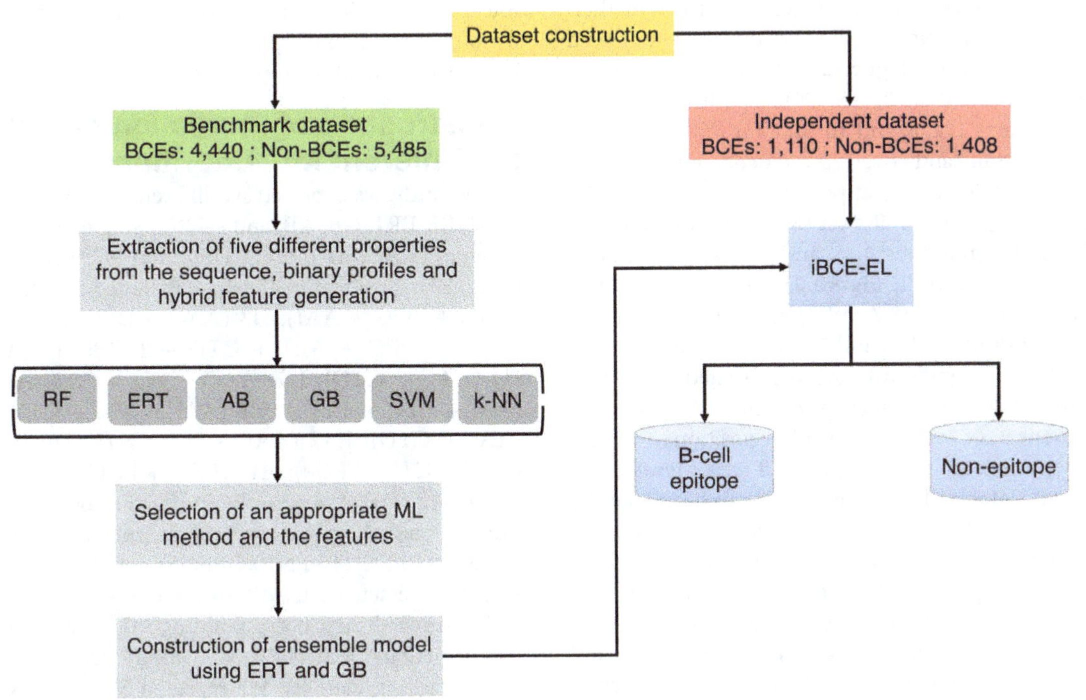


**FIGURE 1** | Overall framework of the proposed predictor. iBCE-EL development involved the following steps: (1) dataset curation, (2) feature extraction, (3) exploration of six different ML algorithms and selection of an appropriate algorithm and the corresponding features, and (4) construction of ensemble model.

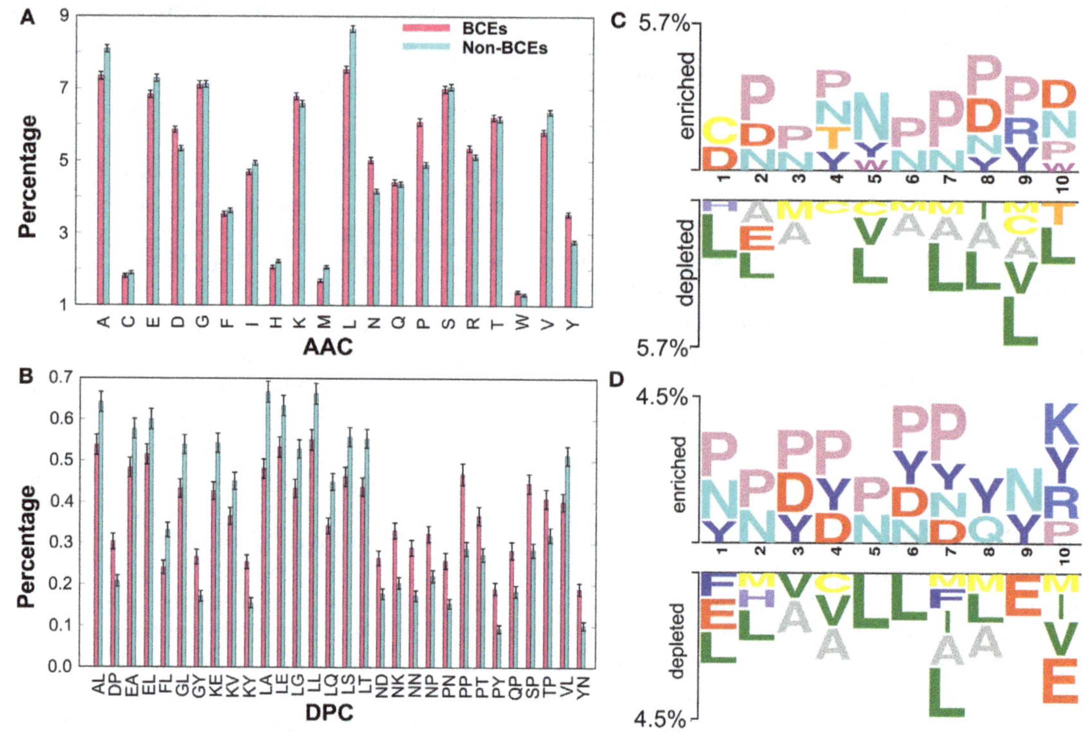


**FIGURE 2** | Compositional and positional preference analysis. **(A)** and **(B)** respectively represent the amino acid and dipeptide preferences of BCEs and non-BCEs. **(B)** Shows significant differences in top 30 dipeptides. **(C,D)** Represent positional conservation of 10 residues at the N- and C-terminals, respectively, between BCEs and non-BCEs, generated using two sample logos. In **(A,B)**, error bar is the SE that indicates the reliability of the mean. A smaller SE indicates that the sample mean is more accurate reflection of the actual population mean.

sample logos (http://www.twosamplelogo.org). To test their statistical significance, the height of the peptide logos was scaled (*t*-test; $P < 0.05$). As shown in **Figure 2C**, at the N-terminal, Pro (P) at positions 2, 3, 4, and 6–10; Asn (N) at positions 2–8 and 10; Asp (D) at positions 1, 2, 8, and 10; and Tyr (Y) at positions 4, 5, 8, and 9 were significantly overrepresented, compared with other amino acids, while Leu (L) at positions 1, 2, 5, and 7–10; Ala (A) at positions 2, 3, and 6–9; Met (M) at positions 3, 6, 7, and 9; and Cys (C) at positions 4, 5, and 9 were significantly underrepresented. As shown in **Figure 2D**, at the C-terminal, Pro (P) at positions 1–7 and 10; Asn (N) at positions 1, 2, 5–7, and 9; Asp (D) at positions 3, 4, 6, and 7; and Tyr (Y) at positions 1, 3, 4, and 6–10 were significantly overrepresented, compared with other amino acids, while Leu (L) at positions 1, 2, and 5–8; Ala (A) at positions 3, 4, 7, and 8; Glu (E) at positions 1, 9, and 10; and Met (M) at positions 2, 7, 8, and 10 were significantly underrepresented. Notably, the predominant amino acids in the non-BCEs (particularly Leu, Val, and Met) were expected to be inside the proteins and if exist on the surface were likely to be present on the protein–protein interfaces. Conversely, the amino acids enriched in BCEs were mostly expected to be present on the protein surface. Overall, these results showed that BCEs and non-BCEs have contrasting amino acid preferences, which is consistent with the compositional analysis. Furthermore, positional preference analysis will be useful for researchers to design *de novo* BCEs by substituting amino acids at the specific position for increasing peptide efficacy. Interestingly, the properties of linear epitopes described here based on our data set are different from conformational epitopes (27), which is mainly due to the local arrangement of amino acids.

## Construction of Prediction Models Using Six Different ML Algorithms

In this study, we explored six different ML algorithms, including SVM, RF, ERT, GB, AB, and *k*-NN, using five different encoding schemes (AAC, AAI, CTD, DPC, and PCP) and their combinations (17 hybrid features), which included H1 (AAC + AAI); H2 (AAC + DPC + AAI); H3 (AAC + DPC + AAI + CTD); H4 (AAC + DPC + AAI + CTD + PCP); H5 (AAC + DPC); H6 (AAC + CTD); H7 (AAC + PCP); H8 (AAI + DPC); H9 (AAI + DPC + CTD); H10 (AAI + DPC + CTD + PCP); H11 (AAI + CTD); H12 (AAI + PCP); H13 (DPC + CTD); H14 (DPC + CTD + PCP); H15 (DPC + PCP); H16 (CTD + DPC); and H17 (AAC + AAI + PCP). Furthermore, we used six features set based on binary profiles, including BPFN5, BPFC5, BPFN5 + BPFC5, BPFN10, BPFC10, and BPFN10 + BPFC10. For each feature set, we used six different ML algorithms as inputs and optimized their corresponding ML parameters (Table S1 in Supplementary Material) using 5-fold cross-validation on the benchmarking data set. We repeated 5-fold cross-validation 10 times by randomly portioning the benchmarking data set and considering median ML parameters and average performance measures. The average performances of these six methods in terms of MCC is shown in **Figure 3**. RF, ERT, and GB performed

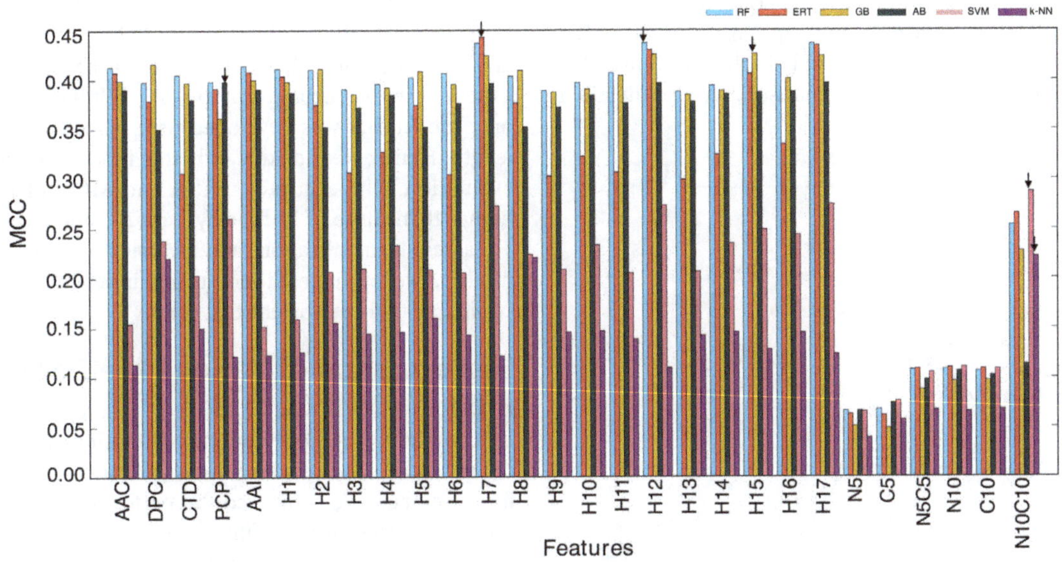


**FIGURE 3** | Performance of six different ML-based classifiers. Performance of various classifiers in distinguishing between B-cell epitopes (BCEs) and non-BCEs. A total of 27 classifiers were evaluated using 10 independent 5-fold cross-validation techniques, and their average performances in terms of AUC is shown. The final selected model for each ML-based method is shown with arrows. Abbreviations: AAC, amino acid composition; DPC, dipeptide composition; CTD, chain-transition-distribution; AAI, amino acid index; PCP, physicochemical properties; H1: AAC + AAI; H2: AAC + DPC + AAI; H3: AAC + DPC + AAI + CTD; H4: AAC + DPC + AAI + CTD + PCP; H5: AAC + DPC; H6: AAC + CTD; H7: AAC + PCP; H8: AAI + DPC; H9: AAI + DPC + CTD; H10: AAI + DPC + CTD + PCP; H11: AAI + CTD; H12: AAI + PCP; H13: DPC + CTD; H14: DPC + CTD + PCP; H15: DPC + PCP; H16: CTD + DPC; H17: AAC + AAI + PCP; N5: BPFN5; C5: BPFC5; N5C5: BPFN5 + BPFC5; N10: BPFN10; C10: BPFC10; and N10C10: BPFN10 + BPFC10.

consistently better than other ML-based methods (SVM, AB, and *k*-NN), regardless of the input features, indicating that decision tree-based methods are better suited for BCE prediction. Next, we investigated the features that produced the best performance for each ML algorithm. We found that SVM and *k*-NN performed best when using N10C10 binary profile as input feature; ERT, RF, GB, and AB performed best when H7, H12, H15, and PCP were used as input features, respectively. This analysis showed that the use of PCP-containing hybrid features as inputs could improve the performance of the ML method. Among the 6 ML methods, surprisingly, RF, ERT, and GB showed similar performances with MCC of 0.437, 0.443, and 0.426, respectively, which was significantly better than MCC of other 3 ML methods (SVM: 0.287, AB: 0.398, and *k*-NN: 0.221).

## Construction of iBCE-EL

An ensemble model (EM) refers to a combination of several prediction models to make the final prediction (28). The major advantage of EMs over single models is the reported increase in robustness and accuracy (29). Here, we generated six ensemble models by combining different ML-based models, EM1 (GB + ERT); EM2 (GB + ERT + RF); EM3 (GB + ERT + RF + SVM); EM4 (GB + ERT + RF + SVM + AB); EM5 (GB + ERT + RF + SVM + AB + NN); and EM6 (GB + SVM + ERT). EM was calculated as follows: $EM = \frac{1}{n}\sum_{i=1}^{n} P_i$, where $n$ is the number of ML-based models and $P$ is the predicted probability value. Notably, we optimized the probability cut-off values ($P$) with respect to MCC using the grid search to define the class (BCEs or non-BCEs), which is a quite common approach and has been applied in various methods (30, 31). A model that produced the highest MCC was considered as the optimal one for each ensemble model. Surprisingly, all these ensemble models showed similar performances (Figure S1A in Supplementary Material) and hence it seems difficult to pick the best one. However, we checked its transferability on an independent data set and selected a model that showed consistent performance both on benchmarking and independent data sets (Figure S1B in Supplementary Material). According to this criterion, EM1 was selected as the best model and was labeled as iBCE-EL. To compare the performance of iBCE-EL with other ML-based models developed in this study, same optimization procedure was applied (**Figure 4**). Our results showed that iBCE-EL, RF, ERT, GB, AB, SVM, and *k*-NN produced the highest MCC with an optimal cut-off of 0.35, 0.47, 0.45, 0.26, 0.50, 0.41, and 0.41, respectively.

## Performance of Various Methods on Benchmarking Data Set

We compared the performance of iBCE-EL with that of the other 6 ML-based methods (RF, ERT, SVM, GB, AB, and *k*-NN). The results are shown in **Table 1**, where the methods are ranked according to the MCC associated with predictive capability. iBCE-EL had the highest MCC, accuracy, and AUC of 0.454, 0.729, and 0.782, respectively. Interestingly, MCC, accuracy, and AUC of iBCE-EL were 0.8–15.9, 0.4–9.5, and 0.6–21.9% higher than those of the other six ML-based methods (RF, ERT, SVM, GB, AB, and *k*-NN). McNemar's Chi-square test (32) was used to evaluate the statistical significance of the differences in the performances of methods. At a $P$-value threshold of 0.05, iBCE-EL significantly outperformed SVM, k-NN, and AB and performed better than RF, ERT, and GB, thus indicating the superiority of iBCE-EL. To the best of our knowledge, iBCE-EL is the first ensemble approach for BCE prediction. For comparison, we also included LBtope (LBtope_variable_nr) cross-validation performance on an nr data set published previously (17). Although four variants are available for LBtope (LBtope_variable, LBtope_confirm, LBtope_variable_nr and LBtope_nr), LBtope_variable_nr is the only model that was developed using nr data set with variable length. Hence, we included only this model for comparison and evaluation. The accuracy, AUC, and MCC of iBCE-EL were higher than those of LBtope by ~6, 12.4, and 5.2%, respectively. To assess generalization and practical applicability of these models, we evaluated them using independent data set and compared their performances.

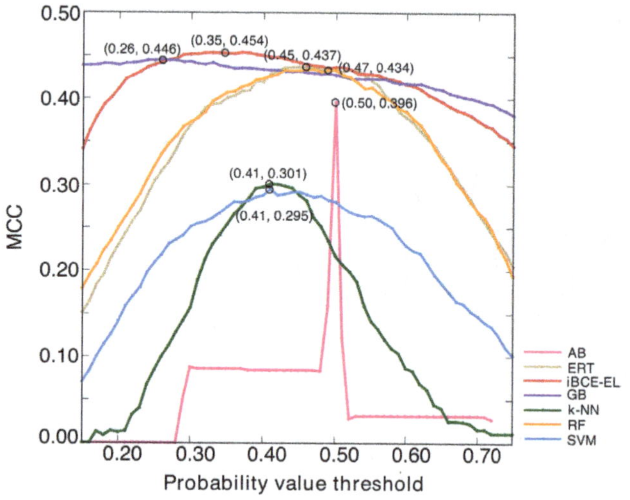


**FIGURE 4** | Optimization of probability value threshold. The x- and y-axes, respectively, represent the probability value threshold and Matthews correlation coefficient. The optimal value selected for each method is shown with a circle.

## Performance of Various Methods on Independent Data Set

By comparing the newly developed method with existing algorithms on the same data set, we could estimate the percentage of improvement. We compared the performance of iBCE-EL with those of LBtope and six other ML-based models. As shown in **Table 2**, iBCE-EL showed MCC, accuracy, and AUC of 0.463, 0.732, and 0.789, respectively. Indeed, the MCC, accuracy, and AUC of iBCE-EL were ~2.0–19.4, ~0.5–11.7, and ~1.0–10.4% higher than those of the other methods, thus indicating the superiority of iBCE-EL.

At a P-value threshold of 0.05, iBCE-EL significantly outperformed SVM, AB, k-NN and LBtope, and performed better than ERT, RF and GB, thus indicating that our approach is indeed a significant improvement over the pioneering approaches

**TABLE 1** | Performance comparison of iBCE-EL with other ML-based methods on the benchmarking data set.

| Method | Matthews correlation coefficient (MCC) | Accuracy | Sensitivity | Specificity | AUC | P-value |
|---|---|---|---|---|---|---|
| iBCE-EL | 0.454 | 0.729 | 0.716 | 0.739 | 0.782 | – |
| GB | 0.446 | 0.725 | 0.712 | 0.735 | 0.773 | 0.051 |
| ERT | 0.437 | 0.718 | 0.734 | 0.705 | 0.776 | 0.205 |
| RF | 0.434 | 0.718 | 0.717 | 0.719 | 0.770 | 0.051 |
| AB | 0.396 | 0.702 | 0.662 | 0.722 | 0.737 | **1.2E−16** |
| k-NN | 0.301 | 0.644 | 0.715 | 0.591 | 0.691 | **1.1E−9** |
| SVM | 0.295 | 0.634 | 0.634 | 0.602 | 0.696 | **<2.2E−16** |
| LBtope | 0.330 | 0.667 | 0.660 | 0.672 | 0.730 | – |

*The first column represents the methods developed in this study. The columns 2–6 respectively represent the MCC, accuracy, sensitivity, specificity, and AUC value. The last column represents McNemar's Chi-squared test was used to evaluate the performance between iBCE-EL and other methods. A P value <0.05 was considered to indicate a statistically significant difference between iBCE-EL and the selected method (shown in bold). For comparison, we have also included LBtope (LBtope_variable_nr) cross-validation performance on non-redundant data set.*

**TABLE 2** | Performance comparison of the iBCE-EL with other methods on independent data set.

| Method | Matthews correlation coefficient (MCC) | Accuracy | Sensitivity | Specificity | AUC | P-value |
|---|---|---|---|---|---|---|
| iBCE-EL | 0.463 | 0.732 | 0.742 | 0.724 | 0.789 | – |
| GB | 0.445 | 0.727 | 0.717 | 0.734 | 0.776 | 0.596 |
| RF | 0.434 | 0.718 | 0.718 | 0.718 | 0.777 | 0.839 |
| ERT | 0.440 | 0.719 | 0.742 | 0.703 | 0.780 | 0.476 |
| AB | 0.385 | 0.697 | 0.660 | 0.725 | 0.742 | **2.4E−05** |
| LBtope | 0.328 | 0.652 | 0.759 | 0.567 | 0.781 | **7.4E−06** |
| k-NN | 0.275 | 0.615 | 0.787 | 0.479 | 0.685 | **4.9E−05** |
| SVM | 0.269 | 0.624 | 0.721 | 0.548 | 0.694 | **1.4E−05** |

*The first column represents the method employed in this study. The columns 2–6, respectively, represent the MCC, accuracy, sensitivity, specificity, and AUC value. The last column represents McNemar's Chi-squared test was used to evaluate the performance between iBCE-EL and other methods. A P value <0.05 was considered to indicate a statistically significant difference between iBCE-EL and the selected method (shown in bold). LBtope (LBtope_variable_nr) used SVM threshold of −0.1 to define the class as reported in Ref. (17).*

in predicting linear BCEs. Interestingly, iBCE-EL performed consistently in both benchmarking and independent data sets (**Figure 5**) among the methods developed in this study suggesting its suitability for BCE prediction, despite the complexity of the problem. We made significant efforts to curate a large nr data set, explore various ML algorithms, and select an appropriate one for constructing an ensemble model thus resulting in consistent performance.

### Comparison of iBCE-EL With LBtope Methodology

We compared our method and LBtope (LBtope_variable_nr) in terms of algorithm characteristics. Since the variation in the number of B-cell experiments were considered to classify the peptides (positive or negative), LBtope used ~2-fold larger benchmarking data set than iBCE-EL. Moreover, we tested for significant differences in the data set using positional information analysis. However, we did not observe any significant differences between these two methods (Figure S2 in Supplementary Material). The choice of ML algorithm is different between these two methods, i.e., SVM used in LBtope, however, a combination of ERT and GB (ensemble model) were used in iBCE-EL. Interestingly, three features such as AAC, PCP, and DPC provide the most discriminative power for identifying BCEs; however, only DPC was used in LBtope.

### Web Server Implementation

Prediction methodologies available as web servers will be helpful for experimentalists, and several web servers for protein function predictions have been reported (23, 33–38). A web server has been developed to implement the iBCE-EL method and made publicly accessible at www.thegleelab.org/iBCE-EL for the use of the wider research community. Python, JAVA script, and HTML languages were employed to construct the web server. Users can submit amino acid sequences in the FASTA format. The output of the web server contains the class and predicted BCE probability values. The data set used in this study can also be downloaded from the iBCE-EL web server.

## DISCUSSION

Computational identification of BCEs is one of the hot research topics in bioinformatics. An increasing number of experimentally validated BCEs is growing exponentially in IEDB, where most BCEs are found to be derived from protein sequences. To identify BCEs from a given protein sequence, experimental methods seem to be time-consuming, highly expensive, and complex to be utilized in a high-throughput manner. Therefore, recent efforts have focused on the development of computational methods to accelerate the identification of BCEs (12–15, 17, 39–46). Most existing BCE prediction methods were developed using very small data sets, with negative ones derived from randomly chosen peptides that are not experimentally validated (13–15, 17, 40, 42). This practice is quite common in other peptide-based prediction methods, including those for anticancer, antifungal, and cell-penetrating peptides (30, 47, 48). Among existing methods, LBtope is the latest publicly available tool with three different prediction models (17). It was developed using an nr data set that produced an accuracy of 66.7%, which is far from satisfactory. Hence, a novel method with better accuracy is necessitated. In this study, we developed a novel software called iBCE-EL, which allowed us to predict BCEs from a given primary peptide sequence based on the features derived from a set of experimentally validated BCEs and non-BCEs.

To the best of our knowledge, the data set we utilized was the most stringent redundancy-reduced data set with variable length

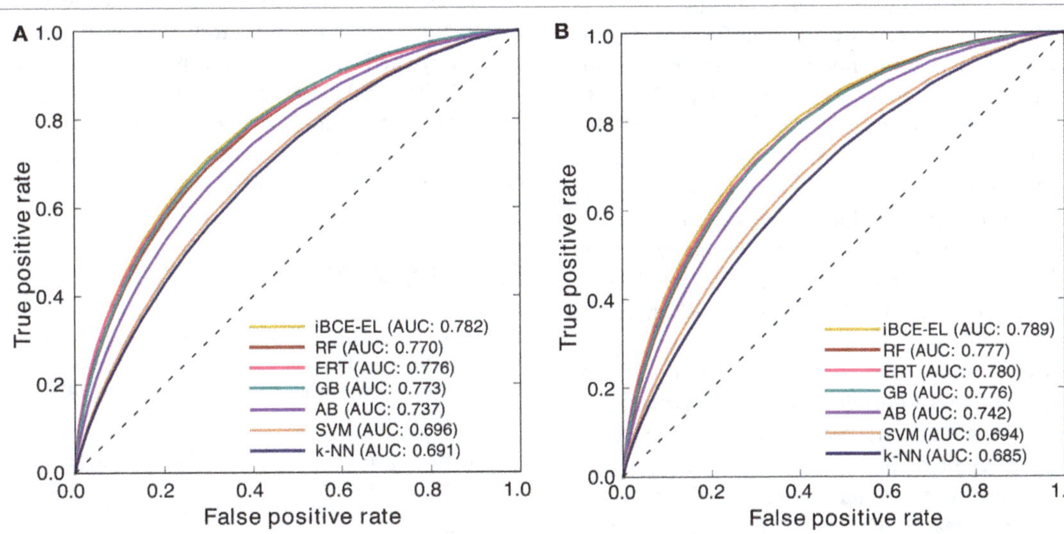


**FIGURE 5** | Receiver operating characteristic curves of the various prediction models. Results of 5-fold cross-validation on **(A)** a benchmarking data set and **(B)** independent data set.

of epitopes (12–25 amino acid residues). Recent studies demonstrated that BCEs with shorter lengths (7–12 amino acids) bind antibodies poorly (49). Therefore, such shorter peptides were not considered in our data set. In general, models developed using such high-quality data sets would have a wide range of applications in modern biology (50). Before developing the prediction model, we analyzed our data set to understand the compositional and positional preferences of BCEs and non-BCEs. We found that Pro and Asn were highly abundant in BCEs, compared to non-BCEs. These observations were consistent with the results of previous reports, where immunoglobulin binding antigenic regions were found to be rich in Pro/Gly (51, 52) residues. Future studies should focus on the experimental validation of the biological significance of various dipeptides we found to be involved in B-cell induction.

It is essential to explore different ML algorithms using the same data set and then select the best one, instead of arbitrarily selecting an ML algorithm (47, 53–58). We explored six different ML algorithms (SVM, RF, ERT, AB, GB, and *k*-NN) and 23 different features encoding schemes for classifying BCEs and non-BCEs. All the features and ML algorithms used in this study have been successfully applied in various sequence-based classification methods (53–55, 59–61); however, only SVM and DPC were used in LBtope (17). To the best of our knowledge, this is the first study to evaluate several ML algorithms for BCE prediction. Our systematic evaluation of features and ML algorithms revealed that RF, ERT, and GB showed similar performances, respectively, with a combination of PCP and AAI, a combination of PCP and AAC, and a combination of DPC and PCP as input features. Subsequently, we constructed an ensemble method called iBCE-EL by fusing ERT and GB. iBCE-EL performed better than individual component classifiers. The ensemble approach has been successfully applied for various problems, including signal peptide prediction (62), membrane protein type classification (63), protein subcellular location (64), and DNase I hypersensitive site prediction (65). However, this is the first instance where this approach has been utilized for BCE prediction. iBCE-EL performed significantly better than the existing method and six other methods developed in this study, when objectively evaluated on an independent data set. Interestingly, the performance of iBCE-EL was consistent on both benchmarking and independent data sets, thus indicating its ability to classify unseen peptides well when compared to other methods. The superior performance of iBCE-EL was primarily due to the larger size of the benchmarking data set, rigorous optimization procedures to select the final ML parameters, and the choice of ML methods to construct the ensemble model. Future studies should focus on identifying novel features that can be combined with the current feature set to further improve prediction performance. Furthermore, we expect that our proposed algorithm could also be applied to other fields of peptide or protein function prediction. Several authors still query whether BCE could be considered as a discrete feature of a protein molecule or not. Indeed, van Regenmortel suggests that an epitope is not an intrinsic feature of a protein molecule, but is a relational entity that can be defined only by its ability to react with the paratope of an antibody molecule (6, 27, 43, 49, 66).

In conclusion, we proposed a novel ensemble method called iBCE-EL to classify a given primary peptide sequence as BCE or non-BCE. The essential component of this study is the generation of high-quality data sets with several manually curated BCEs and non-BCEs. iBCE-EL showed consistent performance with both benchmarking and independent data sets, thus indicating its effectiveness and robustness. We have also created a user-friendly web interface, allowing researchers to use our prediction method. iBCE-EL is the second publicly available method for predicting BCEs, and its accuracy is remarkably higher than that of currently available methods. We anticipate that iBCE-EL will become a very useful tool for BCE prediction.

## AUTHOR CONTRIBUTIONS

BM and GL conceived and designed the experiments. BM and RG performed the experiments. BM, RG, and TS analyzed the data. GL and MK contributed reagents/materials/software tools. BM, RG, and GL wrote the manuscript. All authors reviewed the manuscript and agreed to its submission in its present form.

## ACKNOWLEDGMENTS

The authors thank Ms. Saraswathi Nithyanantham for her support in data set preparation and Ms. Da Yeon Lee for secretarial assistance in the preparation of the manuscript.

## FUNDING

This work was supported by the Basic Science Research Program through the National Research Foundation (NRF) of Korea funded by the Ministry of Education, Science, and Technology (2018R1D1A1B07049572 and 2009-0093826) and the Brain Research Program through the National Research Foundation of Korea (NRF) funded by the Ministry of Science, ICT, and Future Planning (2016M3C7A1904392).

## SUPPLEMENTARY MATERIAL

**FIGURE S1** | Optimization of probability value threshold. The *x*- and *y*-axes, respectively, represent the probability value threshold and MCC. The optimal value selected for each method is shown with a circle. **(A)** A benchmarking data set and **(B)** independent data set.

**FIGURE S2** | Comparison of position preference analysis using iBCE-EL and LBtope data set. **(A,B)** Represent positional conservation of 10 residues at N- and C-terminal, respectively, using iBCE-EL data set. **(C,D)** Represent positional conservation of 10 residues at N- and C-terminal, respectively, using LBtope data set.

## REFERENCES


1. Getzoff ED, Tainer JA, Lerner RA, Geysen HM. *The Chemistry and Mechanism of Antibody Binding to Protein Antigens. Advances in immunology. 43.* Elsevier (1988). p. 1–98.
2. Katsumata M. Promotion of intramuscular fat accumulation in porcine muscle by nutritional regulation. *Anim Sci J* (2011) 82(1):17–25. doi:10.1111/j.1740-0929.2010.00844.x
3. Webster SD, Galvan MD, Ferran E, Garzon-Rodriguez W, Glabe CG, Tenner AJ. Antibody-mediated phagocytosis of the amyloid beta-peptide in microglia is differentially modulated by C1q. *J Immunol* (2001) 166(12): 7496–503. doi:10.4049/jimmunol.166.12.7496
4. Feldmann M, Maini RN. Anti-TNF alpha therapy of rheumatoid arthritis: what have we learned? *Annu Rev Immunol* (2001) 19:163–96. doi:10.1146/annurev.immunol.19.1.163
5. Potocnakova L, Bhide M, Pulzova LB. An introduction to B-cell epitope mapping and in silico epitope prediction. *J Immunol Res* (2016) 2016:6760830. doi:10.1155/2016/6760830
6. Van Regenmortel MH. Immunoinformatics may lead to a reappraisal of the nature of B cell epitopes and of the feasibility of synthetic peptide vaccines. *J Mol Recognit* (2006) 19(3):183–7. doi:10.1002/jmr.768
7. Hopp TP, Woods KR. Prediction of protein antigenic determinants from amino acid sequences. *Proc Natl Acad Sci U S A* (1981) 78(6):3824–8. doi:10.1073/pnas.78.6.3824
8. Barlow DJ, Edwards MS, Thornton JM. Continuous and discontinuous protein antigenic determinants. *Nature* (1986) 322(6081):747–8. doi:10.1038/322747a0
9. Caoili SE. Hybrid methods for B-cell epitope prediction. *Methods Mol Biol* (2014) 1184:245–83. doi:10.1007/978-1-4939-1115-8_14
10. Abbott WM, Damschroder MM, Lowe DC. Current approaches to fine mapping of antigen–antibody interactions. *Immunology* (2014) 142(4):526–35. doi:10.1111/imm.12284
11. Saha S, Raghava GP. Prediction methods for B-cell epitopes. *Methods Mol Biol* (2007) 409:387–94. doi:10.1007/978-1-60327-118-9_29
12. Jespersen MC, Peters B, Nielsen M, Marcatili P. BepiPred-2.0: improving sequence-based B-cell epitope prediction using conformational epitopes. *Nucleic Acids Res* (2017) 45(W1):W24–9. doi:10.1093/nar/gkx346
13. Sweredoski MJ, Baldi P. COBEpro: a novel system for predicting continuous B-cell epitopes. *Protein Eng Des Sel* (2009) 22(3):113–20. doi:10.1093/protein/gzn075
14. Saha S, Raghava G. Prediction of continuous B-cell epitopes in an antigen using recurrent neural network. *Proteins* (2006) 65(1):40–8. doi:10.1002/prot.21078
15. Yao B, Zhang L, Liang S, Zhang C. SVMTriP: a method to predict antigenic epitopes using support vector machine to integrate tri-peptide similarity and propensity. *PLoS One* (2012) 7(9):e45152. doi:10.1371/journal.pone.0045152
16. Gupta S, Ansari HR, Gautam A; Open Source Drug Discovery Consortium, Raghava GP. Identification of B-cell epitopes in an antigen for inducing specific class of antibodies. *Biol Direct* (2013) 8:27. doi:10.1186/1745-6150-8-27
17. Singh H, Ansari HR, Raghava GP. Improved method for linear B-cell epitope prediction using antigen's primary sequence. *PLoS One* (2013) 8(5):e62216. doi:10.1371/journal.pone.0062216
18. Schisler NJ, Palmer JD. The IDB and IEDB: intron sequence and evolution databases. *Nucleic Acids Res* (2000) 28(1):181–4. doi:10.1093/nar/28.1.181
19. Vita R, Overton JA, Greenbaum JA, Ponomarenko J, Clark JD, Cantrell JR, et al. The immune epitope database (IEDB) 3.0. *Nucleic Acids Res* (2015) 43(Database issue):D405–12. doi:10.1093/nar/gku938
20. Song J, Wang H, Wang J, Leier A, Marquez-Lago T, Yang B, et al. PhosphoPredict: a bioinformatics tool for prediction of human kinase-specific phosphorylation substrates and sites by integrating heterogeneous feature selection. *Sci Rep* (2017) 7(1):6862. doi:10.1038/s41598-017-07199-4
21. Song J, Tan H, Wang M, Webb GI, Akutsu T. TANGLE: two-level support vector regression approach for protein backbone torsion angle prediction from primary sequences. *PLoS One* (2012) 7(2):e30361. doi:10.1371/journal.pone.0030361
22. Dubchak I, Muchnik I, Holbrook SR, Kim S-H. Prediction of protein folding class using global description of amino acid sequence. *Proc Natl Acad Sci U S A* (1995) 92(19):8700–4. doi:10.1073/pnas.92.19.8700
23. Manavalan B, Basith S, Choi YM, Lee G, Choi S. Structure-function relationship of cytoplasmic and nuclear IkappaB proteins: an in silico analysis. *PLoS One* (2010) 5(12):e15782. doi:10.1371/journal.pone.0015782
24. Kawashima S, Pokarowski P, Pokarowska M, Kolinski A, Katayama T, Kanehisa M. AAindex: amino acid index database, progress report 2008. *Nucleic Acids Res* (2007) 36(Suppl_1):D202–5. doi:10.1093/nar/gkm998
25. Saha I, Maulik U, Bandyopadhyay S, Plewczynski D. Fuzzy clustering of physicochemical and biochemical properties of amino acids. *Amino Acids* (2012) 43(2):583–94. doi:10.1007/s00726-011-1106-9
26. Mathura VS, Kolippakkam D. APDbase: amino acid physico-chemical properties database. *Bioinformation* (2005) 1(1):2–4. doi:10.6026/97320630001002
27. Kringelum JV, Nielsen M, Padkjaer SB, Lund O. Structural analysis of B-cell epitopes in antibody:protein complexes. *Mol Immunol* (2013) 53(1–2):24–34. doi:10.1016/j.molimm.2012.06.001
28. Mendes-Moreira J, Soares C, Jorge AM, Sousa JFD. Ensemble approaches for regression: a survey. *ACM Computing Surveys (CSUR)* (2012) 45(1):10. doi:10.1145/2379776.2379786
29. García-Pedrajas N, Hervás-Martínez C, Ortiz-Boyer D. Cooperative coevolution of artificial neural network ensembles for pattern classification. *IEEE Trans Evol Comput* (2005) 9(3):271–302. doi:10.1109/TEVC.2005.844158
30. Agrawal P, Bhalla S, Chaudhary K, Kumar R, Sharma M, Raghava GP. In Silico approach for prediction of antifungal peptides. *Front Microbiol* (2018) 9:323. doi:10.3389/fmicb.2018.00323
31. Sicho M, de Bruyn Kops C, Stork C, Svozil D, Kirchmair J. FAME 2: simple and effective machine learning model of cytochrome P450 regioselectivity. *J Chem Inf Model* (2017) 57(8):1832–46. doi:10.1021/acs.jcim.7b00250
32. McNemar Q. Note on the sampling error of the difference between correlated proportions or percentages. *Psychometrika* (1947) 12(2):153–7. doi:10.1007/BF02295996
33. Basith S, Manavalan B, Gosu V, Choi S. Evolutionary, structural and functional interplay of the IkappaB family members. *PLoS One* (2013) 8(1):e54178. doi:10.1371/journal.pone.0054178
34. Basith S, Manavalan B, Govindaraj RG, Choi S. In silico approach to inhibition of signaling pathways of toll-like receptors 2 and 4 by ST2L. *PLoS One* (2011) 6(8):e23989. doi:10.1371/journal.pone.0023989
35. Govindaraj RG, Manavalan B, Basith S, Choi S. Comparative analysis of species-specific ligand recognition in toll-like receptor 8 signaling: a hypothesis. *PLoS One* (2011) 6(9):e25118. doi:10.1371/journal.pone.0025118
36. Govindaraj RG, Manavalan B, Lee G, Choi S. Molecular modeling-based evaluation of hTLR10 and identification of potential ligands in Toll-like receptor signaling. *PLoS One* (2010) 5(9):e12713. doi:10.1371/journal.pone.0012713
37. Manavalan B, Govindaraj R, Lee G, Choi S. Molecular modeling-based evaluation of dual function of IkappaBzeta ankyrin repeat domain in toll-like receptor signaling. *J Mol Recognit* (2011) 24(4):597–607. doi:10.1002/jmr.1085
38. Manavalan B, Murugapiran SK, Lee G, Choi S. Molecular modeling of the reductase domain to elucidate the reaction mechanism of reduction of peptidyl thioester into its corresponding alcohol in non-ribosomal peptide synthetases. *BMC Struct Biol* (2010) 10:1. doi:10.1186/1472-6807-10-1
39. EL-Manzalawy Y, Dobbs D, Honavar V. Predicting linear B-cell epitopes using string kernels. *J Mol Recogn* (2008) 21(4):243–55. doi:10.1002/jmr.893
40. Lian Y, Ge M, Pan XM. EPMLR: sequence-based linear B-cell epitope prediction method using multiple linear regression. *BMC Bioinformatics* (2014) 15:414. doi:10.1186/s12859-014-0414-y
41. El-Manzalawy Y, Dobbs D, Honavar V. Predicting flexible length linear B-cell epitopes. *Comput Syst Bioinformatics Conf* (2008) 7:121–32. doi:10.1142/9781848162648_0011
42. Larsen JE, Lund O, Nielsen M. Improved method for predicting linear B-cell epitopes. *Immunome Res* (2006) 2:2. doi:10.1186/1745-7580-2-2
43. Ponomarenko J, Bui HH, Li W, Fusseder N, Bourne PE, Sette A, et al. ElliPro: a new structure-based tool for the prediction of antibody epitopes. *BMC Bioinformatics* (2008) 9:514. doi:10.1186/1471-2105-9-514
44. Zhang W, Xiong Y, Zhao M, Zou H, Ye X, Liu J. Prediction of conformational B-cell epitopes from 3D structures by random forests with a distance-based feature. *BMC Bioinformatics* (2011) 12:341. doi:10.1186/1471-2105-12-341
45. Kringelum JV, Lundegaard C, Lund O, Nielsen M. Reliable B cell epitope predictions: impacts of method development and improved benchmarking. *PLoS Comput Biol* (2012) 8(12):e1002829. doi:10.1371/journal.pcbi.1002829
46. Qi T, Qiu T, Zhang Q, Tang K, Fan Y, Qiu J, et al. SEPPA 2.0 – more refined server to predict spatial epitope considering species of immune host and

subcellular localization of protein antigen. *Nucleic Acids Res* (2014) 42(Web Server issue):W59–63. doi:10.1093/nar/gku395
47. Manavalan B, Basith S, Shin TH, Choi S, Kim MO, Lee G. MLACP: machine-learning-based prediction of anticancer peptides. *Oncotarget* (2017) 8(44): 77121–36. doi:10.18632/oncotarget.20365
48. Gautam A, Chaudhary K, Kumar R, Raghava GP. Computer-aided virtual screening and designing of cell-penetrating peptides. *Methods Mol Biol* (2015) 1324:59–69. doi:10.1007/978-1-4939-2806-4_4
49. Rahman Kh S, Chowdhury EU, Sachse K, Kaltenboeck B. Inadequate reference datasets biased toward short non-epitopes confound B-cell epitope prediction. *J Biol Chem* (2016) 291(28):14585–99. doi:10.1074/jbc.M116.729020
50. Porto W, Pires A, Franco O. Computational tools for exploring sequence databases as a resource for antimicrobial peptides. *Biotechnol Adv* (2017) 35(3):337–49. doi:10.1016/j.biotechadv.2017.02.001
51. Hedén LO, Frithz E, Lindahl G. Molecular characterization of an IgA receptor from group B streptococci: sequence of the gene, identification of a proline-rich region with unique structure and isolation of N-terminal fragments with IgA-binding capacity. *Eur J Immunol* (1991) 21(6):1481–90. doi:10.1002/eji.1830210623
52. Jerlström P, Chhatwal G, Timrnis K. The IgA-binding β antigen of the c protein complex of group B streptococci: sequence determination of its gene and detection of two binding regions. *Mol Microbiol* (1991) 5(4):843–9. doi:10.1111/j.1365-2958.1991.tb00757.x
53. Chen W, Feng P, Yang H, Ding H, Lin H, Chou K-C. iRNA-3typeA: identifying 3-types of modification at RNA's adenosine sites. *Mol Ther Nucleic Acids* (2018) 11:468–74. doi:10.1016/j.omtn.2018.03.012
54. Manavalan B, Shin TH, Kim MO, Lee G. AIPpred: sequence-based prediction of anti-inflammatory peptides using random forest. *Front Pharmacol* (2018) 9:276. doi:10.3389/fphar.2018.00276
55. Manavalan B, Shin TH, Lee G. PVP-SVM: sequence-based prediction of phage virion proteins using a support vector machine. *Front Microbiol* (2018) 9:476. doi:10.3389/fmicb.2018.00476
56. Manavalan B, Shin TH, Lee G. DHSpred: support-vector-machine-based human DNase I hypersensitive sites prediction using the optimal features selected by random forest. *Oncotarget* (2018) 9(2):1944–56. doi:10.18632/oncotarget.23099
57. Manavalan B, Subramaniyam S, Shin TH, Kim MO, Lee G. Machine-learning-based prediction of cell-penetrating peptides and their uptake efficiency with improved accuracy. *J Proteome Res* (2018). doi:10.1021/acs.jproteome.8b00148
58. Su ZD, Huang Y, Zhang ZY, Zhao YW, Wang D, Chen W, et al. iLoc-lncRNA: predict the subcellular location of lncRNAs by incorporating octamer composition into general PseKNC. *Bioinformatics* (2018) bty508. doi:10.1093/bioinformatics/bty508
59. Bhadra P, Yan J, Li J, Fong S, Siu SWI. AmPEP: sequence-based prediction of antimicrobial peptides using distribution patterns of amino acid properties and random forest. *Sci Rep* (2018) 8(1):1697. doi:10.1038/s41598-018-19752-w
60. Rayhan F, Ahmed S, Shatabda S, Farid DM, Mousavian Z, Dehzangi A, et al. iDTI-ESBoost: identification of drug target interaction using evolutionary and structural features with boosting. *Sci Rep* (2017) 7(1):17731. doi:10.1038/s41598-017-18025-2
61. Lee J, Basith S, Cui M, Kim B, Choi S. In silico prediction of multiple-category classification model for cytochrome P450 inhibitors and non-inhibitors using machine-learning method. *SAR QSAR Environ Res* (2017) 28(10):863–74. doi:10.1080/1062936X.2017.1399925
62. Chou KC, Shen HB. Signal-CF: a subsite-coupled and window-fusing approach for predicting signal peptides. *Biochem Biophys Res Commun* (2007) 357(3):633–40. doi:10.1016/j.bbrc.2007.03.162
63. Chou KC, Shen HB. MemType-2L: a web server for predicting membrane proteins and their types by incorporating evolution information through Pse-PSSM. *Biochem Biophys Res Commun* (2007) 360(2):339–45. doi:10.1016/j.bbrc.2007.06.027
64. Lin WZ, Fang JA, Xiao X, Chou KC. iLoc-animal: a multi-label learning classifier for predicting subcellular localization of animal proteins. *Mol Biosyst* (2013) 9(4):634–44. doi:10.1039/c3mb25466f
65. Liu B, Long R, Chou KC. iDHS-EL: identifying DNase I hypersensitive sites by fusing three different modes of pseudo nucleotide composition into an ensemble learning framework. *Bioinformatics* (2016) 32(16):2411–8. doi:10.1093/bioinformatics/btw186
66. Ponomarenko JV, Bourne PE. Antibody-protein interactions: benchmark datasets and prediction tools evaluation. *BMC Struct Biol* (2007) 7:64. doi:10.1186/1472-6807-7-64

# 9

# Beyond Hot Spots: Biases in Antibody Somatic Hypermutation and Implications for Vaccine Design

*Chaim A. Schramm* and Daniel C. Douek**

*Vaccine Research Center, National Institute of Allergy and Infectious Diseases, NIH, Bethesda, MD, United States*

***Correspondence:**
*Chaim A. Schramm*
*chaim.schramm@nih.gov;*
*Daniel C. Douek*
*ddouek@mail.nih.gov*

The evolution of antibodies in an individual during an immune response by somatic hypermutation (SHM) is essential for the ability of the immune system to recognize and remove the diverse spectrum of antigens that may be encountered. These mutations are not produced at random; nucleotide motifs that result in increased or decreased rates of mutation were first reported in 1992. Newer models that estimate the propensity for mutation for every possible 5- or 7-nucleotide motif have emphasized the complexity of SHM targeting and suggested possible new hot spot motifs. Even with these fine-grained approaches, however, non-local context matters, and the mutations observed at a specific nucleotide motif varies between species and even by locus, gene segment, and position along the gene segment within a single species. An alternative method has been provided to further abstract away the molecular mechanisms underpinning SHM, prompted by evidence that certain stereotypical amino acid substitutions are favored at each position of a particular *V* gene. These "substitution profiles," whether obtained from a single B cell lineage or an entire repertoire, offer a simplified approach to predict which substitutions will be well-tolerated and which will be disfavored, without the need to consider path-dependent effects from neighboring positions. However, this comes at the cost of merging the effects of two distinct biological processes, the generation of mutations, and the selection acting on those mutations. Since selection is contingent on the particular antigens an individual has been exposed to, this suggests that SHM may have evolved to prefer mutations that are most likely to be useful against pathogens that have co-evolved with us. Alternatively, the ability to select favorable mutations may be strongly limited by the biases of SHM targeting. In either scenario, the sequence space explored by SHM is significantly limited and this consequently has profound implications for the rational design of vaccine strategies.

**Keywords: somatic hypermutation, hot spot motifs, affinity maturation, substitution profiles, vaccine design**

## INTRODUCTION

In order to combat an arbitrarily large number of unknown pathogens, the humoral immune system relies on three mechanisms to generate diversity in antibody variable domains. In the primary repertoire, combinatorial diversity is created by the random joining of germline-encoded *V*, *D*, and *J* heavy chain or *V* and *J* light chain gene segments. During this process, junctional diversity is also introduced through the action of exonucleases and terminal deoxynucleotidyl transferase. This results in an estimated $10^{15}$–$10^{18}$ possible unique naive B cell (1, 2). Furthermore, upon encountering cognate antigen, a naive B cell can enter a germinal center and begin to undergo somatic hypermutation (SHM), increasing the number of realizable antibodies by several additional orders of magnitude. However, the total number of circulating B cells in a human is only ~$10^9$ (3, 4), meaning that if all possible antibodies were equally likely to be made, the odds of correctly producing one capable of binding to and clearing a particular antigen would be minuscule. In fact, precisely such arguments were initially used to argue against the "somatic" theory of antibody diversity predicting the existence of SHM (5). Hood and Talmage even pointed out that potential number of wasted mutations alone (i.e., those leading to non-functional antibodies and cell death) would far exceed the total number of cells thought to be produced over a human lifetime (6).

Nonetheless, the immune system has also evolved mechanisms for biasing the generation of diversity in ways, which presumably optimize the search for effective antibodies. For instance, different *V* gene segments are used at different frequencies (7, 8) and certain *D* genes may be more often recombined with specific *J* genes (9, 10). Many studies have shown that the parameters governing recombination vary dramatically from a uniform distribution and are generally reproducible between individuals (2, 11–14). Indeed, they appear to be optimized to produce B cells that can pass tolerance checkpoints and mature into naive B cells (2).

The SHM process is similarly biased. Soon after the first experimental confirmations of SHM (15, 16), it was quickly noted that mutations are more clustered together than random expectation (17) and fall into intrinsic hot spots (18, 19). Since the discovery of activation-induced cytidine deaminase (AID), the enzyme that initiates SHM by deaminating cytidine to uridine (20–22), much progress has been made in understanding the molecular origins of these biases. Many factors have been described that participate in targeting AID activity to the Ig loci by associating it with enhancer transcription and polymerase stalling [reviewed in Ref. (23–25)]. Studies of the specificity loop of AID (26–28) have elucidated the basis for the preferential deaminations of cytidines within specific microsequence motifs. Finally, investigations of uracil-DNA glycosylase, MutSα, DNA polymerase η, and many other components of the base excision and mismatch repair pathways have revealed some of the mechanisms behind patterns of mutations other than the C→T transitions generated directly by AID [reviewed in Ref. (25, 29, 30)].

The study of AID and other molecular components of the SHM machinery has always been complemented and even driven by computational approaches. For instance, the two-phase model of SHM (deamination by AID, followed by removal of the resulting uracil and error-prone repair) was first proposed in response to the observation that SHM is more focused on RGYW (where R is A or G; Y is C or T; and W is A or T) hot spots in MSH2-deficient mice (31). Similarly, the role of DNA polymerase η was deduced in part by comparing the motifs mutated by that enzyme to the WA hot spot motifs observed in SHM (32).

In addition, computational analysis can be clarifying, abstracting away molecular details to reveal higher level patterns such as the canonical RGYW hot spot motif itself. Recent work has suggested that the repertoire of nucleotide mutations generated by SHM can be further abstracted to amino acid substitution profiles (33, 34). These profiles point toward a new, simpler avenue for predictive analyses of the immune system, such as understanding potential responses to a specific vaccine immunogen. Here, we review the history, use, and limitations of microsequence motifs for predicting the targeting of SHM; the evidence that evolution has focused the SHM machinery toward producing specific types of amino acid changes at specific positions; the emerging use of substitution profiles and other similar predictive frameworks (FWR) for amino acid usages, along with their potential challenges and limitations; and how substitution profiles might find use in rational vaccine design.

## MICROSEQUENCE MOTIFS

The idea that the diversity of antibody specificities could be attributed to ongoing accumulation of genetic mutations in proliferating lymphocytes was first proposed by Lederberg (35). Brenner and Milstein then suggested a mechanism based on DNA cleavage targeted to specific genetic loci, followed by exonuclease activity and error-prone repair (36). After the emergence of experimental support for this hypothesis (17, 37), analogy to the action of known mutagenic agents led Rogozin and Kolchanov to examine the possible influence of neighboring bases on the occurrences of mutations in antibodies. This resulted in the discovery of the now-canonical RGYW/WRCY hot spot motif (where the underline indicates the mutated base), as well as the apparently equally mutable TAA motif (38). Later, a disfavored cold spot motif of SYC (where S is C or G) was also reported (39).

However, despite the usefulness of the WRCY and TAA motifs, only about 30% of observed SHMs fall into such hot spots (38). Moreover, it quickly became clear that not all 8 WRCY sequences were equally "hot," with AGCT being favored (19, 40–42) and AGCC or TGCG being disfavored (43, 44). At various times, WRCH (where H is A, C, or T) (45), WRCR (46), and WRCW (47) have been suggested as more accurate motifs, with the WRC thought to be the core motif (39, 46), with the last base possibly influencing the choice of repair pathways (45). Similarly, the originally proposed TAA motif was later refined to WA (32). In addition, other potential hot spot motifs have been suggested, such as CRCY and ATCT (48).

Another approach has been to explicitly calculate mutation rates for each possible nucleotide sequence of a given length. In the first such study, Smith estimated the relative mutability for all possible di- and trinucleotide motifs using downstream Jκ sequences from mouse hybridoma lines, concluding that the dinucleotides explained most of the variation in mutational targeting (40). They later extended this analysis to mouse and human heavy chains (49) and human kappa chains (50), using non-productive rearrangements instead of intronic sequences to calculate mutabilities in humans (49, 50). They found broad similarity between species and between heavy and kappa (49, 50), while a later analysis of non-productive human IgL sequences with higher mutation levels suggested substantial differences from IgH (51). Ohm-Laursen used non-productive rearrangements of

$V_H$3-23 with $J_H$4 or $J_H$6 to derive a quartet model and showed that the frequency of mutation at specific motifs in the D and J genes correlated well with those in the V gene (43). A different quartet model used the V gene region of all publicly available antibody sequences and modeled the effects of the flanking nucleotides as independent from the position of the mutation itself (52). These authors found a high correlation of observed quartet mutation frequencies (~0.7) between heavy and light chains and between human and mouse antibodies. However, the full model could only explain around half of the variation in mutation frequencies in the real data (52).

More recently, with the advent of high-throughput sequencing technologies, attempts have been made to build out more finely discriminatory models. Yaari constructed a 5 nucleotide motif model using only synonymous mutations from functional sequences (44). The frequency at which each motif was targeted was highly correlated between individuals (~0.9), but the correlation between expected and observed mutations was only 0.67. Moreover, 46% of possible 5-mer motifs were not observed directly and had to be estimated from other similar motifs (44). The same group also immunized mice transgenic for the B1-8 heavy chain with (4-hydroxy-3-nitrophenyl)acetyl, which produces a response heavily biased toward λ chain usage (53). They sequenced the non-productive kappa chains from these animals and confirmed that the 5-mer mutation frequencies from functional and non-functional sequences correlated well with each other (48). They also built 5-mer models for mouse heavy chains and human light chains, finding an overall correlation of only 0.63 between the species. Specifically, C:G base pairs were observed to be more likely to mutate in mice and also to have a higher probability to result in a transition substitution than in humans (48).

To overcome the limitation of motifs that do not appear in the repertoire of germline Ig sequences, Elhanati et al. constructed a 7-nucleotide position weight matrix (PWM) that treats each position independently, finding a correlation of 0.8 between predicted and observed mutations frequencies (2). A later refinement of this model also calculated 7-mer PWMs for *D* and *J* gene-derived nucleotides, finding that those differed sharply from the PWMs learned for *V* genes (54). Another new approach, termed "samm," uses a proportional hazards model with a lasso penalty and a flexible motif dictionary to extract the most important features and construct motifs accordingly (55). When used to build a 5-mer motif model and compared directly to Cui et al. (48), the results are similar, but samm tended to discount the effect of the final nucleotide, inferring only 382 unique mutability values instead of 1,015 (55).

In addition to calculating the frequency of mutations at each motif, many groups have investigated the resulting mutation spectrums, or the relative rates of mutation to each possible destination nucleotide. Although a preference for transitions over transversions was first reported in the early 1990s (19, 56), Cowell and Kepler were the first to report a dependency on neighboring bases for mutations spectrums (57). They found that both nucleotides in a homodimer have an increased propensity for transitions, while AT and TA dinucleotides have a preference to mutate to AA or TT homodimers (57). Ohm-Laursen calculated mutation spectrums for all 4-nucleotide motifs (43), but did not specifically analyze the effects of context. The quartet model of Cohen calculated mutation frequencies independently for each possible destination nucleotide, finding that the particular substitution had as much impact on the variability of mutation frequencies as did the microsequence context (52). Several other groups have calculated mutation spectrums, as well (2, 44, 48, 54) though those authors all deemphasized mutation spectrums compared to mutation frequencies or general properties of the antibody repertoire. This is due to the fact that mutation spectrums are considered less computationally tractable, as the underlying molecular machinery is significantly more complex and less well understood. In addition, they have been thought to be less useful, as the observed substitutions are presumed to be heavily influenced by selection for antigen binding, which acts on the amino acid sequence. One attempt has been made to parameterize an amino acid substitution matrix for antibodies (58), which does not compare favorably to real data when used to simulate SHM (33).

Even extended to 5- and 7-nucleotide motifs, microsequence context can only account for 70–80% of variability in mutation frequencies (2, 44, 52, 54). Much of the residual variation appears to be due to positional effects within the antibody sequence. Differences between FWR and complementarity determining regions (CDR) have been reported (49, 50, 52, 59), and regional variation can be observed even in non-Ig transgenes (59). In addition, mutation frequencies for the same sequence decay exponentially with distance from the transcription start site (60). In addition, differences between the heavy, kappa, and lambda chain loci are consistently observed (48, 49, 51, 52). The complex interdependence among all of these factors suggests that an evolutionary balancing has optimized the types and distributions of mutations produced by SHM.

## EVOLUTIONARY OPTIMIZATION OF SHM

One of the primary selective pressures driving antibody gene evolution is the need for functional diversity. Antibody genes were originally thought to be subject to "coincidental" or "concerted" evolution, as seen for other multigene families like ribosomal RNA and histone genes, with diversity generated by unequal crossing over and/or gene conversion (61, 62). However, an early study of the phylogenetic relationships between mouse and human $V_H$ genes suggested that the rate of $V_H$ gene duplication would have to be over 100-fold lower than for other multigene families (63). Later, studies with access to more sequences from more species were able to show that V gene evolution is instead governed by a "birth-and-death" process, which results in a more dynamic and diverse repertoire between species (64, 65). Within $V_H$ genes, moreover, the germline sequences of the CDRs, but not FWRs, are under diversifying selection (63, 66). In addition, SHM is itself an evolutionarily ancient diversification mechanism, preceding the emergence of combinatorial *V(D)J* joining and the full diversification of $V_H$ genes (67). SHM has been observed *in vivo* in the horn shark (67), and AID orthologs with *in vitro* deaminase activity have been isolated from cartilaginous fish (68) and even jawless vertebrates (69). Although all of the AID orthologs tested retained a general preference for WRC motifs over non-WRC substrates, the exact microsequence specificity varied substantially (68), suggesting co-evolution of the SHM machinery with antibody gene sequences to optimize the humoral immune response.

The interplay between evolution of the primary sequences of the germline repertoire and the biased mechanisms of SHM can also be seen in the fact that the codon composition of CDRs make them more prone to replacement mutations, while the structurally important FWRs use codons that are biased toward silent mutations (70–72). Similarly, Wagner et al. found that highly mutable AGY codons are preferentially used to encode serines in CDRs, while less mutable TCN codons tend to appear in FWRs (73). Kepler reported a general difference in codon usage between CDRs and FWRs, which was strongly correlated with differential mutability (74). Moreover, both the specific serine bias (75–77) and the general codon bias (78) appear to be phylogenetically conserved, emphasizing the importance of plasticity in the CDRs. In fact, recent work has demonstrated that AGC hot spot triplets in the CDRs are specifically conserved in the serine reading frame (79). These codons are exceptionally plastic, and mutated AGY serine codons are disproportionately involved in antigen contacts seen in crystal structures (79).

Shaping of the action of SHM extends beyond differences between CDRs and FWRs. For instance, Zheng et al. showed that C→T transitions are predominantly silent, and that those which would lead to replacement mutations are found primarily in cold spots (80). A similar, though less strict, distribution was reported for G→A transitions. Those authors speculate that this pattern might have evolved to keep mutations created directly by AID from overwhelming those caused by error-prone repair in phase II (80).

Somatic hypermutation is also targeted to be able to introduce gross structural changes to antibodies in a favorable way. For instance, mutations are frequently observed in human Vκ1-derived antibodies at two FWR positions, which affect inter-domain dynamics and enhance thermostability (81). Similarly, sequences that can give rise to an NxS/T glycosylation motif with only one nucleotide change are concentrated in the antigen-proximal loops of the variable domains (82).

Evolution appears to shape the naive repertoire, as well. Recent work has demonstrated that observed biases in the usages of various V gene segments correlates with the predisposition of each gene to focus SHM toward its CDRs (72). More generally, the likelihood that the antibody encoded by an immature B cell can survive central tolerance and get selected into the naive repertoire correlates with the likelihood of that sequence being generated by the recombination machinery in the first place (2). In a similar vein, mouse antibodies have substantially less $D_H$ gene variation and junctional diversity than humans, which has been hypothesized to overcome the limitations of a numerically small B cell population by focusing the naive repertoire on the most critical specificities (83).

Even in humans, these biases allow the development of stereotyped antibodies, specific recombinations using particular genetic elements that can be reproducibly elicited by a particular antigen (12). These stereotyped antibodies can even target complex antigens such as influenza HA (84–86) and HIV Env (87, 88). In addition to stereotyped genes, the antibody response can reproducibly make use of specific amino acid substitutions generated by SHM. This had been observed in both mice (18, 89) and humans (84, 85, 90), and even when the mutation in question occurs in a cold spot of AID activity (91). Moreover, substitutions that appeared in $V_H$1-46-derived antibodies targeting the CD4-binding site of HIV Env from multiple donors were also observed in $V_H$1-46-derived antibodies from HIV-uninfected donors (92). This demonstrates that shared substitutions can occur in the selected functional repertoire even without a common antigen and may reflect the way that the SHM machinery has evolved to sample the mutations that are most likely to be useful.

## SUBSTITUTION PROFILES

It seems counterintuitive that *a priori* predictions can be made about the state of the selected functional repertoire without reference to the antigens that have driven that selection. However, the number of unique clones in which a particular position has been substituted is correlated with the diversity of germline amino acids available at that position, in both CDRs and FWRs (93). Strikingly, the diversity of substitutions at changed positions is also correlated with germline diversity, though the diversity of the germline amino acids is less than that of the substitutions (93). While this at least partially reflects the structural constraints of the antibody domain, the physicochemical properties of the observed substitutions did not generally parallel those of the germline residues at the same positions (93).

In fact, the diversity of the observed substitutions is constrained not only by the diversity of all germline genes at a position but specifically by the particular gene from which the antibody was derived (33, 34) (**Figure 1**). As seen in studies of microsequence motifs (44) and *V(D)J* recombination (2, 11, 13, 91, 94), these substitution profiles are stable between individuals and across time (33). Similar findings have been reported both for sequences isolated from peripheral memory B cells (33) and from bone marrow cells (34). Both substitution frequency and the diversity of observed substitutions are generally higher in CDRs than in FWRs, though several FWR positions have substitution profiles similar to those characteristic of CDRs (33, 34). In addition, assorted $V_H$ genes accumulate substitutions in CDRH1 versus CDRH2 at different rates, and similar variations appear in the preferred locations of insertions and deletions (34).

Many expected factors contribute to the observed substitution profiles. For instance, the frequencies of substitution are generally lower at structurally important residues such as the charge cluster (95), though individual genes may display higher rates, as for R95 of $V_H$1-8 (34) [residue numberings are reported using the IMGT convention (96)]. Similarly, when a particular gene carries a residue that is distinct from other genes in its $V_H$ family (e.g., L71 in $V_H$1-18 and T46 of $V_H$1-8), substitutions at that positions are frequently biased toward the germline residue(s) encoded by the other members of the gene's family (in this case, F and P, respectively) (34). The presence or absence of a microsequence hot spot also clearly impacts the observed differential substitution rates at some positions, such as S29 in $V_H$5-51, which forms an

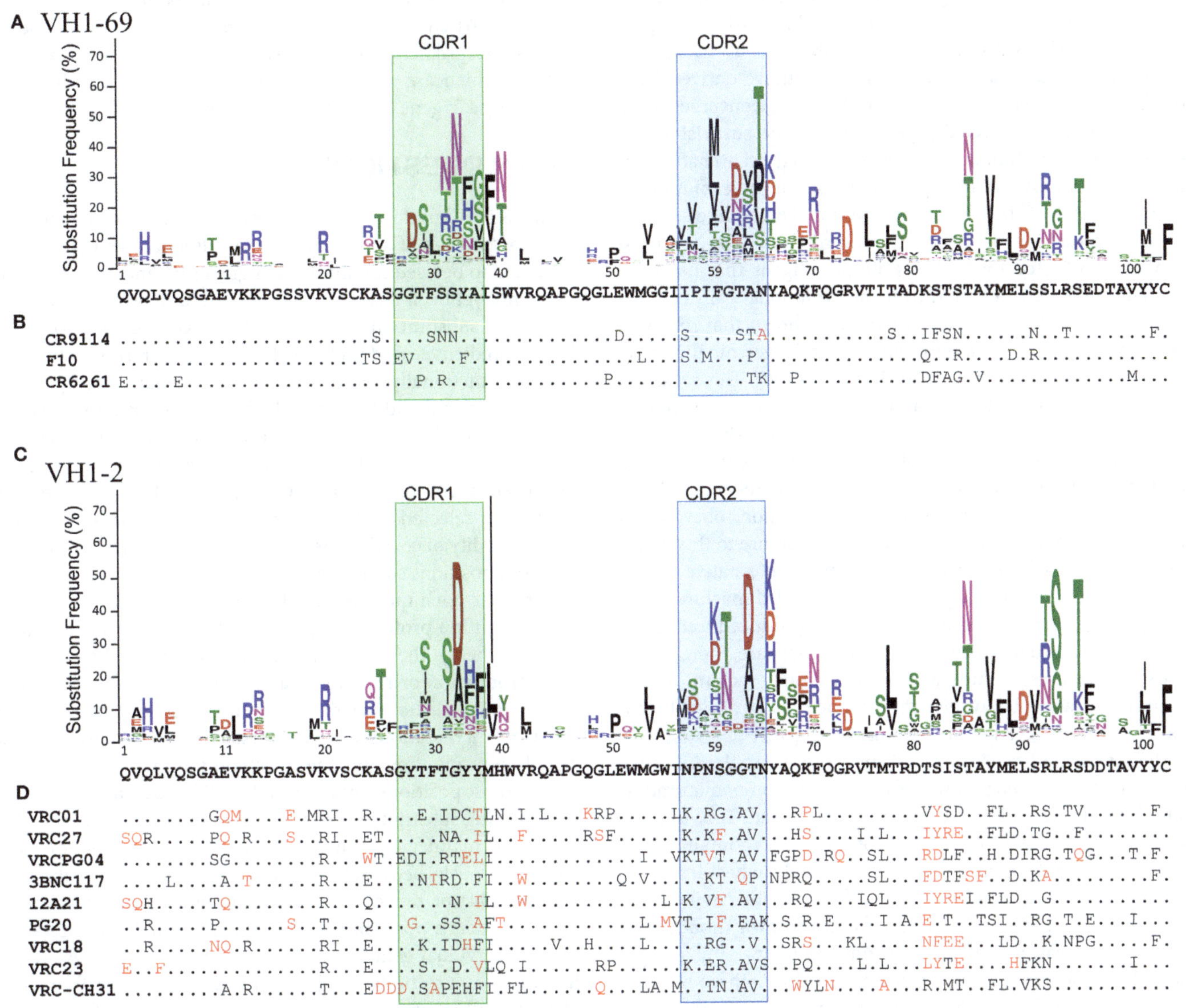


**FIGURE 1** | Substitution profiles and the accumulation of rare mutations. **(A)** Substitution profile of VH1-69 as calculated by Sheng et al. (33). The germline amino acid sequence is shown below the logo plot. **(B)** Sequence alignment of VH1-69-derived influenza antibodies capable of neutralizing multiple subtypes. Dots indicate the germline amino acid and extremely rare substitutions [as defined in Ref. (33)] are shown in red. **(C)** Substitution profile of VH1-2. **(D)** Sequence alignment of VH1-2-derived broadly neutralizing HIV antibodies targeting the CD4 binding site. Each contains greater than ~20% or more extremely rare substitutions.

AGCT hot spot and diversifies extensively, while the same serine in $V_H4$ genes is encoded by a TCC codon and mutates only rarely (34). However, it cannot account for all such differences; for instance, R80 in $V_H1$-8 diversifies extensively despite the absence of a canonical hot spot, while the equivalent arginine in $V_H3$ genes is almost complete conserved, without the presence of an AID cold spot (34). Simulations indicate that microsequence motifs can account for about 70% of the variation in substitution frequencies, similar to previous reports (44), but only about 50% of the variation when the identity of the substitutions is included (33). Another contributing factor to substitution profiles is the fact that observed substitutions are typically those that can be reached by a single nucleotide change. However, the same codon can have substantially different profiles even in a highly similar sequence context. Thus, the TCC codon encoding S83 of $V_H1$-2 is most likely to be substituted to A, followed by T and P, while the most likely substitutions for S83 of $V_H1$-46 are P and F, followed by A (33). Furthermore, while biases in substitutions are somewhat correlated with the physicochemical similarity between the germline amino acid and the observed substitution, many commonly seen substitutions are non-conservative, and even conservative substitutions are frequently asymmetric (e.g., E→D and K→R substitutions are more likely to occur than D→E and R→K substitutions, respectively) (33, 97).

In addition to highly significant similarities in substitution profiles between individuals with presumably distinct antigen-exposure histories, substitution profiles observed in the selected functional repertoire are also correlated to those derived from non-functional passenger alleles (33). This convergence of the selected and unselected repertoires is quite surprising and implies stricter limitations on the action of SHM than had previously been understood. One possibility is that the evolutionary optimizations described above are fine-tuned enough to strongly bias the production of mutations toward those that are most likely to be selected for by the suite of antigens that has been most commonly encountered over the evolutionary history of a species (33). In this vein, recent work has shown that relatively low-affinity antibody lineages can persist in germinal centers responding to complex protein antigens (98–100). This results in a memory response with increased clonal diversity compared to that generated by haptens, and it has been hypothesized that this diversity enhances the capacity of the immune system to respond to future challenges from novel but structurally related antigens (101). It may be that the characteristic substitutions observed in substitution profiles serve to optimize the structure to this diversity. An additional, perhaps complementary, alternative is that the biases in the mutations produced by the SHM machinery are strong enough that most mutations are not produced frequently enough to be acted upon by selection. In either case, there would appear to be drastic implications for rational vaccine design efforts, as certain substitutions may not be reliably available in a typical repertoire, even with an optimal antigen.

More generally, the existence of substitution profiles indicates that there are preferred pathways for antibody affinity maturation that depend powerfully on the germline gene used. This, in turn, suggests that germline-based substitution profiles contain useful information about which substitutions are likely to be tolerated at each position, which can be leveraged for antibody engineering. As most engineering efforts begin from a known monoclonal antibody, a narrower substitution profile, encompassing a single antibody lineage, may be of particular use (102). These lineage-specific substitution profiles are expected to be different from gene-specific substitution profiles (33), but may better reflect the constraints of binding to a specific antigen. They also provide an opportunity to extract information about which substitutions can be tolerated at positions in CDR3 and FWR4, which are absent in V gene-specific profiles. Frequently, however, the antibody that is being engineered is the only known member of its lineage; even when deep repertoire sampling is done with high-throughput sequencing, most lineages are represented by only one or a few members (103).

A new program named SPURF attempts to overcome that limitation by combining several types of substitution profiles derived from a large public data set to predict the substitution profile of an antibody lineage from the sequence of a single member (102). In training the SPURF model, the authors found that the most important sources of information are the *V* gene-specific substitution profile and the inferred naive sequence, in addition to the input sequence itself. They also use a gene-family substitution profile (i.e., derived from all $V_H1$ genes, etc.) and a substitution profile calculated from simulations of neutral mutation of the inferred naive sequence using the S5F model from reference (44, 102). In particular, the inclusion of the inferred naive sequence allows the prediction of a substitution profile for CDR3 and FWR4, which are not encoded by the *V* gene and, therefore, missed by a *V* gene-specific profile alone.

## OPEN QUESTIONS

While SPURF performs well predicting the lineage-specific substitution profiles of an out-of-sample validation set (102) and is designed to be used for antibody engineering and improvement, it has not yet been tested in that context. Similarly, it remains to be seen if substitution profiles can be successfully incorporated into a predictive model of SHM. And while rare substitutions can be functionally important (104), systematic comparisons of the structural and biophysical effects of common versus rare substitutions are ongoing. In addition, substitution profiles treat the mutations observed at each position as being independent. However, recent work suggests that affinity-enhancing mutations may be co-selected with structurally stabilizing ones (105), and the possibility of correlations between the substitution profiles of different positions should be investigated.

Another open question involves the effects of allelic variants on substitution profiles. Even silent polymorphisms could theoretically change the pattern of mutations generated by SHM by the introduction or removal of a microsequence hot spot. More importantly, allelic variants are sometimes distinguished by replacement mutations (e.g., G55 versus R55 in $V_H1$-69). Since the germline residue remains the most commonly observed amino acid at most positions, these variants will have a large impact on the resulting substitution profile. So far, this has been handled in an *ad hoc* manner, by either excluding genes from donors who have previously been determined to be heterozygous for such variants (34) or by collectively excluding all possible germline residues at each position from the substitution profile, irrespective of individual genotype (33). Since the germline residues at homologous positions in closely related genes are frequently observed substitutions (34), a more systematic way of investigating the effects of allelic variants is necessary. This is especially true as it has recently become clear that many such variants remain to be discovered (106–109).

Finally, one of the most striking findings about substitution profiles is the similarity of the selected and unselected repertoires. Yet, this observation rests on mere 650 non-productive rearrangements derived from a single $V_H$–$J_H$ gene pair (33, 110). Although the strong correlations between substitution profiles from different individuals also support the idea that SHM is capable of generating only a limited set of mutations, more data are needed to test this. Meanwhile, it is clear that mutation and selection are distinct biological processes. In order to avoid possible confounding effects of selection, studies of microsequence motifs have typically used sequences derived from introns, transgenes, or non-productive rearrangements; or, if using sequences from functional antibodies subject to selection, have included only silent mutations extracted from those data sets.

Separately, many efforts have been made to detect and quantify the action of selection on affinity maturation. Initially, these evaluated the frequency of replacement mutations observed in CDRs versus FWRs using a binomial (111) or multinomial (112) distribution. The binomial model has also been extended to account for codon biases that lead to a higher neutral rate of replacement mutations CDRs (70) and to account for general differences in mutability driven by microsequence context (113). However, determining the appropriate null distribution of replacement versus silent mutations in antibodies has proven challenging, as the intrinsic biases of SHM can give the appearance of selection (114) even when microsequence motifs are accounted for (113). One strategy for addressing this difficulty has been to use a focused binomial test examining the replacement mutations from only a single CDR or FWR at time, while using the silent mutations from all regions (115, 116). Another strategy exploited a large data set of non-productive rearrangements to normalize the ratio of replacement to silent mutations on a germline- and position-specific basis (94). Other recent advancements include the use of a log-odds ratio of the posterior distribution of the replacement mutation frequency compared to the expected distribution for the germline sequence, to quantify the strength of selection (117); the integration of phylogenetic information (118, 119); and estimation of the null distribution for the number of replacement mutations so that selection effects can be calculated for a single sequence (120).

While there is general agreement that purifying selection typically acts on FWRs, reports have been inconsistent as to whether diversifying selection acting on CDRs can (94, 115, 117) or cannot (114, 121) be detected at the repertoire level. Meanwhile, a review of available structural data found no relation between hot spot motifs and observed substitutions; the latter were instead strongly correlated with antigen contacts and contributions to calculated binding energy (122). In addition, a recent study found that the need to distinguish between closely related foreign and self antigens can drive the expansion of higher affinity clonal variants that remain subdominant in the absence of self antigen (123), demonstrating another way in which selection can influence the observed substitutions in a repertiore. On the other hand, an in-depth analysis of an antibody against influenza hemagglutinin found that mutability and selection synergized, such that replacement mutations expected to occur more frequently under a neutral model were also more like to be selected once generated (124). It is, therefore, clear that more work is needed to resolve when the effects of selection must be explicitly accounted for and when they can be implicitly included by the use of substitution profiles or other similar abstractions. Structural and biophysical characterizations of common versus rare substitutions should help resolve this question and will also be important for understanding the underlying biological mechanisms.

## VACCINE IMPLICATIONS

Reverse vaccinology 2.0 (125, 126) is a strategy for rational vaccine design that starts by characterizing the epitope targeted by an effective natural antibody and selecting or designing an immunogen that can elicit a similar antibody in other individuals. One particular implementation is lineage-based vaccine design, which attempts to find a series of immunogens that can together induce a vaccine-elicited antibody to recapitulate the ontogeny of a known lineage (127–130). Both strategies rest on the assumption that antibody elicitation is fundamentally reproducible. Thus, lineage-based vaccine design for HIV has focused on "classes" of antibodies (128) with similar genetic characteristics that have been observed in multiple donors. Despite genetic and structural similarity, however, several obstacles to the successful design of a vaccine capable of eliciting protective classes of antibodies remain to be overcome.

In particular, antibodies capable of broad neutralization of HIV have particularly high levels of SHM (128, 131, 132) and tend to be enriched for rare substitutions (104, 133, 134) (**Figure 1**). Extraordinary levels of SHM (15–35% nucleotide mutations) are characteristic of antibodies targeting HIV (135), and elevated levels of SHM have also been observed in other types of chronic infection and in systemic autoimmune disorders (136). By contrast, the maximum level of SHM that has been observed in vaccine-responsive antibodies is 8–10% nucleotide mutations, even after multiple doses (137, 138).

Fortunately, however, many mutations found in broadly neutralizing antibodies (bnAbs) against HIV appear to be unnecessary for full function (139, 140). In fact, two HIV bnAbs have recently been reported with at least 50% breadth and less than 10% nucleotide mutation in $V_H$: CAP256-VRC26.25 (141) and DH270.1 (142). Importantly, though, both contain other unusual features. CAP256-VRC26.25 has an extraordinarily long heavy chain CDR3 of 38 amino acids, including a 1 amino acid insertion relative to the inferred naive ancestor (141), while the neutralization activity of DH270.1 depends on a critical Gly64Arg (IMGT numbering) mutation in a canonical SY<u>C</u> cold spot (142). As noted above, such rare mutations are generally enriched in HIV bnAbs compared to flu bnAbs (**Figure 1**) and antibodies from normal repertoires or induced by a vaccine (104). While accumulation of some rare substitutions may be incidental to the overall level of SHM (33, 104), a recent report demonstrated that half of the HIV bnAbs studied have accumulated significantly more rare mutations than expected under a neutral evolutionary model of SHM (104). Similarly, several positions with low intrinsic mutation rates were determined to be significantly enriched in a class of $V_H$1-2-derived HIV bnAbs, based on their recurrence in members of that class (133). These observations suggest that, as for the DH270 lineage, at least some rare mutations may be functionally important. Indeed, this has recently been confirmed for three additional HIV bnAbs (104). The identification of critical rare mutations and strategies to reproduce them will be central to the success of lineage-based vaccine design.

One possible approach is to design immunogens capable of exerting strong selection on rare mutations as soon as they occur (104). However, even mutations that increase the affinity of an antibody 10-fold take much longer to dominate a germinal center reaction than would be expected from a simple model of SHM (91, 143). Moreover, recent work has shown that lower affinity subclones can persist in germinal centers (98–100), which may prevent antibodies with the desired rare substitution from reaching protective levels, even with an optimal immunogen. Indeed, while several recent studies in transgenic mice have elicited B cells enriched for substitutions present in the targeted mature antibody

(144–146), none have yet specifically elicited critical rare substitutions or fully recapitulated the neturalization activity of the target antibodies. Notably, however, the most successful example focuses on PGT121 (146), which contains fewer rare substitutions than many other HIV antibodies (104, 134). It may, therefore, be more prudent to choose lineage-based vaccine design targets by avoiding those with functionally important rare substitutions (33, 134).

## CONCLUSION

The mechanisms of antibody diversification have evolved to achieve a balance between the plasticity needed to successfully bind to unknown novel antigens and the robustness needed to do so in a biologically feasible manner. This results in a series of patterns and variations that can be studied computationally both to illuminate the underlying cellular processes and to predict the response to specific manipulations. As advances in technology have made it possible to collect ever larger datasets, our ability to detect and understand these patterns has grown, as well. The insights provided thus far by substitution profiles and related concepts have already begun to be applied to antibody engineering and vaccine design. Concurrently, work is ongoing to understand the biology behind these patterns and to develop them into predictive models of immune function.

## AUTHOR CONTRIBUTIONS

CS wrote the paper. All authors reviewed, commented on, and approved the manuscript.

## ACKNOWLEDGMENTS

We thank Dr. Zizhang Sheng for helpful comments and assistance with the figure.

## FUNDING

Funding was provided by the intramural program of the Vaccine Research Center, National Institute of Allergy and Infectious Disease, National Institutes of Health.

## REFERENCES

1. Schroeder HW. Similarity and divergence in the development and expression of the mouse and human antibody repertoires. *Dev Comp Immunol* (2006) 30(1):119–35. doi:10.1016/j.dci.2005.06.006
2. Elhanati Y, Sethna Z, Marcou Q, Callan CG, Mora T, Walczak AM. Inferring processes underlying B-cell repertoire diversity. *Philos Trans R Soc Lond B Biol Sci* (2015) 5(1676):370. doi:10.1098/rstb.2014.0243
3. Morbach H, Eichhorn EM, Liese JG, Girschick HJ. Reference values for B cell subpopulations from infancy to adulthood. *Clin Exp Immunol* (2010) 162(2):271–9. doi:10.1111/j.1365-2249.2010.04206.x
4. Perez-Andres M, Paiva B, Nieto WG, Caraux A, Schmitz A, Almeida J, et al. Human peripheral blood B-cell compartments: a crossroad in B-cell traffic. *Cytometry B Clin Cytom* (2010) 78B(S1):S47–60. doi:10.1002/cyto.b.20547
5. Gearhart PJ. Antibody wars: extreme diversity. *J Immunol* (2006) 177(7):4235–6. doi:10.4049/jimmunol.177.7.4235
6. Hood L, Talmage DW. Mechanism of antibody diversity: germ line basis for variability. *Science* (1970) 168(3929):325–34. doi:10.1126/science.168.3929.325
7. Schroeder HW, Hillson JL, Perlmutter RM. Early restriction of the human antibody repertoire. *Science* (1987) 238(4828):791–3. doi:10.1126/science.3118465
8. Suzuki I, Pfister L, Glas A, Nottenburg C, Milner EC. Representation of rearranged VH gene segments in the human adult antibody repertoire. *J Immunol* (1995) 154(8):3902–11.
9. Volpe JM, Kepler TB. Large-scale analysis of human heavy chain V(D)J recombination patterns. *Immunome Res* (2008) 4:3. doi:10.1186/1745-7580-4-3
10. Hansen TØ, Lange AB, Barington T. Sterile DJH rearrangements reveal that distance between gene segments on the human Ig H chain locus influences their ability to rearrange. *J Immunol* (2015) 194(3):973–82. doi:10.4049/jimmunol.1401443
11. Briney BS, Willis JR, Hicar MD, Thomas JW, Crowe JE. Frequency and genetic characterization of V(DD)J recombinants in the human peripheral blood antibody repertoire. *Immunology* (2012) 137(1):56–64. doi:10.1111/j.1365-2567.2012.03605.x
12. Henry Dunand CJ, Wilson PC. Restricted, canonical, stereotyped and convergent immunoglobulin responses. *Philos Trans R Soc Lond B Biol Sci* (2015) 370. doi:10.1098/rstb.2014.0238
13. Ralph DK, Matsen FA. Consistency of VDJ rearrangement and substitution parameters enables accurate B cell receptor sequence annotation. *PLoS Comput Biol* (2016) 12(1):e1004409. doi:10.1371/journal.pcbi.1004409
14. Briney BS, Willis JR, McKinney BA, Crowe JE. High-throughput antibody sequencing reveals genetic evidence of global regulation of the naïve and memory repertoires that extends across individuals. *Genes Immun* (2012) 13(6):469–73. doi:10.1038/gene.2012.20
15. Weigert MG, Cesari IM, Yonkovich SJ, Cohn M. Variability in the lambda light chain sequences of mouse antibody. *Nature* (1970) 228(5276):1045–7. doi:10.1038/2281045a0
16. Bernard O, Hozumi N, Tonegawa S. Sequences of mouse immunoglobulin light chain genes before and after somatic changes. *Cell* (1978) 15(4):1133–44. doi:10.1016/0092-8674(78)90041-7
17. Gearhart PJ, Bogenhagen DF. Clusters of point mutations are found exclusively around rearranged antibody variable genes. *Proc Natl Acad Sci U S A* (1983) 80(11):3439–43. doi:10.1073/pnas.80.11.3439
18. Berek C, Milstein C. Mutation drift and repertoire shift in the maturation of the immune response. *Immunol Rev* (1987) 96:23–41. doi:10.1111/j.1600-065X.1987.tb00507.x
19. Betz AG, Rada C, Pannell R, Milstein C, Neuberger MS. Passenger transgenes reveal intrinsic specificity of the antibody hypermutation mechanism: clustering, polarity, and specific hot spots. *Proc Natl Acad Sci U S A* (1993) 90(6):2385–8. doi:10.1073/pnas.90.6.2385
20. Muramatsu M, Sankaranand VS, Anant S, Sugai M, Kinoshita K, Davidson NO, et al. Specific expression of activation-induced cytidine deaminase (AID), a novel member of the RNA-editing deaminase family in germinal center B cells. *J Biol Chem* (1999) 274(26):18470–6. doi:10.1074/jbc.274.26.18470
21. Muramatsu M, Kinoshita K, Fagarasan S, Yamada S, Shinkai Y, Honjo T. Class switch recombination and hypermutation require activation-induced cytidine deaminase (AID), a potential RNA editing enzyme. *Cell* (2000) 102(5):553–63. doi:10.1016/S0092-8674(00)00078-7
22. Revy P, Muto T, Levy Y, Geissmann F, Plebani A, Sanal O, et al. Activation-induced cytidine deaminase (AID) deficiency causes the autosomal recessive form of the hyper-IgM syndrome (HIGM2). *Cell* (2000) 102(5):565–75. doi:10.1016/S0092-8674(00)00079-9
23. Chandra V, Bortnick A, Murre C. AID targeting: old mysteries and new challenges. *Trends Immunol* (2015) 36(9):527–35. doi:10.1016/j.it.2015.07.003
24. Casellas R, Basu U, Yewdell WT, Chaudhuri J, Robbiani DF, Noia JMD. Mutations, kataegis and translocations in B cells: understanding AID promiscuous activity. *Nat Rev Immunol* (2016) 16(3):164–76. doi:10.1038/nri.2016.2
25. Methot SP, Di Noia JM. Molecular mechanisms of somatic hypermutation and class switch recombination. *Adv Immunol* (2017) 133:37–87. doi:10.1016/bs.ai.2016.11.002
26. Kohli RM, Abrams SR, Gajula KS, Maul RW, Gearhart PJ, Stivers JT. A portable hot spot recognition loop transfers sequence preferences from APOBEC family members to activation-induced cytidine deaminase. *J Biol Chem* (2009) 284(34):22898–904. doi:10.1074/jbc.M109.025536

27. Wang M, Rada C, Neuberger MS. Altering the spectrum of immunoglobulin V gene somatic hypermutation by modifying the active site of AID. *J Exp Med* (2010) 207(1):141–53. doi:10.1084/jem.20092238
28. Pham P, Afif SA, Shimoda M, Maeda K, Sakaguchi N, Pedersen LC, et al. Structural analysis of the activation-induced deoxycytidine deaminase required in immunoglobulin diversification. *DNA Repair* (2016) 43:48–56. doi:10.1016/j.dnarep.2016.05.029
29. Halemano K, Guo K, Heilman KJ, Barrett BS, Smith DS, Hasenkrug KJ, et al. Immunoglobulin somatic hypermutation by APOBEC3/Rfv3 during retroviral infection. *Proc Natl Acad Sci U S A* (2014) 111(21):7759–64. doi:10.1073/pnas.1403361111
30. Zanotti KJ, Gearhart PJ. Antibody diversification caused by disrupted mismatch repair and promiscuous DNA polymerases. *DNA Repair* (2016) 38:110–6. doi:10.1016/j.dnarep.2015.11.011
31. Rada C, Ehrenstein MR, Neuberger MS, Milstein C. Hot spot focusing of somatic hypermutation in MSH2-deficient mice suggests two stages of mutational targeting. *Immunity* (1998) 9(1):135–41. doi:10.1016/S1074-7613(00)80595-6
32. Rogozin IB, Pavlov YI, Bebenek K, Matsuda T, Kunkel TA. Somatic mutation hotspots correlate with DNA polymerase eta error spectrum. *Nat Immunol* (2001) 2(6):530–6. doi:10.1038/88732
33. Sheng Z, Schramm CA, Kong R; NISC Comparative Sequencing Program, Mullikin JC, Mascola JR, et al. Gene-specific substitution profiles describe the types and frequencies of amino acid changes during antibody somatic hypermutation. *Front Immunol* (2017) 8:537. doi:10.3389/fimmu.2017.00537
34. Kirik U, Persson H, Levander F, Greiff L, Ohlin M. Antibody heavy chain variable domains of different germline gene origins diversify through different paths. *Front Immunol* (2017) 8:1433. doi:10.3389/fimmu.2017.01433
35. Lederberg J. Genes and antibodies. *Science* (1959) 129(3364):1649–53. doi:10.1126/science.129.3364.1649
36. Brenner S, Milstein C. Origin of antibody variation. *Nature* (1966) 211(5046):242–3. doi:10.1038/211242a0
37. Selsing E, Storb U. Somatic mutation of immunoglobulin light-chain variable-regiongenes. *Cell* (1981) 25(1):47–58. doi:10.1016/0092-8674(81)90230-0
38. Rogozin IB, Kolchanov NA. Somatic hypermutagenesis in immunoglobulin genes: II. Influence of neighbouring base sequences on mutagenesis. *Biochim Biophys Acta* (1992) 1171(1):11–8. doi:10.1016/0167-4781(92)90134-L
39. Pham P, Bransteitter R, Petruska J, Goodman MF. Processive AID-catalysed cytosine deamination on single-stranded DNA simulates somatic hypermutation. *Nature* (2003) 424(6944):103–7. doi:10.1038/nature01760
40. Smith DS, Creadon G, Jena PK, Portanova JP, Kotzin BL, Wysocki LJ. Di- and trinucleotide target preferences of somatic mutagenesis in normal and autoreactive B cells. *J Immunol* (1996) 156(7):2642–52.
41. Jolly CJ, Wagner SD, Rada C, Klix N, Milstein C, Neuberger MS. The targeting of somatic hypermutation. *Semin Immunol* (1996) 8(3):159–68. doi:10.1006/smim.1996.0020
42. Dörner T, Foster SJ, Farner NL, Lipsky PE. Somatic hypermutation of human immunoglobulin heavy chain genes: targeting of RGYW motifs on both DNA strands. *Eur J Immunol* (1998) 28(10):3384–96. doi:10.1002/(SICI)1521-4141(199810)28:10<3384::AID-IMMU3384>3.0.CO;2-T
43. Ohm-Laursen L, Barington T. Analysis of 6912 unselected somatic hypermutations in human VDJ rearrangements reveals lack of strand specificity and correlation between phase II substitution rates and distance to the nearest 3' activation-induced cytidine deaminase target. *J Immunol* (2007) 178(7):4322–34. doi:10.4049/jimmunol.178.7.4322
44. Yaari G, Vander Heiden JA, Uduman M, Gadala-Maria D, Gupta N, Stern JNH, et al. Models of somatic hypermutation targeting and substitution based on synonymous mutations from high-throughput immunoglobulin sequencing data. *Front Immunol* (2013) 4:358. doi:10.3389/fimmu.2013.00358
45. Rogozin IB, Diaz M. Cutting edge: DGYW/WRCH is a better predictor of mutability at G:C bases in Ig hypermutation than the widely accepted RGYW/WRCY motif and probably reflects a two-step activation-induced cytidine deaminase-triggered process. *J Immunol* (2004) 172(6):3382–4. doi:10.4049/jimmunol.172.6.3382
46. Yu K, Huang F-T, Lieber MR. DNA substrate length and surrounding sequence affect the activation-induced deaminase activity at cytidine. *J Biol Chem* (2004) 279(8):6496–500. doi:10.1074/jbc.M311616200
47. Wei L, Chahwan R, Wang S, Wang X, Pham PT, Goodman MF, et al. Overlapping hotspots in CDRs are critical sites for V region diversification. *Proc Natl Acad Sci U S A* (2015) 112(7):E728–37. doi:10.1073/pnas.1500788112
48. Cui A, Niro RD, Heiden JAV, Briggs AW, Adams K, Gilbert T, et al. A model of somatic hypermutation targeting in mice based on high-throughput Ig sequencing data. *J Immunol* (2016) 197(9):3566–74. doi:10.4049/jimmunol.1502263
49. Shapiro GS, Aviszus K, Ikle D, Wysocki LJ. Predicting regional mutability in antibody V genes based solely on di- and trinucleotide sequence composition. *J Immunol* (1999) 163(1):259–68.
50. Shapiro GS, Aviszus K, Murphy J, Wysocki LJ. Evolution of Ig DNA sequence to target specific base positions within codons for somatic hypermutation. *J Immunol* (2002) 168(5):2302–6. doi:10.4049/jimmunol.168.5.2302
51. Boursier L, Su W, Spencer J. Imprint of somatic hypermutation differs in human immunoglobulin heavy and lambda chain variable gene segments. *Mol Immunol* (2003) 39(16):1025–34. doi:10.1016/S0161-5890(03)00033-6
52. Cohen RM, Kleinstein SH, Louzoun Y. Somatic hypermutation targeting is influenced by location within the immunoglobulin V region. *Mol Immunol* (2011) 48(12–13):1477–83. doi:10.1016/j.molimm.2011.04.002
53. Chan OT, Hannum LG, Haberman AM, Madaio MP, Shlomchik MJ. A novel mouse with B cells but lacking serum antibody reveals an antibody-independent role for B cells in murine lupus. *J Exp Med* (1999) 189(10):1639–48. doi:10.1084/jem.189.10.1639
54. Marcou Q, Mora T, Walczak AM. High-throughput immune repertoire analysis with IGoR. *Nat Commun* (2018) 9(1):561. doi:10.1038/s41467-018-02832-w
55. Feng J, Shaw DA, Minin VN, Simon N, Matsen FA IV. Survival analysis of DNA mutation motifs with penalized proportional hazards. *arXiv* (2017) arXiv:1711.04057.
56. Lebecque SG, Gearhart PJ. Boundaries of somatic mutation in rearranged immunoglobulin genes: 5' boundary is near the promoter, and 3' boundary is approximately 1 kb from V(D)J gene. *J Exp Med* (1990) 172(6):1717–27. doi:10.1084/jem.172.6.1717
57. Cowell LG, Kepler TB. The nucleotide-replacement spectrum under somatic hypermutation exhibits microsequence dependence that is strand-symmetric and distinct from that under germline mutation. *J Immunol* (2000) 164(4):1971–6. doi:10.4049/jimmunol.164.4.1971
58. Mirsky A, Kazandjian L, Anisimova M. Antibody-specific model of amino acid substitution for immunological inferences from alignments of antibody sequences. *Mol Biol Evol* (2015) 32:806–819. doi:10.1093/molbev/msu340
59. Yeap L-S, Hwang JK, Du Z, Meyers RM, Meng F-L, Jakubauskaitė A, et al. Sequence-intrinsic mechanisms that target AID mutational outcomes on antibody genes. *Cell* (2015) 163(5):1124–37. doi:10.1016/j.cell.2015.10.042
60. Rada C, Milstein C. The intrinsic hypermutability of antibody heavy and light chain genes decays exponentially. *EMBO J* (2001) 20(16):4570–6. doi:10.1093/emboj/20.16.4570
61. Hood L, Campbell JH, Elgin SC. The organization, expression, and evolution of antibody genes and other multigene families. *Annu Rev Genet* (1975) 9:305–53. doi:10.1146/annurev.ge.09.120175.001513
62. Ohta T. *Evolution and Variation of Multigene Families*. Berlin, Heidelberg: Springer-Verlag (1980).
63. Gojobori T, Nei M. Concerted evolution of the immunoglobulin VH gene family. *Mol Biol Evol* (1984) 1(2):195–212.
64. Ota T, Nei M. Divergent evolution and evolution by the birth-and-death process in the immunoglobulin VH gene family. *Mol Biol Evol* (1994) 11(3):469–82.
65. Nei M, Gu X, Sitnikova T. Evolution by the birth-and-death process in multigene families of the vertebrate immune system. *Proc Natl Acad Sci U S A* (1997) 94(15):7799–806. doi:10.1073/pnas.94.15.7799
66. Tanaka T, Nei M. Positive Darwinian selection observed at the variable-region genes of immunoglobulins. *Mol Biol Evol* (1989) 6(5):447–59.
67. Hinds-Frey KR, Nishikata H, Litman RT, Litman GW. Somatic variation precedes extensive diversification of germline sequences and combinatorial joining in the evolution of immunoglobulin heavy chain diversity. *J Exp Med* (1993) 178(3):815–24. doi:10.1084/jem.178.3.815
68. Quinlan EM, King JJ, Amemiya CT, Hsu E, Larijani M. Biochemical regulatory features of activation-induced cytidine deaminase remain conserved from lampreys to humans. *Mol Cell Biol* (2017) 37(20). doi:10.1128/MCB.00077-17
69. Rogozin IB, Iyer LM, Liang L, Glazko GV, Liston VG, Pavlov YI, et al. Evolution and diversification of lamprey antigen receptors: evidence for

involvement of an AID-APOBEC family cytosine deaminase. *Nat Immunol* (2007) 8(6):647–56. doi:10.1038/ni1463
70. Chang B, Casali P. The CDR1 sequences of a major proportion of human germline Ig VH genes are inherently susceptible to amino acid replacement. *Immunol Today* (1994) 15(8):367–73. doi:10.1016/0167-5699(94)90175-9
71. Hershberg U, Shlomchik MJ. Differences in potential for amino acid change after mutation reveals distinct strategies for kappa and lambda light-chain variation. *Proc Natl Acad Sci U S A* (2006) 103(43):15963–8. doi:10.1073/pnas.0607581103
72. Saini J, Hershberg U. B cell variable genes have evolved their codon usage to focus the targeted patterns of somatic mutation on the complementarity determining regions. *Mol Immunol* (2015) 65(1):157–67. doi:10.1016/j.molimm.2015.01.001
73. Wagner SD, Milstein C, Neuberger MS. Codon bias targets mutation. *Nature* (1995) 376(6543):732. doi:10.1038/376732a0
74. Kepler TB. Codon bias and plasticity in immunoglobulins. *Mol Biol Evol* (1997) 14(6):637–43. doi:10.1093/oxfordjournals.molbev.a025803
75. Golub R, Charlemagne J. Structure, diversity, and repertoire of VH families in the Mexican axolotl. *J Immunol* (1998) 160(3):1233–9.
76. Oreste U, Coscia M. Specific features of immunoglobulin VH genes of the Antarctic teleost *Trematomus bernacchii*. *Gene* (2002) 295(2):199–204. doi:10.1016/S0378-1119(02)00686-8
77. Conticello SG, Thomas CJF, Petersen-Mahrt SK, Neuberger MS. Evolution of the AID/APOBEC family of polynucleotide (deoxy)cytidine deaminases. *Mol Biol Evol* (2005) 22(2):367–77. doi:10.1093/molbev/msi026
78. Oprea M, Kepler TB. Genetic plasticity of V genes under somatic hypermutation: statistical analyses using a new resampling-based methodology. *Genome Res* (1999) 9(12):1294–304. doi:10.1101/gr.9.12.1294
79. Detanico T, Phillips M, Wysocki LJ. Functional versatility of AGY serine codons in immunoglobulin variable region genes. *Front Immunol* (2016) 7:525. doi:10.3389/fimmu.2016.00525
80. Zheng N-Y, Wilson K, Jared M, Wilson PC. Intricate targeting of immunoglobulin somatic hypermutation maximizes the efficiency of affinity maturation. *J Exp Med* (2005) 201(9):1467–78. doi:10.1084/jem.20042483
81. Koenig P, Lee CV, Walters BT, Janakiraman V, Stinson J, Patapoff TW, et al. Mutational landscape of antibody variable domains reveals a switch modulating the interdomain conformational dynamics and antigen binding. *Proc Natl Acad Sci U S A* (2017) 114(4):E486-E495. doi:10.1073/pnas.1613231114
82. van de Bovenkamp FS, Derksen NIL, Ooijevaar-de Heer P, van Schie KA, Kruithof S, Berkowska MA, et al. Adaptive antibody diversification through N-linked glycosylation of the immunoglobulin variable region. *Proc Natl Acad Sci U S A* (2018) 115(8):1901–6. doi:10.1073/pnas.1711720115
83. Collins AM, Jackson KJL. On being the right size: antibody repertoire formation in the mouse and human. *Immunogenetics* (2018) 70(3):143–58. doi:10.1007/s00251-017-1049-8
84. Krause JC, Tsibane T, Tumpey TM, Huffman CJ, Briney BS, Smith SA, et al. Epitope-specific human influenza antibody repertoires diversify by B cell intraclonal sequence divergence and interclonal convergence. *J Immunol* (2011) 187(7):3704–11. doi:10.4049/jimmunol.1101823
85. Jackson KJL, Liu Y, Roskin KM, Glanville J, Hoh RA, Seo K, et al. Human responses to influenza vaccination show seroconversion signatures and convergent antibody rearrangements. *Cell Host Microbe* (2014) 16(1):105–14. doi:10.1016/j.chom.2014.05.013
86. Joyce MG, Wheatley AK, Thomas PV, Chuang G-Y, Soto C, Bailer RT, et al. Vaccine-induced antibodies that neutralize group 1 and group 2 influenza A viruses. *Cell* (2016) 166(3):609–23. doi:10.1016/j.cell.2016.06.043
87. Zhou T, Zhu J, Wu X, Moquin S, Zhang B, Acharya P, et al. Multidonor analysis reveals structural elements, genetic determinants, and maturation pathway for HIV-1 neutralization by VRC01-class antibodies. *Immunity* (2013) 39(2):245–58. doi:10.1016/j.immuni.2013.04.012
88. Zhou T, Lynch RM, Chen L, Acharya P, Wu X, Doria-Rose NA, et al. Structural repertoire of HIV-1-neutralizing antibodies targeting the CD4 supersite in 14 donors. *Cell* (2015) 161(6):1280–92. doi:10.1016/j.cell.2015.05.007
89. Allen D, Cumano A, Dildrop R, Kocks C, Rajewsky K, Rajewsky N, et al. Timing, genetic requirements and functional consequences of somatic hypermutation during B-cell development. *Immunol Rev* (1987) 96:5–22. doi:10.1111/j.1600-065X.1987.tb00506.x
90. Pappas L, Foglierini M, Piccoli L, Kallewaard NL, Turrini F, Silacci C, et al. Rapid development of broadly influenza neutralizing antibodies through redundant mutations. *Nature* (2014) 516(7531):418–22. doi:10.1038/ature13764
91. Radmacher MD, Kelsoe G, Kepler TB. Predicted and inferred waiting times for key mutations in the germinal centre reaction: evidence for stochasticity in selection. *Immunol Cell Biol* (1998) 76(4):373–81. doi:10.1046/j.1440-1711.1998.00753.x
92. Bonsignori M, Zhou T, Sheng Z, Chen L, Gao F, Joyce MG, et al. Maturation pathway from germline to broad HIV-1 neutralizer of a CD4-mimic antibody. *Cell* (2016) 165(2):449–63. doi:10.1016/j.cell.2016.02.022
93. Schwartz GW, Hershberg U. Germline amino acid diversity in B cell receptors is a good predictor of somatic selection pressures. *Front Immunol* (2013) 4:357. doi:10.3389/fimmu.2013.00357
94. McCoy CO, Bedford T, Minin VN, Bradley P, Robins H, Matsen FA. Quantifying evolutionary constraints on B-cell affinity maturation. *Philos Trans R Soc Lond B Biol Sci* (2015) 5:370. doi:10.1098/rstb.2014.0244
95. Honegger A, Malebranche AD, Röthlisberger D, Plückthun A. The influence of the framework core residues on the biophysical properties of immunoglobulin heavy chain variable domains. *Protein Eng Des Sel PEDS* (2009) 22(3):121–34. doi:10.1093/protein/gzn077
96. Lefranc MP. Unique database numbering system for immunogenetic analysis. *Immunol Today* (1997) 18(11):509. doi:10.1016/S0167-5699(97)01163-8
97. Clark LA, Ganesan S, Papp S, van Vlijmen HWT. Trends in antibody sequence changes during the somatic hypermutation process. *J Immunol* (2006) 177(1):333–40. doi:10.4049/jimmunol.177.1.333
98. Tas JMJ, Mesin L, Pasqual G, Targ S, Jacobsen JT, Mano YM, et al. Visualizing antibody affinity maturation in germinal centers. *Science* (2016) 351:1048–54. doi:10.1126/science.aad3439
99. Kuraoka M, Schmidt AG, Nojima T, Feng F, Watanabe A, Kitamura D, et al. Complex antigens drive permissive clonal selection in germinal centers. *Immunity* (2016) 44(3):542–52. doi:10.1016/j.immuni.2016.02.010
100. Reshetova P, van Schaik BD, Klarenbeek PL, Doorenspleet ME, Esveldt RE, et al. Computational model reveals limited correlation between germinal center B-cell subclone abundancy and affinity: implications for repertoire sequencing. *Front Immunol* (2017) 8:221. doi:10.3389/fimmu.2017.00221
101. Baumgarth N. How specific is too specific? B-cell responses to viral infections reveal the importance of breadth over depth. *Immunol Rev* (2013) 255(1):82–94. doi:10.1111/imr.12094
102. Dhar A, Davidsen K, Matsen IVFA, Minin VN. Predicting B cell receptor substitution profiles using public repertoire data. *arXiv* (2018). arXiv:1802.06406
103. Ralph DK, Matsen FA. Likelihood-based inference of B cell clonal families. *PLoS Comput Biol* (2016) 12(10):e1005086. doi:10.1371/journal.pcbi.1005086
104. Wiehe K, Bradley T, Meyerhoff RR, Hart C, Williams WB, Easterhoff D, et al. Functional relevance of improbable antibody mutations for HIV broadly neutralizing antibody development. *Cell Host Microbe* (2018) 23(6):759–65.e6. doi:10.1016/j.chom.2018.04.018
105. Julian MC, Li L, Garde S, Wilen R, Tessier PM. Efficient affinity maturation of antibody variable domains requires co-selection of compensatory mutations to maintain thermodynamic stability. *Sci Rep* (2017) 7. doi:10.1038/srep45259
106. Scheepers C, Shrestha RK, Lambson BE, Jackson KJL, Wright IA, Naicker D, et al. Ability to develop broadly neutralizing HIV-1 antibodies is not restricted by the germline Ig gene repertoire. *J Immunol* (2015) 194(9):4371–8. doi:10.4049/jimmunol.1500118
107. Corcoran MM, Phad GE, Vázquez Bernat N, Stahl-Hennig C, Sumida N, Persson MAA, et al. Production of individualized V gene databases reveals high levels of immunoglobulin genetic diversity. *Nat Commun* (2016) 20(7):13642. doi:10.1038/ncomms13642
108. Luo S, Yu JA, Song YS. Estimating copy number and allelic variation at the immunoglobulin heavy chain locus using short reads. *PLoS Comput Biol* (2016) 12(9):e1005117. doi:10.1371/journal.pcbi.1005117
109. Yu Y, Ceredig R, Seoighe C. A database of human immune receptor alleles recovered from population sequencing data. *J Immunol* (2017) 198(5):2202–10. doi:10.4049/jimmunol.1601710
110. Ohm-Laursen L, Nielsen M, Larsen SR, Barington T. No evidence for the use of DIR, D-D fusions, chromosome 15 open reading frames or VH replacement in the peripheral repertoire was found on application of an improved algorithm, JointML, to 6329 human immunoglobulin H rearrangements. *Immunology* (2006) 119(2):265–77. doi:10.1111/j.1365-2567.2006.02431.x

111. Shlomchik MJ, Marshak-Rothstein A, Wolfowicz CB, Rothstein TL, Weigert MG. The role of clonal selection and somatic mutation in autoimmunity. *Nature* (1987) 328(6133):805–11. doi:10.1038/328805a0
112. Lossos IS, Tibshirani R, Narasimhan B, Levy R. The inference of antigen selection on Ig genes. *J Immunol* (2000) 165(9):5122–6. doi:10.4049/jimmunol.165.9.5122
113. Bose B, Sinha S. Problems in using statistical analysis of replacement and silent mutations in antibody genes for determining antigen-driven affinity selection. *Immunology* (2005) 116(2):172–83. doi:10.1111/j.1365-2567.2005.02208.x
114. Dunn-Walters DK, Spencer J. Strong intrinsic biases towards mutation and conservation of bases in human IgVH genes during somatic hypermutation prevent statistical analysis of antigen selection. *Immunology* (1998) 95(3):339–45. doi:10.1046/j.1365-2567.1998.00607.x
115. Hershberg U, Uduman M, Shlomchik MJ, Kleinstein SH. Improved methods for detecting selection by mutation analysis of Ig V region sequences. *Int Immunol* (2008) 20(5):683–94. doi:10.1093/intimm/dxn026
116. Uduman M, Yaari G, Hershberg U, Stern JA, Shlomchik MJ, Kleinstein SH. Detecting selection in immunoglobulin sequences. *Nucleic Acids Res* (2011) 39(Web Server issue):W499–504. doi:10.1093/nar/gkr413
117. Yaari G, Uduman M, Kleinstein SH. Quantifying selection in high-throughput immunoglobulin sequencing data sets. *Nucleic Acids Res* (2012) 40(17):e134. doi:10.1093/nar/gks457
118. Shahaf G, Barak M, Zuckerman NS, Swerdlin N, Gorfine M, Mehr R. Antigen-driven selection in germinal centers as reflected by the shape characteristics of immunoglobulin gene lineage trees: a large-scale simulation study. *J Theor Biol* (2008) 255(2):210–22. doi:10.1016/j.jtbi.2008.08.005
119. Uduman M, Shlomchik MJ, Vigneault F, Church GM, Kleinstein SH. Integrating B cell lineage information into statistical tests for detecting selection in Ig sequences. *J Immunol* (2014) 192(3):867–74. doi:10.4049/jimmunol.1301551
120. Yaari G, Benichou JIC, Vander Heiden JA, Kleinstein SH, Louzoun Y. The mutation patterns in B-cell immunoglobulin receptors reflect the influence of selection acting at multiple time-scales. *Philos Trans R Soc Lond B Biol Sci* (2015):370. doi:10.1098/rstb.2014.0242
121. MacDonald CM, Boursier L, D'Cruz DP, Dunn-Walters DK, Spencer J. Mathematical analysis of antigen selection in somatically mutated immunoglobulin genes associated with autoimmunity. *Lupus* (2010) 19(10):1161–70. doi:10.1177/0961203310367657
122. Burkovitz A, Sela-Culang I, Ofran Y. Large-scale analysis of somatic hypermutations in antibodies reveals which structural regions, positions and amino acids are modified to improve affinity. *FEBS J* (2014) 281(1):306–19. doi:10.1111/febs.12597
123. Burnett DL, Langley DB, Schofield P, Hermes JR, Chan TD, Jackson J, et al. Germinal center antibody mutation trajectories are determined by rapid self/foreign discrimination. *Science* (2018) 360(6385):223–6. doi:10.1126/science.aao3859
124. Kepler TB, Munshaw S, Wiehe K, Zhang R, Yu J-S, Woods CW, et al. Reconstructing a B-cell clonal lineage. II. Mutation, selection, and affinity maturation. *Front Immunol* (2014) 5:170. doi:10.3389/fimmu.2014.00170
125. Rappuoli R, Bottomley MJ, D'Oro U, Finco O, Gregorio ED. Reverse vaccinology 2.0: human immunology instructs vaccine antigen design. *J Exp Med* (2016) 213(4):469–81. doi:10.1084/jem.20151960
126. Burton DR. What are the most powerful immunogen design vaccine strategies? Reverse vaccinology 2.0 shows great promise. *Cold Spring Harb Perspect Biol* (2017) 9(11):a030262. doi:10.1101/cshperspect.a030262
127. Haynes BF, Kelsoe G, Harrison SC, Kepler TB. B-cell-lineage immunogen design in vaccine development with HIV-1 as a case study. *Nat Biotechnol* (2012) 30(5):423–33. doi:10.1038/nbt.2197
128. Kwong PD, Mascola JR. Human antibodies that neutralize HIV-1: identification, structures, and B cell ontogenies. *Immunity* (2012) 37(3):412–25. doi:10.1016/j.immuni.2012.08.012
129. Kwong PD, Mascola JR. HIV-1 vaccines based on antibody identification, B cell ontogeny, and epitope structure. *Immunity* (2018) 48(5):855–71. doi:10.1016/j.immuni.2018.04.029
130. Doria-Rose NA, Joyce MG. Strategies to guide the antibody affinity maturation process. *Curr Opin Virol* (2015) 11:137–47. doi:10.1016/j.coviro.2015.04.002
131. Wu X, Zhou T, Zhu J, Zhang B, Georgiev I, Wang C, et al. Focused evolution of HIV-1 neutralizing antibodies revealed by structures and deep sequencing. *Science* (2011) 333(6049):1593–602. doi:10.1126/science.1207532
132. Scheid JF, Mouquet H, Ueberheide B, Diskin R, Klein F, Oliveira TYK, et al. Sequence and structural convergence of broad and potent HIV antibodies that mimic CD4 binding. *Science* (2011) 333(6049):1633–7. doi:10.1126/science.1207227
133. Hwang JK, Wang C, Du Z, Meyers RM, Kepler TB, Neuberg D, et al. Sequence intrinsic somatic mutation mechanisms contribute to affinity maturation of VRC01-class HIV-1 broadly neutralizing antibodies. *Proc Natl Acad Sci U S A* (2017) 114(32):8614–9. doi:10.1073/pnas.1709203114
134. Chuang G-Y, Zhou J, Rawi R, Shen C-H, Sheng Z, West AP, et al. Structural survey of HIV-1-neutralizing antibodies targeting Env trimer delineates epitope categories and suggests vaccine templates. *bioRxiv* (2018). doi:10.1101/312579
135. Scheid JF, Mouquet H, Feldhahn N, Seaman MS, Velinzon K, Pietzsch J, et al. Broad diversity of neutralizing antibodies isolated from memory B cells in HIV-infected individuals. *Nature* (2009) 458(7238):636–40. doi:10.1038/nature07930
136. Breden F, Lepik C, Longo NS, Montero M, Lipsky PE, Scott JK. Comparison of antibody repertoires produced by HIV-1 infection, other chronic and acute infections, and systemic autoimmune disease. *PLoS One* (2011) 6(3):e16857. doi:10.1371/journal.pone.0016857
137. Moody MA, Yates NL, Amos JD, Drinker MS, Eudailey JA, Gurley TC, et al. HIV-1 gp120 vaccine induces affinity maturation in both new and persistent antibody clonal lineages. *J Virol* (2012) 86(14):7496–507. doi:10.1128/JVI.00426-12
138. Scherer EM, Smith RA, Simonich CA, Niyonzima N, Carter JJ, Galloway DA. Characteristics of memory B cells elicited by a highly efficacious HPV vaccine in subjects with no pre-existing immunity. *PLoS Pathog* (2014) 10(10):e1004461. doi:10.1371/journal.ppat.1004461
139. Georgiev IS, Rudicell RS, Saunders KO, Shi W, Kirys T, McKee K, et al. Antibodies VRC01 and 10E8 neutralize HIV-1 with high breadth and potency even with Ig-framework regions substantially reverted to germline. *J Immunol* (2014) 192(3):1100–6. doi:10.4049/jimmunol.1302515
140. Jardine JG, Sok D, Julien J-P, Briney B, Sarkar A, Liang C-H, et al. Minimally mutated HIV-1 broadly neutralizing antibodies to guide reductionist vaccine design. *PLoS Pathog* (2016) 12(8):e1005815. doi:10.1371/journal.ppat.1005815
141. Doria-Rose NA, Bhiman JN, Roark RS, Schramm CA, Gorman J, Chuang G-Y, et al. New member of the V1V2-directed CAP256-VRC26 lineage that shows increased breadth and exceptional potency. *J Virol* (2016) 90(1):76–91. doi:10.1128/JVI.01791-15
142. Bonsignori M, Kreider EF, Fera D, Meyerhoff RR, Bradley T, Wiehe K, et al. Staged induction of HIV-1 glycan-dependent broadly neutralizing antibodies. *Sci Transl Med* (2017) 9(381):eaai7514. doi:10.1126/scitranslmed.aai7514
143. Kleinstein SH, Singh JP. Why are there so few key mutant clones? The influence of stochastic selection and blocking on affinity maturation in the germinal center. *Int Immunol* (2003) 15(7):871–84. doi:10.1093/intimm/dxg085.sgm
144. Briney B, Sok D, Jardine JG, Kulp DW, Skog P, Menis S, et al. Tailored immunogens direct affinity maturation toward HIV neutralizing antibodies. *Cell* (2016) 166(6):1459–70.e11. doi:10.1016/j.cell.2016.08.005
145. Tian M, Cheng C, Chen X, Duan H, Cheng H-L, Dao M, et al. Induction of HIV neutralizing antibody lineages in mice with diverse precursor repertoires. *Cell* (2016) 166(6):1471–84.e18. doi:10.1016/j.cell.2016.07.029
146. Escolano A, Steichen JM, Dosenovic P, Kulp DW, Golijanin J, Sok D, et al. Sequential immunization elicits broadly neutralizing anti-HIV-1 antibodies in Ig knockin mice. *Cell* (2016) 166(6):1445–58.e12. doi:10.1016/j.cell.2016.07.030

# 10

# ImmuneDB, A Novel Tool for the Analysis, Storage and Dissemination of Immune Repertoire Sequencing Data

*Aaron M. Rosenfeld*[1], *Wenzhao Meng*[2], *Eline T. Luning Prak*[2] *and Uri Hershberg*[1,3,4*]

[1] School of Biomedical Engineering Science and Health Systems, Drexel University, Philadelphia, PA, United States, [2] Department of Pathology and Laboratory Medicine, Perelman School of Medicine, University of Pennsylvania, Philadelphia, PA, United States, [3] Department of Microbiology and Immunology, College of Medicine, Drexel University, Philadelphia, PA, United States, [4] Department of Human Biology, Faculty of Sciences, University of Haifa, Haifa, Israel

***Correspondence:***
*Uri Hershberg*
*uh25@drexel.edu*

ImmuneDB is a system for storing and analyzing high-throughput immune receptor sequencing data. Unlike most existing tools, which utilize flat-files, ImmuneDB stores data in a well-structured MySQL database, enabling efficient data queries. It can take raw sequencing data as input and annotate receptor gene usage, infer clonotypes, aggregate results, and run common downstream analyses such as calculating selection pressure and constructing clonal lineages. Alternatively, pre-annotated data can be imported and analyzed data can be exported in a variety of common Adaptive Immune Receptor Repertoire (AIRR) file formats. To validate ImmuneDB, we compare its results to those of another pipeline, MiXCR. We show that the biological conclusions drawn would be similar with either tool, while ImmuneDB provides the additional benefits of integrating other common tools and storing data in a database. ImmuneDB is freely available on GitHub at https://github.com/arosenfeld/immunedb, on PyPi at https://pypi.org/project/ImmuneDB, and a Docker container is provided at https://hub.docker.com/r/arosenfeld/immunedb. Full documentation is available at http://immunedb.com.

**Keywords: next-generation sequencing, antibody repertoire analysis, bioinformatics, B-cell receptor, database**

## INTRODUCTION

The study of immune cell populations has been revolutionized by next-generation sequencing. It is now commonplace to have hundreds of thousands or even millions of sequences from a single sample or individual (1, 2). With this increase in experimental data output, many tools have been created for pre-processing sequences (3), germline association and clonal inference (4–7), and post-processing analysis (8, 9). Lacking from this space, however, is a system to store fully-annotated sequences, their inferred germline sequences, clonal associations, and study-specific metadata. This paper describes ImmuneDB (10) and introduces new features added since its original publication including: additional importing & exporting formats, a more flexible metadata system, extra clonal assignment methods, integration of a novel allele detection tool (11), and the ability to analyze other species and light chains. ImmuneDB provides an easy to use immune-receptor sequence database, which has been optimized for and tested with datasets of up to hundreds of millions of sequences (1). It can take as input raw FASTA/FASTQ sequence files, or import pre-annotated sequences from an array of formats including the Change-O data standard (5) and the AIRR data standard currently being implemented and further refined (2). With either method, it can infer clonal associations, calculate selection pressure, generate lineages, and make all resulting information available both from the command line and as a web-interface. For interoperability with other systems, ImmuneDB can output data in AIRR, Change-O, VDJtools, and genbank formats. ImmuneDB's usage of MySQL also allows for rapid querying and data-sharing using a variety of existing tools.

# MATERIALS AND METHODS

The methods below describe the ImmuneDB pipeline in the context of human B-cell heavy chain rearrangements. We then extend the methods to T cells, light chains, and other species (**Figure 1**).

## Computer Hardware and Software Requirements

ImmuneDB is primarily written in Python and can therefore run on most common Unix-based operating systems (including macOS). Local installation of the version described in this paper (v0.24.1) requires Python 3.5+, although legacy versions support Python 2.7. The setup will automatically install all Python library dependencies. Additionally, MySQL (or a drop-in replacement like MariaDB) is required, although it need not run on the same host as ImmuneDB.

Optional steps require installation of additional external tools. Local alignment requires Bowtie 2 (12), lineage construction depends on Clearcut (13), selection pressure calculations utilize BASELINe (9), novel gene detection requires TIgGER (11), and the web-frontend exists in a separate repository[1].

Alternatively, a Docker image[2] is available with all these dependencies pre-installed along with helper scripts, and is therefore the recommended method for using ImmuneDB.

Hardware requirements depend on the input data, but as a general guideline it is recommended that ImmuneDB be run on a machine with enough available memory to store at least three times the largest input sample (e.g., for a 5 Gb input file, 15 Gb of memory should be available). Any number of cores are acceptable and ImmuneDB uses Python's multiprocessing library to utilize as many cores as possible.

## Germline Reference Database

ImmuneDB can use any IMGT aligned V- and J-gene database which it accepts as a pair of FASTA files. We suggest always using the most recent IMGT/GENE-DB (14) database including only functional germlines.

## License

ImmuneDB is released under the GNU General Public License, version 3[3] allowing for unlimited use, modification, and distribution under the same license and with any changes explicitly stated.

[1]https://github.com/arosenfeld/immunedb-frontend
[2]https://hub.docker.com/r/arosenfeld/immunedb/
[3]https://www.gnu.org/licenses/gpl-3.0.en.html

## The ImmuneDB Pipeline

ImmuneDB is comprised of sequential steps, run via the command line, that generate a database with analyzed immune receptor data as shown in **Figure 1**. Before running ImmuneDB, it is recommended that pRESTO (3) be used for quality control and, when applicable, paired-read assembly. ImmuneDB itself begins with V- and J-gene identification and optional local-alignment. Then, duplicate sequences are identified across samples originating from the same subject. These sequences are then grouped into clones using one of three methods of clonal inference (described in section Clonal Inference). Finally, aggregate statistics are generated and results can be exported, explored in a web browser, or further analyzed with an integrated set of downstream-analysis tools.

Each step of the pipeline is detailed in this section along with an example of the command to run. In all cases passing the `--help` flag will list all possible parameters and their default values (if any).

### Raw Data Processing

Before running the ImmuneDB pipeline itself, raw FASTQ reads from a sequencer should be quality controlled using pRESTO. First, sequences are trimmed of poor-quality bases on the end farthest from the primer where base call confidence tends to degrade. Using default parameters, sequences are then trimmed to the point where a window of 10 nucleotides has an average quality score of at least 20. If reads are paired, the next step is to align the R1 and R2 reads into full-length, contiguous sequences. Short sequences, those with less than 100 bases, are then removed from further analysis. Finally, any base with a quality score less than 20 is replaced with an *N* and any sequence containing more than 10 such bases is removed from further analysis. In the case of FASTA input which has no quality information, only paired-end assembly and short sequence removal are recommended. A detailed script for running this process can be found in Rosenfeld et al. (15).

After this process, the remaining filtered sequences are presumed to be of adequate quality for germline inference and clonal assignment.

### Creating a Database

ImmuneDB allows users to separate their datasets into individual ImmuneDB *project*, each with their own database. To create a properly structured MySQL database, the `immunedb_admin` command is used:

```
$ immunedb_admin create db_name ~/configs
```

Running this command with `db_name` replaced with an appropriate name will create a database named `db_name` and create a configuration file in `~/configs` with information for the remainder of the pipeline to access it. Specifically, it records a unique username and password for the database so each project you create is separated from others. Database names must consist of only alphanumeric characters, integers, and underscores.

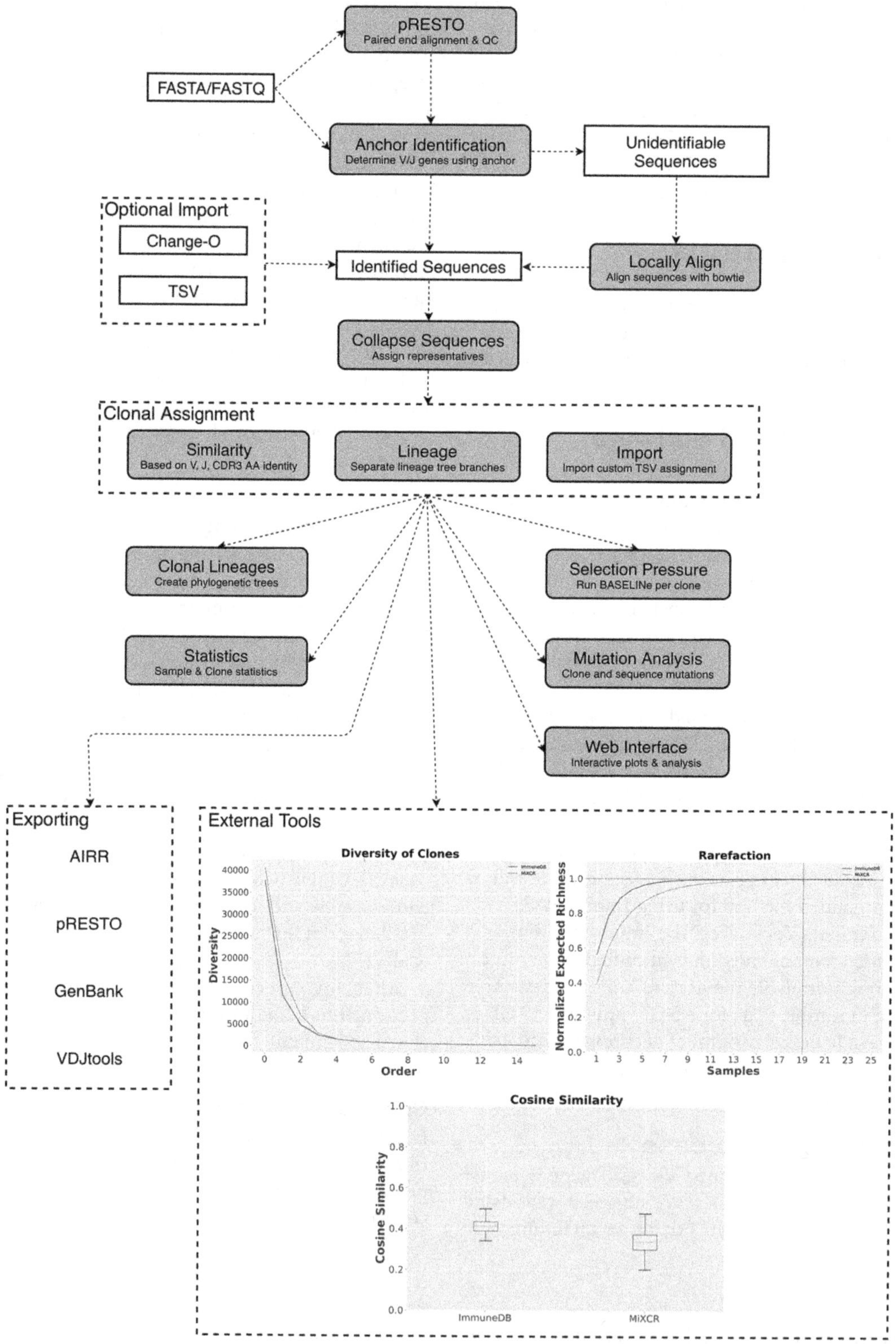


**FIGURE 1 |** A general overview of the ImmuneDB pipeline. To start, sequences are optionally pre-processed with pRESTO to remove poor-quality sequences and mask bases below a user-defined threshold. Next, using a conserved region anchoring method, sequences are either assigned V- and J-genes or labeled as "unidentifiable" which optionally can be corrected by local alignment. After gene assignment, sequences are collapsed across samples and grouped into clones based on one of three methods (see text). Lastly, downstream analyses such as selection pressure, and lineage construction are performed. A web interface is available to browse the resulting data and analyzed data can be exported in a variety of formats. Inset: Examples of downstream analysis: cosine similarity between inferred B-cell rearrangements in tissue samples from an organ donor, diversity (calculated as defined in Equation 1) plotted at different orders from the same tissue samples; rarefaction calculated for B-cell rearrangements amplified from colon samples.

## Sample Metadata Assignment

Each ImmuneDB project is designed to house data across many samples and subjects. It is recommended that each quality-controlled FASTA/FASTQ file contains the sequences from one biologically independent sample. This implies that, if a given sequence is found in multiple independent samples, it actually occurred in multiple cells. Although not recommend, ImmuneDB will still operate normally if samples originated from multiple sequencing runs of the same PCR aliquot. However, many measures of sequence abundance and clone size break down under this conditions [see section Sequence Collapsing (copies, uniques, instances) for discussion].

For the ImmuneDB pipeline, some metadata about each sample are required: a unique sample name and a subject identifier. Samples with the same subject identifier came from the same source organism. Additional custom metadata (e.g., cell subset, tissue) can be attached to each sample, which can be useful for later analysis and grouping.

To generate a template metadata file in the directory with the FASTA/FASTQ files for processing, the user runs:

```
$ immunedb_metadata --use-filenames
```

This will generate a `metadata.tsv` file that should be further edited with the appropriate information, and will be used in the next step of the pipeline. The optional `-use-filenames` flag pre-populates the sample names with the associated filename, stripped of its.`fasta` or.`fastq` extension.

## Germline Assignment (Anchoring, Local Alignment)

The first portion of the ImmuneDB pipeline infers V- and J-genes for each set (sample) of quality-filtered reads using the approach in Zhang et al. (4). This method was chosen because it is quicker than local-alignment and works for the majority of sequences which are not mutated in conserved regions flanking the CDR3. Given a small number of restrictions detailed in the documentation, this method can accept user-defined germlines so long as they are properly IMGT numbered (16). Specifics about the numbering scheme can be found at[4].

For each sequence, the anchor method first searches for a conserved region of the J gene. If it is found, all germline J-gene sequences are compared to the same region in the sequence, and the one with the smallest Hamming distance (17) is assigned as the putative J gene. Since ImmuneDB requires sequences to have a J- and V-gene assignment to be included in clones, if no anchor is found the sequence is marked as unidentifiable and is excluded from V-gene assignment for efficiency.

Then, a conserved region near the 3′ end of the V-segment is used to position each sequence correctly relative to the IMGT numbered germline sequences. As with J-genes, each germline sequence is then compared using Hamming distance, and the one with the smallest distance is assigned as the putative V gene. If the conserved region is not found, the sequence is marked as unidentifiable and excluded from the rest of the anchoring process.

[4]http://www.imgt.org/IMGTScientificChart/Numbering/IMGTIGVLsuperfamily.html

After every sequence is assigned a V and J gene (or marked as unidentifiable) the average mutation frequency and sequence length are calculated. For each sequence, other germline genes which are statistically indistinguishable from the putative genes are added as "gene-ties." Thus, each sequence may have multiple V- and J-gene assignments.

As a post-identification quality control step, ImmuneDB then marks sequences with a low V-germline identity (defaulting to 60%) as unidentifiable. Further, any sequence which has a window of 30 nucleotides with less than 60% germline identity is marked as a "potential insertion or deletion".

To run this step, the user enters the following commands:

```
$ immunedb_identify /path/to/config.json \
       /path/to/v_germlines.fasta \
       /path/to/j_germlines.fasta .
```

After this command finishes, the anchoring portion of alignment is complete. Due to insertions or deletions, mutations in the conserved regions, and other anomalies, there are generally sequences which cannot be identified with this approach. To rectify such sequences, ImmuneDB can then optionally use Bowtie 2 (12) to attempt local-alignment on each of these sequences. Any insertion or deletions that Bowtie 2 finds are also stored with the sequence. The command to locally align sequences is similar to identification:

```
$ immunedb_local_align /path/to/config.json \
       /path/to/v_germlines.fasta \
       /path/to/j_germlines.fasta .
```

## Sequence Collapsing (Copies, Uniques, Instances)

After sequences are assigned V and J genes, sequences that differ only at N positions—those which had low quality calls from the sequencer—are collapsed within each sample resulting in one set of unique sequences per sample. Each unique sequence maintains a count called "copy number" of how many duplicates occurred in the sample. Then, all the sample-level unique sequences within the same subject are compared to one another and duplicates are marked and collapsing information is stored.

After this process, each subject-level unique sequence has two fields associated with it: *total copies* and *instances*. When samples are biologically distinct, which is recommended in section Sample Metadata Assignment, the instance count of a sequence is the number of samples in which that sequence occurred (which can be interpreted as the lower bound on number of cells that contained that sequence) and the total copies is the number of duplicates across all samples. Although the latter is subject to PCR artifacts, it can give an indication of true sequence abundance. Alternatively, when samples are *not* biologically independent, the instances of a sequence no longer give a bound on cell count and the copy number of a sequence may be inflated, leading to skewed sequence and clone abundance calculations.

An overview of the terms copy number, instances, and unique sequences is provided in **Table 1**.

**TABLE 1** | Summary of terms for sequence collapsing.

| Term | Description |
|---|---|
| Unique Sequence | A distinct sequence across an entire subject |
| Instance | A distinct sequence within a single sample |
| Copy number | The number of raw reads that are associated with an instance or unique sequence |

*A description of the three terms used to indicate sequence or clonal sizes.*

To run the collapsing process, run:

```
$ immunedb_collapse /path/to/config.json
```

### Novel Allele Detection and Correction

The ImmuneDB gene identification process assumes the germline allele database provided, from IMGT or another repository, are indeed those present within the subjects being analyzed. Users can add or remove genes as needed by modifying the germline FASTA files input into ImmuneDB. However, in many cases it may not be known *a priori* which genes are or if the subjects have novel germline alleles. To determine which genes are present in a dataset, ImmuneDB may optionally run TIgGER (11) on sequences to identify potential differences from the standard germline database. To do so, the identification and collapsing processes above is run with a presumed germline database followed by:

```
$ immunedb_export /path/to/config.json
        changeo \
        --min-subject-copies 2
$ immunedb_genotype /path/to/config.json \
        /path/to/v_germlines.fasta
```

This exports the sequences, as identified with the presumed germline genes, with at least two copies in the subject and then runs TIgGER. If novel alleles are found, a new set of input germlines is generated, and ImmuneDB can be re-run with these germline reference genes.

### Clonal Inference

ImmuneDB incorporates two methods of clonal inference, all of which start with the same set of sequences: the subject-level unique sequences calculated previously. By default, only such sequences with a copy number of at least two are considered eligible for clonal assignment. This eliminates some of the sequences that potentially arose from sequencing error and could cause spurious construction of clones. After this process, each clone has three defined levels of size. The number of *unique sequences* are the number of distinct sequences that comprise a clone. *Copies* and *instances* are defined as the sum of *copies* and *instances* over the clone's constituent unique sequences. These clone size metrics are reviewed in detail in Rosenfeld et al. (15).

### CDR3 Similarity

The first method of clonal inference is for B cells. It uses CDR3 similarity to group sequences from the same subject with the same gene assignments and CDR3 length into clones. Initially an empty list of clones $C$ is created. Let $S$ be the set of all subject-level unique sequences.

Each sequence $s \in S$ is visited in order of decreasing copy number. If there is a clone $c \in C$ such that every sequence already assigned to $c$ has the same V gene, J gene, CDR3 length in nucleotides, and has 85% CDR3 amino-acid similarity, $s$ is added to the clone $c$. Otherwise, a new clone is added to $C$ containing only $s$. This results in a set of clones such that all the sequences in a clone share the same gene assignments, CDR3 length, and pairwise are at least 85% similar in the CDR3. The percent similarity can be tweaked by the user as necessary.

This method of clonal inference can be run with:

```
$ immunedb_clones /path/to/config.json \
        similarity
```

### Lineage Separation

The newest method of clonal assignment in ImmuneDB is based on (18). For each subject, sequences are placed into buckets based on their V gene, J gene, and CDR3 length in nucleotides. Then, a lineage is made out of each bucket. Working from the root node of the lineage (the germline) each edge is traversed until a specified number (by default four) mutations accumulates. The subtree starting at that point is then grouped into a clone. This method, unlike similarity-based methods, is order-agnostic and can be run with:

```
$ immunedb_clones /path/to/config.json \
        lineage
```

### Selection Pressure

After clonal inference, ImmuneDB can optionally use BASELINe (9) to estimate clonal selection pressure. It first runs on each clone as a whole, providing an overview of selection pressure in the framework and complementary regions. Then, it runs independently on the subset of sequences that occur in each sample. This can be useful when a clone spans multiple samples with various biological features. For example, a clone may appear in samples from different tissues or cell subsets.

To run BASELINe via ImmuneDB, the path to the `Baseline_Main.r` script must be specified.

```
$ immunedb_clone_pressure /path/to/config.json \
        /path/to/Baseline_Main.r
```

### Lineages

ImmuneDB integrates Clearcut (13) to infer clonal lineages using neighbor-joining. For each clone, a lineage is constructed and every node maintains information about its associated sequence, as shown via the web-interface in **Figure 2**. This process can be parameterized in different ways including filtering sequences or mutations that occur less than a set number of times. Generally, it is recommended to run Clearcut excluding mutations that happen exactly once with:

```
$ immunedb_clone_trees
        /path/to/config.json \
        /path/to/clearcut \
        --min-count 2
```

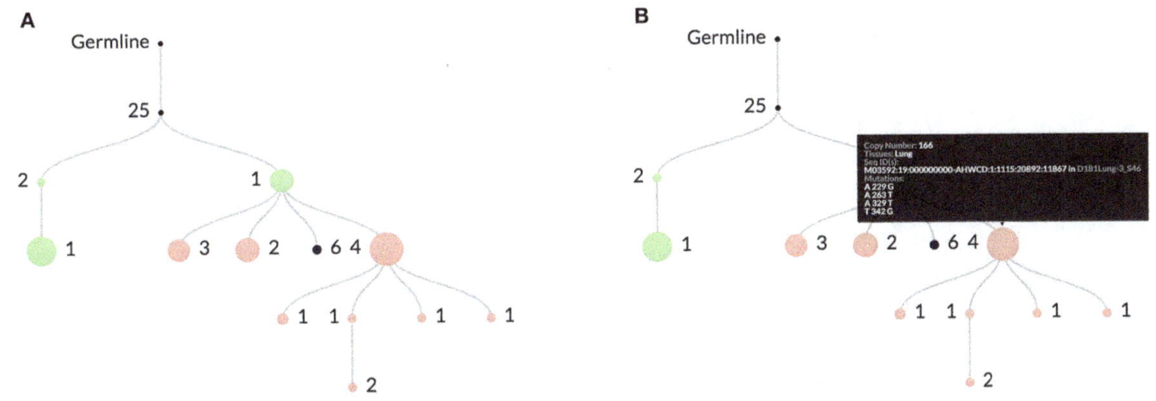


**FIGURE 2 |** In **(A)** an example clonal lineage as viewed through the web interface for ImmuneDB. Node diameter is proportional to the total number of sequence copies at that node and the edge numbers show the number of mutations between the parent and child nodes. The colors indicate the tissue(s) that make up the sequences at the node. In this case green is Bone Marrow, red is Lung, and black is a combination of both. As shown in **(B)**, hovering over a node gives more information such as the specific mutations, copy number, and sequence metadata.

**Figure 3** shows the same clone's lineage constructed with **Figure 3A** no mutation threshold, **Figure 3B** a threshold requiring mutations to occur in at least 2 sequences, and **Figure 3C** a threshold requiring mutations to occur in at least 5 sequences. The large expansion of nodes in **Figure 3A** is likely due to sequencing error. A higher threshold like in **Figure 3C** may be useful when there is high sequencing depth or when clones are extremely large (such as in some hematopoietic malignancies). In these cases it is quite likely that the same sequencing error will occur multiple times. However, thresholding mutations means the lineages may not accurately reflect recent or rare clonal events.

### Web Interface

ImmuneDB comes with a web interface for browsing analyzed data. It allows users to group and filter data to generate interactive plots, view clones, and inspect sequences. It is primarily intended to explore data at a high-level, visualizing individual samples or comparing different samples in various ways. The command line tools can then be used for more fine-grained analysis. An example interface can be found at http://immunedb.com/tissue-atlas.

To utilize the web interface using the Docker container simply run the following and open http://localhost:8080 in a browser:

```
$ serve_immunedb.sh /path/to/config.json
```

Information about running the web interface without the Docker container or with more sophisticated configurations, such as hosting multiple databases, are described in the documentation.

## Importing Gene Assignments and Clonal Inference From Other AIRR Tools

Although ImmuneDB has the features to fully analyze sequences from raw reads through clonal assignment, a concerted effort has been made to allow users to import both identified sequences and clonal assignments from other tools. For pre-identified sequences, ImmuneDB can import files in the Change-O data format (5) with:

```
$ immunedb_import /path/to/config.json \
      /path/to/v_germlines.fasta \
      /path/to/j_germlines.fasta \
      /path/to/changeo_files
```

Note that this requires a metadata file identical to that needed by the identification step.

Clonal assignments can be imported from either ImmuneDB-identified sequences or imported sequences. First, the command below is run to output a template file with a list of clonal-assignment eligible sequences:

```
$ immunedb_clone_import /path/to/config.json \
      --action export sequences.tsv
```

Users then fill in the `clone_id` column in sequences.tsv as they desire and import it back into ImmuneDB with:

```
$ immunedb_clone_import /path/to/config.json \
      --action import sequences.tsv
```

Assuming that no constraints are broken (clones must still have the same V gene and J gene and originate from the same subject), the custom clonal assignment will then be accepted by ImmuneDB.

As members of the AIRR Community (19), the authors will continue to integrate data standards (2) as they are defined.

## Aggregate Analysis and Data Export

ImmuneDB automatically aggregates data for some common analyses in the last step of the pipeline with:

```
$ immunedb_clone_stats /path/to/config.json
$ immunedb_sample_stats /path/to/config.json
```

This auto-generated, aggregate analysis is not exhaustive, and is meant to provide sufficient data for the web-interface and to guide further investigation. To assist with this, ImmuneDB allows users to easily export all portions of the analyzed dataset in useful, common formats. Specifically, ImmuneDB has integrated

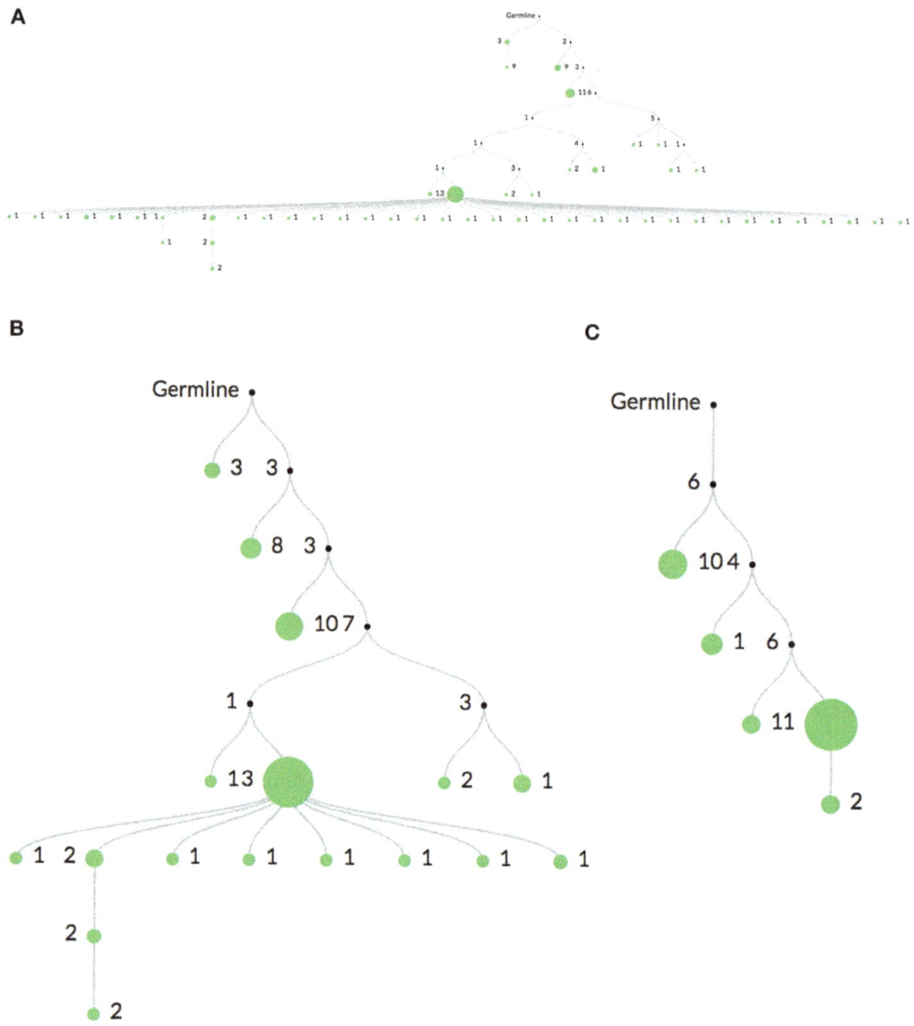


**FIGURE 3 |** Comparison of mutation thresholding on lineage shape. A comparison of a single clonal lineage constructed from bulk IgH V-region sequencing data where **(A)** all mutations are included, **(B)** only mutations found in at least 2 sequences are included, and **(C)** only mutations in at least 5 sequences are included. The drastic elimination of leaf nodes between **(A)** and **(B)** indicate that they are most likely due to sequencing error. In very deeply sequenced samples or in malignancies where clones are very large, an even higher threshold may be required, such as in **(C)**, since the same sequencing error may occur multiple times.

export capabilities for the Change-O (5),vdjtools (8), genbank, and FASTA/FASTQ formats. This enables users to quickly use common downstream analysis tools including VDJtools and those included with the Immcantation Framework[5], or submit their datasets in the AIRR-compliant GenBank format. The basic template for this command is as follows, replacing the term **`format`** with `changeo`, `vdjtools`, or `genbank`:

```
$ immunedb_export /path/to/config.json \
      format
```

## Applications to Other Data Types

### T-cells

ImmuneDB can analyze T-cell receptor sequences, in addition to B-cell receptor sequences. When compared to B-cell analysis, the two changes necessary in the pipeline for T-cell analysis are to use T-cell germline sequences during germline assignment and to specify the T-cell method during clonal inference. The T-cell method groups sequences with the same V gene, J gene, and 100% CDR3 nucleotide identity into clones. Like the B-cell similarity method described in section CDR3 Similarity, the T-cell method does not take into account any mutations in the V- and J genes. In the case of T cells, mutations are assumed to be experimental artifacts as T cell receptors do not undergo somatic hypermutation due to lack of activation-induced cytidine deaminase (AID). Putative T-cell clones may be comprised of sequences which appear to differ in the V- and J-gene sequences. Spurious intra-clonal diversification is likely from sequencing error whereas consistent divergence from the germline within a clone likely arises from allelic differences from the germline database. The latter case can be corrected with TIgGER as described in section Novel Allele Detection and Correction.

[5]https://immcantation.readthedocs.io

### Light Chains

Because ImmuneDB does not attempt to determine D-genes for sequences during germline assignment, light-chains are naturally supported when a proper germline database of the V- and J genes are provided. At the present, the germline genes for kappa and lambda chains must be placed in separate files and run independently. This restriction will be lifted in future versions. Additionally, because of lower junctional diversity, it is recommended that clonal assignment be considered. For example, when using the similarity method, it is likely appropriate to lower the default amino-acid similarity threshold to a value below 85%.

### Other Species

Species other than humans are supported by ImmuneDB, but with two restrictions. First, for the built-in anchoring method for gene identification, germline genes must have conserved anchoring points as described in Zhang et al. (4) and be IMGT aligned. Second, the length of all J genes past the 3′ end of the CDR3 must be fixed, which is the case for all species currently in the IMGT database.

## COMPARISON TO MIXCR

It is difficult to verify the results of clonal and germline association methods as there is no agreed upon gold standard. We attempt to associate different types of diversity to their underlying cause(s), but in the end, this is still just an educated guess. Our methodology, as described above, is based on the best practices described in Yaari and Kleinstein (20): stringent pre-processing, correcting for allelic differences between subjects, identification of insertions and deletions, and multiple clonal assignment methods for different datasets. ImmuneDB also provides the option of varying the stringencies of both data filtering and clonal assignment to ensure reproducible and robust results.

As a final argument for the efficacy of ImmuneDB, we show that repertoires analyzed with ImmuneDB take a form similar to those observed with other tools. In this section we compare ImmuneDB to a commonly used pipeline, MiXCR (6), on two datasets. First, we compare the germline gene assignment and clonal inference of the two methods on five samples, one each from five different tissues, all from one human organ donor. Second, we inspect how similar the overall view of a larger repertoire (19 biological replicates from a single organ donor's colon) appears with each method (1).

### Germline Assignment and Clonal Inference

To determine how similarly MiXCR and ImmuneDB assign germline genes and infer clones, both pipelines were run on five samples from one human subject selected from Meng et al. (1) as listed in **Table 2**. The associated SRA accession information can be found in **Table S1**. This data set has a total of 651,988 reads. Sequences which were considered incorrect or misleading were discarded from both result sets: sequences had to have at least 160 bases in the V gene (at least all of CDR2), between 3 and 96 nucleotides in the CDR3, a functional V-gene assignment (no pseudogenes), and all V-gene calls (V-ties) for a given sequence had to be from the same V-gene family. For clonal comparisons, clones with only one total copy were discarded.

**TABLE 2 |** Input reads for germline assignment comparison.

| Donor | Tissue | Input reads |
|---|---|---|
| D181 | Bone Marrow | 185,057 |
| D181 | Ileum | 140,084 |
| D181 | Jejunum | 117,641 |
| D181 | Lung | 113,325 |
| D181 | Peripheral Blood | 95,881 |
| | Total Reads | 651,988 |

*Total number of input reads for germline assignment comparison between ImmuneDB and MiXCR. The total number of input reads was after pre-processing with pRESTO. The samples were selected from one of the deeply sequenced donors in Meng et al. (1).*

#### Germline Assignment

First, we compared which sequences each method was able to identify given this filtering. MiXCR identified 599,930 while ImmuneDB identified 611,252, and both identified the same 577,750. The corresponding Jaccard index of 0.91 indicates that the two methods identified a similar set of sequences.

Next, we compared how many of the identified sequences were assigned to the same genes. Since both methods allowed multiple assignments for both V genes and J genes, we considered two sequences to have the same gene call if the intersection of their gene calls contained at least one shared gene. For V genes, the two methods agreed on 98% of the sequences, for J-genes 95%, and when considering both genes, 93%. Of the sequences that differed with either gene, less than 1% differed in their gene family calls. Thus, overall both methods generally agreed on which germline genes gave rise to each sequence.

#### Clonal Inference

Next, we compared how similarly the two methods inferred clonotypes for the 19 biologically independent colon sample replicates. The associated SRA accession information can be found in **Table S2**. For this process, we assigned each clone one or more labels from each method:

- If clone *A* from one method contained exactly the same sequences as clone *B* from the other, we labeled both "*identical*".
- If clone *A* from one method contained a strict superset of sequences compared to clone *B* from the other method, we labeled *A* "*superset*" and *B* "*subset*".
- If clone *A* from one method contained a portion of sequences compared to a clone *B* from the other method, we labeled both "*intersecting*".
- If clone *A* from one method was disjoint from all clones from the other method, we labeled it "*disjoint*".

Note that a clone could potentially have both the labels *superset* and *intersecting* simultaneously if it contained all the sequences from a clone inferred by the other method and contained sequences from another clone. Further, a clone could have

**TABLE 3** | Label assignments for clonal inference comparison.

| Clone Type | ImmuneDB | MiXCR |
|---|---|---|
| Identical | 10,788 | 10,788 |
| Subset | 1,665 | 2,819 |
| Superset | 1,155 | 726 |
| Intersecting | 22 | 12 |
| Superset & Intersecting | 72 | 74 |
| Disjoint | 36 | 36 |

*Clonal labels when comparing methods of clonal inference between ImmuneDB and MiXCR. Identical indicates the same set of clones was identified by both methods, subset/superset means the clone constructed by the associated pipeline was a subset/superset of one assigned by the other pipeline, and intersecting means there some sequences from a clone assigned by one pipeline that overlapped sequences assigned by the other pipeline.*

multiple *superset* labels if it contained all the sequences from multiple clones inferred from the other method.

As shown in **Table 3**, ImmuneDB inferred 13,736 clones whereas MiXCR inferred 14,453. Of these 10,786 were identical; that is both methods constructed clones with exactly the same set of sequences. In 1,665 cases, an ImmuneDB clone was a subset of a MiXCR clone. There are two reasons this occurred. First, different amounts of *N* nucleotides in the either the V- or J-region can cause sequences, that are otherwise similar, to be assigned different sets of gene ties and therefore placed in different clones. Second, since ImmuneDB requires *pairwise* 85% similarity of CDR3 amino-acid sequences in clones, some sequences that may actually originate from the same clone are separated. Conversely, 2,819 MiXCR clones are subsets of an ImmuneDB clone. Nearly all of these are due to overly-strict J-gene assignment, resulting in separation of likely clonally related sequences. For example, some sequences that are one nucleotide away from IGHJ1 and two away from IGHJ4 could easily be confused due to sequencing error (4).

## Overall Repertoire Features

Repertoire analysis pipelines should reveal similar overall trends in acceptably large datasets even if the minutiae of sequence assignment and clonal inference differ. Specifically, when looking at sufficiently large clones, the overlap across samples and diversity should lead to similar conclusions. It is generally acceptable to only look at larger clones as smaller clones have likely been under-sampled or are an artifact of sequencing error (21).

To compare repertoire-level metrics generated from ImmuneDB and MiXCR processed data, 19 biologically independent colon replicates were analyzed. We assessed the similarity of the two pipelines by comparing their clone size distributions, diversity measures, rarefaction, and clonal overlap between samples as described in Meng et al. (1).

### Clone Size Distribution

We first looked at clone size distributions from the two pipelines. In **Figure 4**, the left panel shows a comparison of clone sizes as measured by copy number. The overall landscape is similar with both methods, especially when looking only at clones with 10 or more sequence copies. For smaller clones, the difference in clone sizes can be attributed to the more stringent CDR3 similarity measure MiXCR uses compared to ImmuneDB. The right panel shows the same comparison but instead measures the size of clones as the number of instances comprising the clone. Both methods have nearly identical clone size distributions, especially when considering clones with at least 2 instances.

### Diversity

We next considered the diversity of the clones assigned by each method. The diversity index ${}^qD$, as defined by Equation 1 quantifies how many different clones there are.

Equation 1: Diversity index ${}^qD$

$$ {}^qD = \left( \sum_{i=1}^{R} p_i^q \right)^{1/(1-q)} $$

Here, $R$ is the number of clones (richness), $p_i$ is the fraction of the repertoire (either as copies or instances) inferred to be in clone $i$, and $q$ is the order. When the order is zero, the diversity is richness, or total number of clones. Increasing the order, $q$, gives more weight to the larger clones (21, 22). **Figure 5** shows the diversity at orders 1 through 15 for ImmuneDB and MiXCR, measuring clone size both as copies and instances.

It is clear that MiXCR infers more clones than ImmuneDB. However, when the order number is increased (more weight is given to large clones) the diversity of the two methods converges.

### Rarefaction

Rarefaction gives insight into how many clones are estimated to occur given a certain number of samples (biological replicates) from the same source. A rarefaction curve that levels out indicates that fewer new clones will be found with further sampling. **Figure 6** shows the rarefaction curves for ImmuneDB and MiXCR for clones with at least 2, 5, 10, and 20 instances. The x-axis shows the number of samples and the y-axis shows the normalized richness (the richness divided by the richness at 19 samples). The solid lines (up to 19) are calculated from the 19 samples being compared, whereas the dashed lines past sample 19 show the projected number of additional clones if more replicates had been acquired. As only larger clones are considered, the rarefaction curves both begin to level out, indicating that those larger-clone populations have been more adequately sampled. Both pipelines tended to agree on when clones had been sampled enough, even though the overall diversity appears to be higher with MiXCR (indicated by lower fractional richness).

### Sample Overlap

We next evaluated the amount of clonal overlap using the cosine similarity, as defined by Equation (2):

Equation 2: Cosine similarity between vectors $A$ and $B$

$$ C(A,B) = \frac{\sum_{i=1}^{n} A_i B_i}{\sqrt{\sum_{i=1}^{n} A_i^2}\sqrt{\sum_{i=1}^{n} B_i^2}} $$

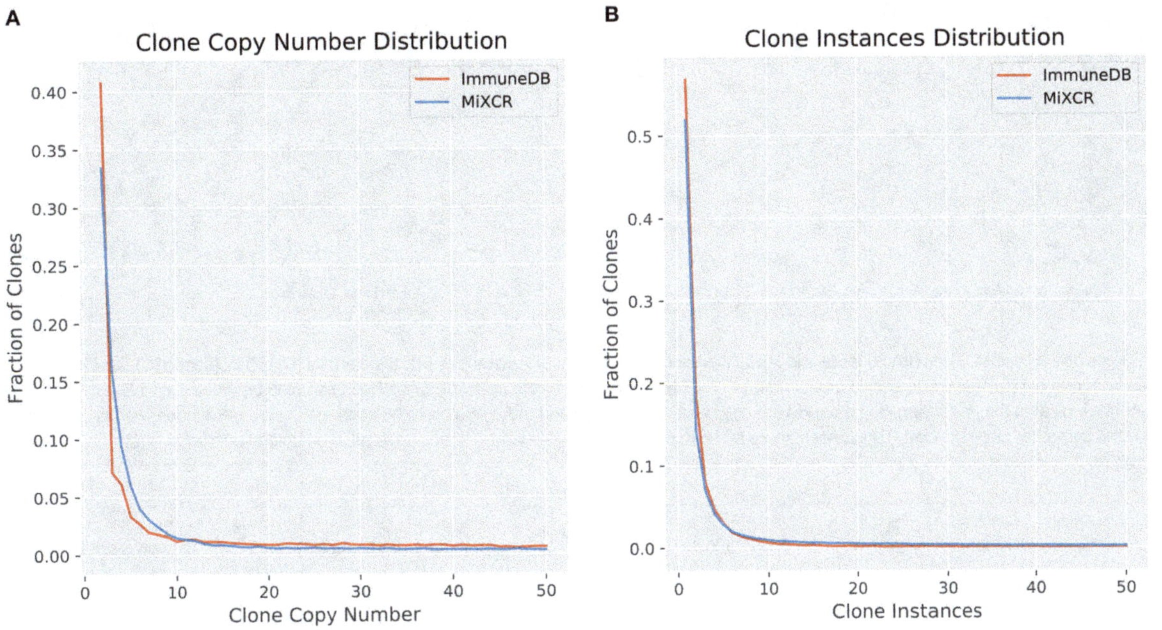


**FIGURE 4 |** Comparison of clone size distributions between ImmuneDB and MiXCR in 19 colon samples subjected to bulk antibody heavy chain V-region sequencing from one organ donor [data from (1)]. Clone size is given as copies in **(A)** and instances in **(B)**. Both plots have been restricted to a maximum X-value of 50, but the trends continue beyond that.

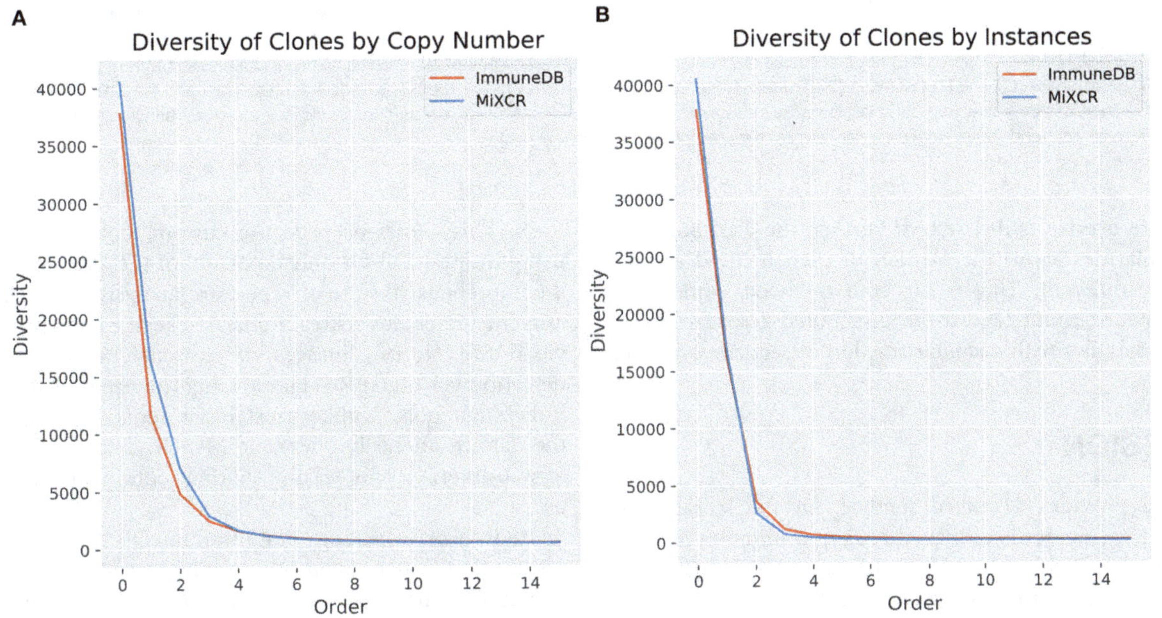


**FIGURE 5 |** Comparison of diversity calculations between ImmuneDB and MiXCR in 19 colon samples from one donor (same data as in **Figure 4**). As order increases, more weight is given to larger clones. For both copies and instances, MiXCR inferred more diverse clonal populations for low order numbers. As order increases, however, the two methods begin to converge.

In this case, $A$ and $B$ are vectors corresponding to two samples both of which have a length equal to the total number of clones in the dataset. The $i$th value in each vector indicates the number of copies of the $i$th clone in the sample represented by the vector.

**Figure 7** shows the cosine similarity for clones with a minimum of 2, 5, 10, and 20 sequence instances. MiXCR infers less overlap between samples, but the general trend between both methods is the same: as expected, with larger

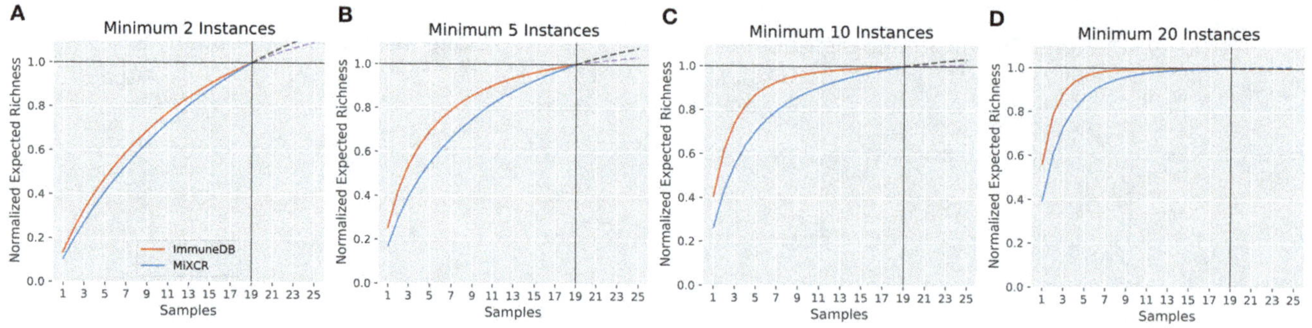

**FIGURE 6 |** Rarefaction analysis for both ImmuneDB and MiXCR for clone size cutoffs of 2 instances **(A)**, 5 instances **(B)**, 10 instances **(C)**, and 20 instances **(D)** in 19 colon samples from one donor. The Y-axis shows the number of predicted clones when the population has been sampled between 1 and 25 times. A rarefaction curve that plateaus indicates the underlying clonal population has been adequately sampled. For all cutoffs, although the overall richness varies, the conclusion drawn would likely be the same: for clones under 10 instances, more sampling is required, while larger clones have been sampled sufficiently.

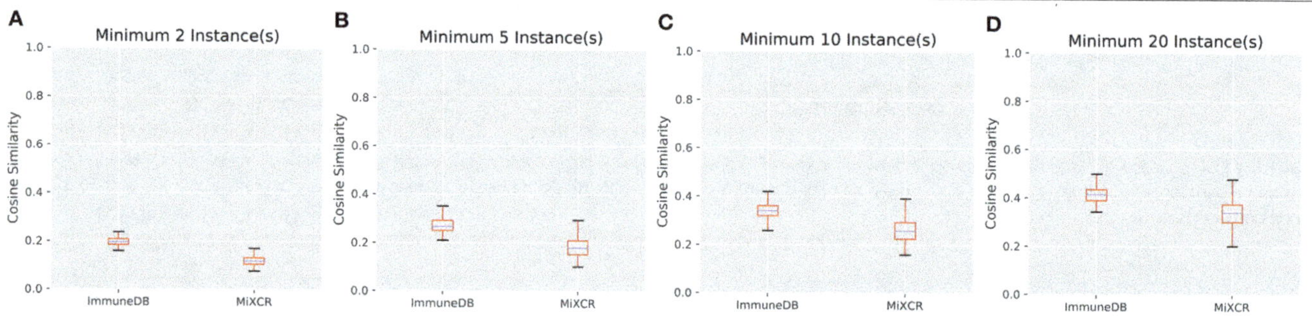

**FIGURE 7 |** The distribution of cosine similarities (a measure of clonal overlap) between each pair of 19 colon samples for clone size cutoffs of 2 instances **(A)**, 5 instances **(B)**, 10 instances **(C)**, and 20 instances **(D)**. The boxes represent the interquartile range, the purple lines are the median, and the whiskers show the range of data. MiXCR finds less overlap across samples, because it has a more stringent CDR3 similarity requirement for clonal sequences than ImmuneDB, but both methods show a similar trend: larger clones overlap across more samples as one may expect.

clones, more overlap is discovered. Further, the distribution of cosine similarities about the median of each method are not significantly different. That is for both methods, clones over a given instance count tend to be distributed across a similar number of samples with a similar fraction of sequences in each sample.

## DISCUSSION

ImmuneDB provides a unified method for the storage and analysis of large amounts of high-throughput immune receptor sequencing data. Like other pipelines such as Change-O (5) and MiXCR (6), it can analyze data from raw reads through clonal assignment. ImmuneDB has two method of germline calculation, anchoring and local-alignment, and provides the option of filtering the data at different QC and copy number cut-offs, which is desirable when samples with different sequencing depths are being compared. In addition, ImmuneDB provides multiple methods of clonal assignment. Combined, these features provide a variety of ways to analyze different types of data.

ImmuneDB is also flexible in that it can import pre-annotated data in a variety of formats supported by other AIRR software tools. This allows users to use custom tools for their dataset, using ImmuneDB for only a portion of the analysis. To provide a comprehensive suite of repertoire analysis tools, ImmuneDB also integrates downstream analyses such as selection pressure via BASELINe (9), lineages via clearcut (13), and novel allele detection via TIgGER (11), reducing the need for users to learn individual tools. Unlike most other tools, ImmuneDB stores the data in an easily queryable MySQL database and provides a web-interface for easily sharing data with non-technical users.

It is worth noting that ImmuneDB does make some assumptions when using other tools, however. For example, it is assumed that sequences in a clone have the same V gene, J gene, and CDR3 length and that they come from the same organism. Although generally this is likely acceptable, there are certain situations where such assumptions may not hold, such as donor/recipient data where a clone may span multiple recipients. As such, it is important to consider the limitations of all tools before using them on non-traditional datasets.

Additionally, since ImmuneDB calculates clones on a per-subject basis, adding new samples to a subject requires clonal inference to be re-run for that subject. However, the rest of the database will remain unchanged.

Finally, in section Comparison to MiXCR we compared ImmuneDB to MiXCR, a pipeline that similarly determines germline usage and infers clonotypes to show that the benefits of using ImmuneDB do not come at the cost of drastically changing conclusions one may draw from the data. Although the methods differ in their approach to clonal assignment, both yield similar clone size distributions, rarefaction plateau points, and sample overlap.

## CONCLUSION AND FUTURE PLANS

In this paper we have provided a comprehensive description of ImmuneDB, a system for the analysis of large-scale, high-throughput immune repertoire sequencing data. ImmuneDB can operate either independently, providing an integrated collection of analysis tools to process raw reads for gene usage, infer clones, aggregate data, and run downstream analyses, or in conjunction with other AIRR tools using its import and export features. Thus, ImmuneDB can be an all-in-one solution for repertoire analysis or serve as an efficient way to visualize and store annotated repertoire data, or both. In either case, the ImmuneDB web-interface can be used to easily interact with the underlying dataset.

ImmuneDB is regularly being updated to address user needs and handle the increasing complexity of adaptive immune receptor repertoire sequencing data. In the future we plan to add a feature to allow users to assess the quality of individual sequencing libraries (replicates) before running the entire pipeline. As pRESTO provides a per-sequence quality control step, this new feature will provide a post-identification quality control step, informing users if their samples have insufficient depth or quality. Further, the CDR3 similarity clonal inference method will receive two additional features. First, it will be extended to allow for different similarity thresholds for different CDR3 lengths. Second, this method will allow users to set a required minimum number of shared V-gene somatic hypermutations for sequences to be grouped into a clone.

## AUTHOR CONTRIBUTIONS

AR developed ImmuneDB and wrote the first draft of this manuscript. WM ran the sequencing experiments generating the data for this manuscript and helped test ImmuneDB. WM, EL, and UH provided input on important features to include in ImmuneDB and in this manuscript. EL and UH both contributed to editing this manuscript.

## FUNDING

This research was sponsored by NIH P01 AI106697, P30 AI0450080, NIH UC4 DK112217, and P30 CA016520.

## ACKNOWLEDGMENTS

The authors thank Jason A. Vander Heiden for his assistance with the GenBank exporting format.

## SUPPLEMENTARY MATERIAL

**Table S1** | SRA accession information for the five samples used in the germline assignment comparison between ImmuneDB and MiXCR.

**Table S2** | SRA accession information for the 19 samples used in the clonal inference comparison between ImmuneDB and MiXCR.

## REFERENCES


1. Meng W, Zhang B, Schwartz GW, Rosenfeld AM, Ren D, Thome JJC, et al. An atlas of B-cell clonal distribution in the human body. *Nat Biotechnol.* (2017) 35:879–86. doi: 10.1038/nbt.3942
2. Rubelt F, Busse CE, Bukhari SAC, Bürckert JP, Mariotti-Ferrandiz E, Cowell LG, et al. Adaptive immune receptor repertoire community recommendations for sharing immune-repertoire sequencing data. *Nat Immunol.* (2017) 18:1274–8. doi: 10.1038/ni.3873
3. Vander Heiden JA, Yaari G, Uduman M, Stern JNH, O'Connor KC, Hafler DA, et al. pRESTO: a toolkit for processing high-throughput sequencing raw reads of lymphocyte receptor repertoires. *Bioinformatics* (2014) 30:1930–2. doi: 10.1093/bioinformatics/btu138
4. Zhang B, Meng W, Luning Prak ET, Hershberg U. Discrimination of germline V genes at different sequencing lengths and mutational burdens: A new tool for identifying and evaluating the reliability of V gene assignment. *J Immunol Methods* (2015) 427:105–16. doi: 10.1016/j.jim.2015.10.009
5. Gupta NT, Vander Heiden JA, Uduman M, Gadala-Maria D, Yaari G, Kleinstein SH. Change-O: A toolkit for analyzing large-scale B cell immunoglobulin repertoire sequencing data. *Bioinformatics* (2015) 31:3356–8. doi: 10.1093/bioinformatics/btv359
6. Bolotin DA, Poslavsky S, Mitrophanov I, Shugay M, Mamedov IZ, Putintseva E V, et al. MiXCR: software for comprehensive adaptive immunity profiling. *Nat Methods* (2015) 12:380–1. doi: 10.1038/nmeth.3364
7. Marcou Q, Mora T, Walczak AM. High-throughput immune repertoire analysis with IGoR. *Nat Commun* (2018) 9:561. doi: 10.1101/141143
8. Shugay M, Bagaev DV, Turchaninova MA, Bolotin DA, Britanova OV, Putintseva EV, et al. VDJtools: Unifying Post-analysis of T Cell Receptor Repertoires. *PLoS Comput Biol.* (2015) 11:e1004503. doi: 10.1371/journal.pcbi.1004503
9. Yaari G, Uduman M, Kleinstein SH. Quantifying selection in high-throughput Immunoglobulin sequencing data sets. *Nucleic Acids Res.* (2012) 40:e134. doi: 10.1093/nar/gks457
10. Rosenfeld AM, Meng W, Luning Prak ET, Hershberg U. ImmuneDB: a system for the analysis and exploration of high-throughput adaptive immune receptor sequencing data. *Bioinformatics* (2017) 33:292–3. doi: 10.1093/bioinformatics/btw593
11. Gadala-Maria D, Yaari G, Uduman M, Kleinstein SH. Automated analysis of high-throughput B-cell sequencing data reveals a high frequency of novel immunoglobulin V gene segment alleles. *Proc Natl Acad Sci USA.* (2015) 112:E862–70. doi: 10.1073/pnas.1417683112
12. Langmead B, Salzberg SL. Fast gapped-read alignment with Bowtie 2. *Nat Methods* (2012) 9:357–9. doi: 10.1038/nmeth.1923
13. Evans J, Sheneman L, Foster J. Relaxed neighbor joining: a fast distance-based phylogenetic tree construction method. *J Mol Evol.* (2006) 62:785–92. doi: 10.1007/s00239-005-0176-2
14. Giudicelli V, Chaume D, Lefranc M-P. IMGT/GENE-DB: a comprehensive database for human and mouse immunoglobulin and T cell receptor genes. *Nucleic Acids Res.* (2005) 33: D256–61. doi: 10.1093/nar/gki010

15. Rosenfeld AM, Chen DY, Zhang B, Granot T, Farber DL, Hershberg U, et al. PROTOCOL: computational evaluation of B-cell clone sizes in bulk populations. *Front Immunol.* (2018) 9:1472. doi: 10.3389/fimmu.2018.01472
16. Lefranc M-P, Pommié C, Ruiz M, Giuducelli V, Foulquier E, Truong L, et al. IMGT unique numbering fro immunoglobulin and T cell receptor variable domains and Ig superfamily V-like domains. *Dev Comp Immunol.* (2003) 27:55–77. doi: 10.1016/S0145-305X(02)00039-3
17. Hamming RW. Error detecting and error correcting codes. *Bell Syst Tech J.* (1950) 29:147–60. doi: 10.1002/j.1538-7305.1950.tb00463.x
18. Liberman G, Benichou J, Tsaban L, Glanville J, Louzoun Y. Multi step selection in Ig H chains is initially focused on CDR3 and then on other CDR regions. *Front Immunol.* (2013) 4:274. doi: 10.3389/fimmu.2013.00274
19. Breden F, Luning Prak ET, Peters B, Rubelt F, Schramm CA, Busse CE, et al. Reproducibility and reuse of adaptive immune receptor repertoire data. *Front Immunol.* (2017) 8:1418. doi: 10.3389/fimmu.2017.01418
20. Yaari G, Kleinstein SH. Practical guidelines for B-cell receptor repertoire sequencing analysis. *Genome Med.* (2015) 7:121. doi: 10.1186/s13073-015-0243-2
21. Colwell RK, Chao A, Gotelli NJ, Lin SY, Mao CX, Chazdon RL, et al. Models and estimators linking individual-based and sample-based rarefaction, extrapolation and comparison of assemblages. *J Plant Ecol.* (2012) 5:3–21. doi: 10.1093/jpe/rtr044
22. Schwartz GW, Hershberg U. Conserved variation: Identifying patterns of stability and variability in BCR and TCR v genes with different diversity and richness metrics. *Phys Biol.* (2013) 10:35005. doi: 10.1088/1478-3975/10/3/035005

# 11

# TCR Analyses of Two Vast and Shared Melanoma Antigen-Specific T Cell Repertoires: Common and Specific Features

*Sylvain Simon*[1,2]*, Zhong Wu*[3]*, J. Cruard*[1,2]*, Virginie Vignard*[1,2,4]*, Agnes Fortun*[1,2]*, Amir Khammari*[1,2,5]*, Brigitte Dreno*[1,2,5]*, Francois Lang*[1,2]*, Samuel J. Rulli*[3] *and Nathalie Labarriere*[1,2,4*]

*[1] CRCINA, INSERM, Université d'Angers, Université de Nantes, Nantes, France, [2] LabEx IGO "Immunotherapy, Graft, Oncology," Nantes, France, [3] Qiagen Sciences, Frederick, MD, United States, [4] Centre Hospitalier Universitaire Nantes, Nantes, France, [5] Department of Dermato-Cancerology of Nantes Hospital, Nantes, France*

***Correspondence:**
*Nathalie Labarriere*
*nathalie.labarriere@inserm.fr*

Among Immunotherapeutic approaches for cancer treatment, the adoptive transfer of antigen specific T cells is still a relevant approach, that could have higher efficacy when further combined with immune check-point blockade. A high number of adoptive transfer trials have been performed in metastatic melanoma, due to its high immunogenic potential, either with polyclonal TIL or antigen-specific polyclonal populations. In this setting, the extensive characterization of T cell functions and receptor diversity of infused polyclonal T cells is required, notably for monitoring purposes. We developed a clinical grade procedure for the selection and amplification of polyclonal CD8 T cells, specific for two shared and widely expressed melanoma antigens: Melan-A and MELOE-1. This procedure is currently used in a clinical trial for HLA-A2 metastatic melanoma patients. In this study, we characterized the T-cell diversity (T-cell repertoire) of such T cell populations using a new RNAseq strategy. We first assessed the added-value of TCR receptor sequencing, in terms of sensitivity and specificity, by direct comparison with cytometry analysis of the T cell populations labeled with anti-Vß-specific antibodies. Results from these analyzes also confirmed specific features already reported for Melan-A and MELOE-1 specific T cell repertoires in terms of V-alpha recurrence usage, on a very high number of T cell clonotypes. Furthermore, these analyses also revealed undescribed features, such as the recurrence of a specific motif in the CDR3α region for MELOE-1 specific T cell repertoire. Finally, the analysis of a large number of T cell clonotypes originating from various patients revealed the existence of public CDR3α and ß clonotypes for Melan-A and MELOE-1 specific T cells. In conclusion, this method of high throughput TCR sequencing is a reliable and powerful approach to deeply characterize polyclonal T cell repertoires, and to reveal specific features of a given TCR repertoire, that would be useful for immune follow-up of cancer patients treated by immunotherapeutic approaches.

**Keywords: TCR sequencing, melanoma, Melan-A, MELOE-1, immunotherapy**

## INTRODUCTION

Among solid tumors, metastatic melanoma is a relevant model for immunotherapeutic approaches because of a high immunogenicity, partly due to a high mutation rate, favoring the development of specific T cell immune responses (1). In previous studies, it has been documented that the specific immune response against melanoma is dominated by two vast T cell repertoires specific for the melanoma antigens Melan-A and MELOE-1, which can be selected and amplified from the peripheral blood of HLA-A2 melanoma patients (2, 3). These two antigens share common features regarding their frequent expression in melanoma tumors, the presence of immunodominant HLA-A2 epitopes and of vast specific TCR repertoires in HLA-A2 melanoma patients. Blood frequencies of Melan-A and MELOE-1 specific T cells are respectively around $10^{-4}$ and $10^{-6}$ among CD8 T cells. In addition, these T cell repertoires also contain high avidity T cells making these T cell repertoires relevant for a use in adoptive transfer.

For a long time, Melan-A has been regarded as a self-antigen, potentially eliciting a suboptimal T-cell repertoire due to negative selection. However, recently it was reported that the immunodominant HLA-A2 Melan-$A_{26-35}$ epitope is not presented by human medullary thymic epithelial cells, due to a misinitiation of gene transcription (4), and leading to the evasion of central self-tolerance toward this epitope. This finding, together with the strong bias documented in Vα usage (5, 6) could explain the abundance of this specific-T cell repertoire and the presence of high avidity T cells among this repertoire.

On the other hand, MELOE-1 antigen is expressed from a polycistronic RNA, whose expression is controlled by specific transcription factors and epigenetic mechanisms in the melanocytic lineage (7). The translation of MELOE-1 from one of the short ORFs of this RNA is controlled by an IRES sequence, exclusively activated in melanoma cells, conferring to this antigen a strict tumor expression profile (8, 9). Like Melan-A specific T cell repertoire, MELOE-1 specific T cell repertoire also contains high avidity T cells, and is also strongly bias toward the preferential usage of a specific TRAV chain (2), probably contributing to the relative high frequency of MELOE-1 specific T cells in the peripheral blood of HLA-A2 individuals. All these features confer to these two antigen-specific-T cell repertoires interesting properties for a use in adoptive transfer setting in a large subgroup of melanoma patients (HLA-A2), contrary to neo-antigen-based therapeutic personalized strategies.

Based on this, we developed a clinical grade method to select and expand *ex-vivo* Melan-A and MELOE-1 specific CD8 T cells from the blood of HLA-A2 patients. This method, relying on the sorting of specific T cells through the use of HLA/peptide-coated magnetic beads (3), is currently used in the MELSORT clinical trial to treat metastatic melanoma patients (NCT02424916, https://clinicaltrials.gov). This standardized procedure allows the production of fully specific, polyclonal and tumor reactive specific T cells. Nonetheless the diversity of these polyclonal populations has been addressed so far through the use of anti-Vß specific antibodies, and we could document that these populations were composed with various Vß subfamilies, but the number of T cell clonotypes present among a given Vß subfamily remained unknown. Furthermore, the available panel of 24 Vß-specific antibodies does not always cover the entire T cell repertoire of all antigen-specific T cell populations.

We thus took advantage of a recent high throughput TCR sequencing method developed by Qiagen, to fully characterize Melan-A and MELOE-1 T cell populations, selected and amplified according our standardized producing method. We first documented the sensitivity and reliability of this method, and we report here an extensive characterization of Melan-A and MELOE-1 specific T cell repertoires. This analysis reveals a high diversity of these antigen-specific sorted T cells that exhibit common and specific TCR features.

Thus, this method enables the complete and accurate characterization of T cell repertoires that is a main issue for immune follow-up purposes, in adoptive transfer setting, but also for other immunotherapeutic approaches including immune-checkpoint blockade (10).

## MATERIALS AND METHODS

### Melan-A and MELOE-1 Specific T Cell Populations

Peripheral blood mononuclear cells (PBMC) were isolated from 40 mL of blood of HLA-A2 metastatic melanoma patients (Unit of Dermato-cancerology, Nantes hospital) after written informed consent (approval number: DC-2011-1399). PBMC were seeded in 96 well/plates at $2 \times 10^5$ cells/well in RPMI 1640 medium supplemented with 8% human serum (HS), 50 IU/mL of IL-2 (Proleukin, Novartis) and stimulated either with 1 μM of Melan-$A_{A27L}$ peptide (ELAGIGILTV) or 10 μM of natural MELOE-$1_{36-44}$ peptide (TLNDECWPA), purchased from Genecust. After 14 days, each microculture was evaluated for the percentage of specific CD8 T lymphocytes by double staining with the relevant HLA-peptide tetramer (from the SFR Sante recombinant protein facility) and anti-CD8 mAb (Clone RPA-T8, Biolegend) using a FACS Canto HTS. Microcultures that contained at least 1% of specific T cells were selected, pooled and sorted with the relevant multimer-coated beads as previously described (3). After a 14-day amplification period on irradiated feeder cells, in presence of PHA-L (1μg/mL) and IL-2 (150U/mL), purity of expanded sorted T cells was assessed by double staining with the relevant HLA-peptide tetramer and anti-CD8 mAb (**Figure S1**).

### Vß Repertoire of Specific T Cells

Vß diversity of sorted Melan-A and MELOE-1 specific T cell lines was analyzed by labeling with 24 anti-Vß mAbs included in the IOTest Beta Mark TCR V Kit (Beckman-Coulter, IM3497). These cytometric analyses were performed on a Facs Canto II (BD Biosciences).

### T-Cell Receptor Sequencing

Total RNA was extracted from 5 × 10^5 antigen specific T cells using QIAGEN RNeasy Kit. RNA from normal PBMC (purchased from Precision for Medicine) was used as a reference control. 10 or 25 ng of RNA was used to build libraries with the QIAseq Immune Repertoire -T-cell Receptor Panel (Catalog 333705- IMHS-001Z). With this kit, RNA is reverse transcribed with a pool of gene specific primers against the C (constant) region for the T cell receptor alpha, beta, gamma, and delta genes. The reverse transcribed cDNA is then used in a 5′ ligation reaction which adds an oligo which contains one side of sample index and unique molecular index. Following reaction cleanup, a single primer extension is used to capture the T-cell receptor using a pool of gene-specific primers. Resulting captured sequences are amplified and purified using QIAseq beads. The libraries then are sample indexed on the other side by using a unique sample index primer and a universal primer. The final dual sample indexed PCR fragment is purified and then quantitated for abundance using real-time qPCR.

For sequecning, each library was diluted to 4 nM, pooled and denatured. 12 pM of denatured library pool was run on a MiSeq using V3 chemistry for 502 cycles with a pair-end 251 base read.

## Read Trimming/Clonotype Calling

FASTQ files were analyzed in the QIAGEN GeneGlobe Data Analysis Center (https://www.qiagen.com/us/shop/genes-and-pathways/data-analysis-center-overview-page/) using the Immune Repertoire Application The web-based read processing service generates clonotype calls and quantity estimates from reads generated by the QIAseq Immune Repertoire Library Kit. The clonotype calls are generated using the IMSEQ software (11). The main tasks of IMSEQ are to align the reads to model V-region and J-region sequences, extract the CDR3 region sequence, and cluster together highly similar CDR3 sequences that likely came from the same input sample clones. A detailed description of the IMSEQ algorithm is at the following URL: http://www.imtools.org.

## Read Processing Steps

### Trim Reads

We first trim from the reads the constant regions generated by the enrichment protocol, and move the UMI sequence to the read identifier line.

Trim 3′ end of reads with less than 18 base quality score.
Trim ligation common oligo AGGACTCCAAT from the 3′ end of R1.
Trim uPCR common oligo CAAAACGCAATACTGTACATT from the 3′ end of R2.

The 12 bp UMI sequence is moved from the start of R2 to the FASTQ read identifier comment region of R1 and R2.

### Down-Sample Reads

When read depth rises above about 8 to 10 read pairs per UMI, very few new real UMIs are observed, but false UMIs caused by PCR or sequencing errors are observed at an increasing rate. The same is true for CDR3 sequences. To control this over-sequencing error in the UMI and CDR3 sequences, we randomly discard the reads until the remaining reads contain about 8 reads per UMI.

### Merge Overlapping R1 and R2 Reads

To accommodate IMSEQ requirement for R1 being entirely VDJ sequence, and R2 being V-only, we merge overlapping R1 and R2 and rename them as R1. The reads are then split by gene (TRAC, TRBC, TRDC, TRGC). To accommodate IMSEQ input requirements, we split reads by gene using "cutadapt" search for the C-region sequence between the 5′-most SPE primer and the start of the J-region.

### Trim V Region

To accommodate the IMSEQ requirement that reads do not overhang the V-region model sequences, we align the reads to the V-region models using BWA mem, and trim overhang regions (e.g., 5′ UTR regions).

### Run IMSEQ

We run IMSEQ with the following parameters: -ev 0.15 -mq 25 -mcq 25 -ma -qc -sc -scme 2 -sfb.

The model V and J sequences used with IMSEQ can be found here: https://storage.googleapis.com/qiaseq-rna-mmrep/QIAseqRNA_immrep_TCR_model_seqs.zip.

We are using two important features of IMSEQ that are designed to minimize false clonotype calls caused by sequencing error. We are using both the "quality-score clustering" and the "simple edit-distance clustering" with edit distance <= 2 (the IMSEQ default). The main idea here is that reads that contain highly similar CDR3 sequences are putatively from the same clone in the sample, so they are grouped together to generate one CDR3 call, as described previously (11).

### Assign Each Read to a Called Clonotype

Although IMSEQ clusters highly similar CDR3 sequences, it does not output detail regarding which reads were clustered together. In part, this is because IMSEQ sometimes counts partial reads, i.e., when a sequence is equal distance from two different CDR3 centroid sequences. To enable UMI counting, we restore the connection between each read and one CDR3 call from IMSEQ, using CD-HIT clustering. We run CD-HIT with the following parameters:

```
cd-hit-v4.6.8-2017-0621/cd-hit-est-2d -n 5 -g 1 -r 0 -d 0 -G 1 -t 0 -c 0.90 -p 1 -S 2 -S2 2.
```

### Filter Low-Evidence Clonotypes

To leverage the power of UMI tagging to reduce NGS errors leading to false clonotype calls, we discard IMSEQ CDR3 calls that do not have at least one UMI supported by three reads. Users can set more stringent filters on reported clonotype calls (such as frequency or minimum number of supporting UMIs) depending on application needs.

## Data and Statistical Analyses

For statistical analyses, clonotypes are defined on the basis of unique amino-acid sequences of CDR3 alpha and CDR3 beta regions. In our set of data, the total number of unique

TCR sequences was identical to the number of clonotypes. The standardized residuals of chi-squared is used to determine if a V or J chain is preferentially used in antigen-specific repertoire, score = $(\text{observed—expected})^2/\text{expected}$, the expected values are calculated from the control sample distribution, the observed values are actually the number of clonotypes using each gene in one given antigen specific repertoire. We considered as significantly used the V or J segment having a score >4.

CDR3 amino acid sequences length has been compared between antigen-specific populations and the control sample using the two-tailed Student's *T*-test. All the calculations were done using R statistical software.

# RESULTS

## TCR Diversity of Melan-A and MELOE-1 Specific T Cell Populations

We analyzed the TCR diversity of 6 Melan-A and 4 MELOE-1 specific CD8+ T cell polyclonal populations, derived from the specific sorting of HLA-A2 patient PBMC stimulated with the cognate peptides (3). These polyclonal populations were fully specific, as assessed by specific tetramer labeling (**Figure S1**) and reactive against their target peptides and HLA-A2 melanoma cell lines.

**Table 1** summarizes the specific richness of these 10 CD8 T cell populations (numbers of CDR3α and CDR3ß amino-acid sequences, thereafter called "clonotypes," detected from libraries prepared from 10 to 25ng of total RNA). The RNAseq library includes unique molecular indexes (UMIs) which are added during library construction to remove amplification duplicates and sequencing errors. For our analysis, we considered data where we had at least 1 UMI and 3 reads per UMI to be a true clonotype. For Melan-A-specific T cell repertoires, we observed high numbers of CDR3α and CDR3ß clonotypes with the highest amount of starting RNA, consistent with increased sensitivity in detecting rare clonotypes when starting with more sample. Concerning MELOE-1 specific T cell repertoires, the differences between the number of clonotypes detected with 10 or 25 ng of RNA are either null or rather modest, in accordance with the fact that MELOE-1 specific T cell repertoires are less diverse than Melan-A-specific ones. Thus, the majority of MELOE-1 specific-T cell clonotypes are already detected with 10 ng of starting RNA.

**Figure 1** illustrates the rank of individual CDR3α and ß clonotypes identified for the 6 Melan-A (1A) and MELOE-1 (1B) specific populations, and the relative abundance of each sequence (number of reads of each sequence associated to a unique UMI), for the two starting RNA quantities. Globally, for Melan-A, and MELOE-1 specific T-cell repertoires, the number of counts for CDR3α (blue circles) and CDR3ß sequences (red circles) was higher when starting with 25 ng (dark circles) vs. 10 ng (light circles) of total RNA. This analysis illustrates the presence of dominant clonotypes within each individual T cell populations, the number of counts for a unique TCR sequence being comprised between 1 and $10^4$. Furthermore, considering the total number of identified clonotypes, we also observed

**TABLE 1** | Number of CDR3 alpha and CDR3 beta clonotypes identified in Melan-A and MELOE-1 specific T cell populations, starting from 10 to 25 ng of total RNA.

| | CDR3 alpha | | CDR3 beta | |
|---|---|---|---|---|
| **Starting RNA** | **10 ng** | **25 ng** | **10 ng** | **25 ng** |
| **MELAN-A SPECIFIC T CELL POPULATIONS** | | | | |
| P1 | 78 | 140 | 72 | 134 |
| P2 | 61 | 112 | 44 | 100 |
| P3 | 24 | 34 | 14 | 28 |
| P4 | 38 | 46 | 27 | 36 |
| P6 | 22 | 41 | 13 | 26 |
| P7 | 27 | 38 | 13 | 31 |
| All samples | 249 | 411 | 183 | 355 |
| **MELOE-1 SPECIFIC T CELL POPULATIONS** | | | | |
| P5 | 49 | 36 | 29 | 29 |
| P8 | 28 | 39 | 23 | 63 |
| P9 | 18 | 20 | 19 | 20 |
| P10 | 62 | 59 | 45 | 41 |
| All samples | 157 | 154 | 116 | 153 |

that scarce CDR3 sequences are not identified for some T cell populations with the lowest RNA quantity (**Figure 1**).

Thus for more diverse populations, higher amounts of RNA will favor the characterization of the complete TCR repertoire, and for less diverse T cell repertoire, RNA quantity will only affect the number of counts for all CDR3 sequences.

## Comparison of TRBV Chain Frequencies Using TCR Sequencing or Specific Antibodies

The proportion of T cells expressing a given Vß chain was determined by flow cytometry within the 10 antigen-specific subpopulations, using a panel of 24 Vß-specific antibodies, covering the most frequently expressed Vß chains. Some of the antibodies cross-react with various TRBV subtypes, such as TRBV4-1, 4-2, and 4-3; TRBV6-5, 6-6 and 6-9; TRBV12-3 and 12-4. In order to compare the frequencies of the different TRBV subfamilies detected either by flow cytometry or sequencing approaches, we gather all TRBV sequences potentially detected by a single anti-Vß antibody and calculated their cumulated frequencies. **Figure 2** illustrates the correlation between frequencies of TRBV chains detected through the sequencing approach (starting from 25ng of total RNA) and antibody-labeling. TRBV chains for whom there is no available Vß-specific antibody are indicated with red circles. These TRBV chains (especially TRBV6 and TRBV7 subfamilies) are rather frequent within the two antigen-specific T cell repertoires and could only be detected through TCR sequencing. With the exception of these particular TRBV chain the correlation between TRBV frequencies detected with the specific antibodies and cumulated frequencies calculated from sequence counts is satisfying, unless the presence of some outliers only detected through sequencing analysis (blue circles). Generally, the

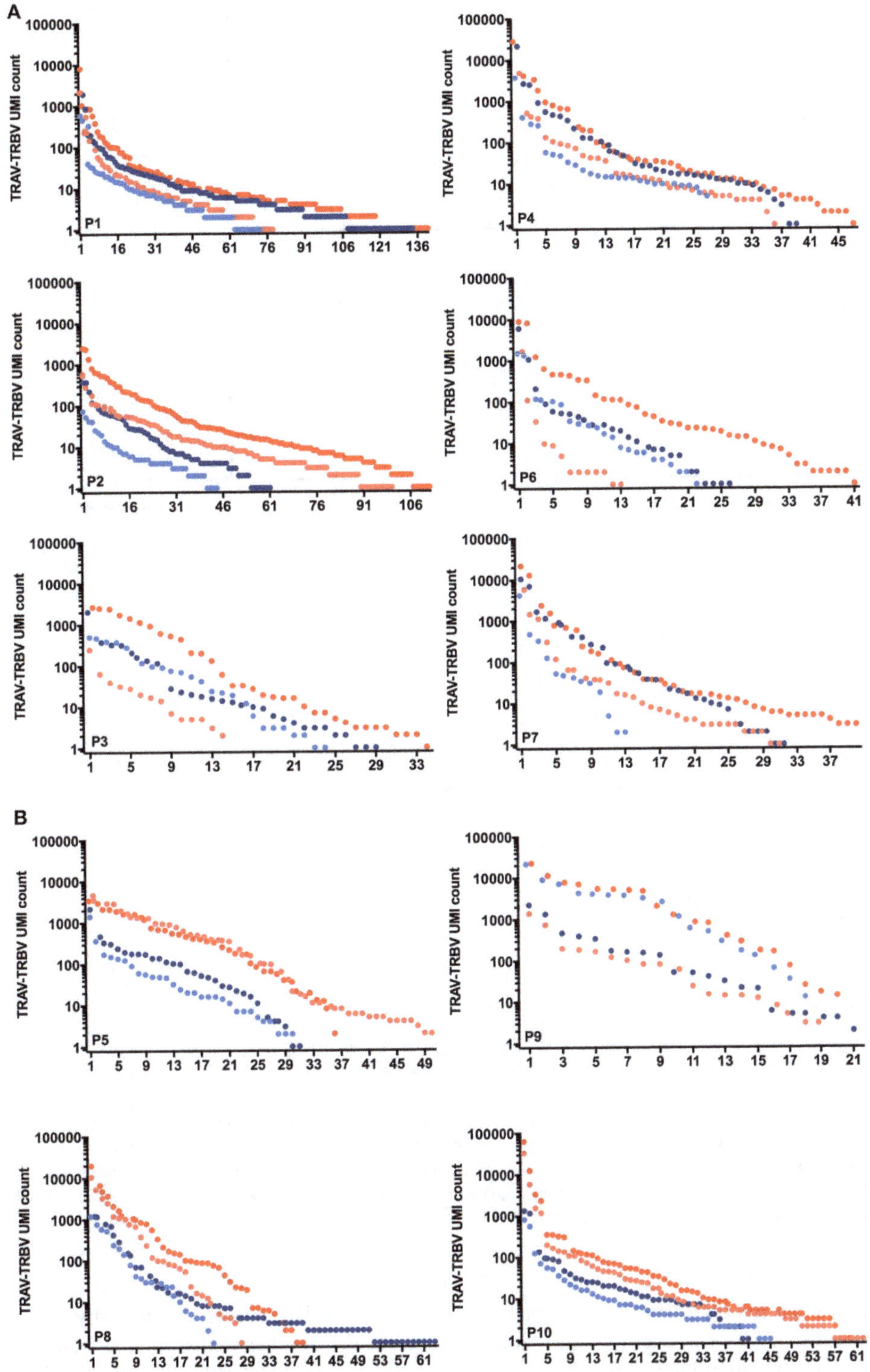

**FIGURE 1 |** Rank and relative abundance of UMI for individual CDR3α (blue circles) and CDR3β clonotypes (red circles) identified for 6 Melan-A specific T-cell populations **(A)** and 4 MELOE-1 specific T-cell populations **(B)**, starting from 10 ng (light circles) or 25 ng (dark circles) of total RNA.

frequency of the concerned TRBV chain is rather low, probably under the detection threshold of specific antibodies. Only the TRBV4-2 chain is detected through TCR sequencing for P7 patient with a high frequency (64%) but is not detected by the specific antibody (**Figure 2A**). Of note, TRBV4-2 chain is supposed to be detected by an antibody also cross-reacting with

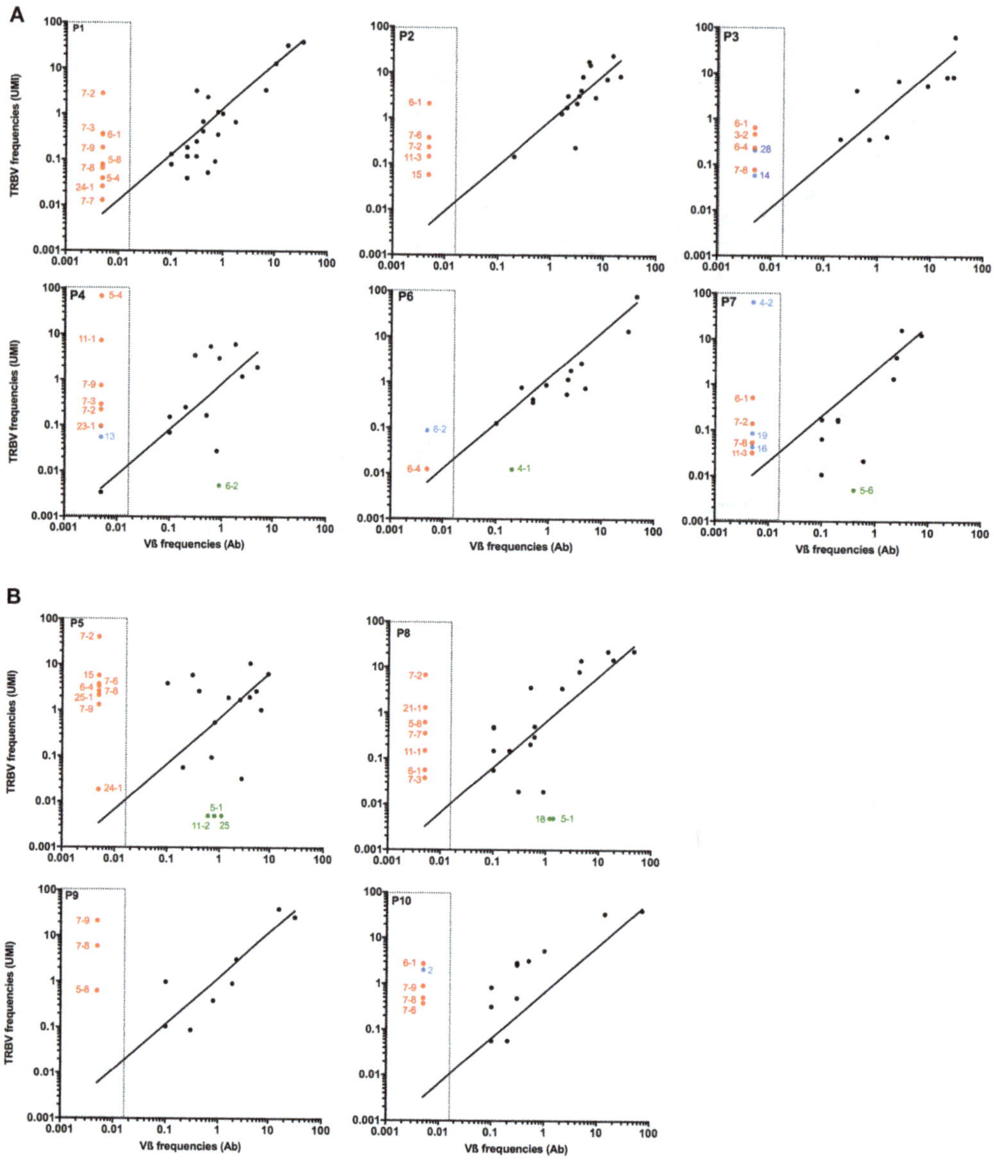


**FIGURE 2 |** Comparison of Vß chain detection with antibody labeling or high throuput sequencing. The frequencies of Vß subfamilies in each polyclonal Melan-A-specific **(A)** and MELOE-1-specific **(B)** T cell populations were documented through labeling with a 24 Vß-specific antibody panel (X axis). CDR3ß clonotypes identified by sequencing were gathered according to their corresponding Vß chain, and their cumulative frequencies are indicated on the Y axis. Red circles represent Vß chains not covered by the antibody panel. Blue and green circles illustrate respectively Vß chain only detected by TCR sequencing despite the use of a specific Ab, and Vß chain only detected by flow cytometry.

TRBV4-1 and 4-3, and we can hypothesize that the reactivity of this antibody against the TRBV4-2 chain is suboptimal. Conversely, some TRBV chains identified through antibody labeling are not detected by the sequencing analyses (green circles on **Figure 2**). Again, these Vß subfamilies represented only small frequencies, and these discrepancies can be attributed to some degree of cross-reactivity of the concerned antibodies.

This comparison validates the reliability of this TCR sequencing method to estimate the proportion of a specific TRBV chain within a given T cell repertoire. This method is undeniably much more powerful than antibody labeling that leads to underestimate the diversity of a polyclonal population, due to the number of distinct clonotypes within the same TRBV subfamily, to the absence of some TRBV-specific antibodies, and to the cross-reactivity of some specific Vß antibodies.

## TRAV and TRBV Usage of Melan-A and MELOE-1 Specific T Cell Repertoires

Melan-A specific T cell repertoire has been largely studied and it is well known that this T cell repertoire present a strong bias in TRAV12-2 gene usage (5, 6). Likewise, a clear TRAV bias toward TRAV19 chain has also been reported for 18 MELOE-1 specific CTL clones (2). With the aim to increase the statistical value of antigen-specific repertoire analyses and to smooth individual variations, we analyzed TRAV and TRBV usage of all the Melan-A and MELOE-1 clonotypes (originating respectively from 6 and 4 HLA-2 metastatic melanoma patients). The same analyses have been conducted for each individual populations and are illustrated by **Figure S2.** We clearly confirm the strong recurrent usage of the TRAV12-2 and TRAV19 chains, used respectively by 185/411 Melan-A-specific CDR3α clonotypes (Chi$^2$ score value= 34.7) and 79/154 MELOE-1-specific CDR3α clonotypes (Chi$^2$ score value = 21) (**Figure 3A**, left panel). These two chains are also frequently used in the control sample, but their preferential usage by Melan-A and MELOE-1-specific T cells remains strongly significant. This strong recurrence is also remarkable for individual populations (**Figures S2A,B**, left panels). We also analyzed TRBV usage for these two specific T cell repertoires. A diverse TRBV usage was previously reported for Melan-A specific T cell repertoire (5, 6, 12, 13), nonetheless with some studies highlighting a frequent usage of TRBV20-1, TRBV27, TRBV28, and TRBV19 (14, 15). Here we documented the significant preferential usage of TRBV19 chain for Melan-A specific T cell repertoire, with 43/355 CDR3ß clonotypes (Chi$^2$ score value = 6.18). The other described recurrent TRBV chains (TRBV20-1, 27, and 27) were also frequently used by Melan-A specific CDR3ß clonotypes, but this usage was not statistically different from that of the control sample (**Figure 3A**, right upper

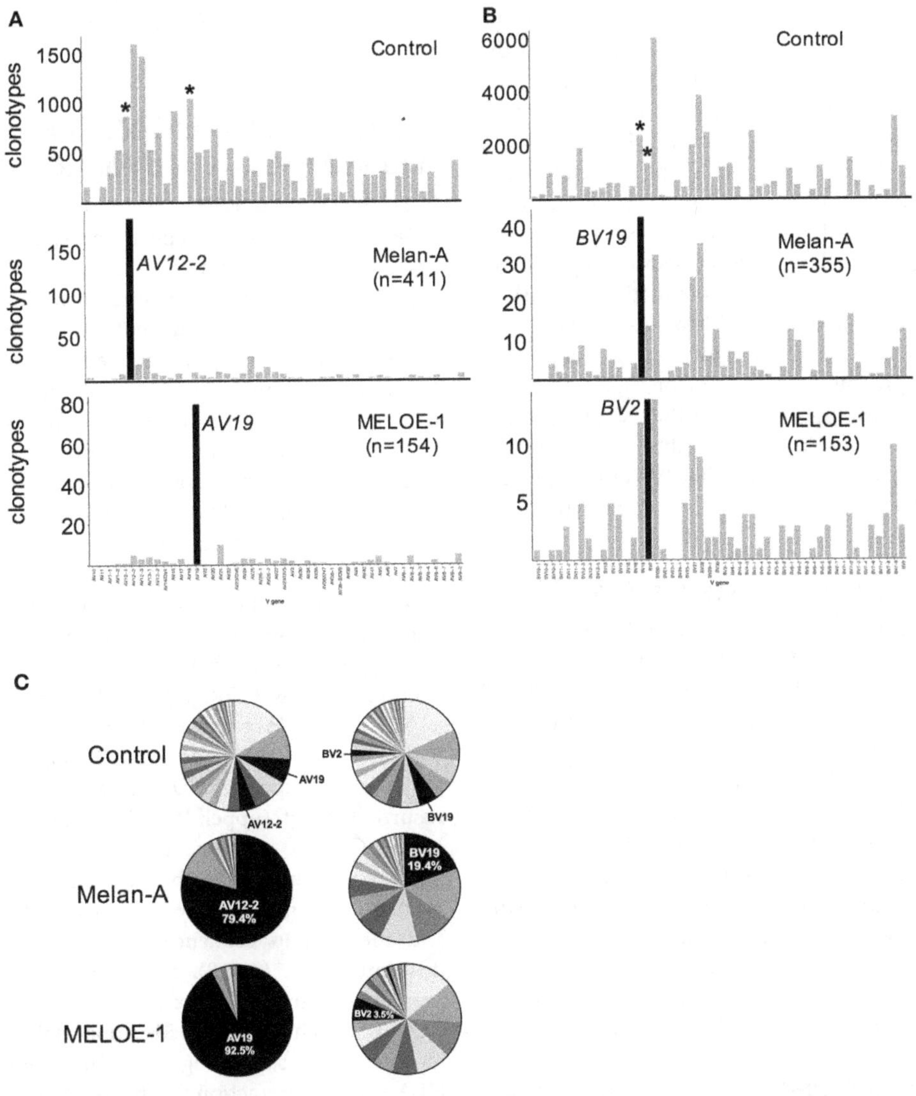


**FIGURE 3 |** TRAV and TRBV usage of specific-T cell populations. Number of clonotypes using individual TRAV **(A)** and TRBV **(B)** chains in control (upper panels); Melan-A-specific T cell repertoire (sum of the clonotypes originating from the 6 populations; middle panels); and MELOE-1-specific T cell repertoire (sum of the clonotypes originating from the 4 populations; lower panels). Black histograms illustrate TRV chains preferentially used in each T cell repertoire, and the same chains are marked with an asterisk in the control sample. **(C)** Cumulative frequencies (UMI) of each TRAV (left panel) and TRBV (right panel) chains in the control sample, Melan-A specific and MELOE-1 specific T cell repertoires.

panel). At individual population level, although frequently used in each population, TRBV19 usage is only dominant in 2/6 Melan-A specific T cell populations (**Figure S2A**, right panel).

No preferential TRBV usage has been reported so far for MELOE-1-specific TCR repertoire, and here we documented a significant bias toward the use of the TRBV2 chain, for this TCR repertoire, with 14/153 CDR3ß clonotypes (Chi$^2$ score value = 4.58). At individual population level (**Figure S2B**, right panel), TRBV2 usage is frequent in each T cell population.

We next analyzed the cumulated frequencies of these preferentially used TRAV and TRBV chains within each specific TCR repertoire (**Figure 3C**). This parameter illustrates the relative abundance of CDR3α and ß clonotypes using these particular TRV genes, within a given repertoire. Within Melan-A and MELOE-1 TCR repertoire, CDR3α clonotypes using respectively the TRAV12-2 and the TRAV19 genes represented almost 80 and 90% of amplified clonotypes, strengthening the crucial role of these TRAV chains in the specificity toward the HLA-peptide complexes. The preponderance of TRAV12-2 and TRAV19 clonotypes, in terms of abundance is also observed in each individual specific-T cell population (**Figures S2A,B**, inserts on left panel). TRBV19 Melan-A specific clonotypes represented the most abundant ones, with almost 20% of amplified Melan-A specific CDR3ß clonotypes, suggesting that this TRBV19 segment also participates to TCR specificity. Indeed, in individual Melan-A-specific T cell populations, TRBV19 clonotypes are overrepresented in 3/6 Melan-A-specific T cell populations (**Figure S2A**, inserts on right panel). Conversely, TRBV2 clonotypes represented only 3.5% of total MELOE-1 specific CDR3ß clonotypes, suggesting that the use of a specific TRBV chain is less crucial for MELOE-1 specific T cell repertoire. Indeed, with the exception of P5 patient, TRBV2 clonotypes are not part of the most abundant ones in individual MELOE-1 specific T cell populations.

## TRAJ and TRBJ Usage of Melan-A and MELOE-1 Specific T Cell Repertoires

Within the Melan-A and MELOE-1 specific repertoires, we looked for the preferential usage of TRAJ and TRBJ segments (**Figure S3**) and to particular TRAV-TRAJ and TRBV-TRBJ combinations (**Figure 4**). We found a significant preferential usage of the TRAJ45 (31/411 clonotypes, Chi$^2$ score value = 4.5, **Figure S3A**) and TRBJ1-5 (67/355 clonotypes, Chi$^2$ score value = 8.05, **Figure S3B**) segments within Melan-A-specific clonotypes. For MELOE-1 specific repertoire, although non-significant, we found some biases in TRAJ usage, with TRAJ22 (9/154 clonotypes, **Figure S3A**) and TRAJ44 (11/154 clonotypes, **Figure S3A**) and we also observed a significant preferential usage of the TRBJ2-1 segment within MELOE-1 repertoire (38/153 clonotypes, Chi$^2$ score value = 4.3, **Figure S3B**).

As these Melan-A and MELOE-1 TCR repertoires are strongly biased toward the use of TRAV12-2 and TRAV19 chains, we further investigated whether these dominant TRAV chains were associated with a given TRAJ segment (**Figure 4A**). For Melan-A-specific repertoire, we confirmed the bias already reported (15, 16) toward the association of the dominant TRAV12-2 chain with the TRAJ45 segment (23/51 TRAV12-2 clonotypes used this segment, i.e., 45%). So far, no specific TRAV-TRAJ association has been reported for MELOE-1-specific T cell repertoire, due to the low number of analyzed T cell clones. Within TRAV19 clonotypes, the preferential use of TRAJ22 (9/51 TRAV19 clonotypes, Chi$^2$ score value = 6.02) and TRAJ44 (9/51, Chi$^2$ score value = 4.61) segments is significant (**Figure 4B**).

We also looked for a preferential TRBV-TRBJ association for the two specificities, represented by heatmaps on **Figure 4C**. For the Melan-A specific repertoire, the significantly preferentially used TRBJ1-5 segment was associated with 21 TRBV chains, that confirms the diversity of Melan-A TRB repertoire. Nonetheless, the most dominant TRBV-TRBJ association was observed with the TRBV19 recurrent BV chain, with 15 CDR3ß clonotypes using the TRBJ1-5 segment among the 43 TRBV19 clonotypes.

For MELOE-1 specific T cell repertoire (**Figure 4C**, lower panel), the frequently used TRBJ2-1 segment was associated with 21 different TRBV chains, with no obvious specific TRBV-association.

## CDR3 Lengths and Motif Recurrence Within Melan-A and MELOE-1 Specific T Cell Repertoires

CDR3 sequences were defined according international criteria, beginning by a cysteine residue at the C-terminal end of the V-gene and ending with a phenylalanine residue coded by the N-terminal end of the J segment (17).

Lengths of CDR3α and ß sequences of Melan-A and MELOE-1 specific clonotypes were first compared with those of the reference sample (**Figure 5A**). The average lengths of CDR3α and CDR3ß sequences are between 13 and 14 aa for the control sample. For Melan-A specific repertoire, the mean length of CDR3α is significantly shorter (Student test, $p = 2.10^{-16}$), with a length centered on 12 amino acids, and the length of CDR3ß is not different from the control sample. The lengths of CDR3α and ß are more heterogeneous and both significantly longer than those of the reference sample for MELOE-1 specific T cell clonotypes, centered on 17 amino acids for CDR3α and 15 amino acids for CDR3ß (CDR3α: $p = 2.10^{-8}$; CDR3ß: $p = 8.10^{-6}$).

We further investigated the presence of a conserved motif within these CDR3α and CDR3ß sequences (**Figure 5B**). For the Melan-A specific CDR3α sequences, we found no clear recurrent motif (upper left). This absence of recurrent motif in the CDR3α sequence is consistent with the fact that the predominant interaction between the TRAV12-2 chain and the HLA-A2/Melan-A peptide is located in the CDR1loop (Gln$^{31}$), and the CDR3α sequence probably does not participate to this interaction (4, 18). Interestingly we also confirmed the presence of the conserved central motif "GLG" for 48/355 CDR3ß sequences (**Figure 5B**, upper right), that has been already reported (15), suggesting a non-negligible role of CDR3ß in HLA-peptide interaction for this repertoire.

The picture is totally inverted for MELOE-1 specific TCR repertoire, with a strong recurrence of a "GP" motif, formed by non-template added nucleotides, in 58/154 CDR3α sequence (position 5-6 of the CDR3α sequence, **Figure 5B**, lower left). This motif was previously found in 5/18 MELOE-1 specific CTL clones (2). This suggests a crucial role of the CDR3α sequence

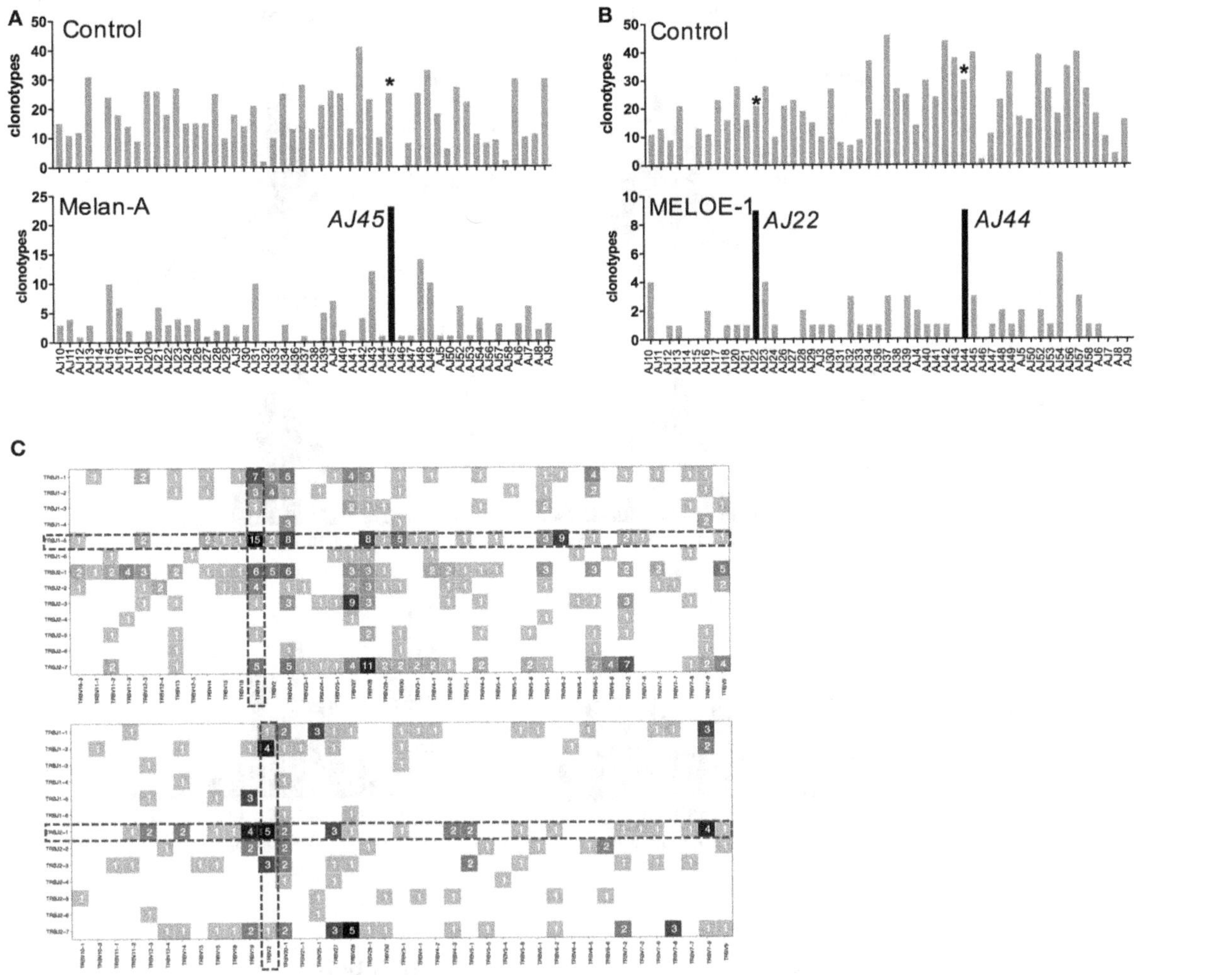


**FIGURE 4 |** TRAJ and TRBJ usage of specific-T cell populations. **(A)** Number of TRAV-12-2 clonotypes using individual TRAJ in the control sample and Melan-A specific T cell repertoire. **(B)** Number of TRAV-19 clonotypes using individual TRAJ in the control sample and MELOE-1 specific T cell repertoire. Black histograms illustrate TRAJ chains preferentially used in each T cell repertoire, and the same chains are marked with an asterisk in the control sample. **(C)** Heatmaps of TRBV-TRBJ combination usage for Melan-A (upper panel) and MELOE-1 (lower panel)-specific T cell repertoires. Numbers of clonotypes using a given combination are indicated in the corresponding square.

for the HLA-peptide interaction. Conversely, no clear recurrent motif was identified in MELOE-1-specific CDR3ß sequences (**Figure 5B**, lower right).

## Particular Features of CDR3 Sequences Harboring a Conserved Amino Acid Motif

The presence of recurrent motifs in CDR3ß and CDR3α clonotypes specific for Melan-A and MELOE-1 antigens prompted us to investigate whether these particular sequences could be associated with specific features. We first analyzed the lengths and the relative abundance of these CDR3 sequences (**Figures 6A,C**). For Melan-A repertoire, CDR3ß sequences harboring the "GLG" motif were mainly of 14 aa-length (41/48), and these 48 clonotypes represented 32% of total CDR3ß sequences, in terms of abundance (**Figure 6A**). For MELOE-1 specific repertoire, the lengths of the 58 CDR3α clonotypes harboring the conserved "GP" motif at positions 5–6, are distributed between 15 and 19 amino acids, centered on a length of 17 amino acids. In terms of abundance, these sequences are the majority of MELOE-1-specific CDR3α repertoire, representing more than 62% of total MELOE-1 CDR3α repertoire (**Figure 6C**).

We further investigated whether these chains harboring a specific motif were associated with particular TRV and TRJ segments. **Figure 6B** illustrates the use of TRBV and TRBJ segments by the 48 Melan-A-specific CDR3ß clonotypes sharing the "GLG" motif in their sequences. As for the global analysis of TRBV-TRBJ association (**Figure 4B**), we observed the dominant usage of the TRBJ1-5 segment (31/48 clonotypes), associated with 9 TRBV chains. Of note, the dominant TRBV19 chain is strictly associated with this TRBJ segment for these particular CDR3ß sequences.

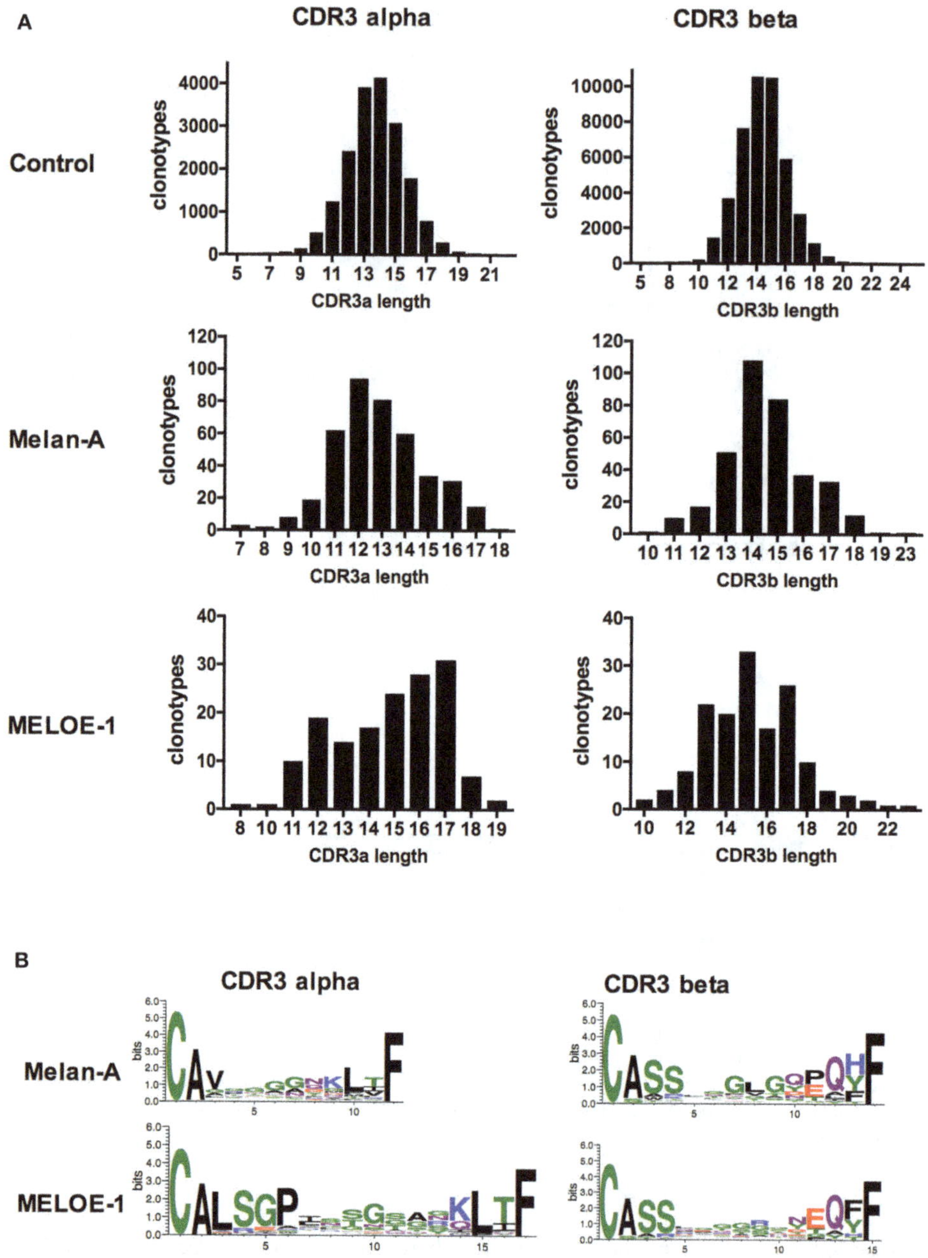


**FIGURE 5 |** CDR3α and CDR3ß lengths and sequence composition of the most abundant CDR3 lengths. **(A)** Amino acid length distribution of CDR3a (left panel) and CDR3ß (right panel) clonotypes, from the control sample and antigen-specific populations. **(B)** Logotypes of amino acid CDR3α (left panel) and CDR3ß (right panel) composition for the most abundant lengths, for antigen-specific T cell clonotypes.

All but one (57/58) CDR3α clonotypes harboring the "GP" conserved motif used the TRAV19 dominant chain, that was found preferentially associated with the two previously identified dominant TRAJ segments: TRAJ44 (9 clonotypes) and TRAJ22 (8 clonotypes; **Figure 6D**).

## Presence of Public Melan-A and MELOE-1 Specific Clonotypes

We finally looked for Melan-A and MELOE-1 CDR3α and CDR3ß specific sequences shared between the different populations that originated from distinct metastatic melanoma patients.

Heatmaps on **Figure 7** illustrate the sequences and the abundance of each shared CDR3 sequences. Numbers indicated in boxes correspond to the frequency of each clonotype, within a given sample. In order to strengthen the value of our results, we reported here CDR3 clonotypes that have been found as shared between patients with both 10 and 25 ng of starting RNA.

Twenty-one semi-public CDR3α clonotypes were identified for Melan-A specific repertoire (**Figure 7A**), among them 17

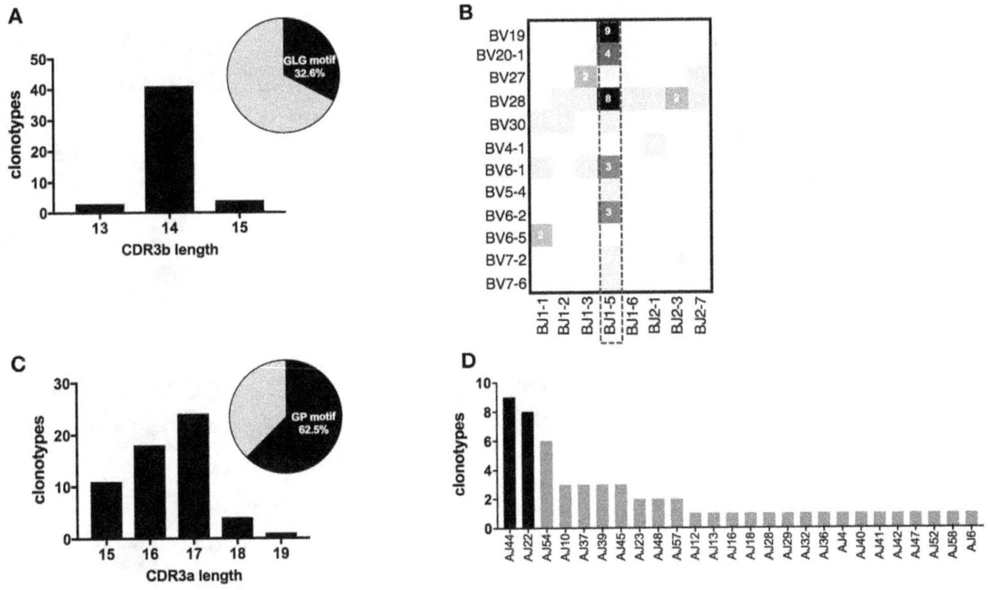


**FIGURE 6 |** CDR3 length distribution and TRJ usage of clonotypes harboring a conserved motif in their CDR3 sequences. **(A)** CDR3ß length distribution for Melan-A-specific clonotypes with the conserved "GLG" motif. Insert in the figure illustrates the abundance of these 48 clonotypes within the global Melan-A specific repertoire (UMI frequency). **(B)** Heatmap illustrating TRBV-TRBJ association of these 48 Melan-A specific clonotypes. **(C)** CDR3α length distribution for MELOE-1-specific clonotypes with the conserved "GP" motif. Insert in the figure illustrates the abundance of these 58 clonotypes within the global MELOE-1 specific repertoire (UMI frequency). **(D)** TRAJ usage of the 57/58 TRAV19 MELOE-1 specific clonotypes, with the conserved "GP" motif.

use the TRAV12-2 dominant chain and 3 of them use the preferential association TRAV-12-2/TRAJ45. The majority of these clonotypes are shared between two distinct Melan-A specific T cell populations, and one of them was identified in 3 populations. Frequencies of these shared clonotypes are highly variable in individual samples, but some of them are substantially represented in terms of abundance, reaching 48% of individual CDR3α Melan-A specific repertoire. To a lesser extent, we also identified CDR3ß sequences fully conserved and shared by two distinct Melan-A specific populations (**Figure 7B**). Among these 5 common CDR3ß sequences, 3 harbored the public "GLG" motif.

Finally, we also performed the same study on the 4 MELOE-1-specific T cell populations, and **Figure 7C** illustrates the characteristics of the 6 CDR3α sequences that are conserved between 2 and 3 patients. All these sequences use the TRAV19 chain, and thus harbor the public motif "GP" in positions 5–6. As for Melan-A-specific CDR3α shared sequences, the frequencies of these common sequences vary from sample to sample, but can reach up to 43% of individual MELOE-1 repertoire in terms of abundance.

## DISCUSSION

In this study, we analyzed the TCR repertoires of CD8$^+$ T cells specific for the immunodominant A2/Melan-A$_{A27L}$ and the A2/MELOE-1$_{36-44}$ melanoma epitopes, originating from the peripheral blood of HLA-A2 melanoma patients, using a recently developed high throughput TCR sequencing method. This method, based on UMI (Unique molecular indexes) technology strongly reduces PCR duplicates and amplification bias, that are major issues in current RNAseq workflows. These molecular barcodes allow the counting of original transcript levels instead of PCR duplicates, thereby enabling digital sequencing and resulting in unbiased and accurate gene expression profiles (19). TCR sequencing was performed on 6 Melan-A and 4 MELOE-1-specific CD8$^+$ T cell populations, amplified *in vitro* after sorting with HLA-peptide coated magnetic beads (3, 10). Libraries prepared from 10 to 25 ng of total RNA revealed that the initial quantity of material is an issue to reveal the entire diversity of the most polyclonal populations, especially for clonotypes present at the lowest frequencies. Indeed, the total number of sequenced CDR3α and CDR3ß clonotypes (cumulated from all populations) increased by nearly half for Melan-A specific repertoire, when starting with the highest RNA quantity. For the less diverse MELOE-1 specific repertoire, the number of total CDR3α and CDR3ß clonotypes is rather similar with the two RNA starting quantities. As expected, and illustrated by **Figure 1**, the highest quantity of starting material allows the detection of the highest number of low frequency clonotypes.

In this study, we also assessed the reliability of this TCR sequencing method comparing the frequencies of CDR3ß clonotypes sharing the same TRBV chain, detected either through TCR sequencing or labeling of polyclonal T cells with Vß-specific antibodies (**Figure 2**). For most TRBV chains, for which a specific antibody is available, there was globally a good correlation between the cumulated frequencies obtained from TCR sequencing and the fraction of Vß positive cells detected by cytometry. Nonetheless, we observed some outliers, detected at

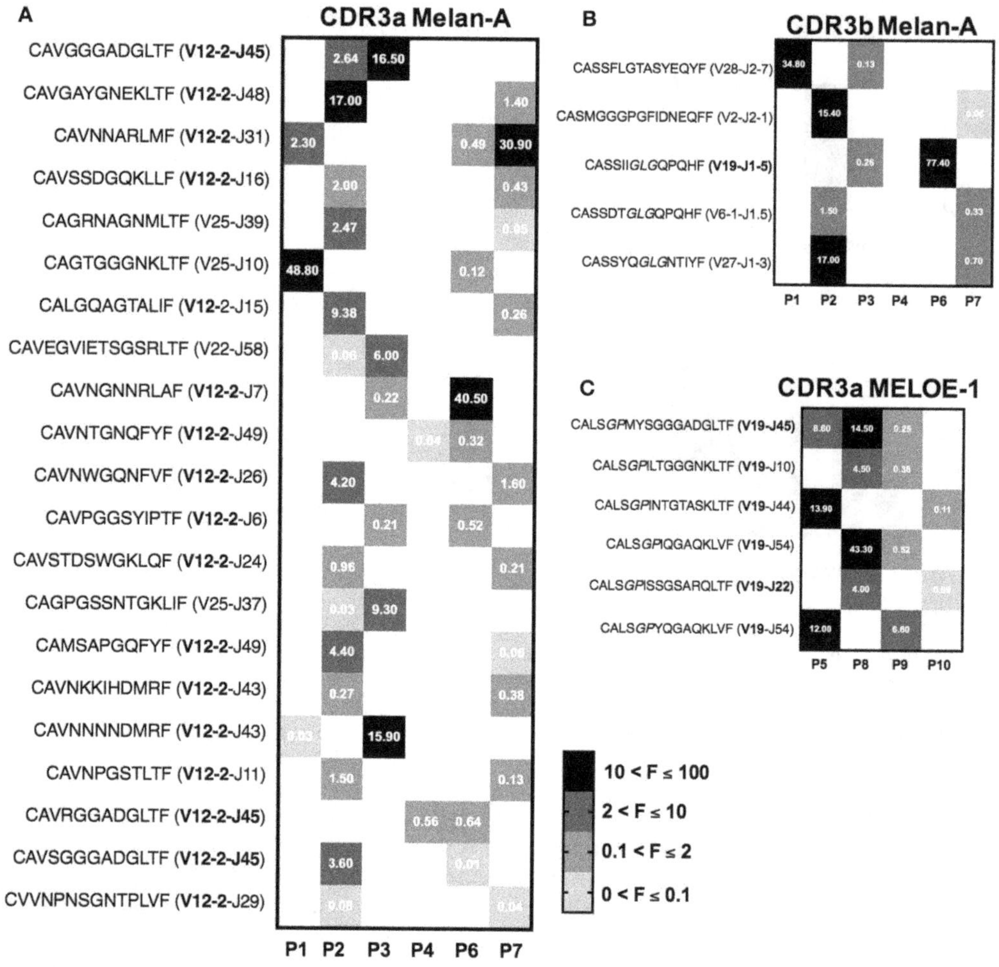


**FIGURE 7 |** Heatmaps illustrating the sequences and frequencies (UMI) of semi-public CDR3 clonotypes shared by melanoma patients. **(A)** Heatmap of the 21 public CDR3α Melan-A specific clonotypes. **(B)** Heatmap of the 5 public CDR3b Melan-A specific clonotypes. The conserved "GLG" motif is indicated in italics in the sequence. **(C)** Heatmap of the 6 public CDR3α MELOE-1 specific clonotypes. The conserved "GP" motif is indicated in italics in the sequence. The frequencies of each clonotype in individual patients are indicated by the numbers in squares.

low frequencies either by TCR sequencing, or antibody labeling. This could be explained by the lower sensitivity of antibody labeling and to some degree of cross-reactivity of some specific antibodies (**Figure 2**). Globally, this TCR sequencing method is a very powerful, sensitive and reliable method to reveal the diversity of polyclonal T cell populations.

The quality of obtained results was also assessed by the confirmation of specific features already described for Melan-A specific T cell repertoire. First, we confirmed a very strong bias in TRAV usage, with the dominant use of TRAV12-2 for Melan-A specific repertoire. This dominance has been widely explored in Melan-A-specific T cells from different origins (TIL, T cell clones originating from tumors or blood from melanoma patients or HLA-A healthy donors), (5, 6, 20). This TRAV12-2 recurrence occurs for T cells specific for the natural epitope Melan-$A_{26-35}$ almost all cross-reactive with the heteroclitic Melan-$A_{A27L}$ peptide, despite the fact that TCR engagement of these two peptides differs in terms of the strength of the interaction (18, 21). Indeed, it has been demonstrated that the TCR is extremely sensitive to minor alterations in peptide conformation and that the use of heteroclictic peptide can skew the natural specific T-cell repertoire (22). Therefore we cannot formally assert that observed features for Melan-$A_{A27L}$-specific T cell repertoire would be observed in the same proportions for Melan-$A_{26-35}$ specific T cell repertoire, although a high degree of similarity between the two repertoires has been reported in structural studies. Indeed, structural analyses of the interaction between HLA-peptide complexes and both Melan-$A_{26-35}$- and Melan-$A_{A27L}$ specific TCR revealed a strong interaction between the TRAV12-2 CDR1 and the Melan-A $_{26-35}$ peptide, presented in the HLA-A2 molecule (4, 23), the CDR1 loop acting as the classical CDR3 loop considering peptide contacts. This unusual TCR binding mode (involving a germline-encoded region) has been proposed to explain the high frequency of naive Melan-A-specific precursors. Supporting this hypothesis, two other T cell repertoires, with a very high frequency of naive precursor, also exhibit a strong bias in TRAV12-2 usage, with a major role of the CDR1 loop: the T cell repertoire specific for the HTLV-1/A2 dominant epitope, (24) and for Yellow fever/A2 dominant one (23). We also confirmed the dominant usage of TRAJ45 segment (16), in the whole Melan-A specific T cell repertoire and even more significant for the TRAV-12-2 expressing clonotypes (**Figure 4A**), also suggesting a combinatorial constraint favoring the association of these two segments for Melan-$A_{A27L}$ repertoire.

A diverse TRBV usage has been reported for Melan-A specific T cell repertoire (5, 6), nonetheless with the recurrence of some TRBV chains, such as TRBV19, BV20-1, BV27 and BV28 (14, 15). It has been documented that TRBV repertoires - specific for the natural and analog Melan-A peptides were overlapping, nonetheless with the preferential usage of TRBV19 by Melan-$A_{A27L}$ specific TCR (16). Our results confirmed this bias, with 43/355 clonotypes using the TRBV19 chain, representing almost 20% of amplified clonotypes. The TRBV20-1, BV27, and BV28 chains are also frequently used, but as these chains are very frequent in the control population, their preferential usage in Melan-A-specific repertoire does not appear significant. Results also confirmed the preferential usage of TRBJ1-5 segment (**Figure S3**), that was also found strongly associated with the dominant TRBV19 chain (15/43 clonotypes, **Figure 4B**). A recurrent usage in TRAJ1-5 segment had been previously reported (15), with a preferential combination with TRBV28 chain. In our study, the combination TRBV28-TRBJ1-5 is also present although less dominant (8/36 TRBV28 clonotypes used this segment) than the TRBV19-TRBJ1-5.

The analysis of CDR3α and ß amino acid composition revealed no specific features concerning CDR3α sequence, but a recurrent central motif "GLG" in CDR3b region (**Figure 5B**) already documented (15, 16). The resolved TCR/HLA-A2-Melan-$A_{A27L}$ structure revealed that the residues "LG" of the CDR3b made interactions with the $Ile^{P7}$ of the Melan-$A_{A27L}$ peptide. Thus, the CDR3ß loop may contribute to the stability of the TCR-Melan-$A_{A27L}$ complex (18). Interestingly, TCR clonotypes harboring this specific motif represented more than 30% of total CDR3ß clonotypes (**Figure 6A**), strengthening the role of this conserved motif for TCR/HLA-peptide interactions. CDR3ß regions harboring this specific motif are mainly of 14 aa-length (41/48 clonotypes), with a clear biased usage of TRBJ1-5 segment (**Figure 6B**). Of note, all the TRBV19 clonotypes harboring this specific motif were associated with this segment, also dominant within TRBV28 clonotypes, in accordance with previous report (15). Our results thus confirmed the existence of a conserved "GLG" amino acid motif in CDR3ß sequences of Melan-A-specific T cells, together with the preferential usage of TRB1-5/TRBV19 combination, and to a lower extent of TRBJ1-5/TRBV28. This strengthens the hypothesis that, besides the well-documented role of the CDR1 region of TRAV12-2 chain, the role of TRB chain, and especially that of the CDR3ß region is far from anecdotal for the sharpness of TCR interaction with Melan-A peptides.

We perform the same analysis on MELOE-1 specific T cell repertoire, that has been far less extensively characterized. Indeed, we reported before that MELOE-1 specific T cell repertoire was also a vast T cell repertoire in HLA-A2 healthy donors and melanoma patients, and that MELOE-1 specific T cells were strongly biased toward TRAV19 usage (2). This initial study was performed on 18 specific T cell clones of diverse origins, and here we clearly confirmed this strong bias on 79/154 clonotypes from 4 different melanoma patients (**Figure 3**). These TRAV19 clonotypes represented more than 90% of total clonotypes, in terms of frequency, strengthening the crucial role of this TRAV chain in the specificity toward the HLA-2-MELOE-$1_{36-44}$ complexes. This TRAV19 chains appears preferentially associated with TRAJ44 and TRAJ22 segments (**Figure 4B**). The analysis of CDR3α sequences reveals interesting features. First, the lengths of CDR3a appeared significantly longer than in the control population, with a mean-length situated around 16–17 amino acids. Furthermore, this analysis also revealed the presence of a very highly conserved motif at the beginning of the CDR3α sequence: CALSGP, in which GP residues are encoded by the diversity. The presence of this conserved motif was previously observed in 12/18 of MELOE-1 specific T cell clones (2), and suggested that, contrary to that described for Melan-A repertoire, the CDR3α region of these TCR could be a key player in the specific interaction with MELOE-$1_{36-44}$ peptide. Of note, all but one clonotypes harboring this specific motif, and representing 62% of total clonotypes in terms of frequency, used the TRAV19 chain (**Figure 6C**). The dominant length of these clonotypes is of 17 amino acids, and in this subgroup, the TRAV19 chain is mainly associated with TRAJ44 and TRAJ22 segments. This study also revealed a preferential usage of the TRBV2 chain with 14/153 clonotypes, nonetheless representing only 3.5% of expanded clonotypes (**Figures 3B,C**). Thus TRBV chain may be less crucial in conferring TCR specificity, also confirmed by the absence of any clear conserved motif in CDR3ß sequences (**Figure 5B**). The most significant feature concerning TRB chain for MELOE-1 specific repertoire was the dominant usage of the TRBJ2-1 segment (38/153 clonotypes), associated with 21 different TRBV chains. This suggest, that TRBJ segment, rather than TRBV chain could be involved in TCR-peptide interaction.

Overall, these data suggest two different structural hypotheses that could explain the high frequencies of Melan-A and MELOE-1 specific T lymphocytes, based either on a specific role of the germline encoded CDR1α and the somatically rearranged CDR3ß regions for Melan-A T cell repertoire, or based on probable interactions within the somatically rearranged CDR3α region, for MELOE-1 specific T cell repertoire, as suggested by the presence of the highly conserved "GP" motif in TRAV19 chain, and also possibly involving the TRBJ2-1 segment.

Based on these particular features, we investigated the presence of public or semi-public clonotypes shared by the different patients from whom these T cells have been derived. Such CDR3α clonotypes have been previously described for Melan-A specific repertoire (5, 6, 16), as also reported for T cells submitted to chronic exposure to antigens (25, 26). Here we found 21 CDR3α semi-public sequences, shared at least by 2 patients (one shared by three patients). Among these clonotypes, 17/22 use the TRBV12-2 chain, and some were highly frequent in individual Melan-A TCR repertoires. Interestingly, 2 of these TRAV12-2 public clonotypes (CAVNNARLMF and CAVGGGADGLTF) have been previously identified from the blood of patients either vaccinated with the natural or the analog Melan-A peptides (16). Nonetheless, no conserved motif was identified within these semi-public clonotypes, strengthening again the fact that CDR3α chain is not involved in TCR-peptide interactions (**Figure 7**). We also observed 5 semi-public CDR3ß sequences, among them 3 harboring the conserved "GLG" motif, and one of these clonotypes (CASSFLGTASYEGYF) being previously reported has a public one (16).

No public CDR3 sequences have been described so far for MELOE-1 specific T cell repertoire, and here we documented the existence of 6 CDR3α sequences shared by 2 distinct melanoma patients. All of them were associated with the TRAV19 chain and harbored the conserved "GP" motif, previously identified. However, no public CDR3ß sequences were found for MELOE-1 repertoire. This final result supports the potential crucial role of CDR3α region in conferring the specificity toward MELOE-1 epitope, and could also explain the lower frequency of MELOE-1 specific T cells (around $10^{-5}$ in $CD8^{+}$) compared to Melan-A specific ones (around $10^{-4}$), whose TCR specificity is mainly conferred by the TRVA12-2 germline encoded CDR1 loop.

Globally this study highlighted common and specific features between T cell repertoires specific for two melanoma antigens, that are relevant targets for immunotherapy. We cannot formally rule out the possibility that *ex-vivo* peptide stimulation, sorting and amplification steps could introduce some biases in the relative abundance of some clonotypes harboring particular features. Nonetheless, results obtained about the dominance of TRAV12-2 and TRAV19 usage, and on specific features of Melan-A-specific CDR3beta sequences, confirmed already reported results, some of them obtained without any culture biases. Therefore, it appears quite plausible to suggest that the new described T cell repertoire features could arise at least partly from *in vivo* amplified T cell repertoires. Beyond these specific results, high throughput TCR sequencing approaches provide reliable and exhaustive T cell repertoire analyses, and will be a real asset to monitor immunotherapy-treated patients, with the aim to improve immunotherapeutic treatments.

## AUTHOR CONTRIBUTIONS

SS, SR, and NL designed the experiments and wrote the manuscript. SS, ZW, AF, and VV performed the experiments. SS, JC, ZW, SR, and NL analyzed the data and prepared the figures. NL, SS, and SR supervised the project. AK and BD provided melanoma patients blood samples and regulatory issues. FL revised the manuscript. All authors read the manuscript carefully.

## FUNDING

This work has been carried out thanks to the support of the LabEx IGO project (n° ANR-11-LABX-0016-01) funded by the Investissements d'Avenir French Government program, managed by the French National Research Agency (ANR), of the Ligue contre Le Cancer (committees 44, 53, 56) and of the Région Pays de la Loire. SS was supported by an allocation from the LabEx IGO program ANR-11-LABX-0016-01.

## ACKNOWLEDGMENTS

We thank the Recombinant Protein Facility (SFR Sante) for HLA-A2/peptide monomers' production and the Cytometry Facility CytoCell (SFR Sante) for expert technical assistance. We thank Hélène Bauby and Julien Pogu for their helpful advices.

## REFERENCES


1. Lawrence MS, Stojanov P, Polak P, Kryukov GV, Cibulskis K, Sivachenko A, et al. Mutational heterogeneity in cancer and the search for new cancer-associated genes. *Nature* (2013) 499:214–8. doi: 10.1038/nature12213
2. Godet Y, Desfrancois J, Vignard V, Schadendorf D, Khammari A, Dreno B, et al. Frequent occurrence of high affinity T cells against MELOE-1 makes this antigen an attractive target for melanoma immunotherapy. *Eur J Immunol.* (2010) 40:1786–94. doi: 10.1002/eji.200940132
3. Labarriere N, Fortun A, Bellec A, Khammari A, Dreno B, Saiagh S, et al. A full GMP process to select and amplify epitope-specific T lymphocytes for adoptive immunotherapy of metastatic melanoma. *Clin Dev Immunol.* (2013) 2013:932318. doi: 10.1155/2013/932318
4. Pinto S, Sommermeyer D, Michel C, Wilde S, Schendel D, Uckert W, et al. Misinitiation of intrathymic MART-1 transcription and biased TCR usage explain the high frequency of MART-1-specific T cells. *Eur J Immunol.* (2014) 44:2811–21. doi: 10.1002/eji.201444499
5. Trautmann L, Labarriere N, Jotereau F, Karanikas V, Gervois N, Connerotte T, et al. Dominant TCR V alpha usage by virus and tumor-reactive T cells with wide affinity ranges for their specific antigens. *Eur J Immunol.* (2002) 32:3181–90. doi: 10.1002/1521-4141(200211)32:11<3181::AID-IMMU3181>3.0.CO;2-2
6. Dietrich PY, Le Gal FA, Dutoit V, Pittet MJ, Trautman L, Zippelius A, et al. Prevalent role of TCR alpha-chain in the selection of the preimmune repertoire specific for a human tumor-associated self-antigen. *J Immunol.* (2003) 170:5103–9. doi: 10.4049/jimmunol.170.10.5103
7. Bobinet M, Vignard V, Florenceau L, Lang F, Labarriere N, Moreau-Aubry A. Overexpression of meloe gene in melanomas is controlled both by specific transcription factors and hypomethylation. *PLoS ONE* (2013) 8:e75421. doi: 10.1371/journal.pone.0075421
8. Carbonnelle D, Vignard V, Sehedic D, Moreau-Aubry A, Florenceau L, Charpentier M, et al. The melanoma antigens MELOE-1 and MELOE-2 are translated from a bona fide polycistronic mRNA containing functional IRES sequences. *PLoS ONE* (2013) 8:e75233. doi: 10.1371/journal.pone.0075233

9. Charpentier M, Croyal M, Carbonnelle D, Fortun A, Florenceau L, Rabu C, et al. IRES-dependent translation of the long non coding RNA meloe in melanoma cells produces the most immunogenic MELOE antigens. *Oncotarget* (2016) 7:59704–13. doi: 10.18632/oncotarget.10923
10. Simon S, Vignard V, Varey E, Parrot T, Knol A-C, Khammari A, et al. Emergence of high-avidity melan-a-specific clonotypes as a reflection of Anti-PD-1 clinical efficacy. *Cancer Res.* (2017) 77:7083–3. doi: 10.1158/0008-5472.CAN-17-1856
11. Kuchenbecker L, Nienen M, Hecht J, Neumann AU, Babel N, Reinert K, et al. IMSEQ–a fast and error aware approach to immunogenetic sequence analysis. *Bioinformatics* (2015) 31:2963–71. doi: 10.1093/bioinformatics/btv309
12. Vignard V, Lemercier B, Lim A, Pandolfino MC, Guilloux Y, Khammari A, et al. Adoptive transfer of tumor-reactive Melan-A-specific CTL clones in melanoma patients is followed by increased frequencies of additional Melan-A-specific T cells. *J Immunol.* (2005) 175:4797–805. doi: 10.4049/jimmunol.175.7.4797
13. Mandruzzato S, Rossi E, Bernardi F, Tosello V, Macino B, Basso G, et al. Large and dissimilar repertoire of Melan-A/MART-1-specific CTL in metastatic lesions and blood of a melanoma patient. *J Immunol.* (2002) 169:4017–24. doi: 10.4049/jimmunol.169.7.4017
14. Valmori D, Dutoit V, Schnuriger V, Quiquerez A-L, Pittet MJ, Guillaume P, et al. Vaccination with a Melan-A peptide selects an oligoclonal T cell population with increased functional avidity and tumor reactivity. *J Immunol.* (2002) 168:4231–240. doi: 10.4049/jimmunol.168.8.4231
15. Serana F, Sottini A, Caimi L, Palermo B, Natali PG, Nisticò P, et al. Identification of a public CDR3 motif and a biased utilization of T-cell receptor V beta and J beta chains in HLA-A2/Melan-A-specific T-cell clonotypes of melanoma patients. *J Transl Med.* (2009) 7:21. doi: 10.1186/1479-5876-7-21
16. Wieckowski S, Baumgaertner P, Corthesy P, Voelter V, Romero P, Speiser DE, et al. Fine structural variations of alphabetaTCRs selected by vaccination with natural versus altered self-antigen in melanoma patients. *J Immunol.* (2009) 183:5397–406. doi: 10.4049/jimmunol.0901460
17. Yousfi Monod M, Giudicelli V, Chaume D, Lefranc M-P. IMGT/JunctionAnalysis: the first tool for the analysis of the immunoglobulin and T cell receptor complex V-J and V-D-J JUNCTIONs. *Bioinformatics* (2004) 20 (Suppl. 1):i379–85. doi: 10.1093/bioinformatics/bth945
18. Cole DK, Yuan F, Rizkallah PJ, Miles JJ, Gostick E, Price DA, et al. Germ line-governed recognition of a cancer epitope by an immunodominant human T-cell receptor. *J Biol Chem.* (2009) 284:27281–9. doi: 10.1074/jbc.M109.022509
19. Xu C, Nezami Ranjbar MR, Wu Z, DiCarlo J, Wang Y. Detecting very low allele fraction variants using targeted DNA sequencing and a novel molecular barcode-aware variant caller. *BMC Genomics* (2017) 18:5. doi: 10.1186/s12864-016-3425-4
20. Mantovani S, Palermo B, Garbelli S, Campanelli R, Robustelli Della Cuna G, Gennari R, et al. Dominant TCR-alpha requirements for a self antigen recognition in humans. *J Immunol.* (2002) 169:6253–260. doi: 10.4049/jimmunol.169.11.6253
21. Dyson J. T-cell receptors: tugging on the anchor for a tighter hold on the tumor-associated peptide. *Eur J Immunol.* (2015) 45:380–2. doi: 10.1002/eji.201445385
22. Madura F, Rizkallah PJ, Holland CJ, Fuller A, Bulek A, Godkin AJ, et al. Structural basis for ineffective T-cell responses to MHC anchor residue-improved "heteroclitic" peptides. *Eur J Immunol.* (2015) 45:584–91. doi: 10.1002/eji.201445114
23. Bovay A, Zoete V, Dolton G, Bulek AM, Cole DK, Rizkallah PJ, et al. T cell receptor alpha variable 12-2 bias in the immunodominant response to Yellow fever virus. *Eur J Immunol.* (2018) 48:258–72. doi: 10.1002/eji.201747082
24. Garboczi DN, Ghosh P, Utz U, Fan QR, Biddison WE, Wiley DC. Structure of the complex between human T-cell receptor, viral peptide and HLA-A2. *Nature* (1996) 384:134–41. doi: 10.1038/384134a0
25. Argaet VP, Schmidt CW, Burrows SR, Silins SL, Kurilla MG, Doolan DL, et al. Dominant selection of an invariant T cell antigen receptor in response to persistent infection by Epstein-Barr virus. *J Exp Med.* (1994) 180:2335–40.
26. McHeyzer-Williams MG, Davis MM. Antigen-specific development of primary and memory T cells *in vivo*. *Science* (1995) 268:106–11.

12

# RepSeq Data Representativeness and Robustness Assessment by Shannon Entropy

Wahiba Chaara[1,2†], Ariadna Gonzalez-Tort[1], Laura-Maria Florez[1], David Klatzmann[1,2], Encarnita Mariotti-Ferrandiz[1,2*†] and Adrien Six[1,2*†]

[1] Sorbonne Université, INSERM, UMR_S 959, Immunology-Immunopathology-Immunotherapy (i3), Paris, France, [2] AP-HP, Hôpital Pitié-Salpêtrière, Biotherapy (CIC-BTi) and Inflammation-Immunopathology-Biotherapy Department (i2B), Paris, France

***Correspondence:**
Encarnita Mariotti-Ferrandiz
encarnita.mariotti-ferrandiz@sorbonne-universite.fr;
Adrien Six
adrien.six@sorbonne-universite.fr

[†]These authors have contributed equally to this work.

High-throughput sequencing (HTS) has the potential to decipher the diversity of T cell repertoires and their dynamics during immune responses. Applied to T cell subsets such as T effector and T regulatory cells, it should help identify novel biomarkers of diseases. However, given the extreme diversity of TCR repertoires, understanding how the sequencing conditions, including cell numbers, biological and technical sampling and sequencing depth, impact the experimental outcome is critical to proper use of these data. Here, we assessed the representativeness and robustness of TCR repertoire diversity assessment according to experimental conditions. By comparative analyses of experimental datasets and computer simulations, we found that (i) for small samples, the number of clonotypes recovered is often higher than the number of cells per sample, even after removing the singletons; (ii) high-sequencing depth for small samples alters the clonotype distributions, which can be corrected by filtering the datasets using Shannon entropy as a threshold; and (iii) a single sequencing run at high depth does not ensure a good coverage of the clonotype richness in highly polyclonal populations, which can be better covered using multiple sequencing. Altogether, our results warrant better understanding and awareness of the limitation of TCR diversity analyses by HTS and justify the development of novel computational tools for improved modeling of the highly complex nature of TCR repertoires.

**Keywords: TCR repertoire, diversity, sampling, normalization, bioinformatics**

## INTRODUCTION

Understanding the specificity of T cells involved in immune responses is of utmost importance in many fields of immunology. T cells are characterized by the expression a unique T cell receptor (TR), which is clonally generated by somatic rearrangement of the V, D, and J genes belonging to the TR genomic locus during thymic T cell differentiation (1). This process leads to the generation of a huge diversity of TR, defining a repertoire of antigen recognition, the hallmark of the adaptive immune response. Immunoscope analysis (also called CDR3 spectratyping) has long been the standard technique for TR repertoire analyses (2). Although immunoscope analysis has been very useful, it misses the key parameters of TR diversity, which include nucleotide sequence, codon usage, and amino acid composition. High-throughput sequencing (HTS) of the adaptive immune receptor rearrangements (RepSeq) expressed in a lymphocyte population now overcomes previous limitations, providing a thorough and multifaceted measure of diversity (3). Several studies have already highlighted the feasibility of HTS for the analysis of TR repertoire diversity in various immune contexts (4–17). However, while the amount of information and the depth of analysis provided by this technique are unprecedented, the representativeness and robustness of the data obtained remain to be established.

First of all, although not addressed in this study, the type of starting material (DNA/RNA) as well as the molecular biology method used to prepare a TR/IG template may impact the resulting diversity observed. Indeed, 5'RACE-PCR and multiplex-PCR, the two major methodologies used for TR/IG template amplification, can both introduce biases. Multiplex-PCR is mainly sensitive to primer competition and does not allow new variant identification, while 5'RACE-PCR will be sensitive to transcript integrity and length (18). An additional issue is the quantification of the species. Unique molecular identifiers have been proposed as a molecular method to trace the origin of identical species, thus distinguishing species arising from different cells or from PCR amplifications (19–22). A comparative study considering UMI on TR sequences obtained by 5'RACE-PCR or not suggested fewer intersample variations in quantification of unique TRB clonotypes based on sequences identified with UMI in comparison with randomly selected sequences (23, 24). However, amplification and sequencing errors in those highly variable short oligonucleotides can still occur and be difficult to assess and correct. In addition, UMI can be used only in 5'RACE-PCR methods. Therefore, not all the commercially available protocols include UMI and tools to handle them may need further improvement (25).

RepSeq is a numbers game (26) particularly dependent on sequencing depth and therefore on sampling. When monitoring T cell leukemia or highly expanded antigen-specific TCRs following an infection, the sampling and depth of sequencing might not be critical parameters. But things are different when studying TR repertoire diversity in physiological conditions, when describing the basics of immune repertoire generation and selection or in immune contexts where subtle or qualitative modifications may be involved in the pathophysiological outcome, such as in complex infectious diseases (27–29), autoimmune disorders (13, 30–35), and transplantation follow-up (36–38). However, RepSeq necessarily implies sampling: (i) only a fraction of the cells from peripheral blood or an organ (or a fragment of that organ in humans) is harvested; (ii) only a fraction of the RNA/DNA extracted from these cells is used for sample preparation; and finally, (iii) only a fraction of the library is used for a sequencing run. These different levels of experimental sampling are likely to affect the observed diversity.

This is a genuine issue described in ecology studies, as "the absence of observation of a species can be either real or the effect of a subsampling" (39). Previous studies showed that the number of clonotypes observed is positively correlated with sampling size (30, 40, 41). This is important, as studies performed in humans are mostly based on peripheral blood, a compartment that represents only around 2% of the total T lymphocyte population. Warren et al. (42) compared TR repertoires from two blood samples from the same individual and found a limited number of shared clonotypes (~10%). They concluded that a considerable proportion of the peripheral blood TR repertoire is unseen when observed randomly (42, 43).

The depth of the sequencing is another confounding factor for TR repertoire diversity studies, since an insufficient number of sequences produced would not adequately assess the molecular diversity of the sample analyzed. To ensure the statistical representativeness of the data produced with regards to the population of interest, two rules should be considered (44): (i) the number of sequences produced must be at least equivalent to the clonal richness of the population of interest and (ii) the rarer a clone, the greater the sequencing depth needed to detect it. Therefore, the RepSeq strategy must be adapted to the nature of the samples and the biological questions investigated (45).

While most studies seek to assess the similarity between the TR repertoires of several samples, without any knowledge of what level of similarity can be observed at best, it seems crucial to determine the limits of this approach in order to be able to interpret the data properly. In this study, we first investigated the impact of the depth of sequencing, in relation to the size of the population analyzed, on the observed TR repertoire diversity. We found that a small sample size is negatively affected by a too high, yet average in common practice, sequencing depth, and proposed an analytical approach to recover the "true" repertoire diversity. We then questioned the representativeness of a single RepSeq experiment by multiple sequencing of the same sample and demonstrated that performing a single sequencing run, even at high depth of sequencing, does not allow exhaustive observation of the existing clones in a polyclonal population. Finally, we addressed these experimental biases by computational simulation on RepSeq data reflecting several levels of clonality and sequencing depth, to have a better assessment of the robustness of the experimental observations.

## MATERIALS AND METHODS

### Mice

Eight- to twelve-week-old female Balb/C Foxp3-GFP (C.129 × 1-Foxp3tm3Tch/J) and 24- to 26-week-old male C57Bl/6 Foxp3-GFP mice, both expressing the green fluorescent protein (GFP) under the promoter of Foxp3 gene, were, respectively, provided by V. Kuchroo, Brigham and Women's Hospital, Boston, MA, USA and B. Malissen of the Centre d'Immunologie de Marseille Luminy (France). All animals were maintained in the Sorbonne Université Centre d'Expérimentation Fonctionnelle animal facility under specific pathogen-free conditions in agreement with current European legislation on animal care, housing, and scientific experimentation (agreement number A751315). All procedures were approved by the local animal ethics committee.

### Cell Preparation

Fresh total cells from spleen were isolated in PBS1X-3% fetal calf serum and stained for 20 min at 4°C with anti-Ter-119-biotin, anti-CD11c-biotin, and anti-B220-biotin antibodies followed by labeling with anti-biotin magnetic beads (Miltenyi Biotec) for 15 min at 4°C. B cells and erythrocytes were depleted on an AutoMACS separator (Miltenyi Biotec) following the manufacturer's procedure. Enriched T cells were stained with anti-CD3 APC, anti-CD4 Horizon V500, anti-CD8 Alexa 700, anti-CD44

PE, and anti-CD62L efluor 450. $6.10^5$ $CD3^+CD4^+GFP^-$ Teff cells were sorted on a BD FACSAria II (BD Biosciences, San Jose, CA, USA) with a purity >99%. Sorted cells were stored in Trizol (Invitrogen) or RNAAquous (Ambion, Inc./Life Technologies, Grand Island, NY, USA) lysis buffer.

## TR Library Preparation

RNA was extracted following the manufacturer's recommendations and cDNA synthesis was performed with the Qiagen OneStep RT-PCR kit (Qiagen Inc., Valencia, CA, USA) and mouse T cell beta receptor primers provided with the mouse TRB iR-Profile Kit (iRepertoire Inc., Huntsville, AL, USA). cDNA was amplified by two rounds of PCR according to the manufacturer's recommendations. The TRB library was sequenced using Illumina on a MiSeqv2 kit.

## RepSeq Data Processing

### Data Annotation

The RepSeq fastq files were demultiplexed by iRepertoire Inc. and then annotated using clonotypeR (46) to identify high-quality productive and non-ambiguous TRB sequences. Clonotypes were defined as unique combinations of TRBV-CDR3-TRBJ segments.

### Sequencing Error Correction

Annotated sequences were clustered per TRBV-TRBJ combination and similar clonotypes collapsed as follows: within each TRBV-TRBJ cluster, the clonotypes observed once (singletons) were separated from the others to constitute two groups. A Levenshtein distance was then calculated between the CDR3 peptide sequences of each clonotype of the two groups. The Levenshtein distance (lev) is a string metric measuring the minimum number of single-character edits (insertions, deletions, or substitutions) required to change one sequence into another (47).

When comparing the CDR3 peptide sequences of singleton with that of a "non-singleton" sequences, if $lev_{seq1,seq2} = 1$, their respective nucleotide sequences are then compared. If the two corresponding nucleotide sequences are also distant by 1, the singleton is considered as erroneous and considered as the "non-singleton" clonotype.

### Dataset Normalization

Using the function *rrarefy* from the Vegan R package (48), randomly rarefied datasets were generated to given sample sizes. Random rarefaction was done without replacement.

## Diversity Profiles

Rényi entropy is a generalization of Shannon entropy, initially developed for information theory. We applied this mathematical function to clonotype frequencies to assess their diversity within each dataset. Rényi entropy is function of a parameter α, a strictly positive real number that differs from 1 and allows the definition of a family of diversity metrics spanning from (i) the species richness ($\alpha = 0$), which corresponds to the number of clonotypes regardless of their abundance, to (ii) the clonal dominance ($\alpha \to +\infty$), corresponding to the frequency of the most predominant clonotype. For $\alpha = 1$, the Shannon diversity index is computed. The exponential of the Rényi entropy defines a generalized class of diversity indices called Hill diversities, which can be interpreted as the effective number of clonotypes in the datasets (49) and thereby is used to build a diversity profile.

## RepSeq Simulation Algorithm

A. $2{\cdot}10^6$ clonotype library construction with the tcR package

Based on the estimated total number of clonotypes in a mouse, a $2{\cdot}10^6$ TRB CDR3 library was generated with the tcR package following the probability rules of V(D)J rearrangement established in Murugan et al. (50):

$$\Omega = \{\omega_1;\omega_2;\ldots\omega_\Lambda\}, \text{ with } \Lambda = 2\cdot10^6$$
$$\forall i, \omega_i \text{ is a clonotype generated by the tcR package}$$
$$\forall i, j, \omega_i \neq \omega_j$$

B. Construction of $6{\cdot}10^5$ sequence datasets following particular Zipf distributions

Based on the demonstration by Greiff et al. (41) that clonotype frequencies determined from RepSeq datasets generally follow a Zipf distribution with a particular $\alpha \in [0, 1]$ parameter, we chose to use the Zipf–Mandelbrot law implemented in the zipfR R package (51) to simulate clonotype distributions. The probability density function used for simulations is given by

$$g(\pi) := \begin{cases} C\cdot\pi^{-\alpha-1} & 0 \le \pi \le B \\ 0 & \text{otherwise} \end{cases}$$

with two free parameters: $\alpha \in [0, 1]$ and $B \in [0, 1]$ and a normalizing constant $C$. $B$ corresponds to the probability $\pi1$ of the most frequent species (clonotype).

Seven Zipf distributions were generated with the following Zipf parameters:

$$A\ (=1/\alpha) \in \{2, 3, 4, 5, 10, 20, 100\} \text{ and } B = 0.2$$

For each Zipf parameter combination, a list $Z_A$ is randomly generated as follows:

$$Z_A = \{z_{A,1};z_{A,2};\ldots z_{A,NA}\},$$
$$\text{with } \forall i,\ z_{A,i} \in \mathbb{R}^{+*}$$
$$\forall i,j, \text{ if } i \le j \text{ then } z_{A,i} \ge z_{A,j}$$
$$N_A = 2\cdot10^6$$

$Z_A$ elements follow a Zipf distribution of $A$ (= 1/α) parameter.

| A | 2 | 3 | 4 | 5 | 10 | 20 | 100 |
|---|---|---|---|---|---|---|---|
| $\sum_{i=1}^{N_A} z_{A,i}$ | $1{\cdot}31{\cdot}10^8$ | $2{\cdot}10{\cdot}10^7$ | $1{\cdot}60\ 10^7$ | $1{\cdot}44{\cdot}10^7$ | $1{\cdot}23{\cdot}10^7$ | $1{\cdot}16{\cdot}10^7$ | $1{\cdot}11{\cdot}10^7$ |
| $N_A$ | $2{\cdot}10^6$ | $2{\cdot}10^6$ | $2{\cdot}10^6$ | $2{\cdot}10^6$ | $2{\cdot}10^6$ | $2{\cdot}10^6$ | $2{\cdot}10^6$ |

C. For each $A$ parameter, the $2{\cdot}10^6$ $Z_A$ values were randomly assigned to the clonotype collection to obtain seven TRB clonotype repertoires.

D. To obtain the final seven datasets, each of them was rarefied using the function *rrarefy* from Vegan R package to datasets of with a size of $6{\cdot}10^5$ sequences.

### Rarefaction at Increasing Sizes

Each of the seven simulated datasets was rarefied into a series of six datasets of size $D \in \{500, 1{,}000, 5{,}000, 5{\cdot}10^4, 5{\cdot}10^5, 1{\cdot}10^6\}$. For each value of $D$, subsamples of TRB sequences were randomly produced using the *vegan:rrarefy* function (without replacement). This process was iteratively repeated 100 times with replacement. For each resulting series of subsamples, clonotype counts were calculated and used to assess the median and 95% CI values of Morisita–Horn index [MH; (52)] between them and the original dataset (representativeness) and between each other (robustness).

Subsample compositions were also compared to evaluate the level of overlap between three subsamples according to the dataset size.

For each $D$, combinations of 3 $Z_A$ dataset subsamples were randomly selected to determine the proportion of clonotypes observed once, twice or in the three subsamples. This process was performed 100 times to calculate the median and 95% CI of each result.

Since the 95% CI values obtained for MH and overlap proportion were similar to the medians, they are not indicated in the corresponding figures and tables.

## RESULTS

### Impact of Sequencing Depth on the Representativeness of the Repertoire Diversity

With advances in HTS technologies, the minimum number of outputs in RepSeq studies is often a million sequences per sample. Besides, small samples are often studied. Thus, to determine the minimum number of sequences required for a representative repertoire, we first explored how the number of raw reads could affect the repertoire description according to the sample size. We chose to analyze a mouse sample with high diversity and used the CD4$^+$Foxp3-GFP$^-$ cell population (Teff) previously described as very diverse (4). $6{\cdot}10^5$ Teff cells from female Balb/C Foxp3 < GFP > splenocytes were sorted. RNA was extracted from these cells and diluted in order to obtain aliquots containing the RNA amount equivalent to what would be obtained from 50,000, 5,000, 1,000, or 500 cells (**Figure 1A**). Two replicates per dilution were prepared. For simplicity in the text, the sample size will be defined according to the theoretical equivalent cell number for each aliquot. Sequencing was performed on RNA amplified by multiplex-PCR using a commercially available kit. We made this choice for three reasons: (1) a commercially available kit is standardized, avoiding pipetting errors in master mix preparation, (2) multiplex-PCR are template-target based, therefore we know what we are supposed to obtain in terms of V genes, and (3) the bias toward genes should be constant.

On average, 1.13 (±0.16) million reads were produced for each aliquot (Table S1 in Supplementary Material), which is in the average range of common practice (18, 44, 53). As summarized in **Figure 1B**, $0.99{\cdot}10^6$ ($\pm 0.15{\cdot}10^6$) TRB sequences were identified per aliquot regardless of the sample size. The point here is to determine whether the sample size will impact the resulting repertoire distribution.

Thus, we analyzed the diversity of the observed repertoires according to sample size. It is noteworthy that the number of unique clonotypes (i.e., unique combination of TRBV-CDR3pep-TRBJ) per sample was always higher than the number of cells per sample. This discrepancy was more marked for small size samples, with approximately 20- to 2-fold more clonotypes per sample than cells with the "500-" and "50,000-cell" samples, respectively. In each dataset, about 50% (±6%) of the clonotypes were observed once (singletons). After removing the singletons, as it is commonly done (44), this bias was reduced for the large samples, while the numbers of clonotypes remained much higher than the actual number of cells in small samples (**Figure 1B**). Still, overall richness remained equivalent between all sample sizes.

In order to refine the diversity assessment of these TRB repertoires, we computed their diversity profile (**Figure 1C**) applying Rényi entropy to the clonotype relative frequencies within each dataset. This function is used in ecological science to quantify the diversity, uncertainty, and randomness of a given system (54, 55). As the α order increases, it defines metrics spanning from (i) the species richness to (ii) the clonal dominance that progressively discards the scarcest species. The exponential of these metrics provides comparable effective numbers of species, used here to build a diversity profile. Analysis of the Rényi profiles for the eight aliquots showed that TRB repertoire diversity strongly decreases when the Rényi order α value increases. While richness was comparable between all sample sizes, diversity drops in proportion to sample size when progressively discarding scarce clonotypes to reach a plateau of clonotype counts below the initial number of cells.

### Shannon Entropy as a Threshold to Filter the Clonotypes

To avoid bias related to sample size, we normalized each dataset to 700,000 sequences, a value corresponding to the smallest sample size (Table S1 in Supplementary Material). Therefore, we randomly selected 700,000 sequences, ranked the unique clonotypes from the most to the least predominant (clonotype rank) and plotted their abundance (clonotype count) to assess their distribution (**Figure 2A**). It is noteworthy that, while all the aliquots come from the same sample, the clonotype distributions within each dataset are different. The smaller a sample, the higher the most predominant clonotype counts, making it difficult to apply a filtering rule based on the count values. The Rényi profiles (**Figure 1C**) showed that the repertoire diversity collapses at a Rényi order α of 1, which corresponds to the Shannon diversity index (56). Since the number of clonotypes assessed by the Shannon index (**Table 1**) correlates best with sample size (Pearson coeff = 0.966, $p = 9.62{\cdot}10^{-5}$ and MH = 0.877 on original clonotype number and Pearson coeff = 0.995, $p = 2.92{\cdot}10^{-7}$ and MH = 0.996 after clonotype number determined by Shannon index), we chose to use this metric as a threshold to discard scarce "uninformative" clonotypes (SUC) that could result from experimental noise (shown in gray in **Figure 2A**) and keep only "informative" ones. As shown in **Figure 2B**, the clonotype relative distribution within each dataset is not significantly altered by this filtering. Interestingly, as shown in **Figure 2C**, regardless of the initial number of cells, this transformation regularizes the values of the Piélou evenness index, a measure of clonotype evenness (57) (filled squares),

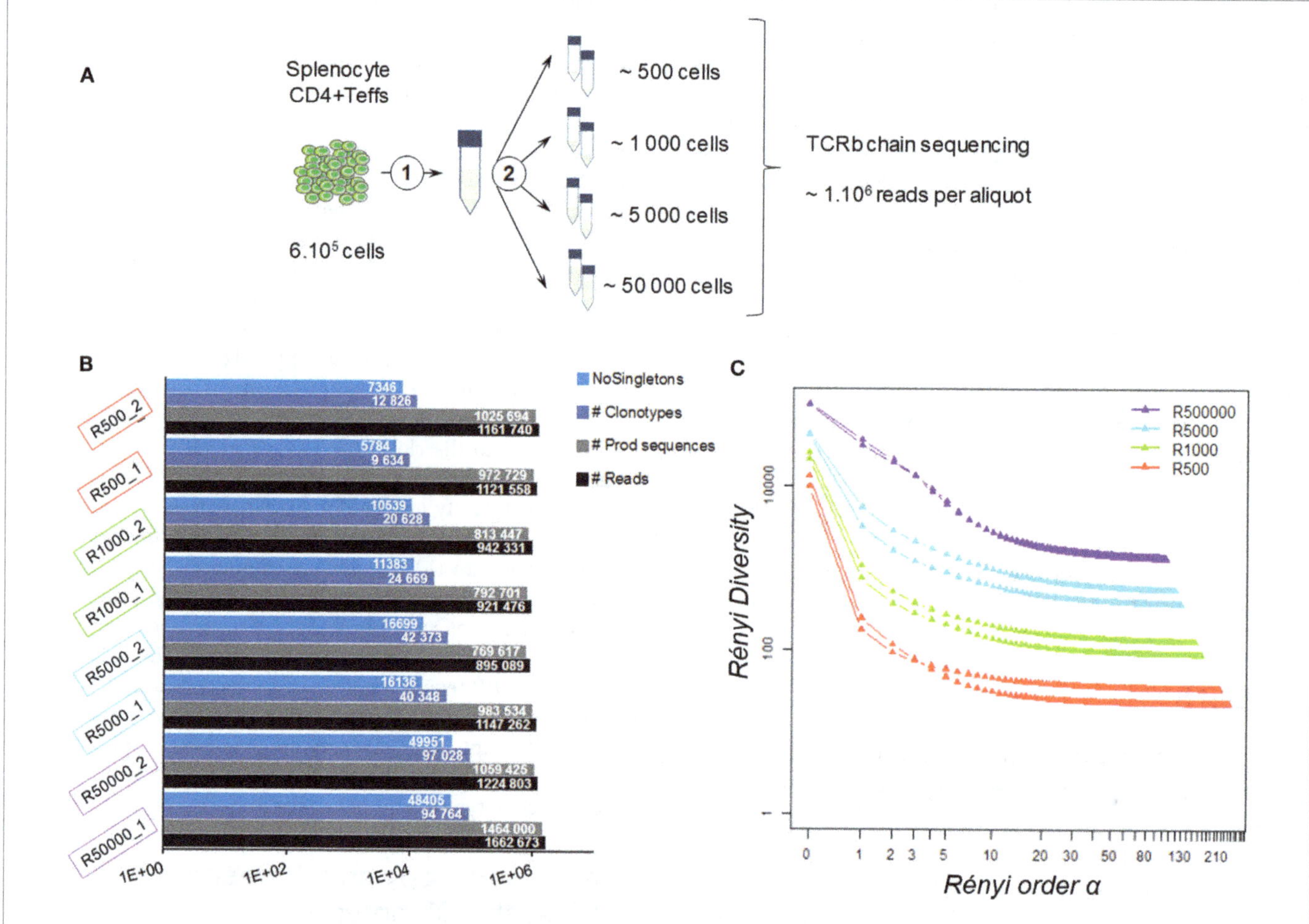


**FIGURE 1** | Impact of sequencing depth on measured diversity. **(A)** Experimental design: 600,000 CD4$^+$Foxp3-GFP$^-$ cells were sorted from female Balb/C Foxp3 splenocytes. RNA was extracted (1) and split into aliquots equivalent to the amount of mRNA of 500, 1,000, 5,000, and 50,000 cells (2). Two aliquots were produced for each amount of RNA. The eight prepared aliquots were processed for TRB chain deep sequencing. **(B)** Dataset summaries. Histograms show, for each resulting dataset, the number of reads (black), productive TRB sequences (gray), observed clonotypes (blue), and clonotypes observed more than once (NoSingletons; light blue). **(C)** Diversity profiles. For each dataset, a Rényi diversity profile was computed: diversity metrics using clonotype frequencies were calculated for increasing values of Rényi order α until stabilization of the resulting diversity. For α = 1, the Shannon entropy was computed.

which otherwise strongly decreases for unfiltered datasets when the clonotype number/cell number ratio increases, revealing that a too high sequencing depth for small samples alters clonotype distributions (**Figure 2C**, empty circles).

To confirm that the filtering does not bias the overall repertoire diversity, we computed the Morisita–Horn (MH) similarity index between the datasets before and after filtering; the high similarity values (0.983; 0.997) shown on the matrix diagonal in **Figure 2D** confirm that the datasets are not altered in the process. The similarity matrix also reveals a low similarity between replicates, except for the "50,000-cell" samples, which are big enough to share rare clonotypes. Thus, high sequencing depth does not ensure good coverage of clonotype richness. This led us to question the robustness of RepSeq experiment results.

## Robustness of the TRB Repertoire Diversity Assessment by RepSeq

We sorted $3{\cdot}10^6$ Teff cells from splenocytes, extracted the RNA and split it into three equivalent RNA aliquots, and then sequenced them independently at a high-depth targeting the TRB chain using the iRepertoire® multiplex-PCR technology. On average, for each aliquot, 8.33 (±0.66) million reads were produced and 5.63 (±0.56) million TRB sequences were identified, among which an average of $130{\cdot}10^3$ ($\pm 5{\cdot}10^3$) clonotypes (Table S2 in Supplementary Material). After applying Shannon filtering, the dataset sizes were reduced to 4.7 (±0.6) million TRB sequences for a total of 44,217 (±304) clonotypes. Datasets were rarefied at an equivalent size by randomly selecting $4{\cdot}10^6$ sequences for each sample.

We first analyzed the clonotype distributions within each dataset. The three distributions were similar between replicates (**Figure 3A**). However, when we compared the composition of the three TRB repertoires by clonotype overlap, it appeared that about 36% of the clonotypes observed in each dataset are shared by another replicate, with only 6,599 clonotypes common to the three replicates. Although these shared clonotypes represent only 6% of the 105,332 clonotypes identified overall, their expression accounted for approximately 38% of each repertoire (**Figure 3B**).

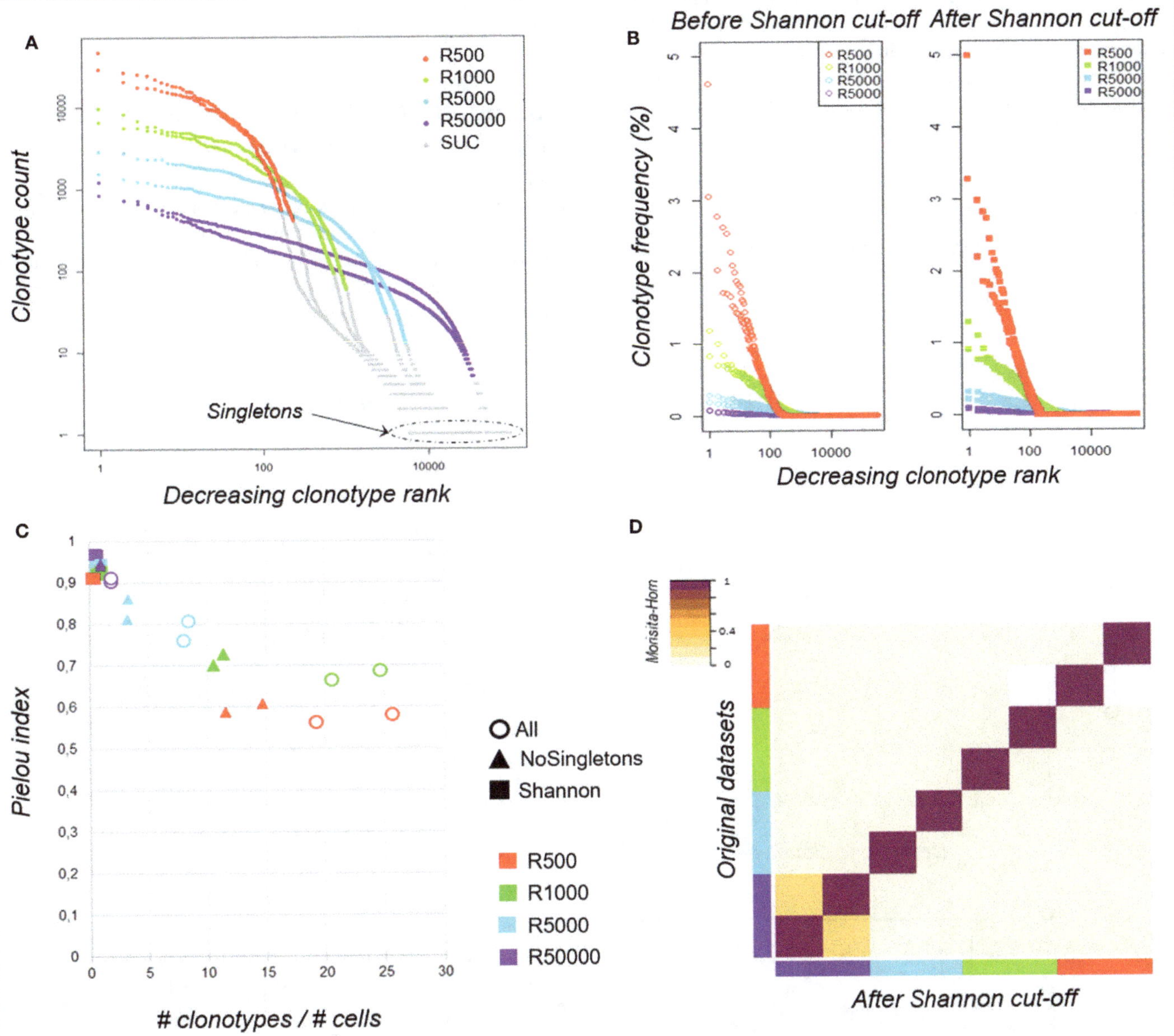


**FIGURE 2** | Clonotype distributions before and after data filtering. **(A)** TRB clonotype counts of the eight aliquots according to sampling size. Within each dataset, clonotypes were ranked according to their counts from the most to the least predominant (decreasing clonotype rank) and their abundance (clonotype count). Both axes are log-scaled. Plots were colored according to the sampling size: "500 cells" in red, "1,000 cells" in green, "5,000 cells" in cyan, and "50,000 cells" in purple. Clonotypes filtered out using the Shannon index (see main text) are colored in gray [scarce uninformative clonotypes (SUC)]. **(B)** TRB clonotype distributions of the eight aliquots before and after data filtering. Before (left) and after (right) filtering each dataset using the Shannon index as threshold, clonotypes were ranked from the most to the least predominant (decreasing clonotype rank) according to their relative frequencies (clonotype frequency). The X-axis is log-scaled. Distributions were colored according to the sampling size as previously. **(C)** Impact of clonotype filtering on the clonotype distribution evenness. The ratio between the number of clonotypes and the number of cells (x-axis) was calculated for each aliquot before (circles) and after clonotype filtering either by removing only singletons (triangles) or using the Shannon index as a threshold (squares). For each dataset, the Piélou evenness index was calculated (y-axis). Aliquots are identified according the sampling size as previously. **(D)** Similarity between datasets before and after Shannon filtering. The Morisita–Horn similarity index between all pairs of datasets is color-coded according to the indicated scale before (lower half-triangle) and after (upper half-triangle) Shannon filtering. Aliquots are identified according to sampling size as previously.

We then decomposed the clonotype collection by labeling the clonotypes as private (not shared between replicates) or shared by two or three replicates. For each dataset, clonotypes were sorted from the most to the least abundant and enrichment curves were built for each category according to the sharing status of each clonotype (**Figure 3C**). The resulting clonotype spectrum revealed that the most predominant clonotypes are shared by the three replicates, while the private clonotypes, which are the more numerous, are enriched for scarce clonotypes, therefore reducing the similarity between technical replicates. These results demonstrate that although the sampling of a large and polyclonal cell population has no impact on the observed clonotype distribution, the repertoire composition is affected: even if the most predominant clonotypes are always captured, a major proportion of the clonotypes observed with a single sequencing are private scarce ones. This observation confirms that the more abundant a clonotype, the more likely it is to be observed by sequencing. However, most rare clonotypes will remain unseen with a single sequencing run.

**TABLE 1** | Shannon diversity calculated for each dataset.

| Shannon diversity | R500 | R1000 | R5000 | R50000 |
|---|---|---|---|---|
| #1 | 171 | 1,034 | 3,124 | 30,432 |
| #2 | 238 | 735 | 5,337 | 35,027 |

## Computational Assessment of the Impact of Sequencing Depth on Observed Diversity

In order to assess the representativeness of the diversity observed when analyzing a clonotype repertoire by RepSeq, it would be necessary to know *a priori* its full diversity and distribution, which is not achievable with a classic experimental approach inherently subject to sampling bias.

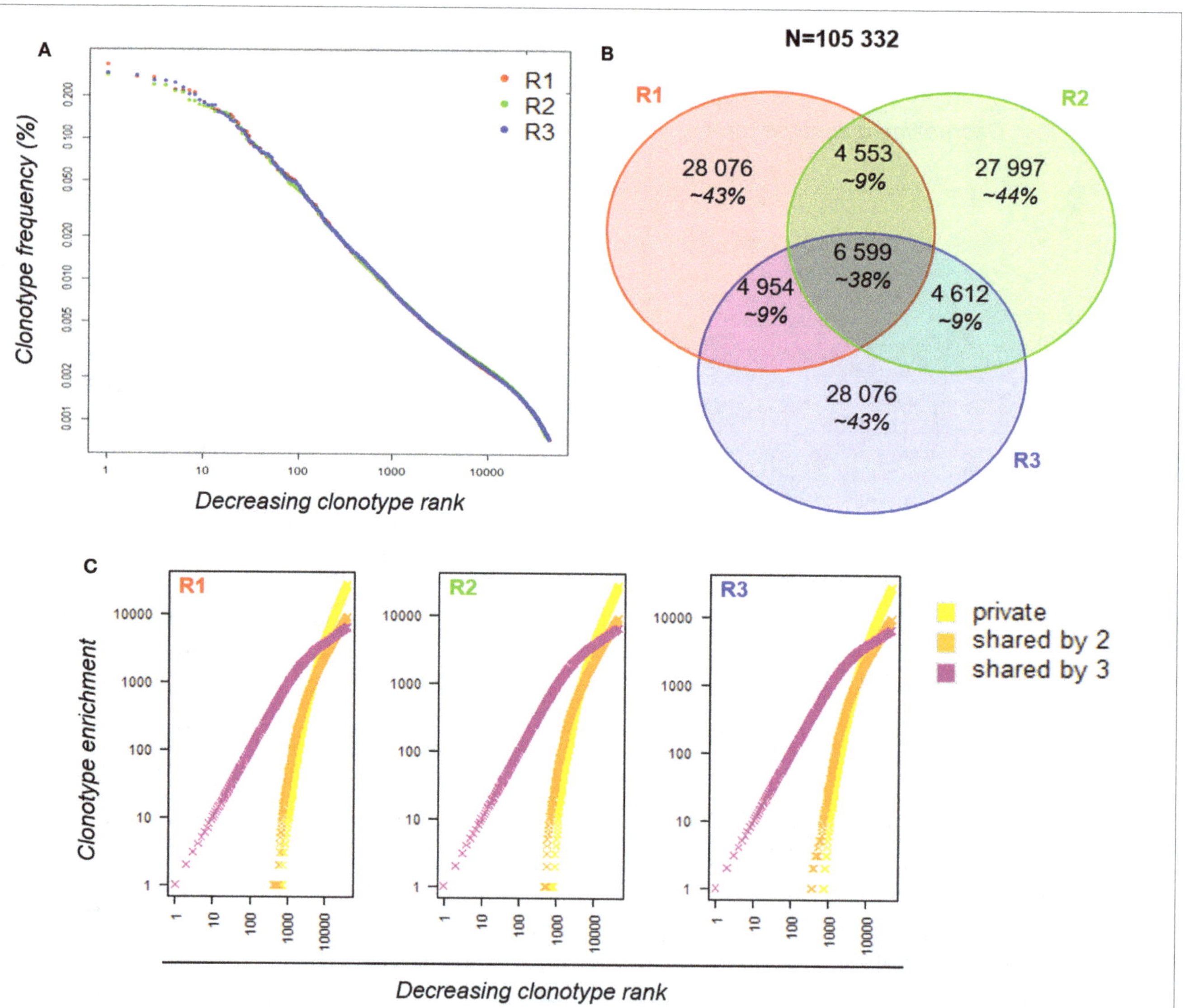


**FIGURE 3** | Robustness of a RepSeq experiment. **(A)** Clonotype distribution of the three replicates within each dataset. Informative clonotypes were ranked decreasingly according to their abundance and their frequency was plotted. The *x*-axis is log-scaled. **(B)** Venn diagram between the three replicates. Out of the 105,332 clonotypes observed in total, only 6,599 are shared by the three replicates; their cumulative frequency covers about 38% of each dataset. **(C)** Spectrum of unshared (yellow) and shared (by two in orange and by three in magenta) clonotypes in each replicate. Within each dataset, clonotypes were ranked according to their counts from the most to the least predominant (decreasing clonotype rank). Since clonotypes are labeled according to their sharing status, the clonotype enrichment (*y*-axis) of each sharing group is incremented (+1) when a corresponding clonotype is found in the ranked list.

Several studies have demonstrated that immune repertoires follow a Zipf-like distribution (58–62), which translates a relation between rank order and frequency of occurrence: the frequency $f$ of a particular observation is inversely proportional to its rank $r$ (63) with:

$$f(r) \propto \frac{1}{r^{\alpha}}$$

for Zipf-α parameter ≈ 1 (64).

In addition, the lower the Zipf-α parameter of a distribution, the more evenly represented the clonotypes involved (59). We applied this observation to build clonotype distributions of a fixed size and known diversity to simulate the sampling effect occurring during a RepSeq experiment.

Seven Zipf distributions of $6{\cdot}10^5$ sequences each were simulated with a parameter A = 1/Zipf-α ranging from 2 to 100. These distributions were then assigned to a list of clonotypes randomly generated using the tcR package (65), leading to seven TRB clonotype repertoires of known diversity.

As observed in **Figure 4A**, the distribution slope varies according to the depth of sequencing of the clonotypes. For example, for the distribution simulated with $A = 2$ (A2), the resulting distribution is skewed in a way that clonotype counts range from 1 to 31,109, whereas when $A = 100$ (A100), clonotype counts do not

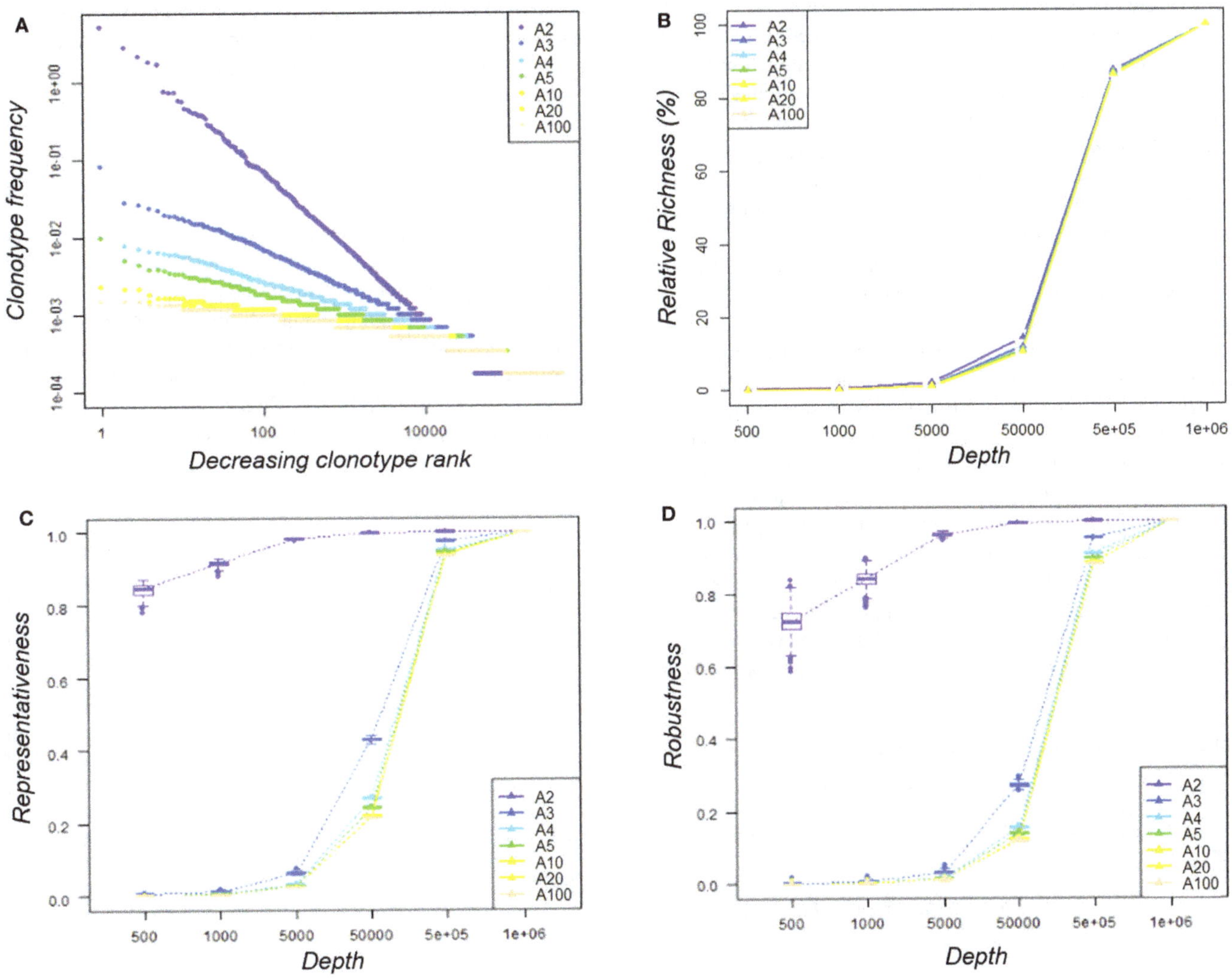


**FIGURE 4** | Impact of sequencing depth on the observed diversity. **(A)** Clonotype distribution within the seven simulated datasets—within each *A*-dataset, clonotypes were ranked decreasingly according to their abundance and their frequency was plotted. Both axes are log-scaled. Distributions are colored according to the *A* parameter used to simulate it. **(B)** Impact of sequencing depth on the observed clonotype richness—for a given *A*-dataset, clonotype richness was measured within the 100 subsamples produced for each depth and divided by that of the original dataset. The median value by depth is represented for each condition. The 95% CI was calculated but cannot be seen since it merged with the median value. **(C)** Representativeness of the sequencing—the Morisita–Horn similarity index was calculated between each subsample and its original dataset. Boxplots across the 100 subsamples of a given depth are color-coded according to the *A* condition. **(D)** Reproducibility of the sequencing—for each *A*-dataset, the Morisita–Horn similarity index was calculated between paired subsamples of a given depth. Boxplots across the 100 subsamples of a given depth are color-coded according to the *A* condition.

exceed 9. These different distributions lead to datasets of varying richness, as summarized in **Table 2**.

For each of our seven "known" repertoire distributions, we generated 100 subsamples at 6 sample sizes (from 500 to $1{\cdot}10^6$ sequences) reflecting several levels of sequencing depth. The clonotype richness observed within each subsample increased according to the depth, as expected (**Figure 4B**). We used the MH similarity index to assess (i) representativeness (**Figure 4C**) by comparing the diversity captured for each subsample with the original repertoire diversity and (ii) reproducibility (**Figure 4D**) for the 100 subsamples for a given depth. When comparing the seven distributions at a given sequencing depth ($5{\cdot}10^4$ sequences, representing 8% of the original repertoire), the representativeness of the diversity between distributions was different (**Figure 4C**), yet with similar relative richness values. For the "A2" condition, the similarity index between this subsample and the original repertoire was above 0.8, while it varied from 0.2 to 0.5 for the other conditions (**Figure 4C**). A dataset of $5{\cdot}10^5$ sequences (80% of the original repertoire size) is needed to reach a 0.9 similarity for the latter. However, a suitable representativeness does not ensure good reproducibility of the observations. With 500 or 1,000 sequences, even if the diversity observed for the "A2" condition is quite representative (MH ~ 0.8), the high variability between the subsamples implies a low reproducibility and thus an inability to observe exhaustively all the clonotypes (**Figure 4D**).

We sought to identify which simulated distribution would be the most representative of our experimental datasets. To this end, we compared the slope at the steepest descent point of each simulated distribution with those of all the experimental data analyzed in this study. The experimental distribution slopes are most comparable with the "A3" and "A5" distributions, with the exception of that of the R500_2 sample (Table S3 in Supplementary Material). Thus, we chose the "A3" distribution dataset as the most representative. In order to understand the low overlap observed between experimental replicates in **Figure 3B**, for each size we compared the "A3" simulated subsamples to determine the proportion of clonotypes shared by three independent subsamples, as performed experimentally in **Figure 3**. As summarized in **Table 3**, the proportion of private and shared clonotypes varies according to the coverage of the initial repertoire stretch. For subsamples with sizes representing less than 1% of that of the initial dataset, almost all the clonotypes observed are private (only captured in one subsample). For the "$5{\cdot}10^4$ sequence" subsamples, the size of which represents 8% of the original repertoire size, 16% of the clonotypes observed are captured at least twice. These proportions correspond to the observations we made in **Figure 3** between the three experimental replicates. Finally, using subsamples of size close (80%) to that of the original, 95% of the observed clonotypes are shared by at least two replicates. In addition, as represented in **Figure 5**, at this depth, while one sample only captures about 12% of the overall existing clonotypes, three replicates cover a third of the overall richness. These observations suggest that multiple sequencing experiments can ensure greater clonotype exhaustiveness than a unique very deep sequencing.

**TABLE 2** | Summary of the simulated Zipf distributions.

| A | 2 | 3 | 4 | 5 | 10 | 20 | 100 |
|---|---|---|---|---|---|---|---|
| $\sum_{i=1}^{N_A} z_{A,i}$ | 6E + 05 | 6E + 05 | 6E + 05 | 6E + 05 | 6E + 05 | 6E + 05 | 6E + 05 |
| $N_A$ | 155,495 | 394,784 | 435,528 | 450,625 | 469,974 | 476,829 | 480,919 |

**TABLE 3** | Sharing proportion between three replicates.

| Median proportion of clonotypes observed | Dataset sizes | | | | | |
|---|---|---|---|---|---|---|
| | $5{\cdot}10^2$ | $1{\cdot}10^3$ | $5{\cdot}10^3$ | $5{\cdot}10^4$ | $5{\cdot}10^5$ | $1{\cdot}10^6$ |
| Private | 99.7 | 99.4 | 97.5 | 83.7 | 5.2 | – |
| Shared by two | 0.3 | 0.6 | 2.4 | 14.3 | 27.2 | – |
| Shared by three | – | – | 0.1 | 2 | 67.6 | 100 |
| Total number across three replicates | 1,493 | 2,973 | 14,456 | 117,634 | 393,434 | 394,784 |

## DISCUSSION

RepSeq offers new opportunities to identify biomarkers of health or disease by monitoring adaptive immune cell diversity at unprecedented high resolution. Continuing improvements in molecular biology protocols and sequencing technologies are increasing the accuracy of clonotype detection (66). Still, clear evaluation of the reproducibility and representability of the observed diversity is missing. This is particularly true when considering bulk sequencing on small size samples such as small cell subsets or cells from

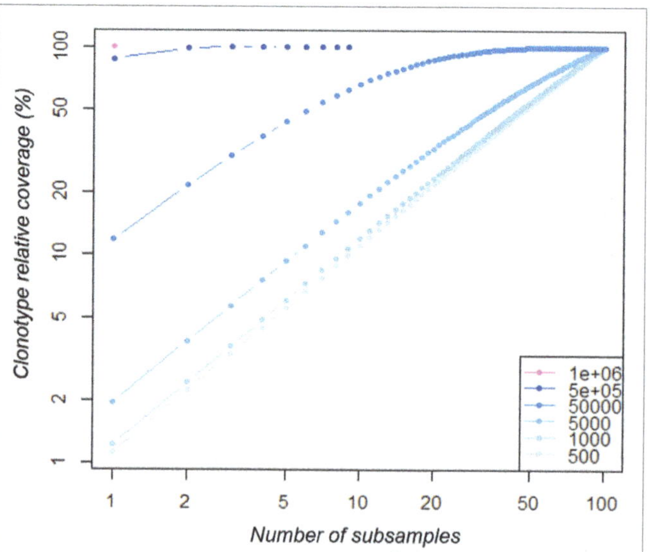


**FIGURE 5** | Clonotype coverage of A3-dataset richness increases with multiple subsamples. The A3-datasets were subsampled at increasing depth (from 500 to $1{\cdot}10^6$ sequences as indicated in the legend from light to dark blue). For each depth, 100 subsamples were produced. Within each subsample series, an increasing number of subsamples (*x*-axis) were randomly selected and their cumulative clonotype richness was calculated relative to the original dataset richness (clonotype richness coverage).

biopsies, though of utmost interest when studying TCR repertoires. Although over-sequencing has been recommended to ensure the identification of rare clonotypes (53), it does increase the risk of generating uninformative, possibly artifactual clonotypes such as duplicate reads and chimeric reads (67). Indeed, when sequencing samples of varying sizes at a commonly used depth, we found that small datasets contained 20 times more clonotypes than would be expected regarding the sample size. This figure decreases when the starting material is increased, demonstrating that over-sequencing small samples dramatically generates noise that cannot be corrected by removing only singletons. Although the relationship between sample size and sequencing depth that we used may appear extreme, it can commonly occur when studying small cell subsets involved in immunological processes. These observations demonstrate the drawbacks of discarding clonotypes based only on their counts and the need for objective approaches in order to assess the actual richness of a repertoire effectively. Single-cell sequencing technologies are an alternative to accurate study of the repertoire of small cell subsets and therefore will surely not require the use of Shannon filtering, because the number of expected unique TR sequences will be at most two per single cell. However, currently the number of required cells is still regularly higher than actually recovered in particularly low-input samples.

Here, we provide a bioinformatics approach to assess accurately the number of unique clonotypes in a large and complex cell population, even when over-sequenced. When analyzing the diversity profiles of repertoires from subsamples of varying sizes of a unique starting sample, we identified Shannon entropy as a reliable threshold to eliminate clonotypes arising from technical noise (SUC) and to focus on informative TR clonotypes (**Figures 1C** and **2A**). This filtering strategy has no impact on the overall clonotype distribution (**Figure 2B**). Importantly, this approach was validated on subsamples originating from a single starting sample. Therefore, the representability of the smallest subsample was questioned. While the distribution evenness was sample size-dependent when considering all the reads, filtering by the Shannon entropy index removed this variability between replicates (**Figure 2C**). This proposed strategy therefore offers an accurate assessment of clonotype identification and representability, even in extreme situations. We applied our method to data produced following multiplex-PCR amplification on bulk polyclonal CD4$^+$ T cells, for which the targeted genes and bias should be constant from one experiment to another. Although the number of uninformative clonotypes should be assessed when analyzing datasets prepared by different molecular methods, we believe that the Shannon index should reflect the true diversity by excluding uninformative clonotypes. Once single-cell sequencing becomes standardized and applicable to a range of very small to very large sample sizes, such correction metrics may not be necessary anymore.

Our results strongly suggest that sequencing depth must be adapted to the initial cell amount. We show that "50,000-cell" replicates are closer to each other than lower input pairs of samples (**Figure 2D**). This observation emphasizes the need to adapt the sample size to the population of interest. All aliquots analyzed here were obtained from a rich and polyclonal cell population. In order to be reliable, a sample needs to be large enough to ensure that most of the clones are represented. Here, about 20% of the clonotypes observed in the two replicates (6,766 out of 30,422 and 35,020 clonotypes) are shared.

Altogether these results show how complex defining a RepSeq strategy can be in guaranteeing the representativeness of the repertoire diversity. If sequencing depth is not adapted to the population size, it can negatively affect the resulting observed diversity, in particular if data are not properly analyzed. This is particularly crucial since the clonality of a population is rarely known before its sequencing, leading to misinterpretation of the results. Since the sequencing depth used was much higher than the size of the samples we analyzed, one would expect good, if not exhaustive, coverage of the overall clonotypes. Conversely, we show that this is by no means the case, with only part of clonotypes being observed with confidence. These observations led us to question the robustness of the results of RepSeq experiments.

Multiple sequencing of the same sample revealed very low overlap between technical replicates, even after filtering out uninformative TR clonotypes, and merely captures the most frequent clonotypes. Rare clonotypes were at best shared by two replicates. As already suggested by Greiff et al. (44), our results are in favor of multiple sequencing when considering very diverse samples. This can be explained by the experimental sampling enforced by the different RepSeq steps (from RNA amplification to library sequencing). In order to validate these experimental observations and propose guidelines for RepSeq studies, we simulated different repertoire distributions and found that the representativeness of a very evenly distributed repertoire, which could be likened to a polyclonal repertoire, is more sensitive to the sequencing depth. The number of sequences produced (by multiple sequencing) needs to be equivalent to the population size to ensure a good assessment of the original diversity (**Figure 4C**). This is particularly true for small samples for which too deep a sequencing can favor the erroneous sequences possibly generated during library preparation (68) and thereby introduce experimental noise.

Altogether, we provide here a method that accurately discards uninformative clonotypes for small and large samples based on the application of Shannon diversity index threshold filtering, as well as guidelines for RepSeq experimental design. In addition, we show how computational simulation of diversity can improve adaptive repertoire analysis assessment where controlled reference repertoires with known actual diversity can be modeled and subject to experimental design and annotation tool flaws. We believe these will be useful in ensuring better RepSeq analyses when looking at rare or unknown cell populations participating in pathophysiological processes and will facilitate the discovery of HTS-based biomarkers.

## AUTHORS NOTE

The RNA sequences presented in this study have been submitted to Sequence Read Archive (SRA; https://www.ncbi.nlm.nih.gov/sra) as Bioproject PRJNA408306, under accession numbers SRR6068973, SRR6068972, and SRR6068975 (Biosample SAMN07682929) and SRR6068974, SRR6068969, SRR6068968, SRR6068971, SRR6068970, SRR6068967, SRR6068966, and SRR6068976 (Biosample SAMN07682930).

## AUTHOR CONTRIBUTIONS

WC performed all the bioinformatics analyses. AG-T and L-MF prepared the samples. WC, EM-F, AS, and DK conceived the studies, designed the experiments, and analyzed the results. WC, EM-F, AS, and DK wrote the first draft of the manuscript, with input from all authors. DK initiated and obtained funding for the study. EM-F and AS contributed equally to the work.

## ACKNOWLEDGMENTS

We are grateful to B. Gouritin for his help in cell sorting. We thank iRepertoire® for providing us with the required data format to implement our analysis pipeline.

## FUNDING

L-MF was funded by a "DIM Région Ile-de-France" doctoral fellowship. The work of WC, DK, EM-F, and AS is funded by the Assistance Publique-Hôpitaux de Paris, INSERM, and Sorbonne Université. The study is part of the LabEx Transimmunom (ANR-11-IDEX-0004-02) and ERC Advanced Grant TRiPoD (322856) funding obtained by DK.

## REFERENCES


1. Davis MM, Bjorkman PJ. T-cell antigen receptor genes and T-cell recognition. *Nature* (1988) 334:395–402. doi:10.1038/334395a0
2. Boudinot P, Mariotti-Ferrandiz ME, Pasquier LD, Benmansour A, Cazenave P-A, Six A. New perspectives for large-scale repertoire analysis of immune receptors. *Mol Immunol* (2008) 45:2437–45. doi:10.1016/j.molimm.2007.12.018
3. Six A, Mariotti-Ferrandiz ME, Chaara W, Magadan S, Pham H-P, Lefranc M-P, et al. The past, present, and future of immune repertoire biology—the rise of next-generation repertoire analysis. *Front Immunol* (2013) 4:413. doi:10.3389/fimmu.2013.00413
4. Bergot A-S, Chaara W, Ruggiero E, Mariotti-Ferrandiz E, Dulauroy S, Schmidt M, et al. TCR sequences and tissue distribution discriminate the subsets of naïve and activated/memory Treg cells in mice: molecular immunology. *Eur J Immunol* (2015) 45:1524–34. doi:10.1002/eji.201445269
5. Dash P, Fiore-Gartland AJ, Hertz T, Wang GC, Sharma S, Souquette A, et al. Quantifiable predictive features define epitope-specific T cell receptor repertoires. *Nature* (2017) 547:89–93. doi:10.1038/nature22383
6. Dong M, Artusa P, Kelly SA, Fournier M, Baldwin TA, Mandl JN, et al. Alterations in the thymic selection threshold skew the self-reactivity of the TCR repertoire in neonates. *J Immunol* (2017) 199:965–73. doi:10.4049/jimmunol.1602137
7. Freeman JD, Warren RL, Webb JR, Nelson BH, Holt RA. Profiling the T-cell receptor beta-chain repertoire by massively parallel sequencing. *Genome Res* (2009) 19:1817–24. doi:10.1101/gr.092924.109
8. Glanville J, Huang H, Nau A, Hatton O, Wagar LE, Rubelt F, et al. Identifying specificity groups in the T cell receptor repertoire. *Nature* (2017) 547:94–8. doi:10.1038/nature22976
9. Kuang M, Cheng J, Zhang C, Feng L, Xu X, Zhang Y, et al. A novel signature for stratifying the molecular heterogeneity of the tissue-infiltrating T-cell receptor repertoire reflects gastric cancer prognosis. *Sci Rep* (2017) 7:7762. doi:10.1038/s41598-017-08289-z
10. Langerak AW, Brüggemann M, Davi F, Darzentas N, van Dongen JJM, Gonzalez D, et al. High-throughput immunogenetics for clinical and research applications in immunohematology: potential and challenges. *J Immunol* (2017) 198:3765–74. doi:10.4049/jimmunol.1602050
11. Maceiras AR, Almeida SCP, Mariotti-Ferrandiz E, Chaara W, Jebbawi F, Six A, et al. T follicular helper and T follicular regulatory cells have different TCR specificity. *Nat Commun* (2017) 8:15067. doi:10.1038/ncomms15067
12. Madi A, Poran A, Shifrut E, Reich-Zeliger S, Greenstein E, Zaretsky I, et al. T cell receptor repertoires of mice and humans are clustered in similarity networks around conserved public CDR3 sequences. *Elife* (2017) 6:e22057. doi:10.7554/eLife.22057
13. Marrero I, Hamm DE, Davies JD. High-throughput sequencing of islet-infiltrating memory CD4+ T cells reveals a similar pattern of TCR Vî² usage in prediabetic and diabetic NOD mice. *PLoS One* (2013) 8:e76546. doi:10.1371/journal.pone.0076546
14. Poschke I, Flossdorf M, Offringa R. Next-generation TCR sequencing—a tool to understand T-cell infiltration in human cancers. *J Pathol* (2016) 240:384–6. doi:10.1002/path.4800
15. Sims JS, Grinshpun B, Feng Y, Ung TH, Neira JA, Samanamud JL, et al. Diversity and divergence of the glioma-infiltrating T-cell receptor repertoire. *Proc Natl Acad Sci U S A* (2016) 113:E3529–37. doi:10.1073/pnas.1601012113
16. Thapa DR, Tonikian R, Sun C, Liu M, Dearth A, Petri M, et al. Longitudinal analysis of peripheral blood T cell receptor diversity in patients with systemic lupus erythematosus by next-generation sequencing. *Arthritis Res Ther* (2015) 17:132. doi:10.1186/s13075-015-0655-9
17. Thomas N, Best K, Cinelli M, Reich-Zeliger S, Gal H, Shifrut E, et al. Tracking global changes induced in the CD4 T-cell receptor repertoire by immunization with a complex antigen using short stretches of CDR3 protein sequence. *Bioinformatics* (2014) 30:3181–8. doi:10.1093/bioinformatics/btu523
18. Rosati E, Dowds CM, Liaskou E, Henriksen EKK, Karlsen TH, Franke A. Overview of methodologies for T-cell receptor repertoire analysis. *BMC Biotechnol* (2017) 17:61. doi:10.1186/s12896-017-0379-9
19. Bolotin DA, Mamedov IZ, Britanova OV, Zvyagin IV, Shagin D, Ustyugova SV, et al. Next generation sequencing for TCR repertoire profiling: platform-specific features and correction algorithms: new technology. *Eur J Immunol* (2012) 42:3073–83. doi:10.1002/eji.201242517
20. Egorov ES, Merzlyak EM, Shelenkov AA, Britanova OV, Sharonov GV, Staroverov DB, et al. Quantitative profiling of immune repertoires for minor lymphocyte counts using unique molecular identifiers. *J Immunol* (2015) 194:6155–63. doi:10.4049/jimmunol.1500215
21. Kivioja T, Vähärautio A, Karlsson K, Bonke M, Enge M, Linnarsson S, et al. Counting absolute numbers of molecules using unique molecular identifiers. *Nat Methods* (2012) 9:72–4. doi:10.1038/nmeth.1778
22. Ma K-Y, He C, Wendel BS, Williams CM, Xiao J, Yang H, et al. Immune repertoire sequencing using molecular identifiers enables accurate clonality discovery and clone size quantification. *Front Immunol* (2018) 9:33. doi:10.3389/fimmu.2018.00033
23. Britanova OV, Putintseva EV, Shugay M, Merzlyak EM, Turchaninova MA, Staroverov DB, et al. Age-related decrease in TCR repertoire diversity measured with deep and normalized sequence profiling. *J Immunol* (2014) 192:2689–98. doi:10.4049/jimmunol.1302064
24. Izraelson M, Nakonechnaya TO, Moltedo B, Egorov ES, Kasatskaya SA, Putintseva EV, et al. Comparative analysis of murine T-cell receptor repertoires. *Immunology* (2018) 153:133–44. doi:10.1111/imm.12857

25. Smith T, Heger A, Sudbery I. UMI-tools: modeling sequencing errors in unique molecular identifiers to improve quantification accuracy. *Genome Res* (2017) 27:491–9. doi:10.1101/gr.209601.116
26. Benichou J, Ben-Hamo R, Louzoun Y, Efroni S. Rep-Seq: uncovering the immunological repertoire through next-generation sequencing: Rep-Seq: NGS for the immunological repertoire. *Immunology* (2012) 135:183–91. doi:10.1111/j.1365-2567.2011.03527.x
27. Emerson RO, DeWitt WS, Vignali M, Gravley J, Hu JK, Osborne EJ, et al. Immunosequencing identifies signatures of cytomegalovirus exposure history and HLA-mediated effects on the T cell repertoire. *Nat Genet* (2017) 49:659–65. doi:10.1038/ng.3822
28. Heather JM, Best K, Oakes T, Gray ER, Roe JK, Thomas N, et al. Dynamic perturbations of the T-cell receptor repertoire in chronic HIV infection and following antiretroviral therapy. *Front Immunol* (2016) 6:644. doi:10.3389/fimmu.2015.00644
29. Mariotti-Ferrandiz E, Pham H-P, Dulauroy S, Gorgette O, Klatzmann D, Cazenave P-A, et al. A TCRβ repertoire signature can predict experimental cerebral malaria. *PLoS One* (2016) 11:e0147871. doi:10.1371/journal.pone.0147871
30. Madi A, Shifrut E, Reich-Zeliger S, Gal H, Best K, Ndifon W, et al. T-cell receptor repertoires share a restricted set of public and abundant CDR3 sequences that are associated with self-related immunity. *Genome Res* (2014) 24:1603–12. doi:10.1101/gr.170753.113
31. Marrero I, Aguilera C, Hamm DE, Quinn A, Kumar V. High-throughput sequencing reveals restricted TCR Vβ usage and public TCRβ clonotypes among pancreatic lymph node memory CD4+ T cells and their involvement in autoimmune diabetes. *Mol Immunol* (2016) 74:82–95. doi:10.1016/j.molimm.2016.04.013
32. Pugliese A. Autoreactive T cells in type 1 diabetes. *J Clin Invest* (2017) 127:2881–91. doi:10.1172/JCI94549
33. Rossetti M, Spreafico R, Consolaro A, Leong JY, Chua C, Massa M, et al. TCR repertoire sequencing identifies synovial Treg cell clonotypes in the bloodstream during active inflammation in human arthritis. *Ann Rheum Dis* (2017) 76:435–41. doi:10.1136/annrheumdis-2015-208992
34. Seay HR, Yusko E, Rothweiler SJ, Zhang L, Posgai AL, Campbell-Thompson M, et al. Tissue distribution and clonal diversity of the T and B cell repertoire in type 1 diabetes. *JCI Insight* (2016) 1:e88242. doi:10.1172/jci.insight.88242
35. Zhao Y, Nguyen P, Ma J, Wu T, Jones LL, Pei D, et al. Preferential use of public TCR during autoimmune encephalomyelitis. *J Immunol* (2016) 196:4905–14. doi:10.4049/jimmunol.1501029
36. van Heijst JWJ, Ceberio I, Lipuma LB, Samilo DW, Wasilewski GD, Gonzales AMR, et al. Quantitative assessment of T cell repertoire recovery after hematopoietic stem cell transplantation. *Nat Med* (2013) 19:372–7. doi:10.1038/nm.3100
37. Lai L, Wang L, Chen H, Zhang J, Yan Q, Ou M, et al. T cell repertoire following kidney transplantation revealed by high-throughput sequencing. *Transpl Immunol* (2016) 39:34–45. doi:10.1016/j.trim.2016.08.006
38. Theil A, Wilhelm C, Kuhn M, Petzold A, Tuve S, Oelschlägel U, et al. T cell receptor repertoires after adoptive transfer of expanded allogeneic regulatory T cells: T cell receptor repertoires post-T $_{reg}$ cell therapy. *Clin Exp Immunol* (2017) 187:316–24. doi:10.1111/cei.12887
39. Magurran A. *Measuring Biological Diversity*. Oxford, UK: Wiley (2004).
40. Robins HS, Srivastava SK, Campregher PV, Turtle CJ, Andriesen J, Riddell SR, et al. Overlap and effective size of the human CD8+ T-cell receptor repertoire. *Sci Transl Med* (2010) 2:47ra64. doi:10.1126/scitranslmed.3001442
41. Shugay M, Bolotin DA, Putintseva EV, Pogorelyy MV, Mamedov IZ, Chudakov DM. Huge overlap of individual TCR beta repertoires. *Front Immunol* (2013) 4:466. doi:10.3389/fimmu.2013.00466
42. Warren RL, Nelson BH, Holt RA. Profiling model T-cell metagenomes with short reads. *Bioinformatics* (2009) 25:458–64. doi:10.1093/bioinformatics/btp010
43. Fisher RA, Steven-Corbet A, Williams CB. The relation between the number of species and the number of individuals in a random sample of an animal population. *J Anim Ecol* (1943) 12:42–58. doi:10.2307/1411
44. Greiff V, Miho E, Menzel U, Reddy ST. Bioinformatic and statistical analysis of adaptive immune repertoires. *Trends Immunol* (2015) 36:738–49. doi:10.1016/j.it.2015.09.006
45. Bashford-Rogers RJM, Palser AL, Idris SF, Carter L, Epstein M, Callard RE, et al. Capturing needles in haystacks: a comparison of B-cell receptor sequencing methods. *BMC Immunol* (2014) 15:29. doi:10.1186/s12865-014-0029-0
46. Plessy C, Mariotti-Ferrandiz E, Manabe R-I, Hori S. clonotypeR—high throughput analysis of T cell antigen receptor sequences. *Biorxiv* (2015). doi:10.1101/028696
47. Levenshtein VI. Binary codes capable of correcting deletions, insertions, and reversals. *Sov Phys Dokl* (1966) 10:707–10.
48. Oksanen J, Blanchet FG, Kindt R, Legendre P, Minchin PR, O'hara RB, et al. *Package 'Vegan.' Community Ecol. Package Version 2* (2013).
49. Hill MO. Diversity and evenness: a unifying notation and its consequences. *Ecology* (1973) 54:427–32. doi:10.2307/1934352
50. Murugan A, Mora T, Walczak AM, Callan CG. Statistical inference of the generation probability of T-cell receptors from sequence repertoires. *Proc Natl Acad Sci U S A* (2012) 109:16161–6. doi:10.1073/pnas.1212755109
51. Evert S, Baroni M. zipfR: word frequency distributions in R. *Proceedings of the 45th Annual Meeting of the ACL on Interactive Poster and Demonstration Sessions (Association for Computational Linguistics)*. Stroudsburg, PA (2007). p. 29–32.
52. Horn HS. Measurement of "overlap" in comparative ecological studies. *Am Nat* (1966) 100:419–24. doi:10.1086/282436
53. Mamedov IZ, Britanova OV, Zvyagin IV, Turchaninova MA, Bolotin DA, Putintseva EV, et al. Preparing unbiased T-cell receptor and antibody cDNA libraries for the deep next generation sequencing profiling. *Front Immunol* (2013) 4:456. doi:10.3389/fimmu.2013.00456
54. Ricotta C. On parametric evenness measures. *J Theor Biol* (2003) 222:189–97. doi:10.1016/S0022-5193(03)00026-2
55. Schroeder HW. The evolution and development of the antibody repertoire. *Front Immunol* (2015) 6:33. doi:10.3389/fimmu.2015.00033
56. Rényi A. On measures of entropy and information. *Proc Fourth Berkeley Symp Math Stat Probab*. (Vol. 1), Berkeley, CA: University of California Press (1961). p. 547–61.
57. Pielou EC. The measurement of diversity in different types of biological collections. *J Theor Biol* (1966) 13:131–44. doi:10.1016/0022-5193(66)90013-0
58. Burgos JD, Moreno-Tovar P. Zipf-scaling behavior in the immune system. *Biosystems* (1996) 39:227–32. doi:10.1016/0303-2647(96)01618-8
59. Greiff V, Bhat P, Cook SC, Menzel U, Kang W, Reddy ST. A bioinformatic framework for immune repertoire diversity profiling enables detection of immunological status. *Genome Med* (2015) 7:49. doi:10.1186/s13073-015-0169-8
60. Mora T, Walczak A. Quantifying lymphocyte receptor diversity. *BioRxiv* (2016). doi:10.1101/046870
61. Schwab DJ, Nemenman I, Mehta P. Zipf's law and criticality in multivariate data without fine-tuning. *Phys Rev Lett* (2014) 113:068102. doi:10.1103/PhysRevLett.113.068102
62. Sepúlveda N, Boucontet L, Pereira P, Carneiro J. Stochastic modeling of T cell receptor gene rearrangement. *J Theor Biol* (2005) 234:153–65. doi:10.1016/j.jtbi.2004.11.018
63. Aitchison L, Corradi N, Latham PE. Zipf's law arises naturally when there are underlying, unobserved variables. *PLoS Comput Biol* (2016) 12:e1005110. doi:10.1371/journal.pcbi.1005110
64. Piantadosi ST. Zipf's word frequency law in natural language: a critical review and future directions. *Psychon Bull Rev* (2014) 21:1112–30. doi:10.3758/s13423-014-0585-6
65. Nazarov VI, Pogorelyy MV, Komech EA, Zvyagin IV, Bolotin DA, Shugay M, et al. tcR: an R package for T cell receptor repertoire advanced data analysis. *BMC Bioinformatics* (2015) 16:175. doi:10.1186/s12859-015-0613-1
66. Friedensohn S, Khan TA, Reddy ST. Advanced methodologies in high-throughput sequencing of immune repertoires. *Trends Biotechnol* (2017) 35:203–14. doi:10.1016/j.tibtech.2016.09.010
67. Head SR, Komori HK, LaMere SA, Whisenant T, Van Nieuwerburgh F, Salomon DR, et al. Library construction for next-generation sequencing: overviews and challenges. *Biotechniques* (2014) 56:61–4. doi:10.2144/000114133
68. Heather JM, Ismail M, Oakes T, Chain B. High-throughput sequencing of the T-cell receptor repertoire: pitfalls and opportunities. *Brief Bioinform* (2017). doi:10.1093/bib/bbw138

# 13

# Regulatory T Cells Suppress Effector T Cell Proliferation by Limiting Division Destiny

*Mark R. Dowling*[1,2*], *Andrey Kan*[1,2], *Susanne Heinzel*[1,2], *Julia M. Marchingo*[1,2‡], *Philip D. Hodgkin*[1,2†] *and Edwin D. Hawkins*[1,2†]

[1] *Immunology Division, The Walter and Eliza Hall Institute of Medical Research, Parkville, VIC, Australia,* [2] *Department of Medical Biology, The University of Melbourne, Parkville, VIC, Australia*

***Correspondence:**
*Mark R. Dowling*
*dowling@wehi.edu.au*

[†] *These authors have contributed equally to this work*

**‡Present Address:**
*Julia M. Marchingo, Division of Cell Signalling and Immunology, School of Life Sciences, University of Dundee, Dundee, United Kingdom*

Understanding how the strength of an effector T cell response is regulated is a fundamental problem in immunology with implications for immunity to pathogens, autoimmunity, and immunotherapy. The initial magnitude of the T cell response is determined by the sum of independent signals from antigen, co-stimulation and cytokines. By applying quantitative methods, the contribution of each signal to the number of divisions T cells undergo (division destiny) can be measured, and the resultant exponential increase in response magnitude accurately calculated. $CD4^+CD25^+Foxp3^+$ regulatory T cells suppress self-reactive T cell responses and limit pathogen-directed immune responses before bystander damage occurs. Using a quantitative modeling framework to measure T cell signal integration and response, we show that Tregs modulate division destiny, rather than directly increasing the rate of death or delaying interdivision times. The quantitative effect of Tregs could be mimicked by modulating the availability of stimulatory co-stimuli and cytokines or through the addition of inhibitory signals. Thus, our analysis illustrates the primary effect of Tregs on the magnitude of effector T cell responses is mediated by modifying division destiny of responding cell populations.

**Keywords: T cells, regulatory T cells (Tregs), modeling and simulation, cytokines, immunity**

## INTRODUCTION

$CD4^+CD25^+Foxp3^+$ regulatory T cells (Tregs) play a critical role in immune homeostasis. However, the precise mechanism of regulatory function on effector T cells remains contentious. Important roles for modulation of co-stimulation by dendritic cells (1–4), absorption of cytokines such as IL-2 (5–8), secretion of inhibitory cytokines such as TGF-β, IL-10 and IL-35 (9–13) and direct cell-contact dependent mechanisms (9, 14) have all been demonstrated in a variety of *in vitro* and *in vivo* systems (15–18). The relative quantitative importance of these different mechanisms is unknown and may depend on context. Apart from suppressing proliferation, Tregs are also known to modulate the function of effector T cells. For example, Maeda et al. recently showed that Tregs can induce self-reactive human $CD8^+$ T cells (Melanin-A specific) to adopt a $CCR7^+CTLA\text{-}4^+$ anergic phenotype in response to peptide stimulation *in vitro*, as well as reducing their proliferation via modulation of dendritic cell co-stimulation (19).

Recent work by Marchingo et al. has defined a quantitative framework for understanding signal integration by T cells (20). A key concept is the notion of "division destiny"—the number of divisions a cell undergoes before ceasing proliferation and reverting to a quiescent state, first described in B cells (21–23). The mean division destiny of $CD8^+$ T cells was shown to be the linear sum of independent contributions from antigen, co-stimulation and cytokines, allowing quantitative prediction of the magnitude of the T cell response from knowledge of the individual stimuli. Heinzel et al. subsequently demonstrated that this quantitative signal integration to determine division destiny can be inferred by levels of Myc within T cells and B cells, providing a molecular mechanism for this phenomenon (24).

We tested whether the calculus of division destiny could be used to quantify the action of Tregs during suppression of effector T cell proliferation. We hypothesized that Tregs may potentially function in an opposing mechanism to T cell co-stimulation, and thus manifest suppression of effector T cell proliferation via a reduction in division destiny in the effector T cell population. Here, using quantitative methods, we illustrate that the dominant action of Tregs is through "subtracting" division destiny in responding T cells in a dose-dependent manner, in comparison to inducing more rapid death or slowing proliferation. These results provide a quantitative framework for studying different mechanisms of suppression in immune responses including genetic polymorphisms associated with autoimmunity or inflammation. Furthermore, they highlight that division destiny is a universal cellular parameter central to not only positive regulation of immune responses, but also effector response suppression.

## MATERIALS AND METHODS

### Mice

All experiments were performed using C57BL/6 mice bred and maintained under specific pathogen-free conditions in the Walter and Eliza Hall Institute (WEHI) animal facilities (Parkville, Victoria, Australia) and used between 6 and 12 weeks of age. All experiments were performed under the approval of the WEHI Animal Ethics Committee.

### CD4+CD25+ Treg and CD4+CD25-CD62L+ Teff Cell Purification

$CD4^+CD25^-CD62L^+$ effector T cells (Teff) were isolated from pooled mouse lymph nodes (inguinal, axillary, brachial, superficial cervical, and lumbar) and spleens by negative and positive selection using the mouse naïve CD4+ T cell isolation kit (Miltenyi). $CD4^+CD25^+$ Tregs were prepared from pooled spleen and total lymph nodes (inguinal, axillary, brachial, superficial cervical, and lumbar) of C57BL/6 mice. Cell suspensions were stained with anti-$CD4^-$PerCP-Cy5.5, anti-CD25-FITC, and enriched for $CD25^+$ cells using anti-FITC beads (Miltenyi). Cells were then sorted for $CD4^+$ $CD25^{hi}$ on a BD FACSAria. Treg purity was checked using intracellular staining for Foxp3 and in all experiments was >90%. Irradiated splenocytes were prepared by red cell lysis of whole spleen suspension and irradiated at 3,000Gy.

### Celltrace Oregon Green Labeling

For division tracking, Teffs were labeled with a final concentration of 20 μM Cell Trace Oregon Green (Invitrogen) by incubation for 10 min at 37°C at a cell density of $10^7$ cells/mL in phosphate-buffered saline (PBS) with 10% bovine-serum albumin (BSA).

### Cell Culture

Cells were cultured in RPMI 1640 medium (Invitrogen) supplemented with non-essential amino acids, 1 mM Sodium-pyruvate, 10 mM HEPES, 100 U/mL Penicillin, 100 μg/mL Streptomycin (all Invitrogen), 50 μM 2-mercaptoethanol, 2 mM L-glutamine (both Sigma) and 10% FCS (JRH Biosciences and Invitrogen). Cells were incubated in a humidified environment at 37°C in 5% $CO_2$.

The *in vitro* Treg suppression assay was set-up as follows (25). Twenty thousand Teffs were co-cultured with 80,000 irradiated splenocytes and 2 μg/mL anti-CD3 (clone 2C11, WEHI antibody facility, Australia) and a varying ratio of Tregs. Proliferation was analyzed by flow cytometry for the next 4 days.

For experiments mimicking suppression the following reagents were added to cultures: CTLA4-Ig (prepared from COS cells, provided by Peter Lane), anti-mouse IL-2 monoclonal antibody (purified from hybridoma cell line S4B6, WEHI), TGF-β (eBioscience), recombinant murine IL-10 (purified from baculovirus-transfected Sf21 insect cell supernatant, DNAX).

### Flow Cytometry Analysis

Triplicate wells were harvested at each time point after addition of a known number of CaliBRITE microbeads (BD) to facilitate quantification of absolute cell numbers. Cells were analyzed on a BD FACSCanto.

### BrdU Labelling

Detection of intracellular BrdU was performed using a BrdU staining kit (BD Pharmingen) as per manufacturer instructions.

### Calculation of Cell Numbers Per Division, Cohort Number and Mean Division Number of Dividing Cells

The number of cells per division, $n_i$, $i = 0, 1, \ldots, 7, 8^+$, was determined by flow cytometry with gating for 2-fold dilution of Cell Trace Oregon Green intensity and the ratio of analyzed cells to the known number of microbeads (division number >7 could not be resolved above background autofluorescence, and $8^+$ refers to all cells gated as having divided 8 or more times).

The number of undivided cells is $n_0$, and the number of dividing cells is:

$$N_{div} = \sum_{i=1}^{8+} n_i \quad (1)$$

Following (26), the precursor cohort numbers for each division, $c_i$, were calculated by dividing the cell number per division by two to the power of division number, in order to remove the expected expansion of cell number with division in the absence of death:

$$c_i = \frac{n_i}{2^i} \tag{2}$$

The total cohort number, $C$, is the sum of the cohort numbers over all divisions:

$$C = \sum_{i=0}^{8^+} c_i \tag{3}$$

The cohort number would remain equal to the starting cell number if there were no cell death in the system, and therefore comparison of differences in cohort number over time according to a varying condition can be used to identify effects on survival (20, 24, 26–28).

Plots of mean division number against harvest time can be used to estimate proliferation features, including average time to first division, subsequent division rate and division destiny (20, 26, 28, 29). A number of methods have been used to calculate mean division number. Here, as not all anti-CD3 stimulated T cells enter division, we averaged the dividing cells only. This value, mean division number of dividing cells ($MDN_{div}$), is calculated as:

$$MDN_{div} = \frac{\sum_{i=1}^{8^+} i c_i}{\sum_{i=1}^{8^+} c_i} \tag{4}$$

A plateau in $MDN_{div}$ can indicate that the cells have stopped dividing having reached their division destiny.

# RESULTS

## Regulatory T Cells Do Not Reduce Survival or Activation of Effector T Cells *in vitro*

In principle, regulatory T cells may suppress effector T cells by directly inducing death, by reducing activation and recruitment into division, by slowing the division rate, or by reducing division destiny. To decipher the effects on these different parameters, we analyzed an *in vitro* suppression assay using the established precursor cohort method (26, 29). This approach uses quantitative graph-based methods to track the fate of founder cells seeded in culture during *in vitro* proliferation assays and allocate effects to changes in division rate, division destiny or overall cell survival. We designed our experimental approach using a suppression assay that reflects the majority of assays used in studies of Treg biology. Teffs labeled with the division tracking dye Cell Trace Oregon Green were co-cultured with varying ratios of Tregs, irradiated splenocytes as antigen-presenting cells (APCs), and anti-CD3 as a polyclonal T-cell-receptor stimulus (25). Addition of counting beads at the time of harvest allowed quantification of absolute cell numbers per division.

**Figure 1A** demonstrates the suppressive effect of Tregs on division of Teff over the time course of T cell stimulation as measured by dilution of cell division tracking dyes. When two ends of the spectrum are compared (no Tregs vs. a high Treg:Teff ratio), the progression through division of the Teff population is significantly reduced. In this system not all T cells are activated to enter division, and cells that are not activated display different survival kinetics than activated cells (27, 30). We first asked whether the suppressive effect of Tregs could be ascribed to a reduction in either the survival of undivided cells or in the proportion of cells induced to divide, as either conclusion could be reached by comparing division profiles shown in **Figure 1A.** Either of these processes would affect the number of undivided cells measured in culture over time. **Figure 1B** shows that the number of undivided cells is unaffected by the Treg ratio over the course of the experiment. Thus, contrary to the above expectation, survival of undivided cells and recruitment into division is not affected by Tregs, and an alternate explanation must be sought.

Next, we examined total cell numbers in culture. **Figure 1C** quantifies the response of Teffs in culture over time as represented by total cell numbers in the context of varying the Treg ratio. The peak of the response was ~60 to 70 h post stimulation for all Treg ratios, followed by a decline thereafter. Late in the culture, after 70 h, the highest cell numbers were observed in the absence of Tregs, and the addition of Tregs reduced the Teff number in a dose-dependent manner, as expected. Interestingly, between ~40 and 60 h we noted an increase in cell number at intermediate ratios of Tregs (1:16, 1:8, 1:4), compared with lower or higher ratios of Tregs, which was unexpected and did not correlate with the overall trend seen in cell numbers at the end of the experiment.

We investigated how the Teff response was altered in the presence of increasing numbers of Tregs by applying the precursor cohort method (20, 26, 27). As described in Methods, the cohort number is defined as the sum of the cell numbers in each division divided by two to the power of division number. Calculating the cohort number removes the effect of cell division on cell number, allowing an analysis of survival of the original cohort of cells placed in culture, independently of other kinetic changes. **Figure 1D** illustrates the effect of Tregs on the cohort number over time. In general, increasing numbers of Tregs did not induce a more rapid decline in the cohort numbers over time, indicating the mechanism of suppression is not via active induction of death of Teffs. This result is also supported by observing survival early in the culture, prior to entry into first division (<50 h—**Figure 1C**), where Teffs appeared to die at a rate that was independent of Treg ratio. The exception is that we observed a small increase in cohort number at ~40–60h with intermediate Treg ratios (as represented by a slight shift in the cohort plot to the right in 1:16, 1:8, 1:4), revealing a small effect on promoting survival. This explains the increased cell numbers seen in **Figure 1C** at this time. As undivided cells were not affected by Tregs (**Figure 1B**), this unexpected survival-enhancing effect of intermediate ratios of Tregs can be ascribed to the activated dividing-cell population.

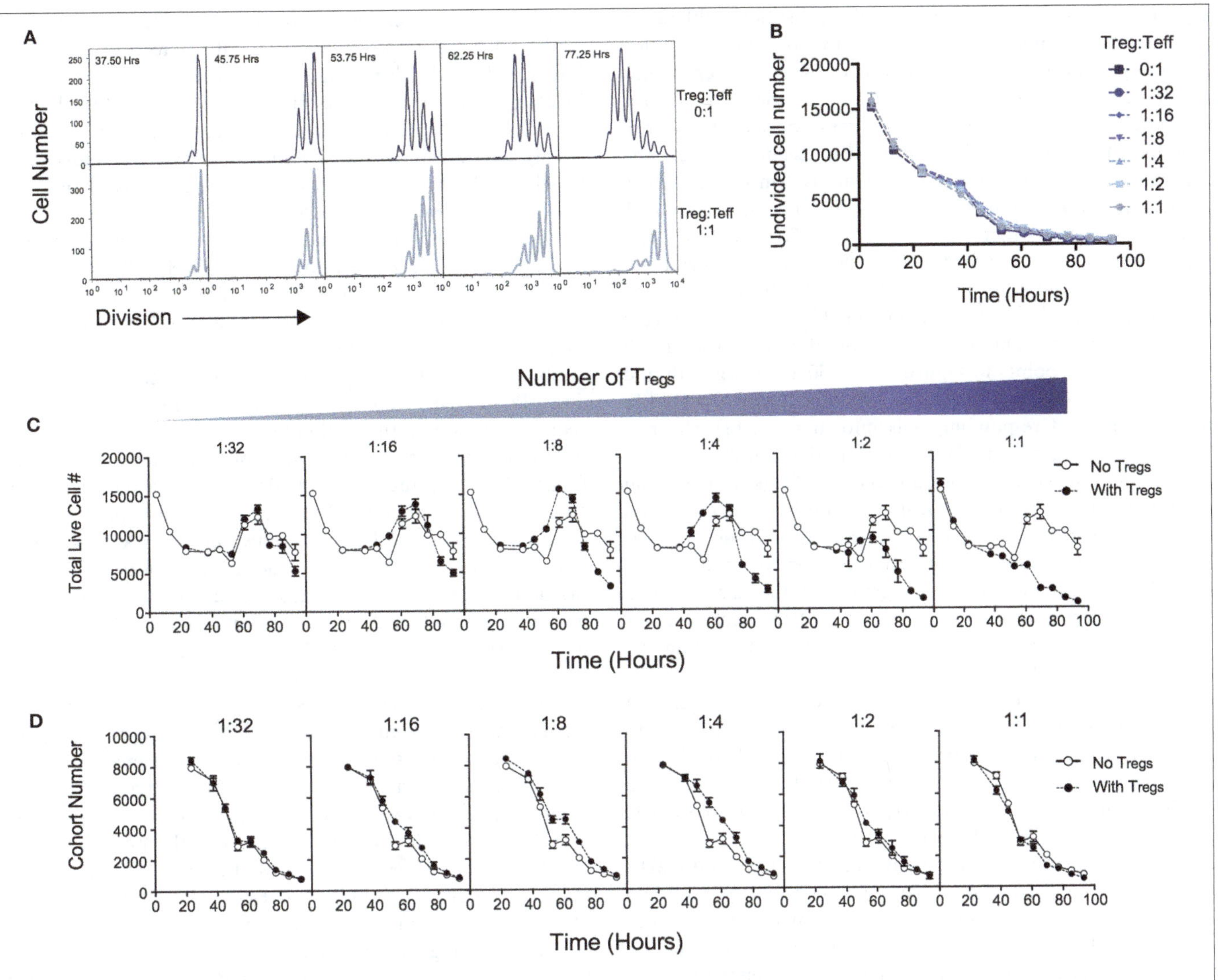


**FIGURE 1** | Quantitative analysis of the effect of Tregs on Teff stimulation. $CD4^+CD25^-CD62L^+$ effector T cells (Teffs) labeled with cell division dyes were co-cultured with varying ratios of Tregs and the response measured. **(A)** Example timecourse of cell division progression in cultures without Tregs (top panel) and with Tregs (lower panel). **(B)** Number of undivided Teff cells in culture over time. Data shown are mean +/− SEM of triplicate samples. One representative data set from three independent experiments is shown. **(C)** The effect of Tregs on the total live cell number of Teffs over time for varying ratios of suppression is shown. For each graph, the Treg ratio (closed circles) is overlaid with the control culture with no Tregs added (open circles). **(D)** The cohort number over time of Teff cells is shown for varying ratios of Tregs. For each graph, the Treg ratio (closed circles) is overlaid with the control culture with no Tregs added (open circles).

## Regulatory T Cells Subtract From the Mean Division Destiny Reached by Activated Effector T Cells in a Dose-Dependent Manner

Late in the culture (after 70 h), there is a clear dose-dependent effect of Tregs on Teff cell number (**Figure 1C**), which represents the predominant suppressive effect of Tregs, and is the time at which *in vitro* Treg assays are typically measured. The number of times cells divide before they return to quiescence (division destiny) has recently been demonstrated as a critical component of T cell responses (20, 24). Division destiny is observed in cohort analysis as a plateau in the mean division number over time. We hypothesized that the suppressive effect of Tregs might be explained by regulation of division destiny or other features of cell division rate.

**Figure 2A** shows the effect on cell division for varying Treg ratios illustrating a progressive reduction in T cell proliferation as Treg numbers are increased. The consequence of this effect on expansion of cell numbers is highlighted by the significant effect on the number of cells in each division (**Figure 2B**). Given the absence of Treg induced cell death (**Figure 1D**), we used the cohort method to investigate other potential kinetic influences that could explain the reduced division progression associated with increasing Treg numbers, namely time to first division, subsequent division rate (after first division) and division destiny.

**Figure 2C** illustrates how changes to these distinct proliferation parameters (i.e., time to first division, division rate or division destiny) will affect cohort plots of mean division number vs. time (20, 21, 24, 27, 28, 31, 32). **Figure 2D** shows the effect of Treg co-culture on $MDN_{div}$, the calculated mean division number of cells that have entered into division (i.e., excluding undivided cells) using the cohort method. This analysis demonstrates three important points of interest regarding the effect of Tregs on T cell stimulation: (1) Increasing the ratio of Tregs had no effect on the mean time taken for the Teff cell population to respond to stimulation and enter the first division (as indicated by the overlapping line for early divisions on the y-axis for all Treg ratios—**Figure 2D**). This is consistent with division tracking data from early time points in **Figure 1A** (37.50 h) shown with and without high Treg exposure. Here, no difference is observed in the first entry of responding cells into division; (2) The rate of division (the gradient of the mean division number vs. time curve) was unaffected by the presence of Tregs, but division destiny was reached earlier, consistent with a timed regulation of division destiny (24); and, (3) Increasing the ratio of Tregs reduced the maximum mean division number reached by Teff in a dose-dependent manner. Together, in the absence of a significant effect observed in all other parameters measured, this suggests that the predominant effect of Tregs is limiting the division potential of responding effector T cells.

To further demonstrate the quantitative effect of regulation of division destiny, we calculated the expected reduction in cell number that can be attributed to the diminished division destiny. This calculation is illustrated in **Figure 2E**. We compared proliferation in the absence of Tregs (ratio 0:1), to the highest ratio of Tregs (1:1). The difference in mean division destiny (dark blue vs. light blue lines) was determined to be 1.1 (**Figure 2D**); thus the expected reduction in cell number is $2^{1.1} = 2.14$. We compared the number of divided cells vs. mean division number of divided cells (**Figure 2E**). Here, the dark blue horizontal line indicates the peak response measured in the absence of Tregs, while the light blue horizontal line represents the predicted reduction in cell number. Strikingly, the vast majority of the effect of adding Tregs to stimulating T cell conditions can be explained by changes in division destiny alone.

To confirm the effect of Tregs on proliferation, we investigated cell cycle turnover by measuring BrdU incorporation. As expected, the presence of Tregs reduced BrdU incorporation in a dose-dependent manner indicating fewer cells were actively dividing at higher Treg:Teff ratios at 63 h post stimulation when measured at either the total population (**Figure 2F**) or per division basis (**Figure 2G**). Thus, while consistent with *in vitro* Treg assays, our analyses provide further detail regarding suppressive mechanisms that regulate Teff kinetics.

### The Quantitative Effect of Tregs on Teff Proliferation Can Be Mimicked by Known Mechanisms of Suppression

Many mechanisms of suppression by Tregs have been demonstrated in a range of different *in vitro* and *in vivo* systems (16, 17). We therefore investigated whether the observed reduction in division destiny could be replicated by previously-studied mechanisms. In **Figure 3**, the effect of previously implicated mechanisms on the kinetics of Teff responses is investigated using the same quantitative assays outlined above. Total cell number (left panel), cohort number (survival—middle panel) and mean division number (Division analysis—right panel) is displayed for each experiment in order to illustrate effects on cell death and division destiny.

The availability of IL-2 has been shown to increase division destiny in a dose-dependent manner in T cells (20). Absorption of IL-2 by Tregs, and therefore reducing the access to free IL-2 has been described as a mechanism of Treg suppression (5–8). To mimic this effect, we added an anti-IL2 blocking antibody (S4B6) to cultures of Teffs stimulated with anti-CD3 and APCs (**Figure 3A**). Similar to the effect of Tregs, anti-IL-2 reduced division destiny without affecting cohort number. Next, we mimicked the effect of inhibition of co-stimulation, by adding CTLA4-Ig to cultures (**Figure 3B**). CTLA4-Ig binds to CD80 and CD86 and competitively blocks engagement of CD28 on T cells (33). Again, similar to the effect of Tregs, CTLA4-Ig did not affect cohort number but had a clear effect on reducing division destiny. There was also a small reduction in time to first division consistent with the effect of CD28 co-stimulation in the presence of IL-2 (29). By contrast, the number of APCs added to Teff cultures affected predominantly cohort number (**Figure 3C**). APC ratios between 1:1 and 8:1 did not appear to regulate division destiny. Thus, the APCs in this system appear to be important for survival of Teffs, through a mechanism that is not fully recapitulated by inhibition of IL-2 or co-stimulation.

Finally, we analyzed the effect of inhibitory cytokines, TGF-β and IL-10 (9, 10, 12–14). TGF-β modestly increased cohort number while reducing division destiny in a dose-dependent manner (**Figure 3D**, middle and right panels). The net effect of TGF-β was suppressive, as indicated by a decrease in total cell number (**Figure 3D**, left panel). This suppressive effect is interesting and unusual, as previous studies have shown that the addition of cytokines or increasing the level of receptor stimulation leads to an increase in division destiny as opposed to the direct subtraction observed here (20). Similar to TGF-β, addition of IL-10 modestly increased cohort number, however there was no effect on division destiny (**Figure 3E**, middle and right panels). Therefore, the net effect of IL-10 was to increase total cell number (**Figure 3E**, left panel). Thus IL-10 was not directly suppressive in this *in vitro* system. While surprising, a similar lack of suppression has been previously reported using a quantitative *in vitro* CD8+ T cell system (20).

## DISCUSSION

Our results demonstrate that the predominant effect of Tregs is on reducing the division destiny of effector T cells, rather than directly reducing survival or division rate. This finding underscores the importance of division destiny as a key mechanism regulating the T cell expansion in activating as well as suppressive conditions.

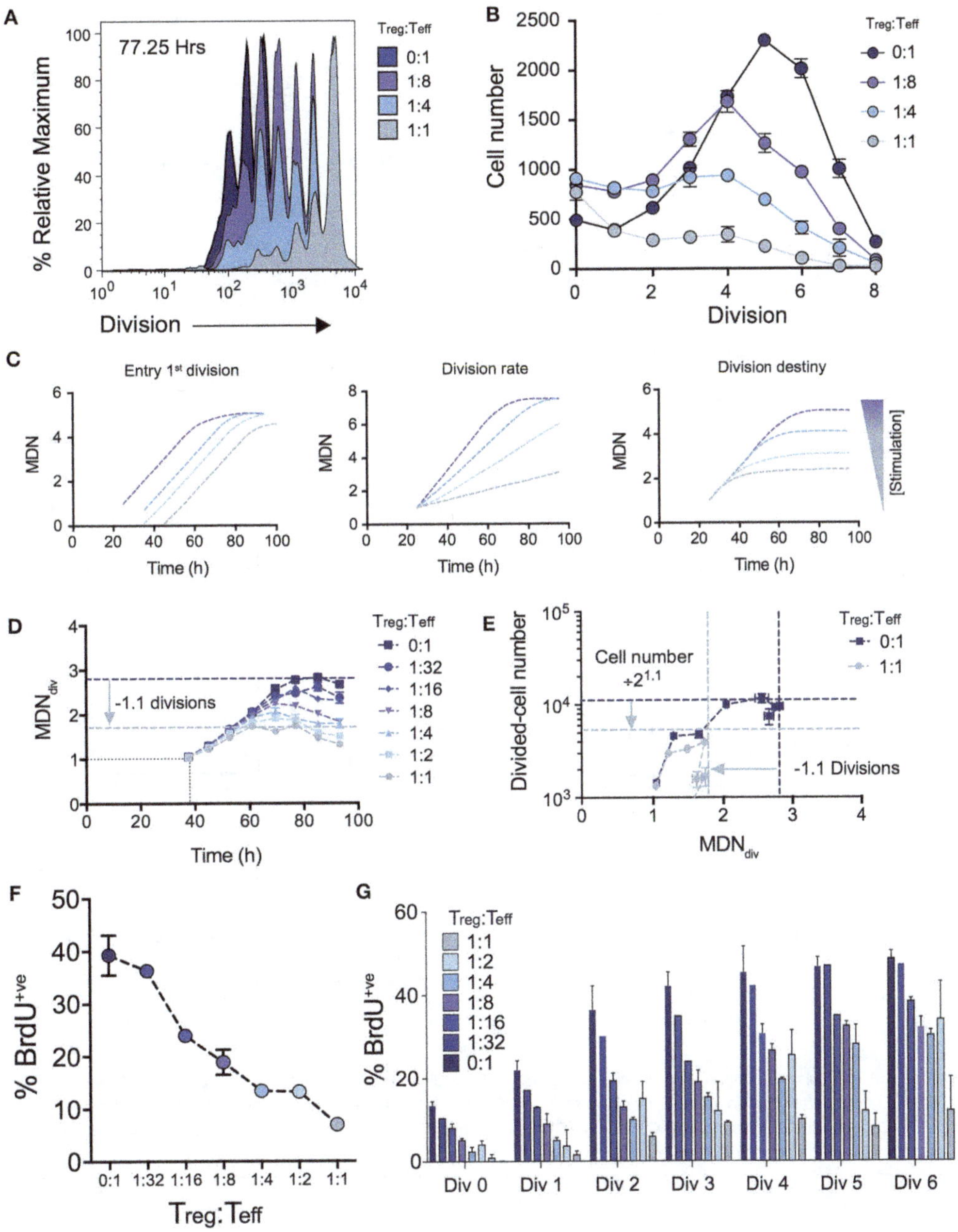


**FIGURE 2 |** Using cohort analysis to dissect the effect of Tregs on Teff cell division. **(A)** Cell division profiles of Teff cells at 77.25 hours with varying ratios of Tregs. **(B)** Cell numbers per division at 77.25 h as determined by quantification to a known number of added beads. **(C)** Cohort plot examples illustrating how trends in graphs are altered by changes in mean time to 1st division, the subsequent division rate and division destiny, as labeled. MDN - mean division number. **(D)** Cohort analysis plot of Mean division number of divided Teff cells over time (cohort method, excluding undivided cells). **(E)** Divided Teff cell number (excluding undivided cells) vs. mean division number of divided cells (cohort method) in the presence and absence of Tregs. The darker horizontal and vertical dashed lines indicate division destiny in the absence of Tregs, the lighter dashed lines indicate the reduction in division destiny at the maximum ratio of Tregs:Teffs (1:1), and the predicted reduction in total live cell number. BrdU incorporation at 63 h as a function of Treg:Teff ratio for the total culture **(F)** and per division basis **(G)** during a 2 h BrdU pulse. Data shown are mean +/– SEM of triplicate samples. One representative data set from three independent experiments is shown.

We propose a "log-dampener" model of Treg suppression as illustrated in **Figure 4**. As shown in (20), contributions of antigen (signal 1), co-stimulation (signal 2) and cytokines (signal 3) to T cell division destiny can be summed linearly to predict the magnitude of the response (**Figure 4A**), thus providing a quantitative basis for classic two- and three-signal theories (34–37). **Figure 4B** shows the effect of Tregs in removing or reducing some of the positive signals (left panel), as well as supplying negative signals (right panel). Examples of reducing positive signals include CTLA4 binding to CD80/86 and inhibition of

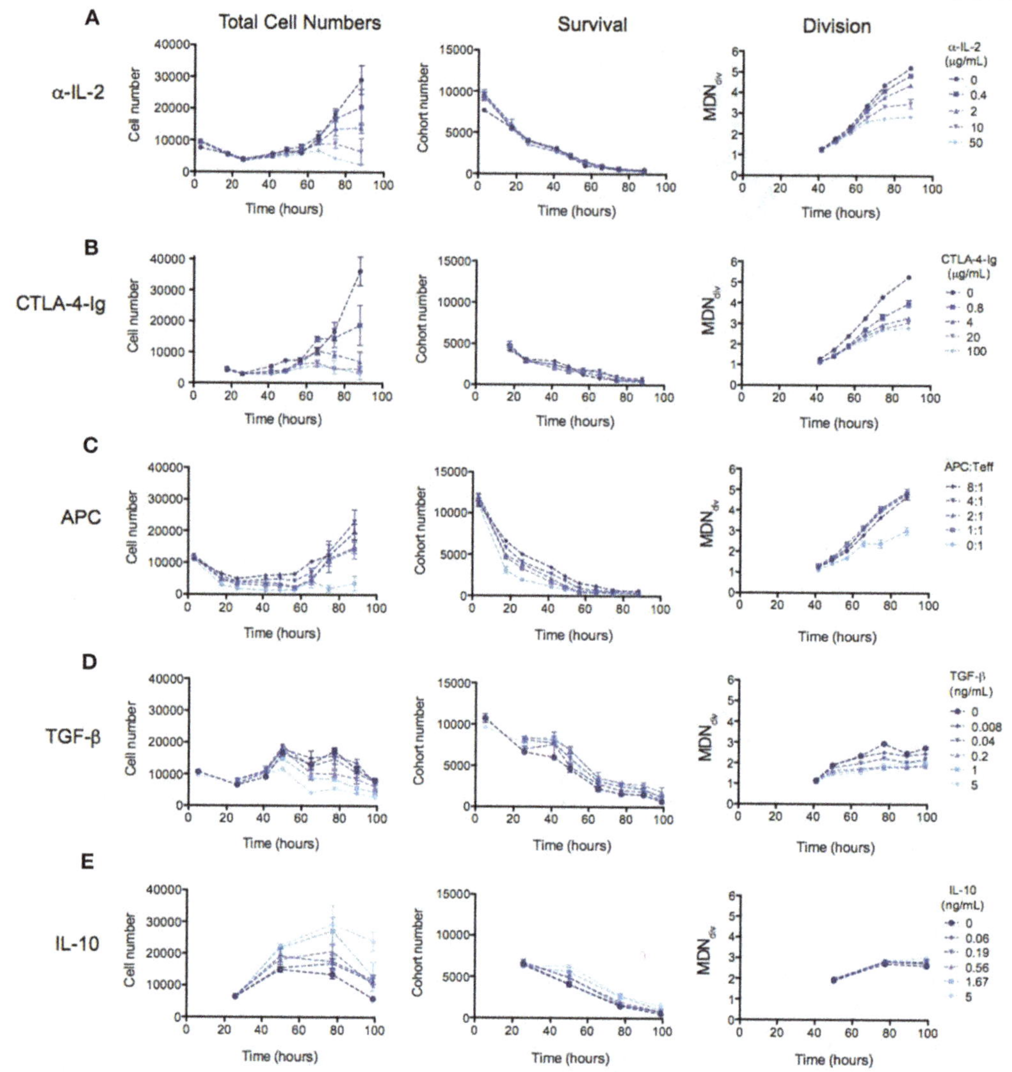


**FIGURE 3 |** The kinetic effects of Treg suppression may be mimicked by some, but not all, known mechanism of Treg action. Teffs were stimulated with irradiated splenocytes (APCs) and anti-CD3. **(A)** Titration of an anti-IL-2 blocking antibody (S4B6)—total cell number (left panel), cohort number (middle panel) and mean division number of divided cells ($MDN_{div}$, right panel). Titration of **(B)** CTLA4-Ig, **(C)** APC number, **(D)** TGF-β and **(E)** Titration of IL-10. Data shown are mean +/− SEM of triplicate samples. One representative data set from two independent experiments is shown.

IL-2 by absorption or decreased production. Tregs also reduce CD80/86 directly on APCs to regulate co-stimulation strength (2, 38–40). Examples of addition of negative signals include TGF-β produced by Tregs acting on effector T cells. We were not able to show a similar mechanism for IL-10 in the *in vitro* system, suggesting a more complex mechanism of action to induce suppression *in vivo*, rather than a direct effect on the proliferation of effector T cells. **Figure 4C** illustrates the effect of removal of positive signals and addition of negative signals by Tregs on effector T cell numbers over time. As changes in division destiny translate to exponential effects on cell numbers, seemingly small perturbations can result in orders of magnitude difference in the peak number of T cells. Multiple pathways may sum independently to achieve suppression, and it is likely that the different pathways vary in their importance in different *in vivo* systems. **Figure 4D** illustrates the log-dampener model in schematic form. Our data highlights the dominant role of reducing division destiny in Treg action under these commonly employed culture conditions. It remains possible that other features might be targeted under different stimulation conditions (for example, antigen-specific T cells and dendritic cells). We anticipate that our assay methods employed here can be adapted and will prove useful to dissect such alternative cell arrangements.

A corollary of this model is that the classic *in vitro* suppression assay (frequently used for studies of Treg function and mechanism), is finely tuned to demonstrate this suppressive effect. The difference in division destiny of dividing Teffs between no Tregs and an equal ratio of Tregs was only slightly more than a single division cycle (**Figure 1**). The classic assay of tritiated thymidine incorporation on day 3 cannot distinguish between

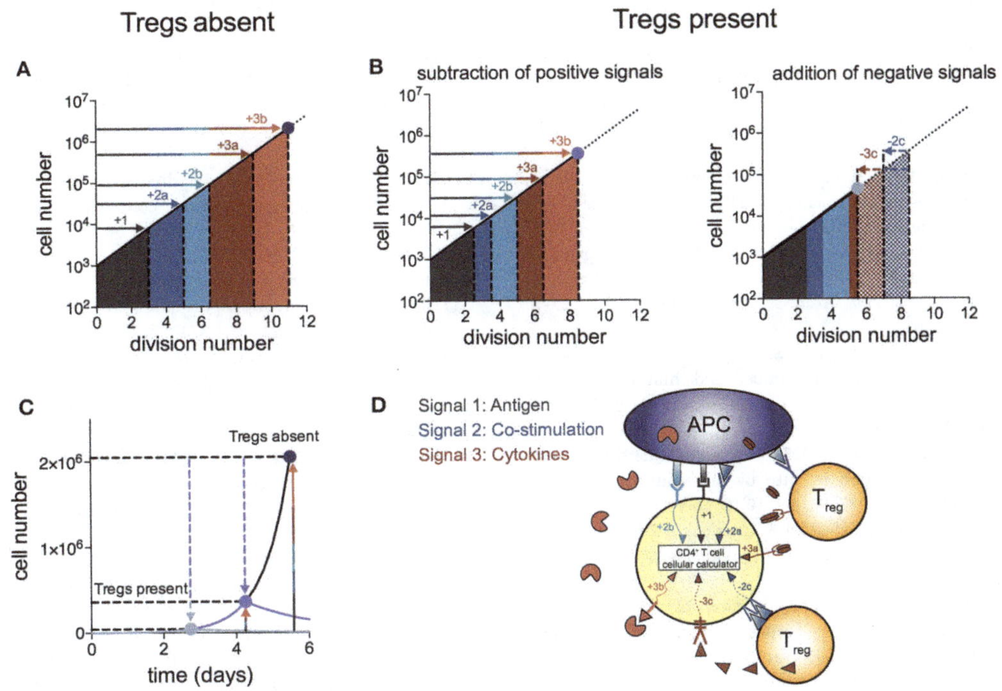

**FIGURE 4 |** Log-dampener model of suppression of CD4$^+$ effector T cell proliferation by Tregs. **(A)** In the absence of Tregs, signals from antigen (signal 1—gray), co-stimulation (signal 2—blue) and cytokines (signal 3—red) sum linearly according to the number of divisions contributed to division destiny by each signal, resulting in an exponential increase in the magnitude of the T cell response (20) (note the log scale on the y-axis). "a" and "b" refer to different types of co-stimulatory and cytokine signals contributing positively to the T cell response. **(B)** Tregs regulate division destiny by reducing positive signals (1, 2a and 3a) and by adding negative signals (2c and 3c). **(C)** Illustration of the effect of Tregs on the size of the effector T cell response (note the linear y-axis). The blue dots represent the peak of the T cell response in the absence of Tregs (dark blue), after subtracting of positive signals (medium blue) and after addition of negative signals (light blue). **(D)** Schematic showing different types of signals being integrated within the CD4$^+$ effector T cell according to the rules of the "cellular calculus".

direct induction of cell death, slowing proliferation rate or reduction in division destiny. Studies of Treg function following genetic manipulation may benefit from using these quantitative methods to study the full kinetics, to assist with drawing conclusions as to the effect of the manipulation on function. Further studies with similar quantitative methods investigating different levels of TCR stimulation/affinity or varied sources of APC may be useful for dissecting whether division destiny is a universal mechanism that is affected by Treg regardless of culture conditions. Our study also indicated the surprising result that at some ratios Tregs enhanced net cell numbers by promoting survival of effector T cells. Two cytokines produced by Treg, TGF-β and IL-10 also promoted survival, potentially explaining this result. Thus, it appears the net outcome of Treg interaction with Teff results from combinations of positive effects on survival and negative influences on division destiny.

In conclusion, our results demonstrate that the complex and multifactorial suppressive effect of Tregs is amenable to study using rigorous quantitative techniques. The many known mechanisms of suppression either remove positive signals or supply negative signals, and combinations act on division destiny according to a simple cellular calculus - addition or subtraction from division destiny. Thus, by reducing division destiny of effector T cells, Tregs act as a "log-dampener" on the magnitude of the Teff response. The net effect is that small changes in division destiny induced by Tregs can have large effects on the peak size of the effector T cell response, with consequences for achieving the balance between protective immunity and tolerance of self.

## AUTHOR CONTRIBUTIONS

MD and EH designed and conducted experiments and wrote the manuscript. SH and JM contributed to data analysis, interpretation, and wrote the manuscript. AK performed mathematical modeling and data analysis. PH designed and supervised experiments and wrote the manuscript.

## FUNDING

MD, PH and EH were supported by National Health and Medical Research Council of Australia (NHMRC) Fellowships. JM was the recipient of an Australian Postgraduate Award, an Edith Moffat Scholarship from The Walter and Eliza Hall Institute and Sydney Parker Smith Postdoctoral Research Fellowship from the Cancer Council of Victoria. This work was supported by the Australian Health and Medical Research Council (program grant 1054925, project grant 105783), Victorian State Government operational infrastructure support and Australian Government NHMRC IRIIS.

## REFERENCES

1. Takahashi T, Tagami T, Yamazaki S, Uede T, Shimizu J, Sakaguchi N, et al. Immunologic self-tolerance maintained by CD25(+)CD4(+) regulatory T cells constitutively expressing cytotoxic T lymphocyte-associated antigen 4. *J Exp Med.* (2000) 192:303–10. doi: 10.1084/jem.192.2.303
2. Wing K, Onishi Y, Prieto-Martin P, Yamaguchi T, Miyara M, Fehervari Z, et al. CTLA-4 control over Foxp3+ regulatory T cell function. *Science* (2008) 322:271–5. doi: 10.1126/science.1160062
3. Onishi Y, Fehervari Z, Yamaguchi T, Sakaguchi S. Foxp3+ natural regulatory T cells preferentially form aggregates on dendritic cells *in vitro* and actively inhibit their maturation. *Proc Natl Acad Sci USA.* (2008) 105:10113–8. doi: 10.1073/pnas.0711106105
4. Wing JB, Ise W, Kurosaki T, Sakaguchi S. Regulatory T cells control antigen-specific expansion of Tfh cell number and humoral immune responses via the coreceptor CTLA-4. *Immunity* (2014) 41:1013–25. doi: 10.1016/j.immuni.2014.12.006
5. Thornton AM, Shevach EM. CD4+CD25+ immunoregulatory T cells suppress polyclonal T cell activation in vitro by inhibiting interleukin 2 production. *J Exp Med.* (1998) 188:287–96. doi: 10.1084/jem.188.2.287
6. de la Rosa M, Rutz S, Dorninger H, Scheffold A. Interleukin-2 is essential for CD4+CD25+ regulatory T cell function. *Eur J Immunol.* (2004) 34:2480–8. doi: 10.1002/eji.200425274
7. D'Cruz LM, Klein L. Development and function of agonist-induced CD25+Foxp3+ regulatory T cells in the absence of interleukin 2 signaling. *Nat Immunol.* (2005) 6:1152–9. doi: 10.1038/ni1264
8. Pandiyan P, Zheng L, Ishihara S, Reed J, Lenardo MJ. CD4+CD25+Foxp3+ regulatory T cells induce cytokine deprivation-mediated apoptosis of effector CD4+ T cells. *Nat Immunol.* (2007) 8:1353–62. doi: 10.1038/ni1536
9. Nakamura K, Kitani A, Strober W. Cell contact-dependent immunosuppression by CD4(+)CD25(+) regulatory T cells is mediated by cell surface-bound transforming growth factor beta. *J Exp Med.* (2001) 194:629–44. doi: 10.1084/jem.194.5.629
10. Green EA, Gorelik L, McGregor CM, Tran EH, Flavell RA. CD4+CD25+ T regulatory cells control anti-islet CD8+ T cells through TGF-beta-TGF-beta receptor interactions in type 1 diabetes. *Proc Natl Acad Sci USA.* (2003) 100:10878–83. doi: 10.1073/pnas.1834400100
11. Collison LW, Workman CJ, Kuo TT, Boyd K, Wang Y, Vignali KM, et al. The inhibitory cytokine IL-35 contributes to regulatory T-cell function. *Nature* (2007) 450:566–9. doi: 10.1038/nature06306
12. Joetham A, Takeda K, Taube C, Miyahara N, Matsubara S, Koya T, et al. Naturally occurring lung CD4(+)CD25(+) T cell regulation of airway allergic responses depends on IL-10 induction of TGF-beta. *J Immunol.* (2007) 178:1433–42. doi: 10.4049/jimmunol.178.3.1433
13. Rubtsov YP, Rasmussen JP, Chi EY, Fontenot J, Castelli L, Ye X, et al. Regulatory T cell-derived interleukin-10 limits inflammation at environmental interfaces. *Immunity* (2008) 28:546–58. doi: 10.1016/j.immuni.2008.02.017
14. Collison LW, Pillai MR, Chaturvedi V, Vignali DA. Regulatory T cell suppression is potentiated by target T cells in a cell contact, IL-35- and IL-10-dependent manner. *J Immunol.* (2009) 182:6121–8. doi: 10.4049/jimmunol.0803646
15. Miyara M, Sakaguchi S. Natural regulatory T cells: mechanisms of suppression. *Trends Mol Med.* (2007) 13:108–16. doi: 10.1016/j.molmed.2007.01.003
16. Vignali DA, Collison LW, Workman CJ. How regulatory T cells work. *Nat Rev Immunol.* (2008) 8:523–32. doi: 10.1038/nri2343
17. Sakaguchi S, Wing K, Onishi Y, Prieto-Martin P, Yamaguchi T. Regulatory T cells: how do they suppress immune responses? *Int Immunol.* (2009) 21:1105–11. doi: 10.1093/intimm/dxp095
18. Miyara M, Sakaguchi S. Human FoxP3(+)CD4(+) regulatory T cells: their knowns and unknowns. *Immunol Cell Biol.* (2011) 89:346–51. doi: 10.1038/icb.2010.137
19. Maeda Y, Nishikawa H, Sugiyama D, Ha D, Hamaguchi M, Saito T, et al. Detection of self-reactive CD8(+) T cells with an anergic phenotype in healthy individuals. *Science* (2014) 346:1536–40. doi: 10.1126/science.aaa1292
20. Marchingo JM, Kan A, Sutherland RM, Duffy KR, Wellard CJ, Belz GT, Lew AM, et al. T cell signaling. Antigen affinity, costimulation, and cytokine inputs sum linearly to amplify T cell expansion. *Science* (2014) 346:1123–27. doi: 10.1126/science.1260044
21. Hawkins ED, Turner ML, Dowling MR, van Gend C, Hodgkin PD. A model of immune regulation as a consequence of randomized lymphocyte division and death times. *Proc Natl Acad Sci USA.* (2007) 104:5032–7. doi: 10.1073/pnas.0700026104
22. Turner ML, Hawkins ED, Hodgkin PD. Quantitative regulation of B cell division destiny by signal strength. *J Immunol.* (2008) 181:374–82. doi: 10.4049/jimmunol.181.1.374
23. Hawkins ED, Markham JF, McGuinness LP, Hodgkin PD. A single-cell pedigree analysis of alternative stochastic lymphocyte fates. *Proc Natl Acad Sci USA.* (2009) 106:13457–62. doi: 10.1073/pnas.0905629106
24. Heinzel S, Binh Giang T, Kan A, Marchingo JM, Lye BK, Corcoran LM, et al. A Myc-dependent division timer complements a cell-death timer to regulate T cell and B cell responses. *Nat Immunol.* (2016) 18:96–103. doi: 10.1038/ni.3598
25. Collison LW, Vignali DA. *In vitro* Treg suppression assays. *Methods Mol Biol.* (2011) 707:21–37. doi: 10.1007/978-1-61737-979-6_2
26. Hawkins ED, Hommel M, Turner ML, Battye FL, Markham JF, Hodgkin PD. Measuring lymphocyte proliferation, survival and differentiation using CFSE time-series data. *Nat Protoc.* (2007) 2:2057–67. doi: 10.1038/nprot.2007.297
27. Hommel M, Hodgkin PD. TCR affinity promotes CD8+ T cell expansion by regulating survival. *J Immunol.* (2007) 179:2250–60. doi: 10.4049/jimmunol.179.4.2250
28. Hawkins ED, Turner ML, Wellard CJ, Zhou JH, Dowling MR, Hodgkin PD. Quantal and graded stimulation of B lymphocytes as alternative strategies for regulating adaptive immune responses. *Nat Commun.* (2013) 4:2406. doi: 10.1038/ncomms3406
29. Gett AV, Hodgkin PD. A cellular calculus for signal integration by T cells. *Nat Immunol.* (2000) 1:239–44. doi: 10.1038/79782
30. Deenick EK, Gett AV, Hodgkin PD. Stochastic model of T cell proliferation: a calculus revealing IL-2 regulation of precursor frequencies, cell cycle time, and survival. *J Immunol.* (2003) 170:4963–72. doi: 10.4049/jimmunol.170.10.4963
31. Rizzitelli A, Hawkins E, Todd H, Hodgkin PD, Shortman K. The proliferative response of CD4 T cells to steady-state CD8+ dendritic cells is restricted by post-activation death. *Int Immunol.* (2006) 18:415–23. doi: 10.1093/intimm/dxh382
32. Waibel M, Christiansen AJ, Hibbs ML, Shortt J, Jones SA, Simpson I, et al. Manipulation of B-cell responses with histone deacetylase inhibitors. *Nat Commun.* (2015) 6:6838. doi: 10.1038/ncomms7838
33. Linsley PS, Wallace PM, Johnson J, Gibson MG, Greene JL, Ledbetter JA, et al. Immunosuppression *in vivo* by a soluble form of the CTLA-4 T cell activation molecule. *Science* (1992) 257:792–5. doi: 10.1126/science.1496399
34. Curtsinger JM, Schmidt CS, Mondino A, Lins DC, Kedl RM, Jenkins MK, et al. Inflammatory cytokines provide a third signal for activation of naive CD4+ and CD8+ T cells. *J Immunol.* (1999) 162:3256–62.
35. Baxter AG, Hodgkin PD. Activation rules: the two-signal theories of immune activation. *Nat Rev Immunol.* (2002) 2:439–46. doi: 10.1038/nri823
36. Bertram EM, Dawicki W, Watts TH. Role of T cell costimulation in anti-viral immunity. *Semin Immunol.* (2004) 16:185–96. doi: 10.1016/j.smim.2004.02.006
37. Zehn D, Lee SY, Bevan MJ. Complete but curtailed T-cell response to very low-affinity antigen. *Nature* (2009) 458:211–4. doi: 10.1038/nature07657

38. Cederbom L, Hall H, Ivars F. CD4+CD25+ regulatory T cells down-regulate co-stimulatory molecules on antigen-presenting cells. *Eur J Immunol.* (2000) 30:1538–43. doi: 10.1002/1521-4141(200006)30:6<1538::AID-IMMU1538>3.0.CO;2-X

39. Hou TZ, Qureshi OS, Wang CJ, Baker J, Young SP, Walker LS, et al. A transendocytosis model of CTLA-4 function predicts its suppressive behavior on regulatory T cells. *J Immunol.* (2015) 194:2148–59. doi: 10.4049/jimmunol.1401876

40. Misra N, Bayry J, Lacroix-Desmazes S, Kazatchkine MD, Kaveri SV. Cutting edge: human CD4+CD25+ T cells restrain the maturation and antigen-presenting function of dendritic cells. *J Immunol.* (2004) 172:4676–80. doi: 10.4049/jimmunol.172.8.4676

14

# The Changing Landscape of Naive T Cell Receptor Repertoire with Human Aging

*Evgeny S. Egorov[1†], Sofya A. Kasatskaya[1,2†], Vasiliy N. Zubov[1], Mark Izraelson[1], Tatiana O. Nakonechnaya[1], Dmitriy B. Staroverov[1], Andrea Angius[3], Francesco Cucca[3], Ilgar Z. Mamedov[1], Elisa Rosati[4], Andre Franke[4], Mikhail Shugay[1,2], Mikhail V. Pogorelyy[1], Dmitriy M. Chudakov[1,2]* and Olga V. Britanova[1]*

[1] Shemyakin and Ovchinnikov Institute of Bioorganic Chemistry, Moscow, Russia, [2] Center of Life Sciences, Skolkovo Institute of Science and Technology, Moscow, Russia, [3] Istituto di Ricerca Genetica e Biomedica, Consiglio Nazionale delle Ricerche, Monserrato, Italy, [4] Institute of Clinical Molecular Biology, Kiel University, Kiel, Germany

***Correspondence:**
Dmitriy M. Chudakov
chudakovdm@mail.ru

† These authors have contributed equally to this work.

Human aging is associated with a profound loss of thymus productivity, yet naïve T lymphocytes still maintain their numbers by division in the periphery for many years. The extent of such proliferation may depend on the cytokine environment, including IL-7 and T-cell receptor (TCR) "tonic" signaling mediated by self pMHCs recognition. Additionally, intrinsic properties of distinct subpopulations of naïve T cells could influence the overall dynamics of aging-related changes within the naïve T cell compartment. Here, we investigated the differences in the architecture of TCR beta repertoires for naïve CD4, naïve CD8, naïve $CD4^+CD25^-CD31^+$ (enriched with recent thymic emigrants, RTE), and mature naïve $CD4^+CD25^-CD31^-$ peripheral blood subsets between young and middle-age/old healthy individuals. In addition to observing the accumulation of clonal expansions (as was shown previously), we reveal several notable changes in the characteristics of T cell repertoire. We observed significant decrease of CDR3 length, NDN insert, and number of non-template added N nucleotides within TCR beta CDR3 with aging, together with a prominent change of physicochemical properties of the central part of CDR3 loop. These changes were similar across CD4, CD8, RTE-enriched, and mature CD4 subsets of naïve T cells, with minimal or no difference observed between the latter two subsets for individuals of the same age group. We also observed an increase in "publicity" (fraction of shared clonotypes) of CD4, but not CD8 naïve T cell repertoires. We propose several explanations for these phenomena built upon previous studies of naïve T-cell homeostasis, and call for further studies of the mechanisms causing the observed changes and of consequences of these changes in respect of the possible holes formed in the landscape of naïve T cell TCR repertoire.

**Keywords: aging, T cell receptor, naive T cells, immunosequencing, Rep-Seq, CDR3 repertoire**

## INTRODUCTION

A diverse set of naïve T cell functions (1) and their antigenic receptors—T-cell receptors (TCRs) (2, 3)—protects us from a multitude of infectious and cancer hazards encountered throughout our lifespan. Furthermore, it essentially provides selection of the appropriate amplitude, type, localization, and duration of immune response. Human aging is associated with profound changes in T cell immunity (2–5), compromising our ability to withstand novel pathogens and manage chronic infections. It also dampens the effect of vaccination (6–8) and can lead to higher cancer susceptibility (9–12). These changes may further result in an imbalanced immune response that can develop into non-specific inflammation, provoking neurodegenerative and cardiovascular disorders, and to the loss of tolerance, leading to autoimmunity (3, 13–15). For the latter, a reduction of regulatory T cell (Treg) diversity (16, 17) could be a one of the causative factors.

With aging, accumulating clonal expansions of memory T cells caused by previously encountered antigens gradually begin to dominate in the available T-cell pool. This leads to a homeostasis characterized by a decreased number of naïve T cells, essentially shrinking the precious reservoir of diverse functions and antigenic specificities (2, 18–23). At the same time, thymus function progressively declines after puberty (24, 25), and drops sharply to a very low level after 40 years of age (4, 26). Along with diminished production of T cell progenitors by the bone marrow (27), this leads to a drop in generation of the so-called recent thymic emigrants (RTE)—the not fully mature (28, 29) form of naïve T cells, and thus in the replenishment of the mature naïve T cell pool (5, 26, 30).

The existing naïve T cells may still support their abundance and diversity for a prolonged period. In humans, both mature naïve T cells and—to a lesser extent—RTE-enriched $CD45RA^+CD31^+$ subset of CD4 T cells (30)—keep ability to proliferate on the periphery (31, 32). However, the number of allowed divisions is not unlimited. Prominent shortening of telomeres is observed in both CD31+ and $CD31^-$ subsets (30) which eventually leads to a gradual, later avalanche, exhaustion of proliferation capacity and depletion of the naïve T cell pool (20, 33). Additionally, prolonged peripheral proliferation could also be associated with the functional deficiency of naïve T cells that fail to differentiate toward memory phenotype upon a specific antigenic challenge (3), although a recent cytokine profile study suggests that naïve T cells derived from elderly individuals retain their functionality and naiveté (26).

How uniform is the naïve T cell proliferation on the periphery remains questionable. Qi et al. demonstrated that both CD4 and CD8 naïve T cells gated as $CCR7^+CD45RA^{high}CD28^+$ gain clonal expansions by the age of 70–85 years (34). This observation suggests that some of the naïve T cell clones are dividing more prominently than others. Furthermore, the most rapidly dividing ones could exhaust and extinguish more rapidly, while those dividing with a moderate rate could form the observed clonal expansions.

Importantly, the peripheral T cell proliferation may be dependent on the so-called "tonic signaling"—recognition of MHC complexes loaded with self antigens while surveying the peripheral lymphoid organs. Such contacts are transient and do not lead to classic T cell activation, but generate sub-threshold signals required for naïve T cell survival and proliferation (35–38).

The desirable (i.e., required to efficiently recognize foreign antigens within MHC) and allowed (i.e., not leading to self-recognition and autoimmunity) TCR affinity to self peptide–MHC complexes is set in the course of positive and negative thymic selection, respectively. The threshold range of such selection is not that narrow, thus naïve T cells that leave the thymus—initially as RTE—have a relatively wide range of self-reactivity. The produced pool of naïve T cells is, therefore, subjected to varying degrees of tonic TCR signaling (38). Therefore, peripheral proliferation of naïve T cells could be potentially biased toward preferential exhaustion of naïve T cell clones carrying TCRs with the highest affinity to MHC. Furthermore, naïve T cells bearing high affinity TCRs could also serve as a preferential source of antigen-responding clones (37) thus being the first one to transit from the naïve T cell pool.

Another factor that could contribute to the dynamics of naïve TCR repertoire landscape is the fate of the specific population of T cells produced in fetal period. We have earlier demonstrated that this subset may survive for decades and contribute to adult TCR repertoire (39). Their TCRs are characterized by a low number of nucleotides that are randomly added by TdT enzyme in the course of VDJ recombination (40, 41). Furthermore, these cells originate from a distinct population of hematopoietic stem cells and are characterized with generally higher proliferation potential (42). However, their fate among other naïve T cells in the elder age remains unexplored.

Altogether, there are number of factors that could shape the landscape of naïve T cell TCR repertoire with aging. To shed light on the nature of ongoing changes, we have focused on the comparative analysis of intrinsic characteristics of the TCR repertoires for the bulk naïve $CD8^+$, bulk naïve $CD4^+$, naïve RTE-enriched $CD31^+CD4^+$, and naïve non-RTE $CD4^+$ T cells derived from the peripheral blood of young versus elderly healthy donors, demonstrating that

1) Characteristics of TCR beta CDR3 repertoires change in both CD4 and CD8, both RTE-enriched and mature naïve CD4 T cell subsets with age.
2) Within the same age group, no significant difference is observed in characteristics of TCR repertoire between RTE-enriched and mature naïve CD4 T cell subsets.
3) TRBV and TRBJ gene segment usage also changes prominently and similarly both within RTE-enriched and mature naïve CD4 T cell subsets of different individuals.
4) Relative "publicity" (i.e., sharing between individuals) of TCR repertoires grows both within RTE-enriched and mature naïve CD4 T cell subsets with age.

The observed changes suggest functional differences of young versus middle-age/old naïve T cell TCR repertoires with respect of potential range and characteristics of recognized antigens.

## MATERIALS AND METHODS

### Donors and Cell Sorting

The study was approved by the local ethics committee and conducted in accordance with the Declaration of Helsinki. All donors were informed of the final use of their blood and signed an informed consent document. The cohort included 18 healthy individuals aged 25–88 years. Individuals with previously diagnosed cancer or autoimmune disease were excluded. Peripheral blood (10–20 ml) was collected into a number of EDTA-treated Vacutainer tubes (BD Biosciences, Franklin Lakes,

NJ, USA), PBMCs extracted using Ficoll-Paque (Paneco, Kirov, Russia) density gradient centrifugation with SepMate™ tubes (STEMCELL Technologies, Vancouver, BC, Canada), and stained according to manufacturer's recommendations. Following antibodies were used: CD3-eFluor450 (eBioscience, clone UCHT1), CD45RA-FITC (eBioscience, clone JS-83), CD27-PC5 (Beckman Coulter, clone O323), CD4-PE (Beckman Coulter, clone 13B8.2), CD25-eFluor450 (eBiosciences, clone BC96), and CD31-PC7 (eBiosciences, clone WM59). T cells of interest were sorted using FACS Aria III (BD Biosciences, Franklin Lakes, NJ, USA), directly in 350 μl of RLT buffer (Qiagen) per 100,000 sorted cells. Total RNA was further isolated using RNeasy Micro kit (Qiagen) and completely used for TCR library preparation. 5′-RACE TCR beta cDNA libraries were prepared according to the previously described protocol (43, 44). See also: https://github.com/repseqio/protocols/blob/master/Human%20TCR%20alpha%20and%20beta%20RNA-based%20RACE%20protocol.md.

Libraries were sequenced with Illumina HiSeq 2000/2500, paired-end 150 + 150 nucleotides.

## TCR Beta Repertoires Profiling and Data Analysis

T-cell receptor beta CDR3 repertoires were extracted using MiXCR software (45), version v2.1.5. Decontamination from memory T cell TCR beta clonotypes and comparative post-analysis were performed using VDJtools software v1.1.7 (46).

Resulting decontaminated TCR beta CDR3 repertoires are available from Figshare:

https://figshare.com/articles/Naive_CD4_CD8_subsets/6548921; https://figshare.com/articles/naive_RTE_and_non-RTE_CD4_T_cells_subsets/6549059.

The obtained repertoires were further filtered to eliminate out-of-frame and stop codon-containing TCR beta CDR3 variants. Averaged physicochemical properties of amino acid residues in the middle portion (5 amino acid residues) of TCR beta CDR3 were calculated using VDJtools, the following metrics were used: strength (47, 48), hydropathy, polarity, and volume (values available from: http://www.imgt.org/IMGTeducation/Aide-memoire/_UK/aminoacids/IMGTclasses.html). During calculation, property values were weighted by the frequency of corresponding clonotypes, so the results favor more frequent clonotypes and do not depend on the sequencing/sampling depth (49). See **Table 1** for the values used for each amino acid property. See **Tables 2** and **3** for the counts of sorted T cells, the number of CDR3 containing sequencing reads, and the number of unique TCR beta CDR3 clonotypes in each sample.

## Statistical Analysis

For comparison of repertoire properties, one-sided *t*-test with unequal variances (Welch's test) was used. Normality of the distribution of sample means was confirmed by performing Shapiro–Wilk tests, and the decision to reject the null hypothesis was made after adjusting for multiple hypothesis testing as in Benjamini–Hochberg. False discovery rate in normality testing was controlled at a level of 0.05 by setting *p*-adjusted upper bound at 0.05. *Z*-score normalization was performed by subtracting the mean value for each TRBV gene segment values and dividing by the SD. Only highly represented TRBV gene segments TRBV9, TRBV7–9, TRBV7–2, TRBV6–5, TRBV29–1, TRBV20–1, and TRBV12–3/12-4, each associated with at least 2% of CDR3 clonotypes in each sample, were taken into analysis.

**TABLE 1** | Values used for CDR3 amino acid properties calculation by VDJtools.

| Amino acid | Hydropathy | Polarity | Volume | Strength |
|---|---|---|---|---|
| A | 1.8 | 0 | 67 | 0 |
| C | 2.5 | 0 | 86 | 1 |
| D | −3.5 | 1 | 91 | 0 |
| E | −3.5 | 1 | 109 | 0 |
| F | 2.8 | 0 | 135 | 1 |
| G | −0.4 | 0 | 48 | 0 |
| H | −3.2 | 1 | 118 | 0 |
| I | 4.5 | 0 | 124 | 1 |
| K | −3.9 | 1 | 135 | 0 |
| L | 3.8 | 0 | 124 | 1 |
| M | 1.9 | 0 | 124 | 1 |
| N | −3.5 | 1 | 96 | 0 |
| P | −1.6 | 0 | 90 | 0 |
| Q | −3.5 | 1 | 114 | 0 |
| R | −4.5 | 1 | 148 | 0 |
| S | −0.8 | 1 | 73 | 0 |
| T | −0.7 | 1 | 93 | 0 |
| V | 4.2 | 0 | 105 | 1 |
| W | −0.9 | 0 | 163 | 1 |
| Y | −1.3 | 1 | 141 | 1 |

# RESULTS

## TCR Repertoires of Both CD4 and CD8 Naïve T Cells Change Properties With Aging

To analyze how the properties of naïve TCR repertoire change with age, we first sorted $CD3^{+}CD4^{+}CD27^{high}CD45RA^{high}$ and $CD3^{+}CD4^{-}CD27^{high}CD45RA^{high}$ T cell subsets gated as shown on **Figure 1** from peripheral blood samples of 4 young (25–35 years old) and 7 middle-age/old (51–88 years old) healthy donors (**Table 2**). TCR beta profiling was performed as described in Ref. (43), extraction of CDR3 repertoires was performed using MiXCR (45). To exclude possible contaminations from memory T cell pool that could occur during cell sorting, we also performed TCR beta repertoires profiling for memory T cells sorted from the same donors (**Figure 1**). Naïve TCR beta repertoires were further decontaminated from the clonotypes present in memory subsets using VDJtools "`Decontaminate`" module with default parameters (20:1 parent-to-child clonotype frequency ratio for contamination filtering). This procedure eliminated from 0.005 to 0.5% of reads and from 0.01 to 0.7% of clonotypes, these numbers did not depend on the donor age group. Despite the low proportion of eliminated reads and clonotypes, such procedure is desirable for accuracy of the whole analysis and general control for cell contamination during sorting.

We complemented our data with multiplex PCR RNA-based TCR profiling data from Ref. (34) for 4 young (20–35 years) and 5 old (70–85 years) healthy donors naïve T cells gated as $CD4^{+}$

**TABLE 2** | CD4 and CD8 naïve and memory cell sorting.

| Donor | Age | Group | Subset | Replica | Number of sorted cells | Number of CDR3 reads | Number of CDR3 clonotypes |
|---|---|---|---|---|---|---|---|
| Donor 1 | 25 | Young | CD4 | 1 | 500,000 | 528,824 | 38,614 |
| | | | | 2 | 500,000 | 475,392 | 240,80 |
| | | | CD8 | 1 | 500,000 | 564,227 | 26,988 |
| | | | | 2 | 500,000 | 648,821 | 19,338 |
| Donor 2 | 26 | | CD4 | 1 | 135,000 | 1,069,588 | 45,098 |
| | | | CD8 | 1 | 251,000 | 633,854 | 28,967 |
| Donor 3 | 35 | | CD4 | 1 | 200,500 | 380,253 | 43,526 |
| | | | | 2 | 231,000 | 223,661 | 23,038 |
| | | | CD8 | 1 | 350,500 | 533,091 | 47,626 |
| Donor 4 | 32 | | CD4 | 1 | 560,000 | 17,494,455 | 165,184 |
| | | | | 2 | 488,000 | 12,525,047 | 113,333 |
| | | | | 3 | 395,000 | 6,077,772 | 54,546 |
| | | | | 4 | 100,000 | 4,353,149 | 24,582 |
| | | | CD8 | 1 | 510,000 | 9,219,066 | 101,096 |
| | | | | 2 | 316,000 | 10,594,890 | 61,022 |
| Donor 5 | 51 | Old | CD4 | 1 | 495,000 | 13,765,788 | 183,873 |
| | | | | 2 | 425,000 | 5,146,822 | 64,134 |
| | | | | 3 | 437,000 | 3,832,144 | 84,458 |
| | | | | 4 | 255,000 | 4,773,131 | 90,459 |
| | | | CD8 | 1 | 509,000 | 7,369,930 | 125,339 |
| | | | | 2 | 200,000 | 2,689,594 | 64,907 |
| | | | | 3 | 343,000 | 517,265 | 20,870 |
| | | | | 4 | 120,000 | 1,945,472 | 32,259 |
| Donor 6 | 88 | | CD4 | 1 | 500,000 | 779,559 | 65,515 |
| | | | CD8 | 1 | 60,000 | 142,639 | 9,991 |
| Donor 7 | 51 | | CD4 | 1 | 100,000 | 28,129 | 5,033 |
| | | | | 2 | 100,000 | 37,556 | 5,455 |
| | | | | 3 | 100,000 | 41,380 | 6,762 |
| | | | CD8 | 1 | 105,000 | 51,463 | 7,434 |
| Donor 8 | 82 | | CD4 | 1 | 100,000 | 46,472 | 8,318 |
| | | | | 2 | 90,000 | 38,109 | 6,694 |
| | | | CD8 | 1 | 12,000 | 6,013 | 846 |
| Donor 9 | 55 | | CD4 | 1 | 100,000 | 82,691 | 7,768 |
| | | | | 2 | 100,000 | 27,215 | 4,740 |
| | | | CD8 | 1 | 100,000 | 51,742 | 5,290 |
| | | | | 2 | 100,000 | 84,532 | 7,666 |
| Donor 10 | 77 | | CD4 | 1 | 254,000 | 677,587 | 24,652 |
| | | | CD4 | 2 | 227,000 | 963,394 | 20,087 |
| | | | CD8 | 1 | 50,000 | 942,430 | 15,033 |
| | | | CD8 | 2 | 105,000 | 553,867 | 19,180 |
| Donor 11 | 53 | | CD4 | 1 | 153,000 | 401,550 | 11,668 |
| | 53 | | CD8 | 1 | 101,000 | 242,248 | 6,857 |

*Donors, replicas, sorted cell counts, and number of extracted T-cell receptor beta CDR3 clonotypes are shown.*

$CCR7^+CD45RA^{high}CD28^+$ and $CD8^+CCR7^+CD45RA^{high}CD28^+$. Repertoire extraction was performed using the same MiXCR version starting from raw data (dbGaP, www.ncbi.nlm.nih.gov/gap, accession no. phs000787.v1.p1). Similarly, we used memory subsets from the same donors in order to decontaminate naïve T cell repertoires from possible contaminations during cell sorting using VDJtools.

Analysis of the normalized Shannon–Wiener diversity index for the joint data confirmed the conclusion by Qi and coauthors that both CD4 and CD8 naïve T cells accumulate clonal expansion with aging (**Figure 2A**). The accuracy of the results for young individuals generally confirmed the validity of combining the data from both experiments, in spite of the fact that different gating was used for the naïve T cell sorting in the two studies.

Multiplex PCR employed in Qi et al. (34) may cause quantitative biases due to the differing efficiency of primers used to amplify different TRBV segments (50, 51). However, such source of bias does not influence the relative frequency of

**TABLE 3** | Recent thymic emigrants (RTEs)-enriched and mature naïve CD4 T cell sorting.

| Donor | Age | Group | Subset | Replica | Number of sorted cells | Number of CDR3 reads | Number of CDR3 clonotypes |
|---|---|---|---|---|---|---|---|
| Donor 12 | 29 | Young | RTE | 1 | 50,000 | 251,199 | 27,208 |
| | | | non-RTE | 1 | 50,000 | 939,999 | 33,389 |
| Donor 13 | 28 | | RTE | 1 | 100,000 | 282,998 | 27,895 |
| | | | non-RTE | 1 | 100,000 | 620,320 | 34,092 |
| Donor 14 | 31 | | RTE | 1 | 50,000 | 144,571 | 30,139 |
| | | | non-RTE | 1 | 50,000 | 622,585 | 29,253 |
| Donor 15 | 30 | | RTE | 1 | 69,000 | 309,070 | 33,233 |
| | | | non-RTE | 1 | 100,000 | 2,844,397 | 63,900 |
| Donor 7 | 51 | Old | RTE | 1 | 100,000 | 14,572 | 5,306 |
| | | | non-RTE | 1 | 105,000 | 17,926 | 4,030 |
| Donor 8 | 82 | | RTE | 1 | 38,000 | 16,033 | 2,835 |
| | | | non-RTE | 1 | 100,000 | 29,970 | 6,244 |
| Donor 9 | 55 | | RTE | 1 | 89,000 | 19,622 | 3,664 |
| | | | non-RTE | 1 | 189,000 | 20,891 | 5,290 |

*Donors, replicas, sorted cell counts, and number of extracted T-cell receptor beta CDR3 clonotypes are shown.*

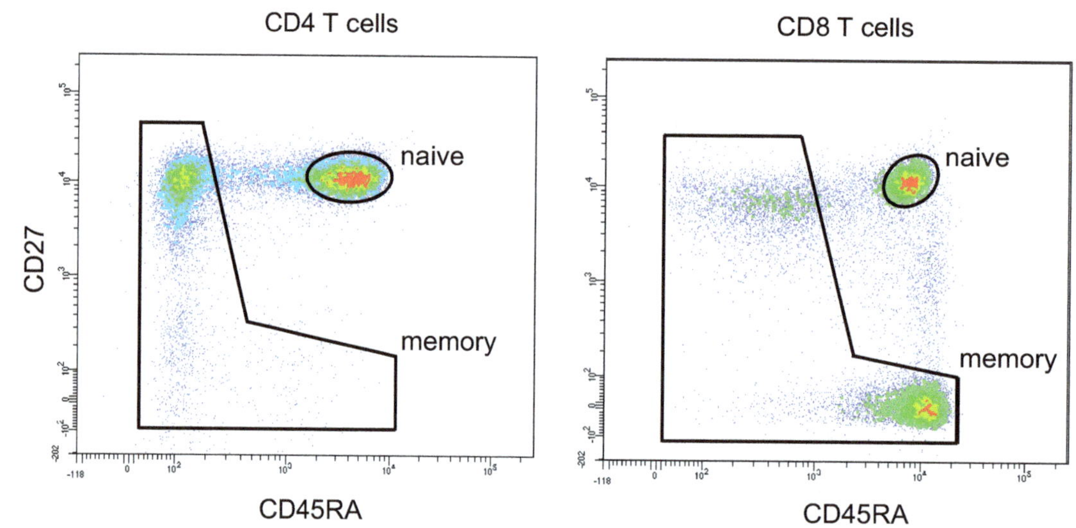


**FIGURE 1** | CD4 and CD8 naïve T cell gating strategy. Naïve CD4 T cells were gated as $CD3^+CD4^+CD27^{high}CD45RA^{high}$. Naïve CD8 T cells were gated as $CD3^+CD4^-CD27^{high}CD45RA^{high}$. 50,000 events were shown.

clonotypes within a particular TRBV segment. Therefore, in order to properly join our 5′RACE and multiplex PCR data from Qi et al., we performed further analysis separately for each of the TRBV gene segments that were abundantly represented in the data.

Notably, this approach has two additional benefits. First, different TRBV genes carry distinct CDR1 and CDR2 regions that participate in TCR–pMHC interaction, and, therefore, could differently influence the averaged properties of CDR3 that we analyze below. Separate analysis of TRBV segments allows to neutralize this bias. Second, distinct TRBV genes correspond to distinct T cell subpopulations allowing for independent evaluation of their properties, that provides better statistics for limited donor cohorts. All analyses were performed "weighted"—per CDR3-covering sequencing read, i.e., accounting for the relative frequency of each clonotype, with *Z*-score normalization used to combine information from different TRBV segments.

The results of comparative analysis of TRB CDR3 repertoire properties with VDJtools software are shown on **Figure 3**. Notably, dispersion of all parameters grows prominently with age, which already reflects the non-uniform proliferation of naïve T cells with age.

CDR3 length, size of NDN insert, and number of randomly added N nucleotides significantly decrease with age both for CD4 and CD8 naïve T cells (**Figure 3A**). Average characteristics of amino acid residues in the middle of CDR3 also change prominently for CD4 naïve T cells (**Figure 3B**).

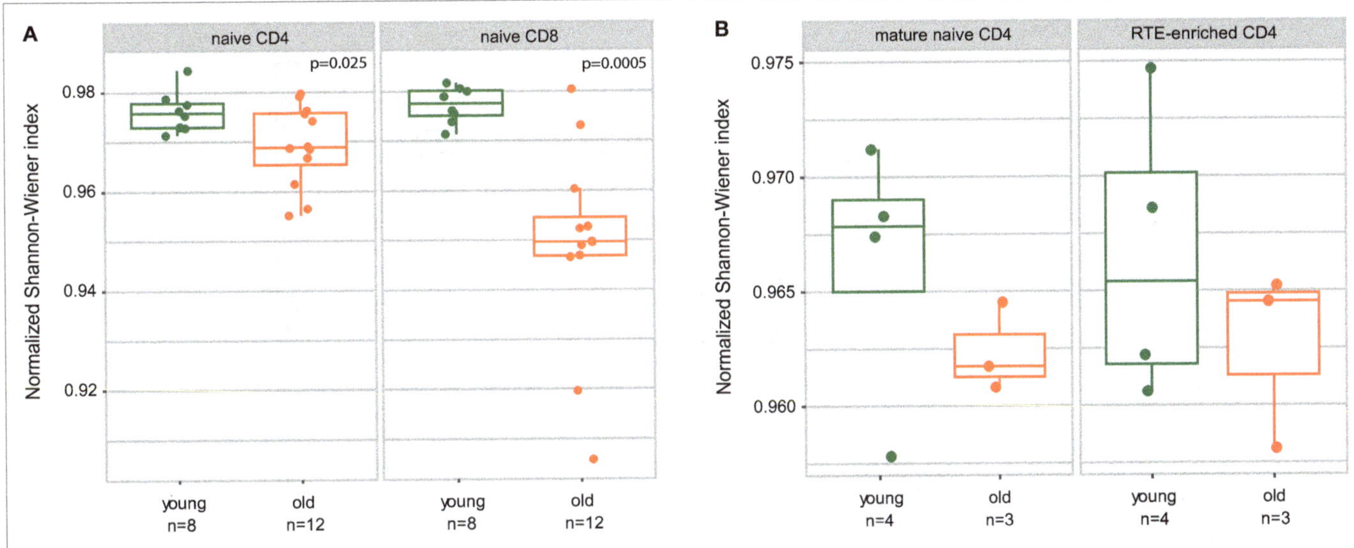


**FIGURE 2** | Both CD4 and CD8 naïve T cell clonality increases with human age. Normalized Shannon–Wiener diversity index for T-cell receptor beta CDR3 repertoires is shown. **(A)** CD4 and CD8 naïve T cells. Joint data from Qi and coauthors and current work. Welch Two Sample *t*-test. **(B)** Recent thymic emigrant (RTE)-enriched and non-RTE naïve CD4 T cells.

## Both RTE and Mature Naïve CD4 T Cells Change Their Properties With Aging

To some extent, both $CD45RA^+CD31^-$ mature naïve $CD4^+$ T cells and RTE-enriched $CD45RA^+CD31^+$ subsets may support their counts by peripheral division: "*CD45RA+CD31+CD4+ subset also undergoes some in vivo proliferation without immediate loss of CD31, resulting in an accumulation of CD45RA+CD31+ proliferative offspring*" (30). Nevertheless, counts of $CD45RA^+CD31^+$ naïve $CD4^+$ T cell notably decrease with time (5, 30). The $CD31^-$ subset is believed to proliferate and support their counts more efficiently than CD31+, although the extent of telomere shortening with aging is prominent and comparable for both subsets (30).

Therefore, one could suggest that characteristics of mature naïve $CD4^+CD31^-$ T cells could change more prominently than those of RTE-enriched $CD4^+CD31^+$ T cell pool. The properties of total naïve $CD4^+$ T cells could change with aging because of the intrinsic differences between the properties of RTE-enriched and mature naïve CD4 T cell TCR repertoires, and decrease of $CD31^+$ cell proportion of all naïve CD4 T cells (5).

To verify the latter hypothesis, we compared TCR beta repertoire characteristics for the sorted $CD4^+CD45RA^{high}CD27^{high}CD31^+$ and $CD4^+CD45RA^{high}CD27^{high}CD31^-$ T cells of 4 young (29–31 years) and 3 elder (aged 51, 55, and 82 years) healthy donors (**Table 3**). Importantly, to exclude the potential influence of naïve Tregs which characteristics essentially differ from conventional CD4 T cells, here we gated out the $CD25^+$ cells from all subsets (**Figure 4**). It should be noted that this strict gating could also cutoff the $CD25^{dull}$ subset of naïve CD4 T cells that was recently reported to accumulate with aging (52), however, these cells were nearly absent (represented less than 2% of naïve CD4 T cells) in our donors.

Analysis of obtained TCR beta CDR3 repertoires revealed that characteristics of $CD4^+CD45RA^{high}CD27^{high}CD25^-CD31^+$ and $CD4^+CD45RA^{high}CD27^{high}CD25^-CD31^-CD4$ T cell TCR repertoires are nearly identical within the same age group, but both prominently differ between the younger and elder donors (**Figures 5A,B**). It should be noted that, since the average CDR3 length decreases with age, larger portions of TRBV and TRBJ segments could be covered by our analysis of the middle 5 amino acid residues of CDR3, which could in turn influence the result amino acid property averages. However, this influence was not prominent since different TRBV segments behaved similarly in our analysis.

Furthermore, young and old naïve CD4 T cell repertoires were characterized by distinct frequencies of TRBV (**Figure 6A**), TRBJ (**Figure 6B**), and paired TRBV–TRBJ (**Figure 6C**) gene segment usage, without any notable differences observed between the RTE-enriched $CD31^+$ and mature naïve CD4 T cell subsets.

Similarly to naïve CD4 and CD8 subsets, RTE-enriched and mature naïve CD4 subsets showed a tendency toward increased clonality in the elder age (**Figure 2B**).

We concluded that observed changes in the characteristics of naïve CD4 T cell TCR beta CDR3 repertoire with aging affect both RTE-enriched and mature subsets, and do not result from the changes in $CD31^+/CD31^-$ subsets ratio.

## Publicity of Naïve CD4 T Cell Repertoire Grows With Aging

Shorter CDR3 length and lower number of randomly added N nucleotides are commonly associated with higher publicity of TCR repertoires (53, 54). To analyze how the relative publicity of naïve CD4 TCR beta repertoires changes with aging, we extracted top-3,000 clonotypes from each dataset, with random sampling of clonotypes having the identical low frequency—a normalization step which is highly desirable to minimize biases in comparison of immune repertoires overlaps. As it could be expected based on

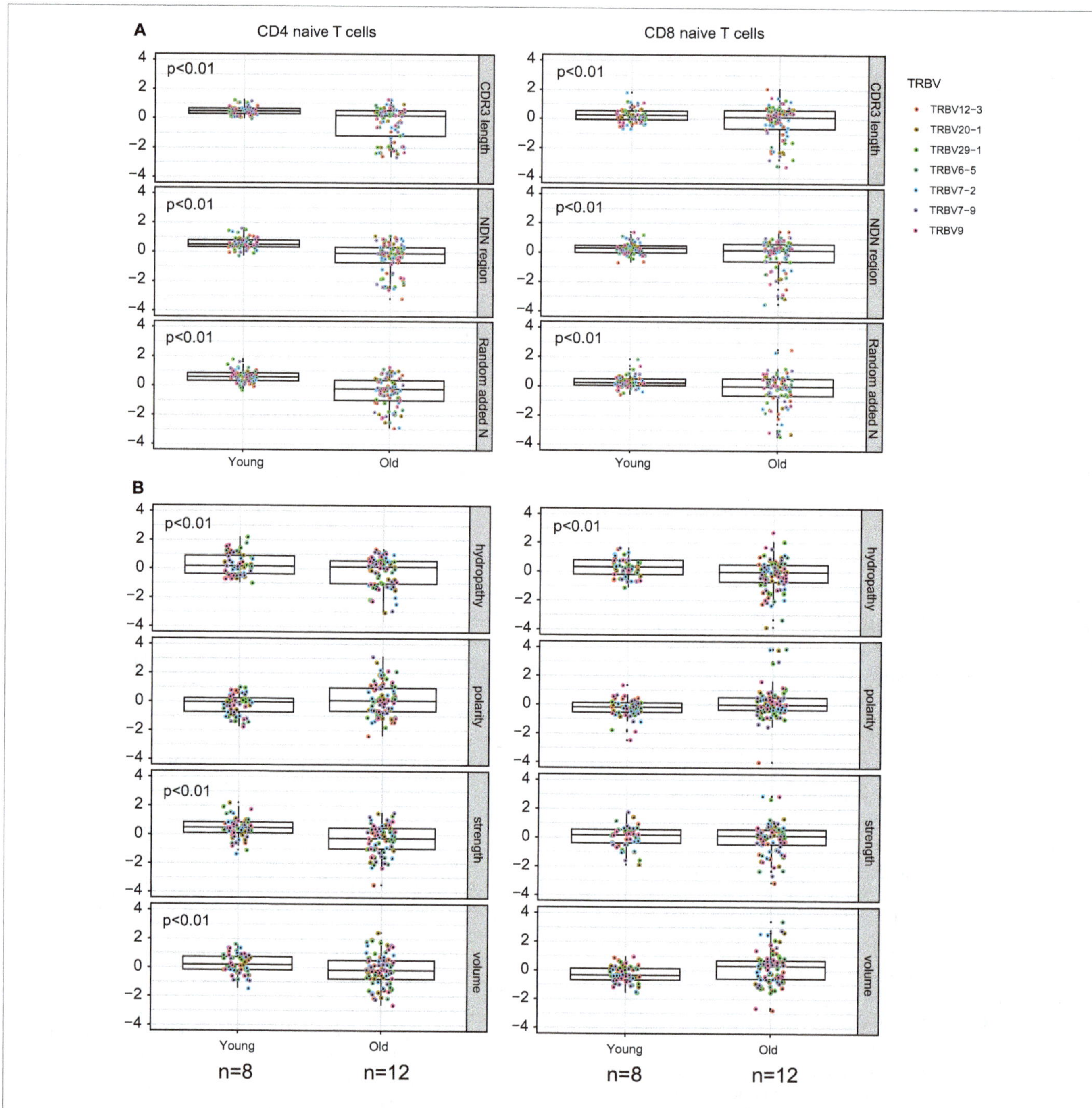


**FIGURE 3** | Properties of naïve T cell T-cell receptor (TCR) beta CDR3 repertoires and aging. Weighted (accounting for clonotype size) analysis of TCR beta repertoires properties for CD4 and CD8 naïve T cells derived from peripheral blood samples of young and old healthy donors. **(A)** Average CDR3 length, size of NDN insert, and count of randomly added N nucleotides. **(B)** Amino acid composition within 5 amino acid residues in the middle of CDR3. Our data and Qi et al. data, $n = 8$ young and 12 old individuals totally. CDR3 repertoires for the seven largest TRBV segments were analyzed separately, with $Z$-score normalization to account for TRBV-specific differences.

CDR3 characteristics (**Figures 5A** and **7A**), analysis of relative overlaps between TCR beta CDR3 repertoires revealed that relative publicity of total CD4 naïve [our data only, excluding the data from Ref. (34)], RTE-enriched CD31$^+$ and mature naïve CD31$^-$ CD4 T cell subsets grows with aging (**Figure 7B**). A moderate overlap was observed between the young and middle-age/old CD4 naïve, RTE-enriched CD31$^+$ and mature naïve CD31$^-$ CD4 T cell subsets. No clear age-related changes in relative publicity were observed for CD8 naïve T cells (our data only).

We used CDR3 sequence similarity graph to analyze whether naïve TCR repertoires form separate networks in young versus old donors. To build the graph, we selected 3,000 most abundant

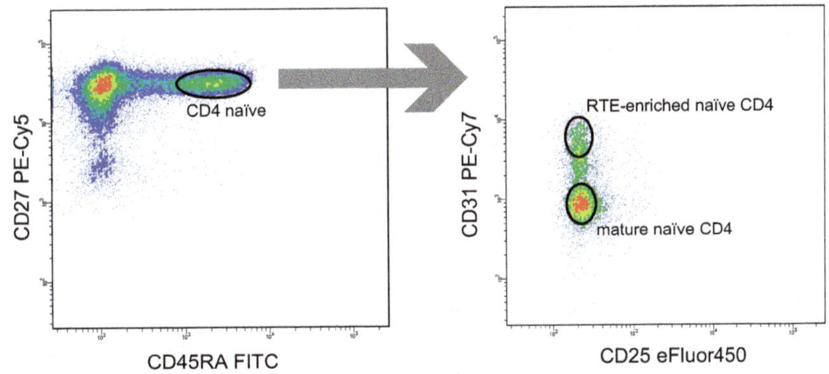


**FIGURE 4** | Recent thymic emigrant (RTE)-enriched and non-RTE naïve CD4 T cell gating strategy. 50,000 events were shown on the left panel.

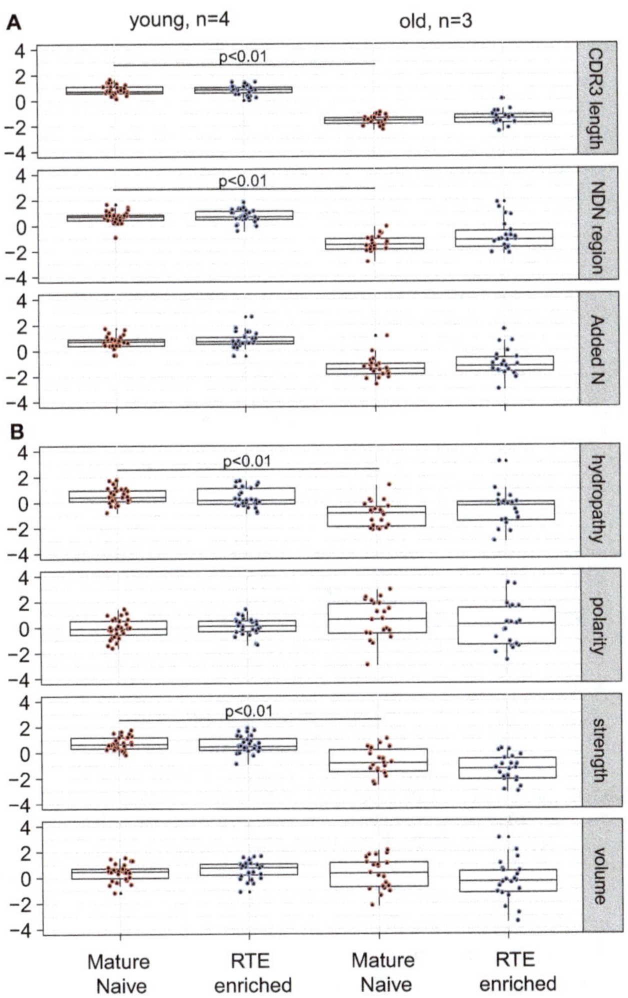


**FIGURE 5** | T-cell receptor beta CDR3 repertoire properties for mature naïve and recent thymic emigrant (RTE)-enriched CD4 T cells. **(A)** Average CDR3 length, size of NDN insert, and count of randomly added N nucleotides. **(B)** Amino acid composition within 5 amino acid residues in the middle of CDR3. CDR3 repertoires for the seven largest TRBV segments were analyzed separately, with *Z*-score normalization to account for TRBV-specific differences.

clonotypes from each donor and pooled them together to form the set of nodes. We connected two clonotypes with an edge if they had the same VJ-combination and CDR3 differed by a single amino acid substitution. Next, we counted the number of edges connecting clonotypes from donors of different age groups (young versus old) and obtained empirical distributions for these counts by running 1,000 random permutations of age group labels.

We found, that in CD8 naive repertoires, the number of edges between clonotypes from young and old donors is larger in data than in simulation in 424 donor age group permutations out of 1,000, so there is no evidence for separate CDR3 networks for young and old donors for this subset. In CD4 naive repertoires, however, there was a weak tendency: only in 95 simulations out of 1,000 (empirical *P*-value of 0.095) we found a lower number of edges between donors of different age, than the one observed in real data. This suggests that repertoires of naive CD4 T cells include distinct communities of homologous TCR variants in young and old individuals. However, this effect was only marginally significant and requires further investigation.

## DISCUSSION

With aging, decreasing thymic output can not efficiently sustain naïve T cell counts, so the homeostatic proliferation becomes the main mechanism to replenish this cell pool in humans. Such proliferation is inevitably associated with certain biases that shape the landscape of naïve T cell TCR repertoire and thus affect the spectrum of the antigens they could recognize.

We have utilized immune repertoire sequencing to study the repertoires of naïve T cells in young and aged donors and revealed notable changes in human TCR repertoires of both CD4 and CD8 peripheral blood naïve T cells with aging:

(1) We confirm the observation of Ref. (34) that relative clonality reflecting the extent of clonal expansion increases both within CD4 and CD8 naïve T cell subsets with age (**Figure 2**).
(2) We demonstrate that average CDR3 length, NDN insert length, and number of randomly added N nucleotides significantly decrease with aging in all subsets of naïve T cells, including CD4, CD8, CD4 RTE-enriched CD25$^{-}$, and CD4

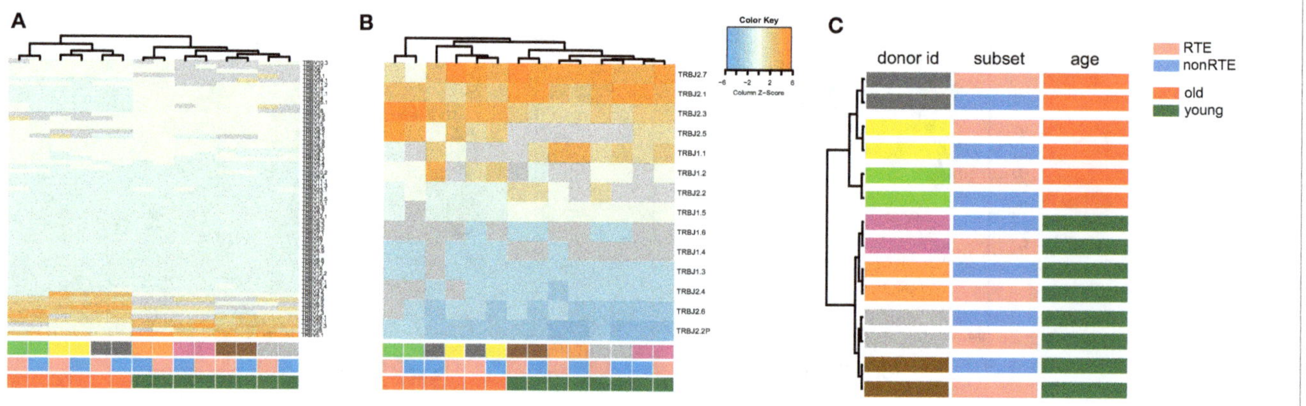

**FIGURE 6** | TRBV and TRBJ gene segment usage in recent thymic emigrant-enriched and mature naïve CD4 T cells of young and old individuals. **(A)** Heatmap and hierarchical clustering dendrogram for weighted TRBV usage. **(B)** Weighted TRBJ usage. **(C)** Hierarchical clustering of TRBV–TRBJ combination frequency (Jensen–Shannon divergence is used as metric). Note that repertoires of young and old individuals cluster separately.

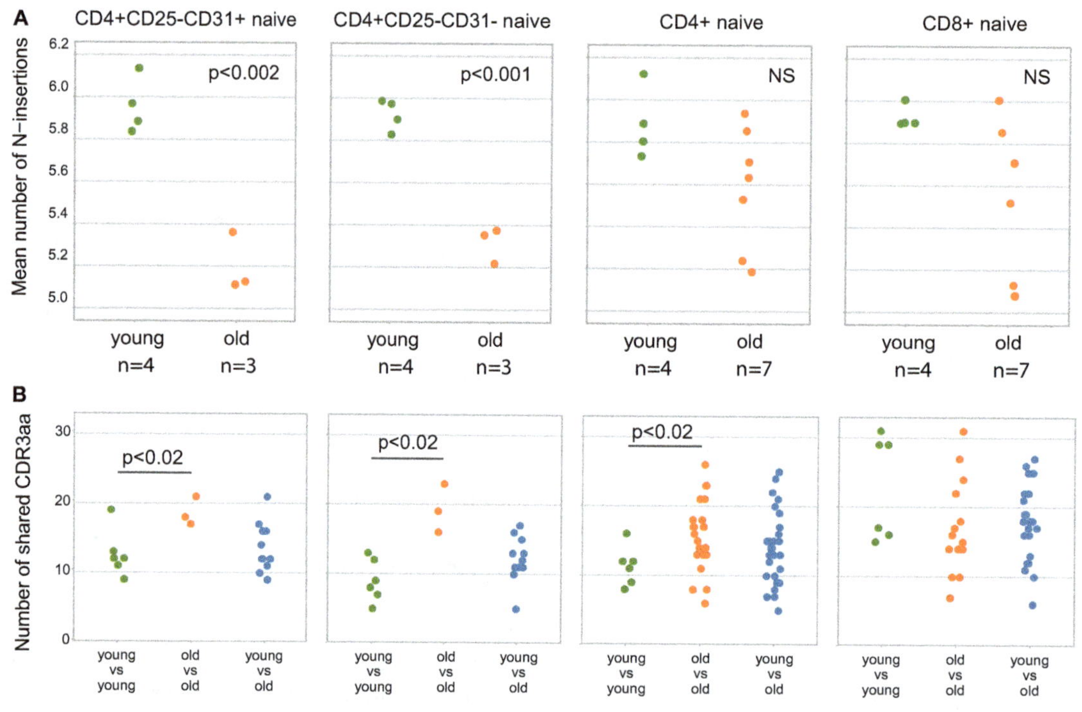

**FIGURE 7** | Relative publicity of naïve T cell T-cell receptor (TCR) beta repertoires. **(A)** Mean number of N-insertions among top-3,000 clonotypes from each sample. Unweighted (per clonotype), only for the clonotypes where TRBD segment borders were identified. **(B)** Repertoire overlaps calculated as the number of TCR beta amino acid CDR3 clonotypes shared between the top-3,000 clonotype repertoires for each pair of individuals. Each dot represents the number of clonotypes shared between a pair of samples. Welch Two Sample *t*-test *p*-values are shown.

mature naïve CD25⁻ subsets (**Figures 3A, 5A** and **7A**). Interestingly, due to spatial restrictions in TCR–pMHC interaction, the length of CDR3 is inversely related to the length of recognized peptide antigen, which affects the spectrum of recognized pMHCs (Shugay et al., manuscript under consideration). The decrease of CDR3 length with aging could, therefore, reflect the averaged properties of pMHCs that are preferentially recognized by naïve T cells in the periphery, and cause better tonic signaling, leading to earlier exhaustion of proliferation capacity of the cells carrying corresponding TCR variants.

(3) As could be expected based on previous works (53, 54), the abovementioned changes favored higher publicity in CD4 naïve T cells (**Figure 7B**). At the same time, we have not observed clear differences in TCR beta CDR3 repertoire publicity for CD8 compartment. These observations differ from the data from Qi et al. (34) suggesting the decrease of CD8 naïve T cell publicity with aging. Further studies

on larger cohorts with thoroughly controlled purity of cell sorting, and proper normalization of the datasets for comparing publicity of repertoires (49) should clarify this point.

(4) Averaged amino acid characteristics in the middle of CDR3 change prominently in CD4, CD8, CD4 RTE-enriched, and CD4 mature naïve subsets (**Figures 3B** and **5B**). In particular, significant decrease is observed for the "strength" metrics, which represents the count of strongly interacting amino acid residues (47, 48). The "strongly interacting" include F, L, I, M, and V that may form hydrophobic contacts, as well as aromatic residues W and Y that are capable of different types of interactions including offset stacked or edge-to-face interactions, thiol–aromatic interactions, and others (55), and may consist of electrostatic, van der Waals, and hydrophobic forces. Correspondingly, similar changes are observed for the "hydropathy" metrics which counts the number of hydrophobic residues in the middle of CDR3.

The "strength" metric efficiently differentiates functional T cell subpopulations, such as Treg and non-Treg CD4 subsets [see Ref. (49, 56) and our data to be published elsewhere]. This metric can be interpreted as an averaged estimation of TCR repertoire affinity to peptide–MHC complexes and in particular to the antigenic peptide, since the middle portion of CDR3 is often in contact with the presented antigen (**Figure 8**).

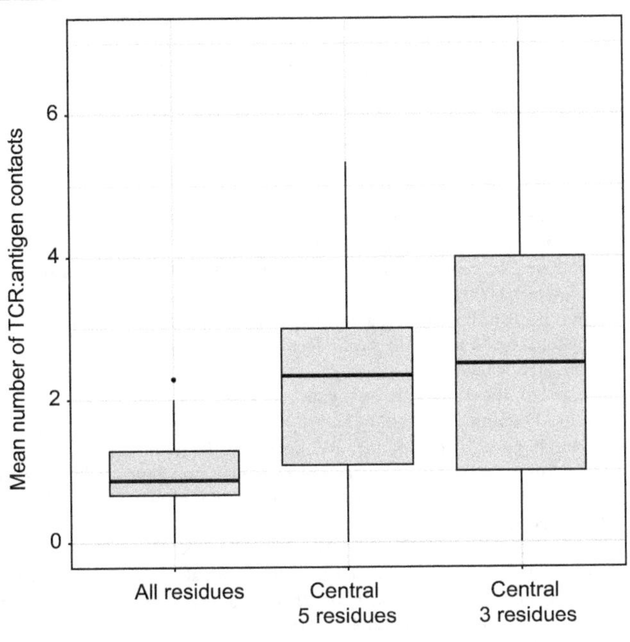


**FIGURE 8** | Number of CDR3:antigenic peptide contacts in structural data. Comparing the mean number of contacts for entire CDR3 (All positions) and its central region (central 5 residues and central 3 residues). ANOVA followed by a *post hoc* Tukey test shows significantly higher number of contacts for the central region: $P < 10^{-8}$ when comparing 5 and 3 central residues to all residues, but no difference between 5 and 3 central residues ($P = 0.42$). The analysis was performed for T-cell receptor (TCR) beta chain using 110 human TCR:pMHC complexes from Protein Data Bank.

The decrease of relative abundance of strongly interacting amino acid residues within TCR beta CDR3 repertoire of naïve T cells with aging may, therefore, reflect more rapid depletion of naïve T cell clones with higher affinity to self pMHC. This could result from more efficient tonic signaling and generally faster proliferation, exhaustion of proliferation capacity, and extinction of such naïve T cells (38).

Notably, similar changes were observed within RTE-enriched $CD31^+$ and mature naïve $CD31^-$ CD4 naïve T cells (**Figures 5–7**). Decrease of the "strength" metric was even more prominent for the RTE-enriched subset (**Figure 5B**), suggesting that the $CD31^+$ naïve CD4 T cell clones bearing TCR variants with high affinity to self pMHC are prominently switching to the $CD31^-$ phenotype due to more efficient TCR signaling.

Complementary explanation for the changes observed in the naïve T cell TCR repertoire characteristics with aging is that the high affinity variants are washed away from the naïve T cell pool in the course of ongoing immune responses. Both $CD4^+$ and $CD8^+$ T cells with strong reaction to self and high tonic signaling dominate in responses to foreign antigens (37, 57, 58). Positive selection in thymus thus favors production of more efficiently responding T cells that should be also more rapidly depleted from the naïve T cell pool. If this is the case, the age-related changes are associated with generation of prominent functional holes in the landscape of naïve T cell receptor repertoire.

An additional factor that could contribute to the observed changes in naïve T cell TCR repertoires is the easier conversion of clones with high affinity to self pMHC to the "memory-like" phenotype, as shown in mice models (59, 60), although such observations have not yet found clear confirmation in humans (3).

Altogether, the observed changes could be interpreted as elimination of generally more "sticky"—having higher affinity to self and non-self peptide–MHC complexes—TCR variants from the naïve T cell pool with aging.

However, there is also an alternative explanation which deserves consideration. Shorter CDR3s, lower numbers of randomly added N nucleotides, and higher publicity are characteristic features of the early wave(s) of naïve T cells generated during fetal period (23, 40, 61–63). Such early wave(s) originate from distinct population(s) of hematopoietic stem cells that may have distinct long-term program including higher proliferation potential (39, 42).

Considering the drop in thymic activity that happens in the middle age (4, 26), one could hypothesize that the counts of conventional naïve T cell decrease after exhaustion of their limited proliferation capacity, while the early-wave naïve T cells of fetal origin with prolonged proliferation capacity persist. Such organization of T cell adaptive immunity in the elderly could be beneficial from the point of more predictable innate-like behavior of the T cells carrying a relatively restricted, more germline-encoded TCR repertoire. To some extent, our network analysis of naïve CD4 T cell TCR repertoires supports this concept.

Summing up, our study sheds light on the intrinsic changes in the naïve T cell TCR repertoire structure with aging, and calls for further functional studies that could clarify the underlying mechanisms.

## AUTHOR CONTRIBUTIONS

EE and DS performed cell sorting. EE, SK, VZ, TN, MS, and MP analyzed the data. EE, MS, and DC prepared the figures. EE, MI, AA, FC, IM, ER, and AF worked on library preparation and sequencing. DC and OB designed the entire study and wrote the manuscript. MS, ER, and AF edited the manuscript. All authors reviewed and approved the final manuscript.

## ACKNOWLEDGMENTS

We thank Minervina A.A. for the help with figures preparation. Cell sorting experiments were carried out using the equipment provided by the IBCH Core facility (CKP IBCH, supported by Russian Ministry of Education and Science, grant RFMEFI62117 × 0018).

## FUNDING

This work was funded by Russian Science Foundation Project 16-15-00149. AF and ER received support from the H2020 EU SYSCID project (grant agreement 733100).

## REFERENCES

1. Marks BR, Nowyhed HN, Choi JY, Poholek AC, Odegard JM, Flavell RA, et al. Thymic self-reactivity selects natural interleukin 17-producing T cells that can regulate peripheral inflammation. *Nat Immunol* (2009) 10:1125–32. doi:10.1038/ni.1783
2. Nikolich-Zugich J. Aging of the T cell compartment in mice and humans: from no naive expectations to foggy memories. *J Immunol* (2014) 193:2622–9. doi:10.4049/jimmunol.1401174
3. Goronzy JJ, Fang F, Cavanagh MM, Qi Q, Weyand CM. Naive T cell maintenance and function in human aging. *J Immunol* (2015) 194:4073–80. doi:10.4049/jimmunol.1500046
4. Kumar BV, Connors TJ, Farber DL, Human T. Cell development, localization, and function throughout life. *Immunity* (2018) 48:202–13. doi:10.1016/j.immuni.2018.01.007
5. van den Broek T, Borghans JAM, van Wijk F. The full spectrum of human naive T cells. *Nat Rev Immunol* (2018) 18(6):363–73. doi:10.1038/s41577-018-0001-y
6. Goodwin K, Viboud C, Simonsen L. Antibody response to influenza vaccination in the elderly: a quantitative review. *Vaccine* (2006) 24:1159–69. doi:10.1016/j.vaccine.2005.08.105
7. Aspinall R, Del Giudice G, Effros RB, Grubeck-Loebenstein B, Sambhara S. Challenges for vaccination in the elderly. *Immun Ageing* (2007) 4:9. doi:10.1186/1742-4933-4-9
8. Pinti M, Appay V, Campisi J, Frasca D, Fulop T, Sauce D, et al. Aging of the immune system: focus on inflammation and vaccination. *Eur J Immunol* (2016) 46:2286–301. doi:10.1002/eji.201546178
9. Fulop T, Larbi A, Kotb R, de Angelis F, Pawelec G. Aging, immunity, and cancer. *Discov Med* (2011) 11:537–50.
10. Foster AD, Sivarapatna A, Gress RE. The aging immune system and its relationship with cancer. *Aging health* (2011) 7:707–18. doi:10.2217/ahe.11.56
11. Fulop T, Larbi A, Witkowski JM, Kotb R, Hirokawa K, Pawelec G. Immunosenescence and cancer. *Crit Rev Oncog* (2013) 18:489–513. doi:10.1615/CritRevOncog.2013010597
12. Stronen E, Toebes M, Kelderman S, van Buuren MM, Yang W, van Rooij N, et al. Targeting of cancer neoantigens with donor-derived T cell receptor repertoires. *Science* (2016) 352:1337–41. doi:10.1126/science.aaf2288
13. Howcroft TK, Campisi J, Louis GB, Smith MT, Wise B, Wyss-Coray T, et al. The role of inflammation in age-related disease. *Aging (Albany NY)* (2013) 5:84–93. doi:10.18632/aging.100531
14. Franceschi C, Campisi J. Chronic inflammation (inflammaging) and its potential contribution to age-associated diseases. *J Gerontol A Biol Sci Med Sci* (2014) 69(Suppl 1):S4–9. doi:10.1093/gerona/glu057
15. Watson N, Ding B, Zhu X, Frisina RD. Chronic inflammation – inflammaging – in the ageing cochlea: a novel target for future presbycusis therapy. *Ageing Res Rev* (2017) 40:142–8. doi:10.1016/j.arr.2017.10.002
16. Li MO, Rudensky AY. T cell receptor signalling in the control of regulatory T cell differentiation and function. *Nat Rev Immunol* (2016) 16:220–33. doi:10.1038/nri.2016.26
17. Feng Y, van der Veeken J, Shugay M, Putintseva EV, Osmanbeyoglu HU, Dikiy S, et al. A mechanism for expansion of regulatory T-cell repertoire and its role in self-tolerance. *Nature* (2015) 528:132–6. doi:10.1038/nature16141
18. Messaoudi I, Lemaoult J, Guevara-Patino JA, Metzner BM, Nikolich-Zugich J. Age-related CD8 T cell clonal expansions constrict CD8 T cell repertoire and have the potential to impair immune defense. *J Exp Med* (2004) 200:1347–58. doi:10.1084/jem.20040437
19. Goronzy JJ, Weyand CM. T cell development and receptor diversity during aging. *Curr Opin Immunol* (2005) 17:468–75. doi:10.1016/j.coi.2005.07.020
20. Naylor K, Li G, Vallejo AN, Lee WW, Koetz K, Bryl E, et al. The influence of age on T cell generation and TCR diversity. *J Immunol* (2005) 174:7446–52. doi:10.4049/jimmunol.174.11.7446
21. Goronzy JJ, Lee WW, Weyand CM. Aging and T-cell diversity. *Exp Gerontol* (2007) 42:400–6. doi:10.1016/j.exger.2006.11.016
22. Britanova OV, Putintseva EV, Shugay M, Merzlyak EM, Turchaninova MA, Staroverov DB, et al. Age-related decrease in TCR repertoire diversity measured with deep and normalized sequence profiling. *J Immunol* (2014) 192:2689–98. doi:10.4049/jimmunol.1302064
23. Britanova OV, Shugay M, Merzlyak EM, Staroverov DB, Putintseva EV, Turchaninova MA, et al. Dynamics of individual T cell repertoires: from cord blood to centenarians. *J Immunol* (2016) 196:5005–13. doi:10.4049/jimmunol.1600005
24. Chinn IK, Blackburn CC, Manley NR, Sempowski GD. Changes in primary lymphoid organs with aging. *Semin Immunol* (2012) 24:309–20. doi:10.1016/j.smim.2012.04.005
25. Palmer DB. The effect of age on thymic function. *Front Immunol* (2013) 4:316. doi:10.3389/fimmu.2013.00316
26. Thome JJ, Grinshpun B, Kumar BV, Kubota M, Ohmura Y, Lerner H, et al. Longterm maintenance of human naive T cells through in situ homeostasis in lymphoid tissue sites. *Sci Immunol* (2016) 1:eaah6506. doi:10.1126/sciimmunol.aah6506
27. Kyoizumi S, Kubo Y, Kajimura J, Yoshida K, Imai K, Hayashi T, et al. Age-associated changes in the differentiation potentials of human circulating hematopoietic progenitors to T- or NK-lineage cells. *J Immunol* (2013) 190:6164–72. doi:10.4049/jimmunol.1203189
28. Haines CJ, Giffon TD, Lu LS, Lu X, Tessier-Lavigne M, Ross DT, et al. Human CD4+ T cell recent thymic emigrants are identified by protein tyrosine kinase 7 and have reduced immune function. *J Exp Med* (2009) 206:275–85. doi:10.1084/jem.20080996
29. Fink PJ. The biology of recent thymic emigrants. *Annu Rev Immunol* (2013) 31:31–50. doi:10.1146/annurev-immunol-032712-100010
30. Kilpatrick RD, Rickabaugh T, Hultin LE, Hultin P, Hausner MA, Detels R, et al. Homeostasis of the naive CD4+ T cell compartment during aging. *J Immunol* (2008) 180:1499–507. doi:10.4049/jimmunol.180.10.6437-a

31. Qi Q, Zhang DW, Weyand CM, Goronzy JJ. Mechanisms shaping the naive T cell repertoire in the elderly – thymic involution or peripheral homeostatic proliferation? *Exp Gerontol* (2014) 54:71–4. doi:10.1016/j.exger.2014.01.005
32. den Braber I, Mugwagwa T, Vrisekoop N, Westera L, Mogling R, de Boer AB, et al. Maintenance of peripheral naive T cells is sustained by thymus output in mice but not humans. *Immunity* (2012) 36:288–97. doi:10.1016/j.immuni.2012.02.006
33. Sauce D, Larsen M, Fastenackels S, Roux A, Gorochov G, Katlama C, et al. Lymphopenia-driven homeostatic regulation of naive T cells in elderly and thymectomized young adults. *J Immunol* (2012) 189:5541–8. doi:10.4049/jimmunol.1201235
34. Qi Q, Liu Y, Cheng Y, Glanville J, Zhang D, Lee JY, et al. Diversity and clonal selection in the human T-cell repertoire. *Proc Natl Acad Sci U S A* (2014) 111:13139–44. doi:10.1073/pnas.1409155111
35. Takeda S, Rodewald HR, Arakawa H, Bluethmann H, Shimizu T. MHC class II molecules are not required for survival of newly generated CD4+ T cells, but affect their long-term life span. *Immunity* (1996) 5:217–28. doi:10.1016/S1074-7613(00)80317-9
36. Azzam HS, Grinberg A, Lui K, Shen H, Shores EW, Love PE. CD5 expression is developmentally regulated by T cell receptor (TCR) signals and TCR avidity. *J Exp Med* (1998) 188:2301–11. doi:10.1084/jem.188.12.2301
37. Stefanova I, Dorfman JR, Germain RN. Self-recognition promotes the foreign antigen sensitivity of naive T lymphocytes. *Nature* (2002) 420:429–34. doi:10.1038/nature01146
38. Myers DR, Zikherman J, Roose JP. Tonic signals: why do lymphocytes bother? *Trends Immunol* (2017) 38:844–57. doi:10.1016/j.it.2017.06.010
39. Pogorelyy MV, Elhanati Y, Marcou Q, Sycheva AL, Komech EA, Nazarov VI, et al. Persisting fetal clonotypes influence the structure and overlap of adult human T cell receptor repertoires. *PLoS Comput Biol* (2017) 13:e1005572. doi:10.1371/journal.pcbi.1005572
40. George JF Jr, Schroeder HW Jr. Developmental regulation of D beta reading frame and junctional diversity in T cell receptor-beta transcripts from human thymus. *J Immunol* (1992) 148:1230–9.
41. Benedict CL, Gilfillan S, Thai TH, Kearney JF. Terminal deoxynucleotidyl transferase and repertoire development. *Immunol Rev* (2000) 175:150–7. doi:10.1111/j.1600-065X.2000.imr017518.x
42. Mold JE, Venkatasubrahmanyam S, Burt TD, Michaelsson J, Rivera JM, Galkina SA, et al. Fetal and adult hematopoietic stem cells give rise to distinct T cell lineages in humans. *Science* (2010) 330:1695–9. doi:10.1126/science.1196509
43. Egorov ES, Merzlyak EM, Shelenkov AA, Britanova OV, Sharonov GV, Staroverov DB, et al. Quantitative profiling of immune repertoires for minor lymphocyte counts using unique molecular identifiers. *J Immunol* (2015) 194:6155–63. doi:10.4049/jimmunol.1500215
44. Egorov E. Human TCR alpha and beta RNA-based RACE protocol with unique molecular barcoding. *Protoc Exch* (2016). doi:10.1038/protex.2016.044
45. Bolotin DA, Poslavsky S, Mitrophanov I, Shugay M, Mamedov IZ, Putintseva EV, et al. MiXCR: software for comprehensive adaptive immunity profiling. *Nat Methods* (2015) 12:380–1. doi:10.1038/nmeth.3364
46. Shugay M, Bagaev DV, Turchaninova MA, Bolotin DA, Britanova OV, Putintseva EV, et al. VDJtools: unifying post-analysis of T cell receptor repertoires. *PLoS Comput Biol* (2015) 11:e1004503. doi:10.1371/journal.pcbi.1004503
47. Miyazawa S, Jernigan RL. Residue-residue potentials with a favorable contact pair term and an unfavorable high packing density term, for simulation and threading. *J Mol Biol* (1996) 256:623–44. doi:10.1006/jmbi.1996.0114
48. Kosmrlj A, Jha AK, Huseby ES, Kardar M, Chakraborty AK. How the thymus designs antigen-specific and self-tolerant T cell receptor sequences. *Proc Natl Acad Sci U S A* (2008) 105:16671–6. doi:10.1073/pnas.0808081105
49. Izraelson M, Nakonechnaya TO, Moltedo B, Egorov ES, Kasatskaya SA, Putintseva EV, et al. Comparative analysis of murine T-cell receptor repertoires. *Immunology* (2018) 153:133–44. doi:10.1111/imm.12857
50. Bolotin DA, Mamedov IZ, Britanova OV, Zvyagin IV, Shagin D, Ustyugova SV, et al. Next generation sequencing for TCR repertoire profiling: platform-specific features and correction algorithms. *Eur J Immunol* (2012) 42:3073–83. doi:10.1002/eji.201242517
51. Carlson CS, Emerson RO, Sherwood AM, Desmarais C, Chung MW, Parsons JM, et al. Using synthetic templates to design an unbiased multiplex PCR assay. *Nat Commun* (2013) 4:2680. doi:10.1038/ncomms3680
52. Pekalski ML, Ferreira RC, Coulson RM, Cutler AJ, Guo H, Smyth DJ, et al. Postthymic expansion in human CD4 naive T cells defined by expression of functional high-affinity IL-2 receptors. *J Immunol* (2013) 190:2554–66. doi:10.4049/jimmunol.1202914
53. Venturi V, Price DA, Douek DC, Davenport MP. The molecular basis for public T-cell responses? *Nat Rev Immunol* (2008) 8:231–8. doi:10.1038/nri2260
54. Murugan A, Mora T, Walczak AM, Callan CG Jr. Statistical inference of the generation probability of T-cell receptors from sequence repertoires. *Proc Natl Acad Sci U S A* (2012) 109:16161–6. doi:10.1073/pnas.1212755109
55. Chakrabarti P, Bhattacharyya R. Geometry of nonbonded interactions involving planar groups in proteins. *Prog Biophys Mol Biol* (2007) 95:83–137. doi:10.1016/j.pbiomolbio.2007.03.016
56. Bolotin DA, Poslavsky S, Davydov AN, Frenkel FE, Fanchi L, Zolotareva OI, et al. Antigen receptor repertoire profiling from RNA-seq data. *Nat Biotechnol* (2017) 35:908–11. doi:10.1038/nbt.3979
57. Mandl JN, Monteiro JP, Vrisekoop N, Germain RN. T cell-positive selection uses self-ligand binding strength to optimize repertoire recognition of foreign antigens. *Immunity* (2013) 38:263–74. doi:10.1016/j.immuni.2012.09.011
58. Fulton RB, Hamilton SE, Xing Y, Best JA, Goldrath AW, Hogquist KA, et al. The TCR's sensitivity to self peptide-MHC dictates the ability of naive CD8(+) T cells to respond to foreign antigens. *Nat Immunol* (2015) 16:107–17. doi:10.1038/ni.3043
59. Rudd BD, Venturi V, Li G, Samadder P, Ertelt JM, Way SS, et al. Nonrandom attrition of the naive CD8+ T-cell pool with aging governed by T-cell receptor:pMHC interactions. *Proc Natl Acad Sci U S A* (2011) 108:13694–9. doi:10.1073/pnas.1107594108
60. Sprent J, Surh CD. Normal T cell homeostasis: the conversion of naive cells into memory-phenotype cells. *Nat Immunol* (2011) 12:478–84. doi:10.1038/ni.2018
61. Feeney AJ. Lack of N regions in fetal and neonatal mouse immunoglobulin V-D-J junctional sequences. *J Exp Med* (1990) 172:1377–90. doi:10.1084/jem.172.5.1377
62. Bogue M, Gilfillan S, Benoist C, Mathis D. Regulation of N-region diversity in antigen receptors through thymocyte differentiation and thymus ontogeny. *Proc Natl Acad Sci U S A* (1992) 89:11011–5. doi:10.1073/pnas.89.22.11011
63. Cherrier M, Cardona A, Rosinski-Chupin I, Rougeon F, Doyen N. Substantial N diversity is generated in T cell receptor alpha genes at birth despite low levels of terminal deoxynucleotidyl transferase expression in mouse thymus. *Eur J Immunol* (2002) 32:3651–6. doi:10.1002/1521-4141(200212)32:12<3651::AID-IMMU3651>3.0.CO;2-D

# 15

# Comparative Analysis of B-Cell Receptor Repertoires Induced by Live Yellow Fever Vaccine in Young and Middle-Age Donors

*Alexey N. Davydov*[1†], *Anna S. Obraztsova*[2,3†], *Mikhail Y. Lebedin*[4†], *Maria A. Turchaninova*[4,5,6†], *Dmitriy B. Staroverov*[4,5], *Ekaterina M. Merzlyak*[4,5], *George V. Sharonov*[4,6], *Olga Kladova*[5], *Mikhail Shugay*[3,4,5,6], *Olga V. Britanova*[4,5,6] and *Dmitriy M. Chudakov*[1,3,4,5,6*]

[1] Adaptive Immunity Group, Central European Institute of Technology, Brno, Czechia, [2] Faculty of Bioengineering and Bioinformatics, Lomonosov Moscow State University, Moscow, Russia, [3] Center of Life Sciences, Skolkovo Institute of Science and Technology, Moscow, Russia, [4] Genomics of Adaptive Immunity Department, Shemyakin and Ovchinnikov Institute of Bioorganic Chemistry, Moscow, Russia, [5] Department of Molecular Technologies, Pirogov Russian National Research Medical University, Moscow, Russia, [6] Laboratory of Genomics of Antitumor Adaptive Immunity, Privolzhsky Research Medical University, Nizhny Novgorod, Russia

***Correspondence:**
Dmitriy M. Chudakov
chudakovdm@mail.ru

† These authors have contributed equally to this work

Age-related changes can significantly alter the state of adaptive immune system and often lead to attenuated response to novel pathogens and vaccination. In present study we employed 5′RACE UMI-based full length and nearly error-free immunoglobulin profiling to compare plasma cell antibody repertoires in young (19–26 years) and middle-age (45–58 years) individuals vaccinated with a live yellow fever vaccine, modeling a newly encountered pathogen. Our analysis has revealed age-related differences in the responding antibody repertoire ranging from distinct IGH CDR3 repertoire properties to differences in somatic hypermutation intensity and efficiency and antibody lineage tree structure. Overall, our findings suggest that younger individuals respond with a more diverse antibody repertoire and employ a more efficient somatic hypermutation process than elder individuals in response to a newly encountered pathogen.

**Keywords: immunoglobulin repertoire, vaccination, age, yellow fever, plasma cell**

## INTRODUCTION

A number of previously published studies suggests that the function of adaptive immunity is impaired in aged individuals (1, 2). The findings include functionally exhausted immune repertoire displaying a substantially lower diversity of T cell and B cell receptors compared to young individuals (3–6), impaired antigen-driven selection mechanisms (7, 8), and attenuated response to vaccines (9–16).

Functional defects of antibody-mediated vaccine-induced immunity in elderly adults are manifested both in the hampered generation of a primary response and in decreased effect of booster vaccination: low production of vaccine-specific antibodies, low affinity and opsonic capacity of generated antibodies, reduced vaccine longevity (9, 13, 14, 17–23). Altogether, this leads to lower protection achieved in the elderly than in young adults. However, the exact reasons of poor vaccine response in old people have not been fully elucidated.

Recent advances in high-throughput sequencing (HTS) allow performing a targeted readout of hundreds of thousands of B-cell receptor (BCR) heavy chain (IGH) sequences from samples of interest (24–30), providing a powerful tool for investigation of age-related changes in B cell immunity. HTS profiling of BCR repertoires reveals contracted clonal diversity both in naive and antigen-experienced B memory subsets, and accumulation of highly mutated immunoglobulin genes and persistent clonal expansions with aging (25, 31, 32). The latter resembles the age-related changes in T cell repertoire (5, 33–35), and altogether these effects can be linked to the decreased efficiency of vaccination in the elderly adults (32, 34, 36).

The HTS approach was also employed for studies of influenza (25, 27), tetanus (37), and hepatitis B (38, 39) vaccines. It was demonstrated that B cell repertoire has the ability to rapidly expand and contract in a highly dynamic mode in response to vaccination (27). Stereotypic changes of B cell repertoires include increase in mutation frequency and decrease in diversity 4–10 days after vaccination, which corresponds to the maximum concentration of mutated plasma cells released into the peripheral blood (38–40). Interestingly, highly homologous "public" BCR variants can be produced in response to the same antigen in different individuals by convergent recombination and selection (27, 41, 42).

There is also an increasing number of data characterizing changes in the antibody repertoires with respect to vaccine immune stimulus and age. We have found three HTS-based studies of BCR repertoires aimed at revealing the age-related differences in vaccine response, all tracking the changes upon influenza vaccine challenge (25, 32, 43).

Wu et al. (43) analyzed cDNA-based BCR repertoires obtained from the peripheral blood mononuclear cells (PBMC) of young (19–25 years) and old (70–89 years) individuals, where responding B cell clones (groups of homologous clonotypes) could be distinguished by their large size at D7 in terms of the number of included clonotypes. In the old individuals, they reported decreased average clone size within IgA isotype, and increased CDR-H3 length and lower mutation frequency for the large IgA and IgM clones.

Jiang et al. (25) analyzed cDNA-based BCR repertoires obtained from PBMC of 8–17, 18–32, and 70–100 years old groups of individuals at D0, D7-8, and D28 (±4) after vaccination. At D7-8, plasmablasts were sorted as CD3–CD19+CD20–CD27+CD38+ cells. The oldest age group was characterized by fewer B cell lineages compared to other age groups both in PBMC samples obtained before and after vaccination and within the vaccine-responding plasmablast repertoire.

de Bourcy et al. (32) analyzed cDNA-based BCR repertoires obtained from the PBMC of young (21–27 years) and old (73–93 years) individuals, where responding B cell lineages were distinguished as those that were detected at both D0 and D7 and increased their transcript abundance between these time points. They reported reduced intralineage mutational diversification, and decreased proportion of radical (prominently changing the amino acid properties) mutations in the clones responding to vaccination in old individuals. These observations may indicate generally impaired affinity maturation in the old age, as well as accumulated original antigenic sin and the requirement of only fine-tuning of the existing flu-specific memory B cell repertoire in old individuals with long history of response to influenza (32).

All these data have highlighted the importance of B cell repertoire dynamics consideration in vaccine studies in the elderly adults, but were limited to tracking the response to a common pathogen with a substantial exposure history. Here we focused on investigation of the age-related differences in BCR repertoire structure of the plasma B cells responding to the live yellow fever (YF) virus vaccine in young (19–26 years old) versus middle-age (45–58 years old) individuals as a model of response to a previously unencountered pathogen.

We utilized our protocol based on 5′-RACE with unique molecular identifiers (UMI) that allows nearly error-free, full-length (FR1-FR4 plus IgD/IgM/IgG/IgE/IgA isotypes identification) sequencing of IGH variable region repertoires (44), with minor modifications. Given that sufficient coverage is achieved in terms of sequencing reads per cDNA molecule, the use of UMIs dramatically increases the quality of long range high-throughput sequencing, and endues the algorithms of PCR errors correction with high power and precision, critical for resolving the true somatic hypermutation events (44–47).

To focus the analysis on the immunoglobulin repertoires specifically responding to vaccination, we isolated CD20-CD19+CD27$^{high}$CD38$^{high}$ plasma B cells from peripheral blood samples obtained from healthy volunteers 9 days after their first vaccination with live YF vaccine. In this time frame, the concentration of plasma B cells in peripheral blood increases dramatically and mainly represents the cells that respond specifically to the vaccine antigens (40, 48).

It should be noted, that a minor portion of peripheral blood plasma B cells analyzed 9 days after vaccination could include clones responding to the current antigens other than the YF, such as self-antigens and antigens arising from commensal microorganisms or chronic infections. Thus the picture of the differences observed in the plasma B cell repertoires of young and middle-age donors after YF immunization could include imprint from the general differences in the ongoing plasma B cell response between the young and middle-age volunteers, as well as differences in memory-track prehistory of these responses. According to our observations, 9 days after YF vaccination, relative abundance of plasma B cells in peripheral blood increased more than 10-fold and reached 15.5% ± 10% of CD19+CD27$^{high}$ B cells (**Supplementary Figure 1**), similar for both age groups, which corresponds well to the previous data with influenza vaccination (48). Thus we estimate the contribution of such non-YF vaccination related B cell clones as ~10% of the analyzed cDNA quantity.

It should be also noted that since our approach to immunoglobulin profiling is RNA-based, the resulting IGH repertoires yield the picture that intrinsically accounts for the difference in the IGH mRNA expression levels, thus favoring B cell clones with high production of immunoglobulins.

In our data analysis, we have focused on three groups of variables that together provide a comprehensive repertoire characterization:

1) V-D-J rearrangement structure and CDR3 physicochemical properties;
2) Antibody lineage structure (clonal trees);
3) Profiles of newly acquired and potentially pre-existing somatic hypermutations.

We reveal a number of antibody repertoire features that were distinct between young and middle-age individuals, highlighting age-related differences in humoral immune response directed against newly encountered antigens, that are already detectable by the age of 50.

# METHODS

## Blood Donors and Samples

This study was approved by the local ethical committee and conducted in accordance with the Declaration of Helsinki. All donors were informed of the final use of their blood and signed an informed consent document. The cohort of healthy donors ($n = 10$, **Table 1**) has been immunized for the first time by the yellow fever vaccine (live freeze-dried preparation of the 17D strain of YFV licensed in Russia, FSUE of Chumakov IPVE, RAMS). Yellow fever is not endemic in Russia and the volunteers have not previously traveled to areas known to be endemic for yellow fever. Peripheral blood (9 ml per sample) was collected on the 9th day after vaccination into EDTA-treated Vacutainer tubes (BD Biosciences). The B cells were stained for surface markers by incubating with following monoclonal antibodies: CD38-PE (clone HB7, eBioscience), CD19-FITC (clone J3-119, Beckman Coulter), CD20-Vio Blue (clone LT20, Miltenyi Biotec), CD27-PC5 (clone O323, eBioscience). The plasma B cells were gated as CD20-CD19+CD27+CD38$^{high}$ and collected directly into RLT buffer (Qiagen) for storage and RNA extraction. The numbers of sorted plasma cells per sample are shown in **Table 1**.

## RNA Extraction, cDNA Libraries Preparation, and Sequencing

UMI-barcoded IGH cDNA libraries for the vaccinated donors were prepared as described previously (44) with minor modifications which allow to introduce Illumina Nextera adapters and indexes during PCR. Briefly, total RNA was extracted from sorted B cells using RNeasy Micro Kit (QIAGEN) and converted to cDNA using 5′ template switch adapter containing UMI. The cDNA was treated with UDG (NEB), and purified using AMPure Beads (Beckman Coulter). A portion of cDNA equivalent to 200 sorted plasma B cells (**Table 1**) was used for further PCR amplification. Appropriate amount of cDNA used for the library preparation is critical in order to achieve sufficient coverage in terms of sequencing reads per UMI, which is a prerequisite for the efficient error correction (44–46). IGH libraries were amplified using a set of IGHC-specific and 5′ template switch adapter-specific primers introducing indexed Nextera sequencing adapters. Please refer to the **Table 2** for the oligonucleotides used. The resulting libraries were analyzed on 2 runs of Illumina MiSeq, paired-end 310+310 nt sequencing. All 10 samples were analyzed within each run, and results of the 2 runs were pooled before further bioinformatic analysis.

## Data Preprocessing and Analysis

UMI extraction and UMI-based consensus assembling was performed using MIGEC software (45), with a 5 reads-per-UMI threshold. Further reads mapping and clonotypes (unique full length IGH nucleotide sequences) assembling was performed using MiXCR as described previously (44) with some changes in MiXCR analysis pipeline (KAligner alignment algorithm was used that allows to detect indels of more than 2 nt). Resulting clonesets deposited at https://figshare.com/articles/Comparative_analysis_of_B-cell_receptor_repertoires_induced_by_live_yellow_fever_vaccine_in_young_and_middle_age_donors/6853961.

All analyses except for depicted in **Figure 5A** were performed using mean values for repertoire features and summary statistics computed for each donor, statistical testing was performed by comparing values for $n = 5$ young and $n = 5$ middle-age donors.

## Antibody Lineage Analysis

Reconstruction of clonal trees was done using in-house algorithm that takes into account VJ assignment and NDN sequence of IGH and can be briefly described as follows. First, IGH clonotypes are

**TABLE 1** | Donor and sample metadata.

| Donor ID | Age range (median), years | Status | Number of sorted plasma cells | Portion of cDNA used | Number of raw paired-end sequencing reads | Number of analyzed IGH cDNA molecules | Number of unique IGH clonotypes extracted |
|---|---|---|---|---|---|---|---|
| P1 | 19–26 (19) | Young | 6,000 | 1/30 | 4,410,583 | 29,052 | 3,913 |
| P2 | | | 6,000 | 1/30 | 3,443,963 | 17,284 | 3,590 |
| P3 | | | 6,000 | 1/30 | 4,254,150 | 10,593 | 2,159 |
| P4 | | | 6,000 | 1/30 | 3,737,681 | 20,665 | 2,916 |
| P5 | | | 6,000 | 1/30 | 2,888,569 | 18,086 | 2,563 |
| P6 | 45–58 (55) | Middle-age | 6,000 | 1/30 | 1,939,674 | 19,111 | 2,529 |
| P7 | | | 5,000 | 1/25 | 3,133,844 | 42,768 | 3,520 |
| P8 | | | 6,000 | 1/30 | 2,731,660 | 21,879 | 2,507 |
| P9 | | | 3,000 | 1/15 | 2,566,472 | 11,154 | 1,761 |
| P10 | | | 3,000 | 1/15 | 1,845,910 | 20,102 | 2,427 |

**TABLE 2** | Oligonucleotides used.

| Primer | Application | Sequence |
|---|---|---|
| **FIRST-STRAND cDNA SYNTHESIS** | | |
| SmartNNNext | 5′-template-switch oligo with sequencing illumina adapter U = dU, rG = riboG | AGATGUGTAUAAGAGACAGNNNNUNNNNUNNNNUCTT(rG)$_4$ |
| **IGH cDNA synthesis primer mix** | | |
| hIGG_r1 | Primer for cDNA synthesis, human IgG heavy-chain mRNA | GAAGTAGTCCTTGACCAGGCA |
| hIGM_r1 | Primer for cDNA synthesis, human IgM heavy-chain mRNA | GTGATGGAGTCGGGAAGGAAG |
| hIGA_r1 | Primer for cDNA synthesis, human IgA heavy-chain mRNA | GCGACGACCACGTTCCCATCT |
| hIGD_r1 | Primer for cDNA synthesis, human IgD heavy-chain mRNA | GGACCACAGGGCTGTTATC |
| hIGE_r1 | Primer for cDNA synthesis, human IgE heavy-chain mRNA | AGTCACGGAGGTGGCATTG |
| **FIRST PCR AMPLIFICATION** | | |
| Common primer | Step-out primer, anneals on the switch adaptor | AGATGTGTATAAGAGACAG |
| **IGH reverse primer mix** | | |
| Common-hIGGE_r2 | Nested primer with sequencing illumina adaptor, human IgG/IgE heavy-chain cDNA | AGATGTGTATAAGAGACAGARGGGGAAGACSGATG |
| Common-hIGA_r2 | Nested primer with sequencing illumina adaptor, human IgA heavy-chain cDNA | AGATGTGTATAAGAGACAGCAGCGGGAAGACCTTG |
| Common-hIGM_r2 | Nested primer with sequencing illumina adaptor, human IgM heavy-chain cDNA | AGATGTGTATAAGAGACAGAGGGGGAAAAGGGTTG |
| Common-hIGD_r2 | Nested primer with sequencing illumina adaptor, human IgD heavy-chain cDNA | AGATGTGTATAAGAGACAGATATGATGGGGAACAC |
| **SECOND PCR AMPLIFICATION** | | |
| F-common | Step-out primer with sequencing and P7 illumina adapters | TCGTCGGCAGCGTCAGATGTGTATAAGAGACAG |
| R- common | Step-out primer with sequencing and P5 illumina adapters | GTCTCGTGGGCTCGGAGATGTGTATAAGAGACAG |
| **THIRD PCR AMPLIFICATION** | | |
| Fc_i7[a] | Step-out primer with index 1 illumina adapter | CAAGCAGAAGACGGCATACGAGAT[i7]GTCTCGTGGGCTCGG |
| Fc_i5[b] | Step-out primer with index 2 illumina adapter | AATGATACGGCGACCACCGAGATCTACAC[i5]TCGTCGGCAGCGTC |

[a,b]*Illumina Nextera index adapters (i5 and i7). See illumina Nextera DNA library preparation reference guide and illumina adapters sequences list for more information.*

clustered into groups containing sequences with matched V and J segments. Then, a pairwise comparison is performed for each group: if the K-mer ($K = 5$) composition of NDN regions of two sequences is highly similar the sequences are considered to originate from one ancestor sequence and connected by an edge on the lineage tree.

An edge connects a pair of clonotypes that are likely to come from a pair of cells, one of which is a hypermutated [bears a B-cell receptor with mutation(s)] sub-variant of another. The direction of edge shows which of the clonotypes is a parent one and which is a child one. As we use full-length immunoglobulin sequencing data, one can infer edge direction using parsimony principle: parent clonotype mutations should be a subset of child mutations.

The similarity is computed by summing the information content of each K-mer (that is, the logarithm of its probability to be found in random VDJ rearrangements), thus K-mers containing many non-template bases are scored the most. The similarity score threshold for drawing an edge was selected according a benchmark performed by *in-silico* mixing Raji hypermutating cell line repertoire and PBMC IGH samples. CDR3 hypermutations were obtained using Smith-Waterman alignment for each pair of connected nodes with different CDR3 sequences. Parsimony principle was applied to remove improbable nodes and infer the direction of edges. In order to eliminate duplicate paths and form a tree structure we next removed all incoming edges except the one with lowest number of mutations. To normalize samples for accurate comparison, we extracted 10,000 randomly sampled IGH cDNA molecules from each dataset.

## CDR3 Physicochemical Property Analysis

Averaged CDR3 physicochemical properties of repertoires accounting for the clonotypes size were computed using custom R script. To estimate the energy of the interaction between CDR3 and a random epitope, we used Miyazawa-Jernigan statistical potential (49), that is based on calculating the frequencies of certain amino acids being in close proximity with each other in available structural data, and assuming that these frequencies follow Boltzmann distribution parameterized by corresponding energy values. For each amino acid among the five positions in the middle of CDR3, we computed the average interaction energy with all 20 amino acids. We then summed values across amino acid residues to estimate the energy of the interaction between CDR3 and a random epitope. Other physicochemical properties were analyzed similarly.

## Selection Strength

The selection strength was estimated using BASELINe framework (50) which compares the observed frequencies of replacement and silent mutations with the expected ones. BASELINe was applied to a subset of Variable segment sequences (FR1-FR3) that do not contain indels and the closest germline alleles as a reference. For each donor, clonal groups of sequences were collapsed to consensus sequences using SHazaM R package (51) as recommended by BASELINe authors. The probability density functions of the selection strength were compared using built-in statistical test.

## RESULTS

### CDR3 Characteristics

Analysis of the averaged CDR3 characteristics was performed for IgA, IgG, and IgM isotypes, weighted by the abundance of each clonotype (i.e., the input of each clonotype was proportional to its frequency within repertoire), and included CDR3 length, added N nucleotides, and physicochemical characteristics for the five amino acid residues located in the middle of CDR3 [having the highest probability to contact with antigen, by analogy with TCRs, (52)]. The latter included averaged statistical potential of CDR3:epitope interactions [the estimated "energy" of interaction between CDR3 and a random epitope (49)], "strength" of interaction [derivative of "energy," VDJtools (53)], hydrophobicity (Kidera factor 4) (54, 55), and "volume" (VDJtools, values from: http://www.imgt.org/IMGTeducation/Aide-memoire/_UK/aminoacids/IMGTclasses.html) for the young versus middle-age individuals (see **Table 3** for the values used for each amino acid property).

The analysis revealed several features that significantly differed between the responding plasma cell IGH repertoires of the two age groups but not between the isotypes (**Figure 1**). Of note, differences in "energy," and hydrophobicity (Kidera factor 4) were previously demonstrated to be critical for antibody affinity and specificity (56). Altogether, observed differences indicated that middle-age individuals tend to respond to a new challenge with IGH variants carrying longer CDR3s [in agreement with (43)], with higher content of bulky, hydrophobic, and strongly interacting amino acid residues in the middle of CDR3.

### Isotype and IGHV Gene Segments Usage

We have not detected prominent differences in IGHV gene segment usage as well as in isotype usage between plasma cell IGH repertoires of young and middle-age individuals vaccinated with YF (**Figures 2A,B**). The list of most commonly used IGHV segments included the IGHV4 (IGHV4-31, IGHV4-34, IGHV4-59, and IGHV4-39) family, IGHV3 (IGHV3-74, IGHV3-30, IGHV3-53, IGHV3-24) family, as well as IGHV1-18 and IGHV5-51.

Note that potential biases in isotype and IGHV gene segment usage are corrected by UMI-based analysis, since sequencing reads that cover the same cDNA molecule (irrespectively to the efficiency of amplification of each particular isotype or gene segment) are clustered together, each cDNA molecule to a single UMI-labeled group of sequencing reads.

**TABLE 3** | Values used for CDR3 amino acid properties calculation.

| Amino acid | Mjenergy | Kf4 | Volume | Strength |
|---|---|---|---|---|
| A | −2.8455 | −0.27 | 67 | 0 |
| C | −3.782 | −1.05 | 86 | 0 |
| D | −2.116 | 0.81 | 91 | 0 |
| E | −2.141 | 1.17 | 109 | 0 |
| F | −5.017 | −1.43 | 135 | 1 |
| G | −2.499 | −0.16 | 48 | 0 |
| H | −2.927 | 0.28 | 118 | 0 |
| I | −4.641 | −0.77 | 124 | 1 |
| K | −1.789 | 1.7 | 135 | 0 |
| L | −5.023 | −1.1 | 124 | 1 |
| M | −4.1915 | −0.73 | 124 | 1 |
| N | −2.349 | 0.81 | 96 | 0 |
| P | −2.443 | −0.75 | 90 | 0 |
| Q | −2.2505 | 1.1 | 114 | 0 |
| R | −2.402 | 1.87 | 148 | 0 |
| S | −2.308 | 0.42 | 73 | 0 |
| T | −2.6145 | 0.63 | 93 | 0 |
| V | −4.093 | −0.4 | 105 | 1 |
| W | −4.1375 | −1.57 | 163 | 1 |
| Y | −3.7505 | −0.56 | 141 | 1 |

### Differences in Immunoglobulin Clonal Lineage Structure

The analysis of antibody repertoires can be extended by grouping IGH clonotypes into clonal lineages (trees) that share a common ancestor (57) and represent a B-cell clone undergoing the affinity maturation process. UMI-based full-length immunoglobulin sequencing (44) and dedicated antibody tree building algorithm (see section Methods) allowed us to accurately infer and analyze clonal lineage structure.

This analysis revealed that basic graph characteristics, such as the Gini inequality coefficient, and number of singletons (clones including only one clonotype) were significantly different between young and middle-age YF-vaccinated donors (**Figure 3A**). The Gini coefficient measures the inequality of tree size (number of nodes) distribution. Large Gini coefficient values mean that large trees with many mutated variants dominate over small trees, i.e., most of the observed immunoglobulin variants come from few B-cell clones. Smaller values mean that more distinct clones enter the affinity maturation process during an immune response. Thus the direction of the observed differences suggests that young individuals have a more diversified responding repertoire, while middle-age individuals display a more biased lineage architecture with larger trees that account for the majority of observed clonotypes (**Figures 3B,C**).

Note that the trees may include impossible lineage relations such as IgA to IgM isotype conversion. This reflects the fact that our analysis is limited by sampling depth and particular time point. We do not observe the whole pre-history of hypermutation process, thus additional unseen IGH sequence variants that can

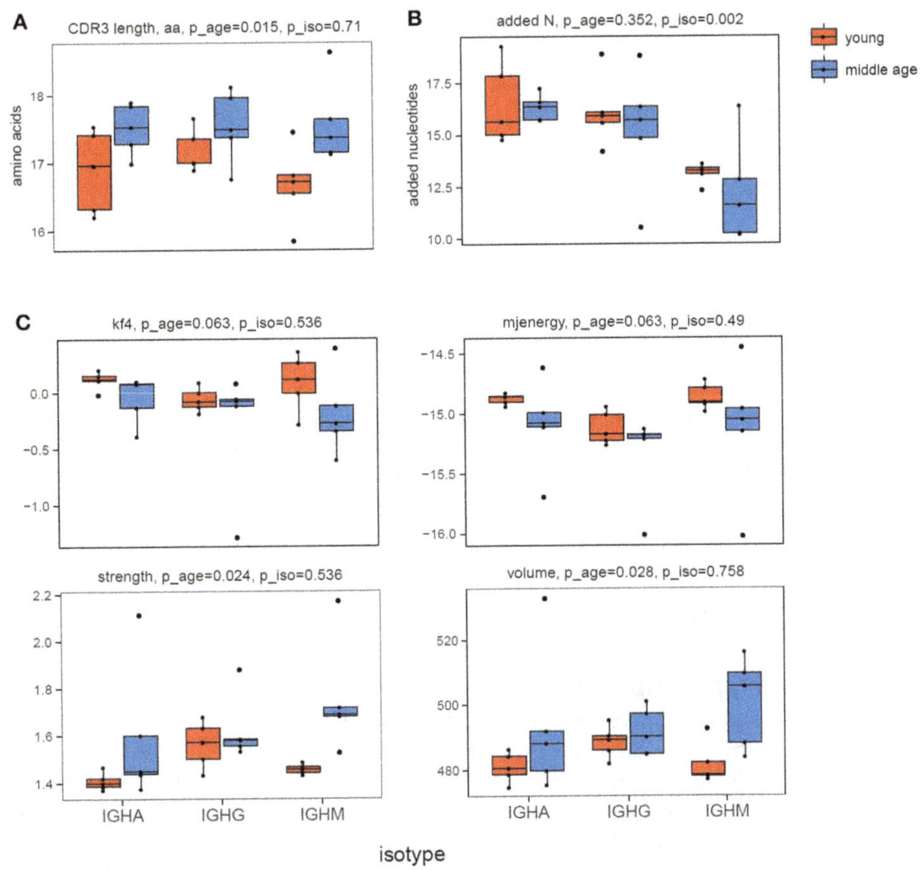


**FIGURE 1 |** CDR3 characteristics. **(A)** CDR3 length, aa. **(B)** Number of non-template added N nucleotides within V-D-J junction. **(C)** Physicochemical properties for the 5 amino acids residues in the middle of CDR3: Kidera factor 4 (hydrophobicity, lower values refer to more hydrophobic amino acids), potential "energy" of interaction (49) (lower values refer to stronger interaction), "strength" and "volume." All characteristics were calculated "weighted"—i.e., accounting for IGH clonotype size. ANOVA *p*-values for age and for isotype adjusted using Benjamini & Hochberg correction are shown on top of each plot.

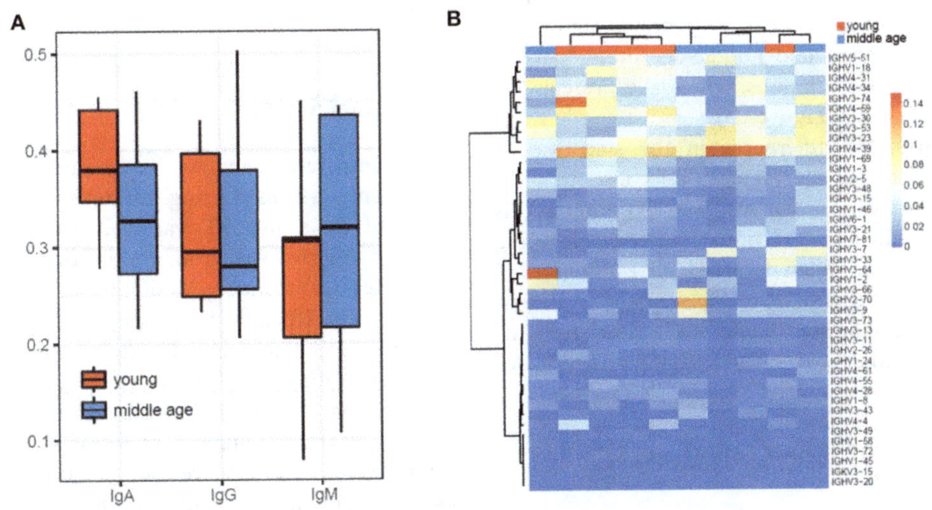


**FIGURE 2 |** Isotype and IGHV segments usage for YF-vaccinated subjects from the two age groups. **(A)** Isotype usage. **(B)** IGHV usage.

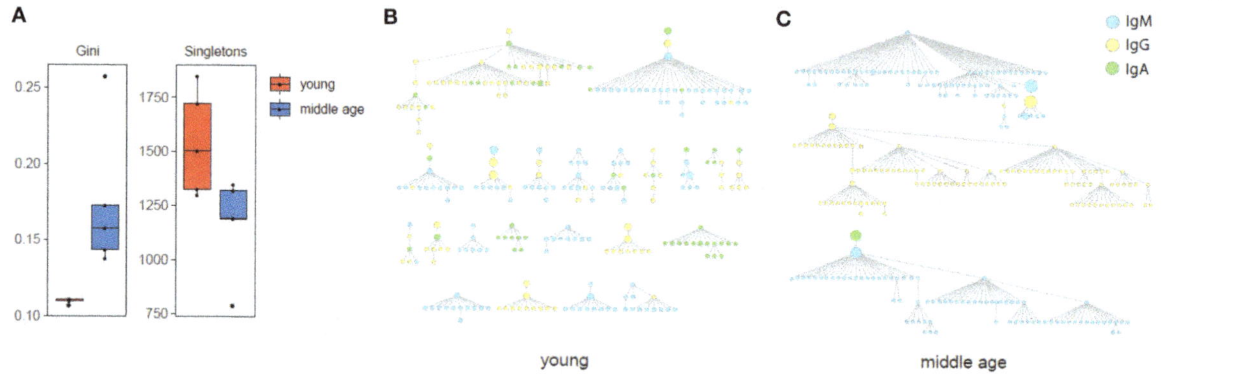


**FIGURE 3 |** Antibody lineage analysis. **(A)** Diversity of antibody lineages: Gini inequality coefficient for the number of nodes (clonotypes) in a tree (clone), and number of "trees" that include only one node. Both parameters are significantly different ($p < 0.05$) between young and middle-age donors. Two-tailed *T*-test, *p*-values adjusted using Benjamini & Hochberg method. **(B,C)** Top IGH trees by size containing equal number of 270 nodes for united data of all young **(B)** and middle-age **(C)** individuals are shown.

resolve this ambiguity may exist, e.g., unseen IgM sequence variant parent to observed IgM and IgA variants.

## Bulk Analysis of Somatic Hypermutations

Bulk load of somatic hypermutations per clonotype obtained without using the information on the trees structure was comparable between young and middle-age plasma cell IGH repertoires (**Figure 4A**). We controlled for isotype which is necessary in such comparisons as there are substantial differences between base mutation burden for each isotype (e.g., mean number of SHMs in an IgG clonotype is about 2 times higher than per IgM clonotype).

In order to estimate the burden of somatic hypermutations that could earlier accumulate within memory B cells clones currently participating in immune response, we analyzed the frequency of hypermutations within the identified roots of the trees—the IGH sequence variants that were closets to germline within each tree. This analysis also has not revealed significant differences between the young and middle-age individuals in a load of root somatic hypermutations, potentially pre-existing within responding IGH clones (**Figure 4B**).

To test for the intrinsic differences in the structure of hypermutations, we estimated the average "selection strength" that drived the accumulation of somatic hypermutations in young versus middle-age individual repertoires using BASELINe framework (50), which is based on estimation of expected versus observed frequencies of replacement and silent mutations. This analysis indicated higher "selection strength" in the young versus middle-age individual IGH repertoires (**Figure 4C**).

## Observed History of Ongoing Somatic Hypermutations

Finally, we focused on the newly generated mutations that are directly observed (identified in the edges of the trees), i.e., hypermutations that are supported by both observed "parent" and "child" clonotypes in the dataset. A dedicated tree building algorithm allowed us to infer the set of currently ongoing hypermutations on the entire length of the immunoglobulin sequence (**Figure 5A**). Note that in the full length analysis of clonal IGH evolution, we are able to identify all hypermutations that occurred within V gene segment, by comparing with the germline. For CDR3 region, we are only able to identify those mutations that differentiate the evolving clones from the identified root. We cannot determine the exact original CDR3 sequence that was generated during IGH recombination and thus cannot identify the hypermutations that have not been sampled by our analysis. This explains the lower proportion of hypermutations observed with CDR3 compared to CDR1 and CDR2 regions.

Middle-age individuals had higher total numbers of the newly acquired unique somatic hypermutations (**Figure 5B**), while the replacement-to-silent (R:S) ratio among such hypermutations was significantly lower compared to the young donors (**Figures 5C,D**).

## DISCUSSION

Our comparative analysis of immune response to a novel pathogen, performed using immune repertoire sequencing and modeled by a live YF vaccine, revealed several differences between the two age groups indicating that humoral adaptive response already undergoes significant changes by the age of 50.

First, physicochemical properties of the hypervariable IGH CDR3 region that are linked to antigen recognition (58, 59) changed significantly (**Figure 1**). Differences in the interaction "energy," Kidera factor 4, "strength" and "volume" indicate the increase of relative number of bulky, hydrophobic and strongly interacting amino acid residues in the middle of CDR3 with aging, potentially associated with increased cross-reactivity (60). In agreement with Wu et al. (43), responding repertoire of the middle-age donors also displayed longer CDR3s.

Second, the analysis of clonal lineages suggests that young individuals produce a more diverse IGH repertoire implying

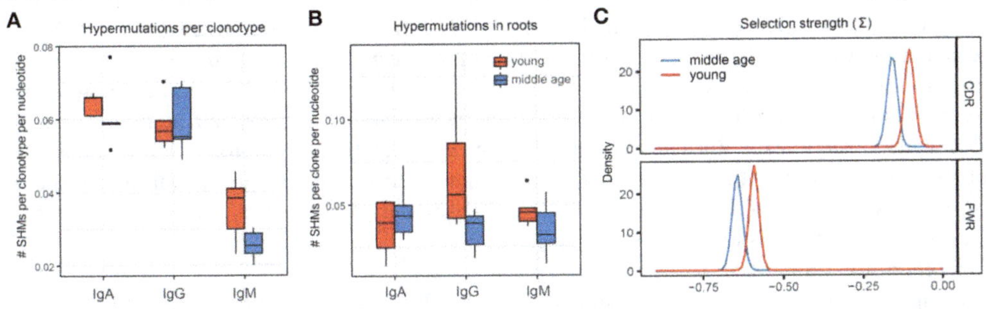


**FIGURE 4 |** Bulk analysis of somatic hypermutations. **(A)** Somatic hypermutations per clonotype, without using trees information (NS, ANOVA). **(B)** Somatic hypermutations within roots of the trees with >2 nodes (NS, ANOVA). **(C)** Selection strength estimated using BASELINe framework. Adjusted $p = 0.011$ for CDR, 0.011 for FWR.

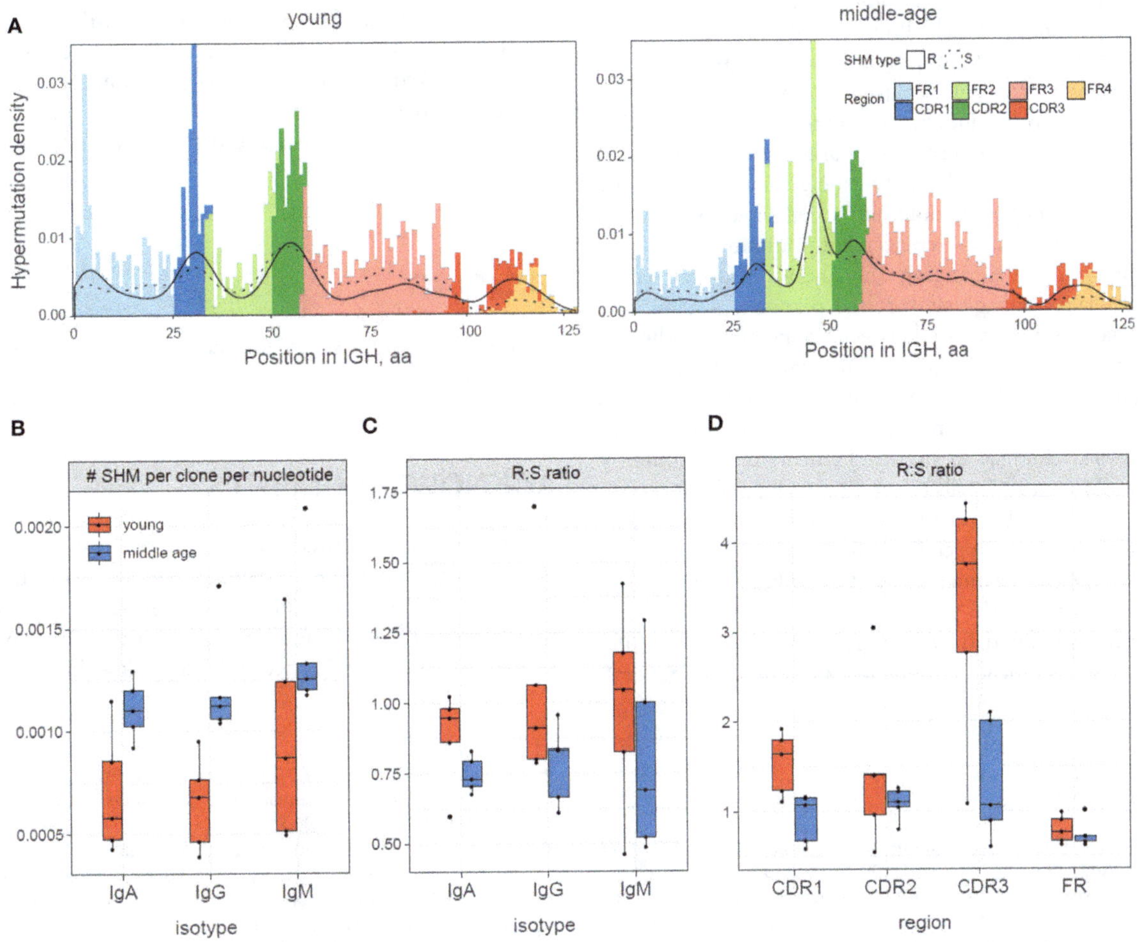


**FIGURE 5 |** Patterns of newly acquired somatic hypermutations in young and middle-age donors vaccinated with YF. **(A)** Summary profile of somatic hypermutations observed in the study. IGH regions are marked with color. The distribution of silent (S) and replacement (R) hypermutations are shown with dashed and solid lines, respectively. For CDR3 region, mutation analysis was done using the root as reference. Data were pooled for all young and all middle-age individuals. **(B)** Frequency of newly acquired somatic hypermutations (SHMs) in young (red) and middle-age (blue) donors. ANOVA $p = 0.0005$ for age, 0.14 for isotype. **(C,D)** Mean replacement:silent ratio (R:S ratio) for newly acquired somatic hypermutations (SHMs) in young and middle-age donors, for isotypes (**C**, ANOVA $p = 0.058$ for age, 0.69 for isotype) and regions (**D**, ANOVA $p =$ 0.0013 for age, 0.00014 for regions).

higher efficiency of the adaptive immune response (61). Middle-age individuals responded to YF vaccination with higher proportion of clonal hypermutating B cell trees of a larger size (**Figure 3**), which echoes the observation that elderly individuals have generally decreased numbers of B-cell lineages (25). Older individuals responded with lower lineage diversity, for which general decrease of B cell diversity with aging, correlating with the health status, could be one of the reasons (6, 62). While the exact reason behind the observed differences in the structure of IGH repertoire responding to novel antigens in young and middle-age individuals is unknown, one can speculate that they could be attributed to overall decrease in circulating B cells (63, 64), including memory B cells that initially recognized unrelated antigens but could respond to YF vaccination, decreased production and counts of naive B-cells (65, 66) and their diminished ability to enter somatic hypermutation (66, 67). All these factors narrow the capability of B cell immunity to select novel immunoglobulin variants.

Third, responding clonal lineages of the middle-age individuals hypermutated more intensely (**Figure 5B**) but less efficiently in terms of replacement-to-silent mutations ratio compared to young individuals (**Figures 4C, 5C,D**). The latter result overlaps with previous works, which show that loss of functional repertoire diversity is determined by not only the reducing the number of different B cell lineages but also by decreased proportion of replacement mutations (68) and mutations prominently changing the amino acid properties (32). This observation suggests that the parameters of affinity maturation may essentially vary between young and middle-age individuals, and is in line with previous works demonstrating impaired ability to produce high affinity protective antibodies against newly encountered antigens in the older individuals (13), and general changes in the mechanisms of IGH affinity maturation and memory B cells generation with aging (66).

Of note, it was earlier demonstrated that AID levels and intensity of hypermutation decrease with aging, but only after the age of 60 (63, 69, 70)—beyond the age of the cohorts that we have studied in the current work.

We have not obtained data on serum titers of YF-specific antibodies due to technical unavailability of samples. In general, it is known that the serum titers are similar for these age groups (71, 72), and are sufficiently high to provide protection for many years: (73). Thus the observed differences in the B cell response to the live YF vaccine between young and middle-age individuals are not detrimental for generation of protective immunoglobulin repertoire. However, these differences reveal the dynamics of changes in humoral response architecture that are already detectable by the age of 50 years.

Further studies involving a larger set of novel antigens and comprehensive longitudinal tracking of the response, as well as studies of vaccinations with vaccine boost, can shed more light on the fine properties of age-related changes in B cell response.

## AUTHOR CONTRIBUTIONS

DS and GS performed cell sorting. AD, AO, ML, and MS analyzed the data. AO, MS, and DC prepared the figures. ML, MT, EM, and OK worked on samples, library preparation, and sequencing. OB and DC designed and managed the entire study. MS and DC wrote the manuscript. All authors reviewed and approved the final manuscript.

## FUNDING

This work was funded by Russian Science Foundation Project 14-14-00533.

## ACKNOWLEDGMENTS

Cell sorting experiments were carried out using the equipment provided by the IBCH core facility (CKP IBCH, supported by Russian Ministry of Education and Science, grant RFMEFI62117X0018). Funding for open access publication: Skolkovo Institute of Science and Technology internal funding.

## REFERENCES

1. Castelo-Branco C, Soveral I. The immune system and aging: a review. *Gynecol Endocrinol.* (2014) 30:16–22. doi: 10.3109/09513590.2013.852531
2. DelaRosa O, Pawelec G, Peralbo E, Wikby A, Mariani E, Mocchegiani E, et al. Immunological biomarkers of ageing in man: changes in both innate and adaptive immunity are associated with health and longevity. *Biogerontology* (2006) 7:471–81. doi: 10.1007/s10522-006-9062-6
3. Nikolich-Zugich J. Aging of the T cell compartment in mice and humans: from no naive expectations to foggy memories. *J Immunol.* (2014) 193:2622–9. doi: 10.4049/jimmunol.1401174
4. Goronzy JJ, Fang F, Cavanagh MM, Qi Q, Weyand CM. Naive T cell maintenance and function in human aging. *J Immunol.* (2015) 194:4073–80. doi: 10.4049/jimmunol.1500046
5. Britanova OV, Shugay M, Merzlyak EM, Staroverov DB, Putintseva EV, Turchaninova MA, et al. Dynamics of individual T cell repertoires: from cord blood to centenarians. *J Immunol.* (2016) 196:5005–13. doi: 10.4049/jimmunol.1600005
6. Gibson KL, Wu YC, Barnett Y, Duggan O, Vaughan R, Kondeatis E, et al. B-cell diversity decreases in old age and is correlated with poor health status. *Aging Cell* (2009) 8:18–25. doi: 10.1111/j.1474-9726.2008.00443.x
7. Dunn-Walters DK. The ageing human B cell repertoire: a failure of selection? *Clin Exp Immunol.* (2016) 183:50–6. doi: 10.1111/cei.12700
8. Martin V, Bryan Wu YC, Kipling D, Dunn-Walters D. Ageing of the B-cell repertoire. *Philos Trans R Soc Lond B Biol Sci.* (2015) 370:20140237. doi: 10.1098/rstb.2014.0237
9. Goodwin K, Viboud C, Simonsen L. Antibody response to influenza vaccination in the elderly: a quantitative review. *Vaccine* (2006) 24:1159–69. doi: 10.1016/j.vaccine.2005.08.105
10. Aspinall R, Del Giudice G, Effros RB, Grubeck-Loebenstein B, Sambhara S. Challenges for vaccination in the elderly. *Immun Ageing* (2007) 4:9. doi: 10.1186/1742-4933-4-9

11. Frasca D, Diaz A, Romero M, Landin AM, Blomberg BB. *Cytomegalovirus* (CMV) seropositivity decreases B cell responses to the influenza vaccine. *Vaccine* (2015) 33:1433–9. doi: 10.1016/j.vaccine.2015.01.071
12. Frasca D, Diaz A, Romero M, Mendez NV, Landin AM, Blomberg BB. Effects of age on H1N1-specific serum IgG1 and IgG3 levels evaluated during the 2011-2012 influenza vaccine season. *Immun Age* (2013) 10:14. doi: 10.1186/1742-4933-10-14
13. Pinti M, Appay V, Campisi J, Frasca D, Fulop T, Sauce D, et al. Aging of the immune system: focus on inflammation and vaccination. *Eur J Immunol.* (2016) 46:2286–301. doi: 10.1002/eji.201546178
14. Park S, Nahm MH. Older adults have a low capacity to opsonize pneumococci due to low IgM antibody response to pneumococcal vaccinations. *Infect Immun.* (2011) 79:314–20. doi: 10.1128/IAI.00768-10
15. Siegrist CA, Aspinall R. B-cell responses to vaccination at the extremes of age. *Nat Rev Immunol.* (2009) 9:185–94. doi: 10.1038/nri2508
16. Del Giudice G, Weinberger B, Grubeck-Loebenstein B. Vaccines for the elderly. *Gerontology* (2015) 61:203–10. doi: 10.1159/000366162
17. Shelly MA, Jacoby H, Riley GJ, Graves BT, Pichichero M, Treanor JJ. Comparison of pneumococcal polysaccharide and CRM197-conjugated pneumococcal oligosaccharide vaccines in young and elderly adults. *Infect Immun.* (1997) 65:242–7.
18. Romero-Steiner S, Musher DM, Cetron MS, Pais LB, Groover JE, Fiore AE, et al. Reduction in functional antibody activity against Streptococcus pneumoniae in vaccinated elderly individuals highly correlates with decreased IgG antibody avidity. *Clin Infect Dis.* (1999) 29:281–8. doi: 10.1086/520200
19. Wolters B, Junge U, Dziuba S, Roggendorf M. Immunogenicity of combined hepatitis A and B vaccine in elderly persons. *Vaccine* (2003) 21:3623–8. doi: 10.1016/S0264-410X(03)00399-2
20. Shi Y, Yamazaki T, Okubo Y, Uehara Y, Sugane K, Agematsu K. Regulation of aged humoral immune defense against pneumococcal bacteria by IgM memory B cell. *J Immunol.* (2005) 175:3262–7. doi: 10.4049/jimmunol.175.5.3262
21. Kaml M, Weiskirchner I, Keller M, Luft T, Hoster E, Hasford J, et al. Booster vaccination in the elderly: their success depends on the vaccine type applied earlier in life as well as on pre-vaccination antibody titers. *Vaccine* (2006) 24:6808–11. doi: 10.1016/j.vaccine.2006.06.037
22. Schenkein JG, Park S, Nahm MH. Pneumococcal vaccination in older adults induces antibodies with low opsonic capacity and reduced antibody potency. *Vaccine* (2008) 26:5521–6. doi: 10.1016/j.vaccine.2008.07.071
23. Lord JM. The effect of ageing of the immune system on vaccination responses. *Hum Vaccin Immunother.* (2013) 9:1364–7. doi: 10.4161/hv.24696
24. Vollmers C, Sit RV, Weinstein JA, Dekker CL, Quake SR. Genetic measurement of memory B-cell recall using antibody repertoire sequencing. *Proc Natl Acad Sci USA.* (2013) 110:13463–8. doi: 10.1073/pnas.1312146110
25. Jiang N, He J, Weinstein JA, Penland L, Sasaki S, He XS, et al. Lineage structure of the human antibody repertoire in response to influenza vaccination. *Sci Transl Med.* (2013) 5:171ra119. doi: 10.1126/scitranslmed.3004794
26. Greiff V, Menzel U, Haessler U, Cook SC, Friedensohn S, Khan TA, et al. Quantitative assessment of the robustness of next-generation sequencing of antibody variable gene repertoires from immunized mice. *BMC Immunol.* (2014) 15:40. doi: 10.1186/s12865-014-0040-5
27. Laserson U, Vigneault F, Gadala-Maria D, Yaari G, Uduman M, Vander Heiden JA, et al. High-resolution antibody dynamics of vaccine-induced immune responses. *Proc Natl Acad Sci USA.* (2014) 111:4928–33. doi: 10.1073/pnas.1323862111
28. Kaplinsky J, Li A, Sun A, Coffre M, Koralov SB, Arnaout R. Antibody repertoire deep sequencing reveals antigen-independent selection in maturing B cells. *Proc Natl Acad Sci USA.* (2014) 111:E2622–9. doi: 10.1073/pnas.1403278111
29. Georgiou G, Ippolito GC, Beausang J, Busse CE, Wardemann H, Quake SR. The promise and challenge of high-throughput sequencing of the antibody repertoire. *Nat Biotechnol.* (2014) 32:158–68. doi: 10.1038/nbt.2782
30. Friedensohn S, Khan TA, Reddy ST. Advanced methodologies in high-throughput sequencing of immune repertoires. *Trends Biotechnol.* (2017) 35:203–14. doi: 10.1016/j.tibtech.2016.09.010
31. Wang C, Liu Y, Xu LT, Jackson KJ, Roskin KM, Pham TD, et al. Effects of aging, *Cytomegalovirus* infection, and EBV infection on human B cell repertoires. *J Immunol.* (2014) 192:603–11. doi: 10.4049/jimmunol.1301384
32. de Bourcy CF, Angel CJ, Vollmers C, Dekker CL, Davis MM, Quake SR. Phylogenetic analysis of the human antibody repertoire reveals quantitative signatures of immune senescence and aging. *Proc Natl Acad Sci USA.* (2017) 114:1105–10. doi: 10.1073/pnas.1617959114
33. Miles JJ, Silins SL, Brooks AG, Davis JE, Misko I, Burrows SR. T-cell grit: large clonal expansions of virus-specific CD8+ T cells can dominate in the peripheral circulation for at least 18 years. *Blood* (2005) 106:4412–3. doi: 10.1182/blood-2005-06-2261
34. Fulop T, Larbi A, Pawelec G. Human T cell aging and the impact of persistent viral infections. *Front Immunol.* (2013) 4:271. doi: 10.3389/fimmu.2013.00271
35. Qi Q, Liu Y, Cheng Y, Glanville J, Zhang D, Lee JY, et al. Diversity and clonal selection in the human T-cell repertoire. *Proc Natl Acad Sci USA.* (2014) 111:13139–44. doi: 10.1073/pnas.1409155111
36. Goronzy JJ, Fulbright JW, Crowson CS, Poland GA, O'Fallon WM, Weyand CM. Value of immunological markers in predicting responsiveness to influenza vaccination in elderly individuals. *J Virol.* (2001) 75:12182–7. doi: 10.1128/JVI.75.24.12182-12187.2001
37. Lavinder JJ, Wine Y, Giesecke C, Ippolito GC, Horton AP, Lungu OI, et al. Identification and characterization of the constituent human serum antibodies elicited by vaccination. *Proc Natl Acad Sci USA.* (2014) 111:2259–64. doi: 10.1073/pnas.1317793111
38. Galson JD, Truck J, Fowler A, Clutterbuck EA, Munz M, Cerundolo V, et al. Analysis of B cell repertoire dynamics following hepatitis B vaccination in humans, and enrichment of vaccine-specific antibody sequences. *EBioMedicine* (2015) 2:2070–9. doi: 10.1016/j.ebiom.2015.11.034
39. Galson JD, Truck J, Clutterbuck EA, Fowler A, Cerundolo V, Pollard AJ, et al. B-cell repertoire dynamics after sequential hepatitis B vaccination and evidence for cross-reactive B-cell activation. *Genome Med.* (2016) 8:68. doi: 10.1186/s13073-016-0322-z
40. Blanchard-Rohner G, Pulickal AS, Jol-van der Zijde CM, Snape MD, Pollard AJ. Appearance of peripheral blood plasma cells and memory B cells in a primary and secondary immune response in humans. *Blood* (2009) 114:4998–5002. doi: 10.1182/blood-2009-03-211052
41. Jackson KJ, Liu Y, Roskin KM, Glanville J, Hoh RA, Seo K, et al. Human responses to influenza vaccination show seroconversion signatures and convergent antibody rearrangements. *Cell Host Microbe* (2014) 16:105–14. doi: 10.1016/j.chom.2014.05.013
42. Truck J, Ramasamy MN, Galson JD, Rance R, Parkhill J, Lunter G, et al. Identification of antigen-specific B cell receptor sequences using public repertoire analysis. *J Immunol.* (2015) 194:252–61. doi: 10.4049/jimmunol.1401405
43. Wu YC, Kipling D, Dunn-Walters DK. Age-related changes in human peripheral blood IGH repertoire following vaccination. *Front Immunol.* (2012) 3:193. doi: 10.3389/fimmu.2012.00193
44. Turchaninova MA, Davydov A, Britanova OV, Shugay M, Bikos V, Egorov ES, et al. High-quality full-length immunoglobulin profiling with unique molecular barcoding. *Nat Protoc.* (2016) 11:1599–616. doi: 10.1038/nprot.2016.093
45. Shugay M, Britanova OV, Merzlyak EM, Turchaninova MA, Mamedov IZ, Tuganbaev TR, et al. Towards error-free profiling of immune repertoires. *Nat Methods* (2014) 11:653–5. doi: 10.1038/nmeth.2960
46. Khan TA, Friedensohn S, de Vries AR, Straszewski J, Ruscheweyh HJ, Reddy ST. Accurate and predictive antibody repertoire profiling by molecular amplification fingerprinting. *Sci Adv.* (2016) 2:e1501371. doi: 10.1126/sciadv.1501371
47. Shugay M, Zaretsky AR, Shagin DA, Shagina IA, Volchenkov IA, Shelenkov AA, et al. MAGERI. Computational pipeline for molecular-barcoded targeted resequencing. *PLoS Comput Biol.* (2017) 13:e1005480. doi: 10.1371/journal.pcbi.1005480
48. Wrammert J, Smith K, Miller J, Langley WA, Kokko K, Larsen C, et al. Rapid cloning of high-affinity human monoclonal antibodies against influenza virus. *Nature* (2008) 453:667–71. doi: 10.1038/nature06890
49. Miyazawa S, Jernigan RL. Residue-residue potentials with a favorable contact pair term and an unfavorable high packing density term, for simulation and threading. *J Mol Biol.* (1996) 256:623–44. doi: 10.1006/jmbi.1996.0114
50. Yaari G, Uduman M, Kleinstein SH. Quantifying selection in high-throughput Immunoglobulin sequencing data sets. *Nucleic Acids Res.* (2012) 40:e134. doi: 10.1093/nar/gks457

51. Gupta NT, Vander Heiden JA, Uduman M, Gadala-Maria D, Yaari G, Kleinstein SH. Change-O: a toolkit for analyzing large-scale B cell immunoglobulin repertoire sequencing data. *Bioinformatics* (2015) 31:3356–8. doi: 10.1093/bioinformatics/btv359
52. Egorov ES, Kasatskaya SA, Zubov VN, Izraelson M, Nakonechnaya TO, Staroverov DB, et al. The changing landscape of naive T cell receptor repertoire with human aging. *Front Immunol.* (2018) 9:1618. doi: 10.3389/fimmu.2018.01618
53. Shugay M, Bagaev DV, Turchaninova MA, Bolotin DA, Britanova OV, Putintseva EV, et al. VDJtools: unifying post-analysis of T cell receptor repertoires. *PLoS Comput Biol.* (2015) 11:e1004503. doi: 10.1371/journal.pcbi.1004503
54. Kidera A, Konishi Y, Oka M. Statistical analysis of the physical properties of the 20 naturally occurring amino acids. *J Protein Chem.* (1985) 4:23–55. doi: 10.1007/BF01025492
55. Rackovsky S. Global characteristics of protein sequences and their implications. *Proc Natl Acad Sci USA.* (2010) 107:8623–6. doi: 10.1073/pnas.1001299107
56. Peng HP, Lee KH, Jian JW, Yang AS. Origins of specificity and affinity in antibody-protein interactions. *Proc Natl Acad Sci USA.* (2014) 111:E2656–65. doi: 10.1073/pnas.1401131111
57. Barak M, Zuckerman NS, Edelman H, Unger R, Mehr R. IgTree: creating Immunoglobulin variable region gene lineage trees. *J Immunol Methods* (2008) 338:67–74. doi: 10.1016/j.jim.2008.06.006
58. Sela-Culang I, Kunik V, Ofran Y. The structural basis of antibody-antigen recognition. *Front Immunol.* (2013) 4:302. doi: 10.3389/fimmu.2013.00302
59. Laffy JMJ, Dodev T, Macpherson JA, Townsend C, Lu HC, Dunn-Walters D, et al. Promiscuous antibodies characterised by their physico-chemical properties: from sequence to structure and back. *Prog Biophys Mol Biol.* (2017) 128:47–56. doi: 10.1016/j.pbiomolbio.2016.09.002
60. Padlan EA. Anatomy of the antibody molecule. *Mol Immunol.* (1994) 31:169–217. doi: 10.1016/0161-5890(94)90001-9
61. Tas JM, Mesin L, Pasqual G, Targ S, Jacobsen JT, Mano YM, et al. Visualizing antibody affinity maturation in germinal centers. *Science* (2016) 351:1048–54. doi: 10.1126/science.aad3439
62. Tabibian-Keissar H, Hazanov L, Schiby G, Rosenthal N, Rakovsky A, Michaeli M, et al. Aging affects B-cell antigen receptor repertoire diversity in primary and secondary lymphoid tissues. *Eur J Immunol.* (2016) 46:480–92. doi: 10.1002/eji.201545586
63. Frasca D, Landin AM, Lechner SC, Ryan JG, Schwartz R, Riley RL, et al. Aging down-regulates the transcription factor E2A, activation-induced cytidine deaminase, and Ig class switch in human B cells. *J Immunol.* (2008) 180:5283–90. doi: 10.4049/jimmunol.180.8.5283
64. Bulati M, Caruso C, Colonna-Romano G. From lymphopoiesis to plasma cells differentiation, the age-related modifications of B cell compartment are influenced by "inflamm-ageing." *Ageing Res Rev.* (2017) 36:125–36. doi: 10.1016/j.arr.2017.04.001
65. Labrie JE III, Borghesi L, Gerstein RM. Bone marrow microenvironmental changes in aged mice compromise V(D)J recombinase activity and B cell generation. *Semin Immunol.* (2005) 17:347–55. doi: 10.1016/j.smim.2005.05.012
66. Frasca D, Diaz A, Romero M, Landin AM, Blomberg BB. Age effects on B cells and humoral immunity in humans. *Ageing Res Rev.* (2011) 10:330–5. doi: 10.1016/j.arr.2010.08.004
67. Banerjee M, Mehr R, Belelovsky A, Spencer J, Dunn-Walters DK. Age- and tissue-specific differences in human germinal center B cell selection revealed by analysis of IgVH gene hypermutation and lineage trees. *Eur J Immunol.* (2002) 32:1947–57. doi: 10.1002/1521-4141(200207)32:7<1947::AID-IMMU1947>3.0.CO;2-1
68. Troutaud D, Drouet M, Decourt C, Le Morvan C, Cogne M. Age-related alterations of somatic hypermutation and CDR3 lengths in human Vkappa4-expressing B lymphocytes. *Immunology* (1999) 97:197–203. doi: 10.1046/j.1365-2567.1999.00779.x
69. Khurana S, Frasca D, Blomberg B, Golding H. AID activity in B cells strongly correlates with polyclonal antibody affinity maturation *in-vivo* following pandemic 2009-H1N1 vaccination in humans. *PLoS Pathog* (2012) 8:e1002920. doi: 10.1371/journal.ppat.1002920
70. Frasca D, Diaz A, Romero M, Phillips M, Mendez NV, Landin AM, et al. Unique biomarkers for B-cell function predict the serum response to pandemic H1N1 influenza vaccine. *Int Immunol.* (2012) 24:175–82. doi: 10.1093/intimm/dxr123
71. Miyaji KT, Avelino-Silva VI, Simoes M, Freire MD, Medeiros CR, Braga PE, et al. Prevalence and titers of yellow fever virus neutralizing antibodies in previously vaccinated adults. *Rev Inst Med Trop Sao Paulo* (2017) 59:e2. doi: 10.1590/s1678-9946201759002
72. Vratskikh O, Stiasny K, Zlatkovic J, Tsouchnikas G, Jarmer J, Karrer U, et al. Dissection of antibody specificities induced by yellow fever vaccination. *PLoS Pathog.* (2013) 9:e1003458. doi: 10.1371/journal.ppat.1003458
73. Collaborative group for studies on yellow fever vaccines. Duration of post-vaccination immunity against yellow fever in adults. *Vaccine* (2014) 32:4977–84. doi: 10.1016/j.vaccine.2014.07.021

# 16

# Computer Simulation of Multi-Color Brainbow Staining and Clonal Evolution of B Cells in Germinal Centers

*Michael Meyer-Hermann*[1,2,3*†], *Sebastian C. Binder*[1,2], *Luka Mesin*[4] *and Gabriel D. Victora*[4]

*[1] Department of Systems Immunology, Braunschweig Integrated Centre of Systems Biology, Helmholtz Centre for Infection Research, Braunschweig, Germany, [2] Institute for Biochemistry, Biotechnology and Bioinformatics, Technische Universität Braunschweig, Braunschweig, Germany, [3] Centre for Individualised Infection Medicine, Hanover, Germany, [4] Laboratory of Lymphocyte Dynamics, The Rockefeller University, New York, NY, United States*

***Correspondence:**
*Michael Meyer-Hermann*
*mmh@theoretical-biology.de*

*† The author share first and senior authorship*

Clonal evolution of B cells in germinal centers (GCs) is central to affinity maturation of antibodies in response to pathogens. Permanent or tamoxifen-induced multi-color recombination of B cells based on the brainbow allele allows monitoring the degree of color dominance in the course of the GC reaction. Here, we use computer simulations of GC reactions in order to replicate the evolution of color dominance *in silico* and to define rules for the interpretation of these data in terms of clonal dominance. We find that a large diversity of clonal dominance is generated in simulated GCs in agreement with experimental results. In the extremes, a GC can be dominated by a single clone or can harbor many co-existing clones. These properties can be directly derived from the measurement of color dominance when all B cells are stained before the GC onset. Upon tamoxifen-induced staining, the correlation between clonal structure and color dominance depends on the timing and duration of the staining procedure as well as on the total number of stained B cells. B cells can be stained with 4 colors if a single brainbow allele is used, using both alleles leads to 10 different colors. The advantage of staining with 10 instead of 4 colors becomes relevant only when the 10 colors are attributed with rather similar probability. Otherwise, 4 colors exhibit a comparable predictive power. These results can serve as a guideline for future experiments based on multi-color staining of evolving systems.

**Keywords: germinal center, multiphoton imaging, sequencing, clonal selection, brainbow, computer simulation, mathematical modeling**

## 1. INTRODUCTION

Permanent multi-color recombination of cells allows monitoring the fate of the stained cells. Cre-dependent recombination of colors based on the Brainbow fluorescent protein reporter construct was applied in the past years to the nervous system (1–4) and to developmental biology (5, 6). As the adopted color is transmitted to the progeny of the cell, this method not only allows to follow the fate of the stained cell itself but also to visualize cell division and the fate of the daughter cells. This particular property of the brainbow allele made it suitable for the study of evolutionary systems like the germinal center (GC) reaction (7), which is an important part of the acute immune response to pathogens (8, 9). While the full repertoire of GC B cells might be assessed in the future at particular time points by sequencing, the brainbow method can be used to monitor the evolution of BC clones in GCs over time (10).

GC reactions are central not only for the clearance of infections but also for generating immune memory. As such they form the basis for the success of vaccinations and are central to the prevention of diseases. The fundamental principle of a GC reaction is an evolutionary process on the scale of a few weeks inside the living organism in lymphoid organs. There, B cells divide and mutate (11) and subsequently undergo a selection process giving rise to high affinity antibodies in response to a pathogenic challenge. The emerging B cells encode a different antibody than their germline counterparts, with better binding properties to the pathogen. The GC reaction is also responsible for a diversification of the pool of antibodies ready to fight against the next infection.

The evolution of B cells in GCs is difficult to monitor. One possibility is sequencing of all B cells at different time points of the reaction (7, 12). Multi-color recombination of B cells bears information of the clonal evolution of the B cells and, thus, would allow us to learn about selection and diversification of B cells. Recent experiments using this approach suggested that B cells are not only optimized for high affinity to the pathogen, as widely accepted, but also for an optimal antibody diversity (7), which was also supported by modeling (13). Here, we analyse the predictive power of the measured color distributions for properties of the GC reaction like clonal dominance and diversification.

## 2. METHODS

The *in silico* GC reactions used as the backbone of the present analysis of B cell clonality is fully described in the **Supplementary Material**. The model architecture is a stochastic event generator with cellular agents in a three-dimensional discretized space. It is complemented by a reaction-diffusion system for chemokines, which are generated and sensed by cellular agents. In addition, each cellular B cell agent carries a position in a shape space, which reflects its similarity to the antibody, which binds optimally to the antigen in question. Somatic hypermutation is modeled as displacement in this shape space. All agents move according to published two-photon measurements. They interact according to the current state-of-the-art model of how GC B cell affinity maturation evolves. Events like movement, division, interaction, and selection are based on rate-derived probabilities per time step, unless stated otherwise (see **Supplementary Material**). Possible fates of B cells are apoptosis, differentiation to output cells, or recycling to the DZ phenotype (14, 15). The simulations reproduce the population kinetics, affinity maturation, and output cell production in agreement with experimental constraints.

The previously published model (16), was corrected by a substantially higher number of founder cells (7) and was extended by a dynamic-number of division (DND), which states that B cells receiving more signals from T follicular helper cells would divide more (16–18).

### 2.1. Increased Number of Founder Cells

By extrapolation from the number of different founder clones found by sequencing of randomly picked GC B cells to the real number of GC founder clones (7), the old picture of an oligoclonal GC (12, 19) was revised. Instead the number of founder clones was estimated in the range of 100 cells (7). The GC simulation (16) needs to be revised correspondingly. Following Meyer-Hermann and Binder and Meyer-Hermann, A continuous influx of new founder cells during the first days after GC onset is assumed (17, 20). Although influx rates of GC founder cells are currently unknown, in our model we assumed 2 cells per hour limited to the first 4 days of the GC reaction, which generated a number of founder cells consistent with Tas et al. (7). This value might also be estimated with a simple ODE model (see **Supplementary Information:** *B cell influx rate*).

### 2.2. Color Probabilities

The brainbow allele as implemented in the *Rosa26*$^{\text{Confetti}}$ allele (1) randomly tags cells with one of 4 different colors. Applying this to both alleles in GC B cells, stains the B cells with one of 10 different color combinations (7). Recombination can be induced prior to the GC reaction or by injection of tamoxifen. In order to simulate the color dynamics in GCs *in silico*, the probability of each color combination was determined as the mean over all GCs in AID-KO experiments, in which mutation and selection are suppressed in GCs (**Table 1**). The probabilities for 4 color stainings *in silico* were assumed. These values were used in all simulations unless stated otherwise.

### 2.3. Delayed Action of Tamoxifen

Injection of tamoxifen induces Cre-lox recombination of one or two alleles. The GC B cell then expresses one of ten possible

**TABLE 1** | Probabilities of staining B cells with one of either 4 or 10 colors.

| Color | 4 color | Tamoxifen | Founder |
|---|---|---|---|
| Black | 0.40 | $5.2\,10^{-1}$ | $1.1\,10^{-1}$ |
| YFP | 0.18 | $1.3\,10^{-1}$ | $1.7\,10^{-1}$ |
| RFP | 0.18 | $1.2\,10^{-1}$ | $1.7\,10^{-1}$ |
| CFP | 0.18 | $1.0\,10^{-1}$ | $1.7\,10^{-1}$ |
| GFP | 0.06 | $5.6\,10^{-2}$ | $5.1\,10^{-2}$ |
| C/R | – | $2.7\,10^{-2}$ | $8.0\,10^{-2}$ |
| C/Y | – | $1.6\,10^{-2}$ | $8.0\,10^{-2}$ |
| Y/R | – | $1.4\,10^{-2}$ | $2.8\,10^{-2}$ |
| G/R | – | $3.2\,10^{-3}$ | $8.0\,10^{-2}$ |
| C/G | – | $1.8\,10^{-3}$ | $2.8\,10^{-2}$ |
| G/Y | – | $1.0\,10^{-3}$ | $2.8\,10^{-2}$ |

*For 10 colors, the probabilities in tamoxifen-induced and founder cell staining experiments were distinguished and derived from AID-KO experiments [(7), renormalized to an amount of black of 52%]. Black denotes the probability of no staining. Values rounded to two digits.*

color combinations. Tamoxifen-activity continues for a finite time. An exponential decay of tamoxifen and, consequently, of the recombination probability was assumed *in silico*. The initial probability $p_{\mathrm{stain},0}$ of tamoxifen-induced recombination is not known. It was chosen such that the experimentally observed fraction of stained cells $f_{\mathrm{stained}}$, which is known from experiment (see **Table 1**, one minus black).

The initial probability of recombination $p_{\mathrm{stain},0}$ after injection of tamoxifen is estimated with the help of a simplifying model. Staining is initiated in the simulation in time steps $\Delta t_{\mathrm{stain}}$. With the tamoxifen decay time $\tau_{\mathrm{tamoxifen}}$, the fraction of stained cells can be approximated as:

$$f_{\mathrm{stained}} = \frac{p_{\mathrm{stain},0}}{\Delta t_{\mathrm{stain}}} \int_0^{\infty} \exp\left(-\frac{t}{\tau_{\mathrm{tamoxifen}}}\right) dt = \frac{p_{\mathrm{stain},0}}{\Delta t_{\mathrm{stain}}} \tau_{\mathrm{tamoxifen}} \,. \quad (1)$$

Note that this holds only for probabilities $p_{\mathrm{stain},0}$, sufficiently small such that double staining can be neglected.

For practical reasons, tamoxifen activity was stopped at time $\tau_{\mathrm{stainstop}}$. This modifies Equation (1) to

$$f_{\mathrm{stained}} = \frac{p_{\mathrm{stain},0}}{\Delta t_{\mathrm{stain}}} \int_0^{\tau_{\mathrm{stainstop}}} \exp\left(-\frac{t}{\tau_{\mathrm{tamoxifen}}}\right) dt = \frac{p_{\mathrm{stain},0}}{\Delta t_{\mathrm{stain}}} \tau_{\mathrm{tamoxifen}} \left(1 - \exp\left(-\frac{\tau_{\mathrm{stainstop}}}{\tau_{\mathrm{tamoxifen}}}\right)\right) . \quad (2)$$

This condition approximates the initial staining probability $p_{\mathrm{stain},0}$ to

$$\frac{p_{\mathrm{stain},0}}{\Delta t_{\mathrm{stain}}} = \frac{f_{\mathrm{stained}}}{\tau_{\mathrm{tamoxifen}} \left(1 - \exp\left(-\frac{\tau_{\mathrm{stainstop}}}{\tau_{\mathrm{tamoxifen}}}\right)\right)} . \quad (3)$$

This relation was used in the simulations in order to fix $p_{\mathrm{stain},0}$ with $\tau_{\mathrm{tamoxifen}} = 24$ h, $\tau_{\mathrm{stainstop}} = 2$ days, and $f_{\mathrm{stained}}$ equal to 1 minus black in **Table 1**. In order to save computation time in the simulations, the staining procedure is called with $\Delta t_{\mathrm{stain}} = 1$ h. In the simulations, a color is only attributed once to a cell, unless stated otherwise, i.e., in the case of an attempt to restain an already stained cell, this attempt is ignored.

## 3. RESULTS

### 3.1. Correlation of Clonal and Color Dominance

It is known that high affinity B cells emerge from the GC reaction in a process of cycles of mutation and selection. The dynamics of clonal selection and shift toward high affinity clones in the course of the reaction was recently analyzed with the help of random attribution of colors to either GC founder cells or to GC B cells in an early phase of the reaction (7). This allowed them to follow GC B cells of a particular color and was interpreted to provide information on the clonal evolution of GC B cells. In particular, the largest fraction of cells stained by a single color, short the *color dominance*, was considered as a measure of the *clonal dominance*, i.e., the largest fraction of GC cells that stem from a single clone (see **Table 2**). A clonal dominance of 100% would correspond to all GC B cells being derived from a single clone, which would be the result of strong selection of an advantageous clone. The smaller the clonal dominance, the more different B cell clones coexist in the same GC.

Here, we replicate these experiments *in silico*, and determine under which conditions the evolution of clonal and color dominance in GCs is correlated and delineate the limits of this correspondance as a guideline for future experiments. The analysis was restricted to the dominant color because, in our hands, the inclusion of the second most dominant color did not improve the results.

### 3.2. Staining of Founder Cells

In a setting in which B cells are stained before the GC reaction, most B cells entering the GC already carry a color (**Table 1** column *founder*). This corresponds to spontaneous recombination of B cells in the Mx1-Cre-mice in Tas et al. (7) and allows monitoring the clonal evolution inside GC reactions based on the evolution of color dominance. However, this relies on a good correlation between clonal and color dominance. We replicated the color dynamics *in silico* (**Figure 1A**). The color dominance starts from a baseline level, which is basically reflecting the probability distribution of getting the different colors (**Table 1**). Around day 5 post GC onset, GCs differ markedly in the fraction of cells expressing the dominant color, which is at the time after B cell expansion when the selection pressure on BCs is getting strong. The diversity of color dominance reaches a saturated level around day 8 post GC onset, which coincides with the time associated of take over of high affinity clones (21), and is kept by the end of the GC reaction.

In the simulations, full information on the clonal evolution is known as well, which puts us in the position to determine the degree of correlation between the color and the clonal dominance (**Figure 1B**). The correlation is sufficiently strong to allow for an association of clonal with color dominance. It was tested whether imposing a threshold staining level for each GC to be included in the analysis would change the correlation. The level of correlation was rather independent of this threshold (**Figure 1B**).

This correlation can be confirmed by the explicit comparison of the color and the clonal dominance (**Figures 1C,D**). During expansion at day 2 post GC onset, the B cells only divided and mutated but only underwent selection processes in rare cases. As a consequence, clonal dominance is rather low and color dominance reflects the staining probabilities. Both peaks are clearly seperated. Later at day 13 post GC onset when affinity maturation is accomplished, both distributions largely overlap. However, it can also be seen that the color dominance has the tendency to over-estimate the clonal dominance.

### 3.3. Tamoxifen-Induced Staining of Cells

Next, we investigated the attribution of colors to B cells at day 2 post GC onset, which corresponds to tamoxifen induced recombinations in AID-CreERT2 mice (7). At day 2 of the reaction, founder clones already expanded and diversified their encoded B cell receptor by somatic hypermutations. This leads to

**TABLE 2** | Definition of the terminology used throughout.

| Term | Symbol | Definition |
|---|---|---|
| Staining | | Cre-lox recombination of the brainbow alleles (one or both) inducing a constitutive expression of a color in the cell that is transmitted to its progeny. In the simulation this corresponds to the simple attribution of a color to a cell object. The probabilities to induce particular colors are listed in **Table 1**. |
| Colors | $C$ | The set of 4 or 10 colors (excluding black) that can be attributed to cells. |
| Clones | $F$ | All GC founder cell define the set of GC clones. |
| Lineages | $L_{t_0}$ | All GC B cells present in the GC at a particular time point $t_0$ (typically the time point of giving tamoxifen) during the GC reaction define the set of GC B cell lineages $L_{t_0}$ with $N(t_0)$ elements. Note that two daughter cells of a clone may give rise to different lineages. |
| Cell numbers | $N(t)$ | The total number of GC B cells at time $t$ of the GC reaction. |
| | $F_i(t)$ | The number of GC B cells at time $t$ that stem from clone $i \in F$. |
| | $L_i(t)$ | The number of GC B cells at time $t > t_0$ that stem from a lineage $i \in L_{t_0}$. |
| | $C_i(t)$ | The number of GC B cells at time $t$ that express a color $i \in C$. |
| Clonal dominance | $F(t) = \max_{i \in F} \left\{ \frac{F_i(t)}{N(t)} \right\}$ | The largest fraction of the GC B cells at particular time points $t$ during the GC reaction that stems from a single clone among all clones. |
| Lineage dominance | $L(t) = \max_{i \in L_{t_0}} \left\{ \frac{L_i(t)}{N(t)} \right\}$ | The largest fraction of the GC B cells at particular time points $t > t_0$ that stems from a single lineage among all lineages. |
| Color dominace | $C(t) = \max_{i \in C} \left\{ \frac{C_i(t)}{N(t)} \right\}$ | The largest fraction of the GC B cells that express a single non-black color. |
| Color density | $D(t) = \sum_{i \in C} C_i(t)$ | The fraction of GC B cells that express any (non-black) color. |
| Staining threshold | $T$ | The staining threshold $T$ restricts the analysis to only those GCs with the property that the color density at the time $t$ of analysis is above the staining threshold, i.e., $D(t) > T$. |
| PDD | $C(t)\, D(t)$ | The product of color dominance and color density. |

a random staining of many copies of cells descendent of the same initial founder clone. Thus, a correlation of cell color with B cell clones is not expected.

The evolution of the color dominance *in silico* and *in vivo* is compared in **Figure 2A**. As in **Figure 1A**, the color dominance starts from a baseline and increases over time. While the overall agreement between theory and experiment is convincing, there is a small subset of GC simulations with a higher color dominance at days 5 and 7 post tamoxifen. This might be a hint to an overestimation of the selection pressure or of the GC diversity *in silico*. Note, that the number of *in silico* GCs is higher than *in vivo* at both days.

B cells stained in the course of a reaction each define a new lineage. The evolution of colors is now interpreted to provide information on the evolution of those lineages. Indeed, a correlation between color and lineage dominance exists (**Figure 2B**, red line). However, it is much weaker than in the case of founder cell staining and limits the interpretation of the data on the evolution of color dominance.

### 3.3.1. A Staining Threshold Guarantees a Correlation of Color and Lineage Dominance

We sought for a possible filter for the *in silico* GC data that improves the correlation between lineage and color dominance. Given that a large proportion, in the range of 50% of lineages, is not stained by tamoxifen *in silico* and *in vivo*, there is a substantial fraction of GCs that are dominated by a black lineage. This results in an underestimation of the lineage dominance by the color dominance. Indeed, the introduction of a staining threshold, i.e., a minimum fraction of total stained cells in each *in silico* GC that has to be reached for inclusion of the GC in the analysis, substantially increases the correlation between lineage and color dominance (**Figure 2B**, blue and magenta lines). However, the level of correlation was still not comparable to that observed when staining founder cells before entering the GC reaction.

The lineage dominance is also (weakly) correlated to the fraction of stained cells in a GC (**Figure S2**), referred to as color density in the following (see **Table 2**), provided a staining threshold is imposed. This is the case because a staining fraction above the initial mean staining level is more likely to occur for GCs with high lineage dominance. We tested the degree of correlation between lineage dominance and the product of color dominance and color density, shortly denoted as *PDD* in the following (**Figure 2C**). PDD approximates the normalized density score (NDS), which was used *in vivo* and is defined as the product of color dominance with the density of colored cells in the dark zone, measured as number of colored cells per 10 $\mu m^2$ (7). While the correlation is even weaker in GCs with low color density (yellow, orange, and red lines), the staining threshold allows to reach the same high degree of correlation as was found for the staining of founder cells. Thus, we recommend to use a staining threshold in the range of 40%. With lower thresholds, the correlation gets weaker. With higher thresholds, the correlation hardly improves. Instead, the statistics get critical because a large fraction of GCs is left out of the analysis.

In order to illustrate how the removal of GCs dominated by black, i.e., not stained, B cells improves the correlation we plot lineage dominance against color density (**Figure 3**). The perfect correlation would correspond to all symbols being concentrated on the diagonal line. The symbols above the diagonal are those with a low color dominance but high lineage dominance. These can be attributed to the cases described above when the staining procedure failed to stain the lineage which became dominant later on during the GC reaction. These GCs are dominantly black.

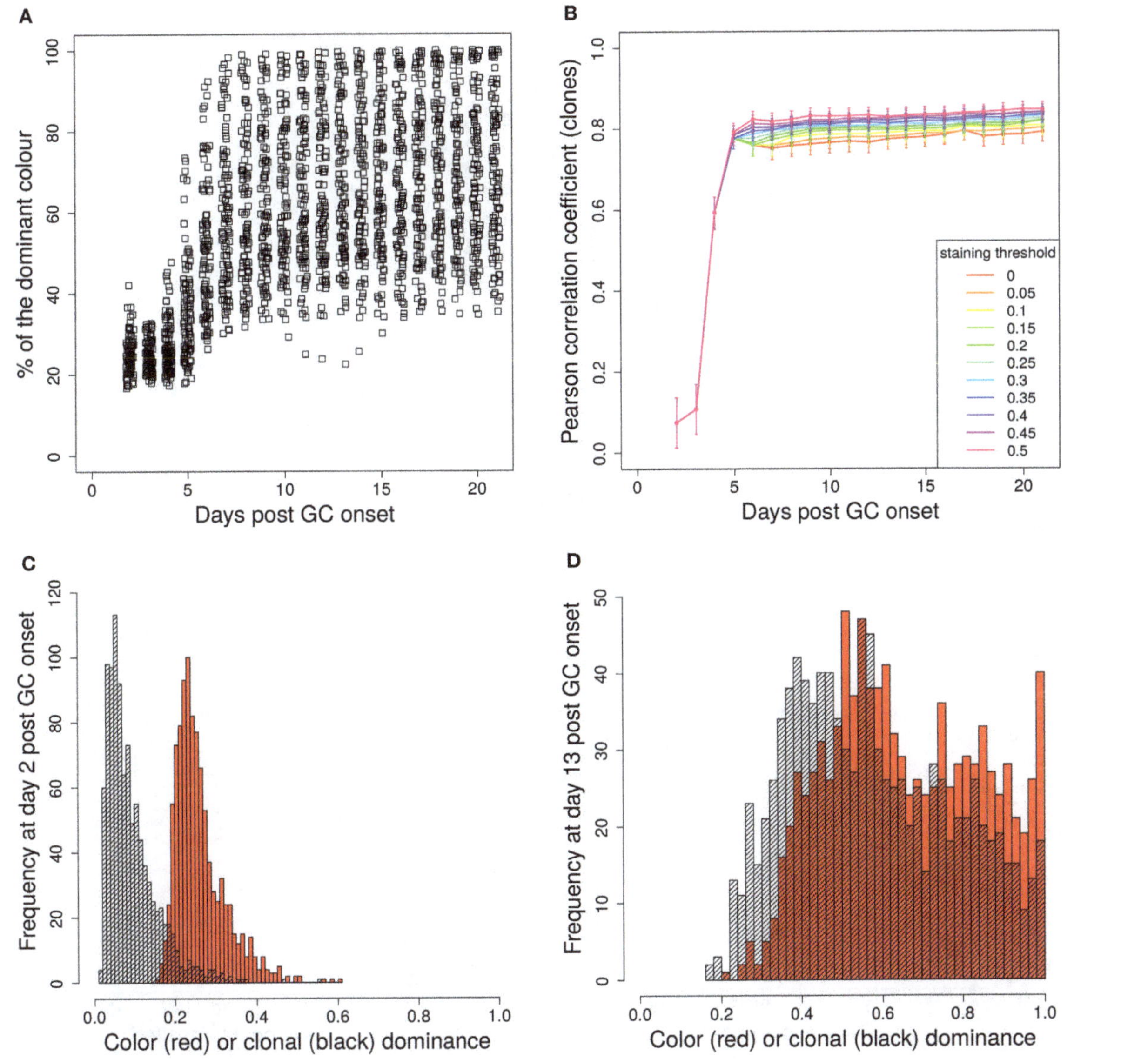


**FIGURE 1 |** Staining of GC founder cells guarantees a good correlation of color and clonal dominance. The GC founder cells were stained with 10 colors before the GC reaction. The size of the largest color **(A)** (first 100 out of 1,000 GC simulations) and its correlation with the clonal dominance **(B)** were monitored over the duration of the GC reactions. The impact of imposing a staining threshold onto the correlation was tested in **(B)** (colors). Pearson correlation coefficient from 1,000 *in silico* GCs. 95% approximate confidence intervals to the Pearson product moment correlation were computed using the Fisher transformation. The distribution of color (red) and clonal (black) dominance are shown at day 2 **(C)** and 13 **(D)** post GC onset.

The introduction of a threshold removes these GCs from the analysis as can be seen by the reduction of the number of GCs above the diagonal line with increasing threshold. Note that a staining threshold of 50% also eliminates a part of the GCs at the day of staining (day 0, red symbols) from the analysis, which by definition exhibit a staining level of 48%. By random fluctuations, there is still a subset of GCs with a staining level above the threshold of 50%. The impact of increasing the threshold from 40 to 50% on later time points of the GC reaction is comparably weak, which explains the minor change in the correlation in **Figure 2C**.

The graph also illustrates that the product of color dominance and color density has the tendency to overestimate lineage dominance. These are the GCs with symbols below the diagonal line in **Figure 3**. Overestimation is a result of different persisting lineages being stained with the same color. If this happens, different lineages contribute to the same color, while the lineage dominance only corresponds to one of those lineages. This effect is less pronounced for large PDD, as was confirmed by sequencing *in vivo* (7). The introduction of a staining threshold to select a subset of GCs for analysis makes the fraction of GCs with an overestimation of the lineage dominance more prominent.

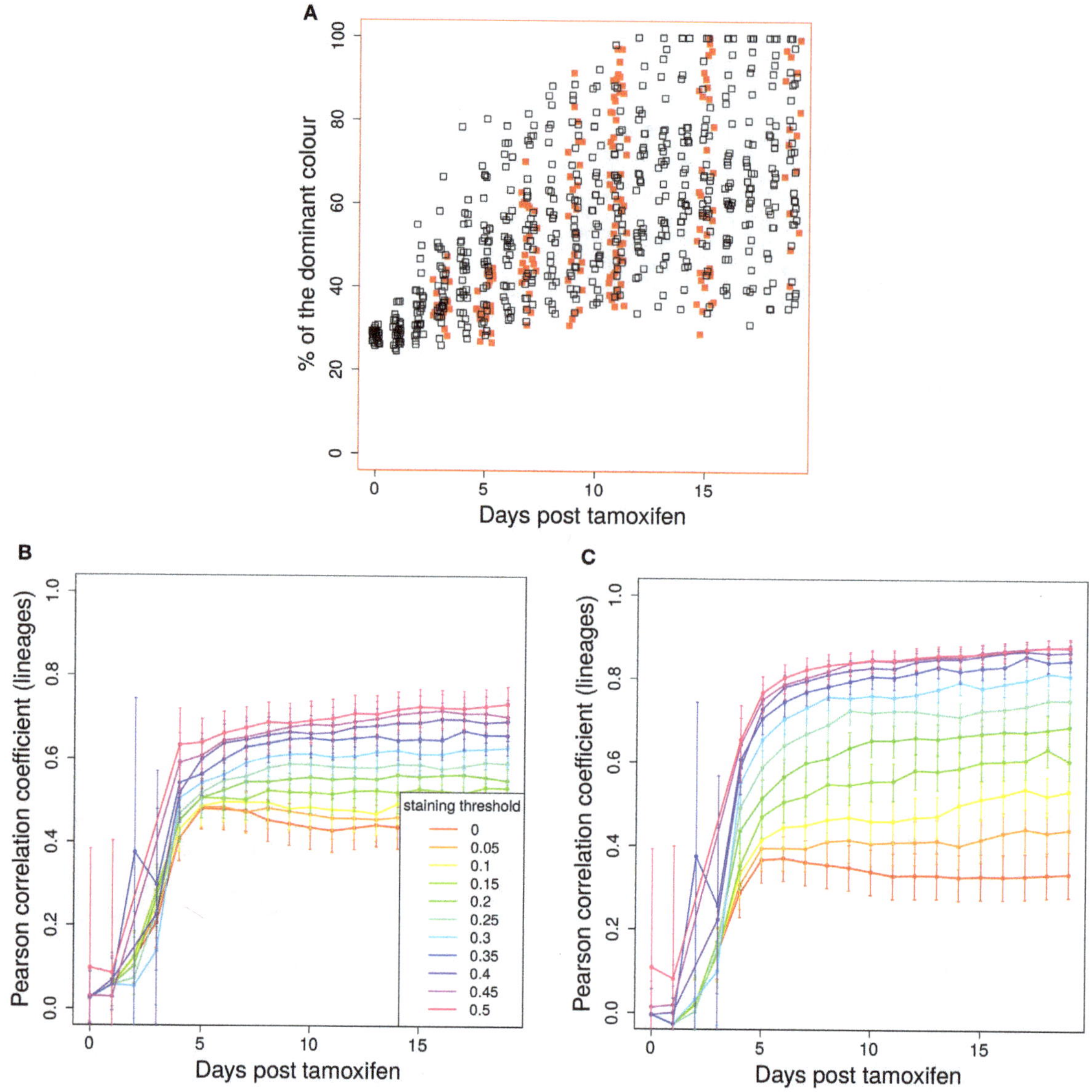


**FIGURE 2 |** Predictivity of tamoxifen-induced staining. **(A)** Evolution of color dominance in response to tamoxifen-induced staining. Thirty simulations (black open squares) are compared to the experimental color dominance behind Figure 3F in Tas et al. (7) (closed red squares). Correlation between lineage dominance and **(B)** color dominance or **(C)** the product of color dominance and color density (PDD). Different staining thresholds were distinguished (line colors). Following tamoxifen induced staining as in **Table 1**, GC B cells were stained at day 2 post GC onset with 10 colors. Pearson correlation coefficient from 1,000 *in silico* GCs. 95% approximate confidence intervals to the Pearson product moment correlation were computed using the Fisher transformation.

### 3.3.2. The Dominant Color Switches During GC Selection

It is possible that the inhomogeneous color distribution to the B cells (**Table 1**) is dominating the subsequent fate of the color dominance. If the color reflects the progression of the selection process during the GC reaction, the dominant color should switch between the time point of staining and the time point of evaluation when the selection of lineages was completed. We assumed that this would be the case at day 11 post staining (21). Indeed, a large fraction of GCs switched the dominant color between the time of staining and day 11 (**Figure 4**). This result further supports that the analysis of color distributions is a suitable measure for the analysis of selection in GCs.

### 3.3.3. The Time of Tamoxifen-Induced Staining Is Important

The time of lineage definition by tamoxifen is critical for the analysis. For one shot stainings it holds that the earlier recombination is induced the better the correlation with the lineage dominance (**Figure 5A**), provided we use a staining threshold of 20% or higher. Two lineages that will survive on long-term might be stained with the same color, which overestimates the lineage dominance. At day 3 or 4 of the GC

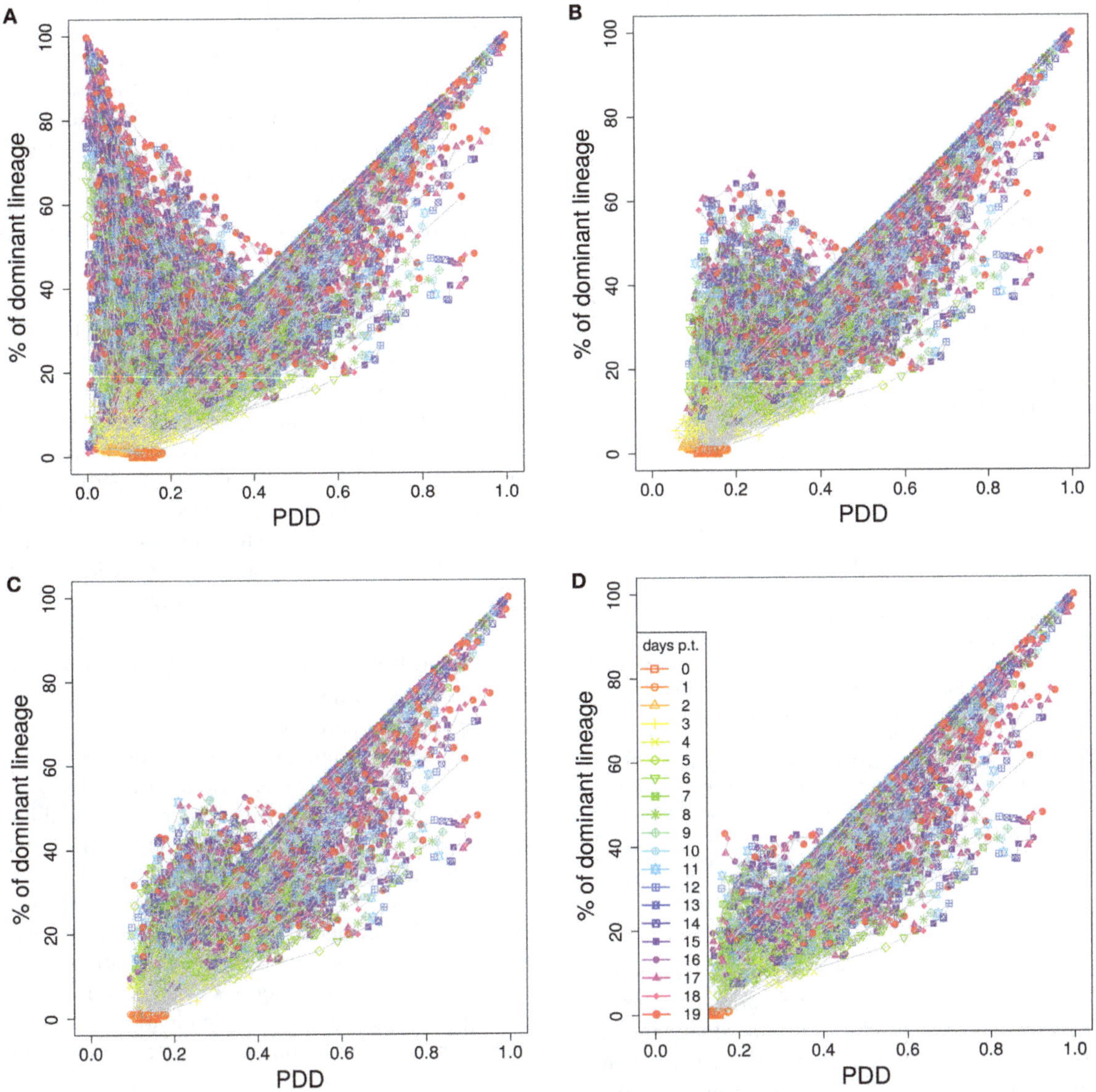


**FIGURE 3 |** Higher staining thresholds eliminate GCs dominated by unstained lineages. Lineage dominance vs. the product of color dominance and staining density (PDD) with a staining threshold of 0 **(A)**, 30 **(B)**, 40 **(C)**, and 50% **(D)**. GC days are distinguished by symbol/line colors. GC B cells were stained at day 2 post GC onset with 10 colors (**Table 1**) in 1,000 *in silico* GCs.

reaction, many low affinity B cells were already eliminated such that the fraction of long-term survivor lineages increases at the time of staining. Hence, an attribution of the same color to different long-term surviving lineages becomes more probable the later the staining is induced.

In addition, lineages become less dominant the later they are defined. This is because similar variants of potentially dominant lineages are defined as different lineages, although neither has a fitness advantage over the other. Hence, it is unlikely that one of them gets lost during further selection. The later staining is induced, the more probable it is to define two similar lineages as different lineages. As a consequence, lineage dominance gets more and more limited the later staining is induced (**Figure S3**). While with a lineage definition at day 1 post GC onset 100% lineage dominance is frequent, at day 4 the largest dominance found in 1,000 GC simulations was at 60%.

## 3.4. Decay of Tamoxifen-Induced Staining of Cells

The staining induced by tamoxifen is not a one shot event. Upon tamoxifen injection, recombination of B cells can be induced for a limited time and the probability of recombination decreases over time. The detailed dynamics of the reduction of the recombination probability is not known. We assumed an exponential decay (Equation 3), which reflects a linear decay of tamoxifen activity. As we are interested in the correlation of the color dominance with the dominance of the lineages existing at the time of tamoxifen injection, we decided to

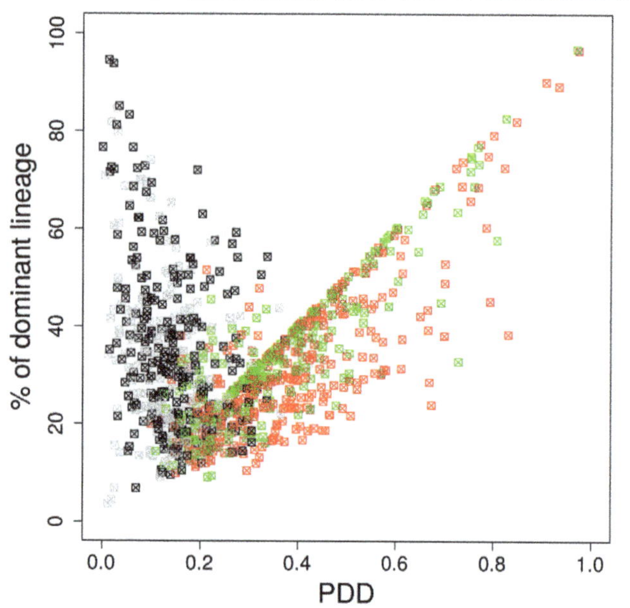


**FIGURE 4 |** The dominant color switches in the course of GC affinity maturation. Lineage dominance vs. the product of color dominance and staining density (PDD) with a staining threshold of 40% at day 11 post staining (subset of data in **Figure 3**). Black and gray squares are GC reactions with a staining level below the threshold, while red and green ones are above the threshold, thus, kept for analysis. Black and red GCs have the property that the initially dominant color was also dominant at day 11 post staining. Thus, in gray and green GCs the dominant color has switched between the time of staining and the time of analysis. GC B cells were stained at day 2 post GC onset with 10 colors (**Table 1**) in 1,000 *in silico* GCs.

define a new lineage not at the time of color attribution but at the time of tamoxifen injection. The correlation between lineage dominance and the product of color dominance and color density is reduced in absolute terms when such staining dynamics are included (**Figures 5A,B**). The comparison of the distribution of lineage dominance and PDD shows how the two distributions approach each other in the course of GC development but stay separate with a substantial fraction of GCs under-estimating the lineage dominance (**Figures 5C,D**). This can be repaired by imposing a staining threshold of 40% (**Figures 5E**).

### 3.4.1. The Set of Lineages Depends on the Time of Tamoxifen Injection

The marking difference to the one-shot staining is the existence of a time point between day 2 and 3 post GC onset at which correlation is maximized. A population of GCs not observed in one-shot stainings and characterized by low lineage dominance and high color dominance emerges. This new GC population exists for early stainings only (day 1 or 2 post GC onset) and is robust against staining thresholds (**Figure S4**). It is associated with founder cells entering the GC reaction after the starting time of staining. Indeed, if these late founder cells are included in the set of lineages, this population of GCs disappears again together with the optimal time of staining (**Figure S1**). At late staining times, correlation is lost due to staining ambiguities. At early staining times, it is lost because of stained cells not belonging to any monitored lineage, giving rise to the observed optimal time point for initiation of B cell lineage staining (**Figure 5B**). This result emphasizes that it is important to consciously chose the time point of tamoxifen injection because it impacts on the resulting set of lineages and may change the interpretation of the experimental results.

### 3.4.2. A Decay of the Staining Probability Effectively Retards Staining

As described for the one-shot staining scenario, there is a general tendency that later staining reduces the correlation. By the decay of tamoxifen-induced staining activity, staining is distributed onto 2 days, which corresponds effectively to a retardation of staining by roughly 1 day. Indeed, inititation at day 3 with tamoxifen decay is effectively rather similar to initiation at day 4 with one-shot staining (**Figure 5**). This effective retardation of staining reduces the overall level of correlation.

### 3.4.3. The Impact of Recombination of Already Recombined Cells

During the time period of tamoxifen activity, it is possible that a cell undergoes multiple recombination events. This would imply that a cell already expressing a color may switch color. Here, we investigated whether this process would impact on the interpretation of color dominance in terms of lineage dominance. When restaining of already stained cells was allowed *in silico*, the resulting correlation between lineage dominance and color dominance is further reduced (**Figures S5A,B**). However, only a small impact was found on the correlation between lineage dominance and PDD (**Figures S5C,D**). While the possibility of ongoing and repetitive recombination makes the resulting color dominance more fuzzy, the correlation with PDD appears robust.

### 3.4.4. A Decay of the Staining Probability Induces a Fuzzy Color Distribution

The resulting distribution of colors at the end of the staining procedure is less well defined compared to the one-shot staining, where the distribution reflects the color probabilities (see **Table 1**). With tamoxifen decay, a lineage stained right at the beginning of the extended staining period will also stain all of the progeny of this lineage. In contrast, for a lineage stained at the end of the staining period, only a small subset of the progeny is stained, for the cell defining the lineage has divided a number of times and only one of these daughter cells is stained together with its progeny. Other progeny from the very same lineage might not be stained or be stained with different colors. As a consequence, the color dominance under-estimates the lineage dominance (**Figure S3**). Thus, at the end of the staining period, the number of stained cells from a lineage does not necessarily reflect the size of the lineage and adds to the uncertainties associated

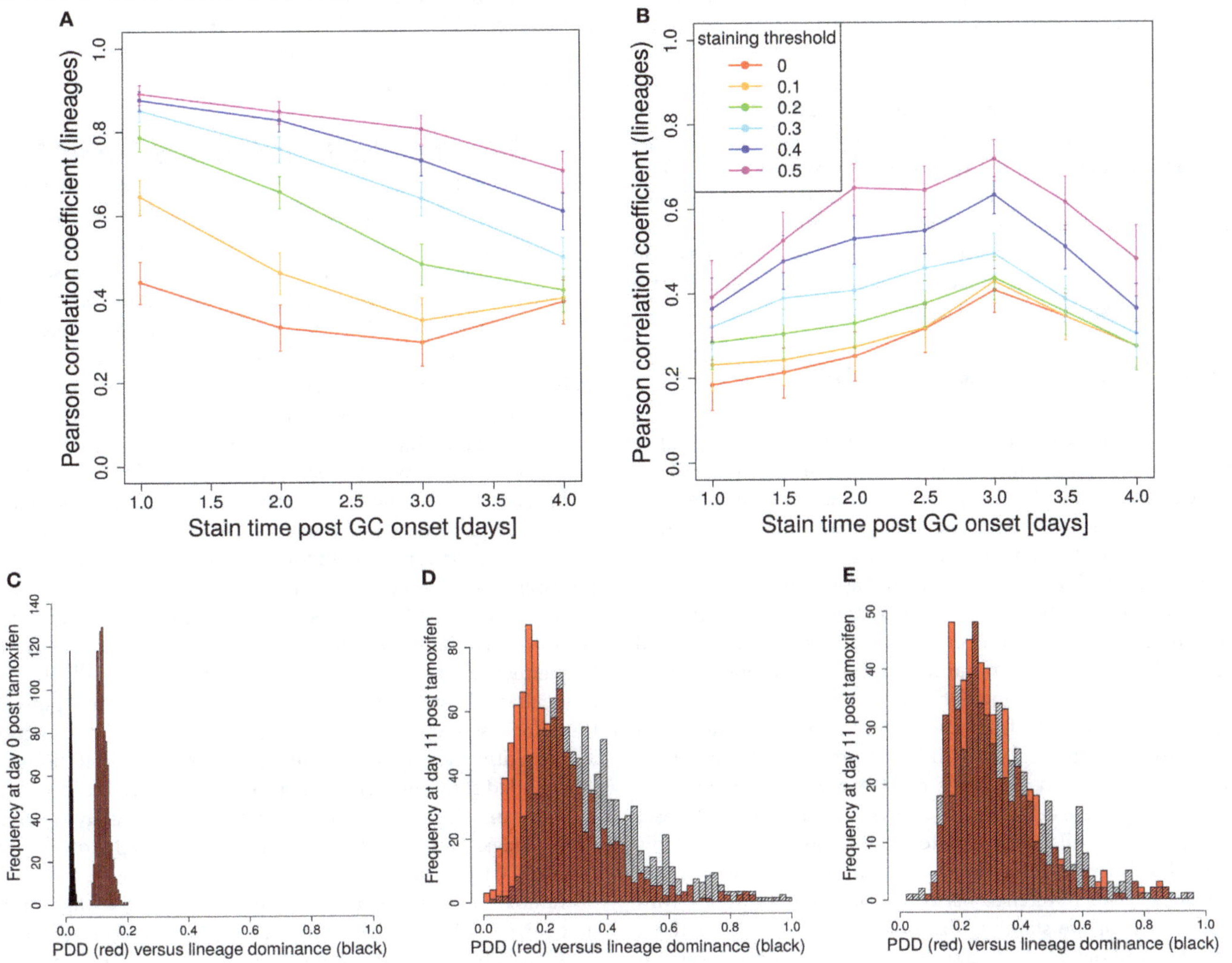


**FIGURE 5 |** The staining time point determines the predictive power. Correlation between lineage and the product of color dominance and color density in dependence on the time point of staining. Simulations with single shot **(A)** or dynamic decay **(B)** of tamoxifen-induced staining with 10 colors (**Table 1**). For dynamic tamoxifen decay in **(B)**, a half life of $\tau_{\text{tamoxifen}} = 24$ h was assumed in Equation (3). Lineages were defined at the time of tamoxifen injection. For lineages complemented by all founder cells entering the GC after injection see **Figure S1**. For dynamic tamoxifen decay with tamoxifen given at day 2 post GC onset, the lineage dominance distribution is compared to the distribution of the product of color dominance and color density (PDD) without threshold at day 2 **(C)** and 13 **(D)** and with a staining threshold of 40% at day 13 post GC onset **(E)**. Data in **(A,B)** show the Pearson correlation coefficient from 1,000 *in silico* GCs at day 11 post tamoxifen with different staining thresholds (line colors). 95% approximate confidence intervals to the Pearson product moment correlation were computed using the Fisher transformation.

with staining different lineages with the same color (over-estimation) or staining the same lineage with different colors (under-estimation). This limitation gets even more important for late initiation of staining, when it gets more likely that two similar parts of a lineages both survive GC selection. The higher variability of the color distributions at the end of the staining process, overall reduces the correlation of color and lineage dominance.

### 3.4.5. A Shortened Tamoxifen Staining Activity Would Improve Color Analysis

Some of these stained GCs under-estimating lineage dominance are removed by the staining threshold (**Figures 5D,E**). As tamoxifen activity was assumed to decay exponentially, in many cases staining happens only one division after the time of initiation of staining, which may still induce a high degree of staining. Also the staining of other progeny from the same lineage with a different color would keep the stained cell fraction high. Thus, a relevant proportion of GCs exists, which exhibits a high fraction of stained cells above the staining threshold but still results in an under-estimate of lineage dominance (**Figure S4**). A slow decay of tamoxifen activity in the range of days, requires a higher staining threshold for the analysis of 50% or higher in order to keep up with the correlation level of one-shot stainings. In view of the reduced statistics (see absolute counts of GCs in **Figures 5D,E**), it would be more advantageous to stop tamoxifen activity at defined time points in experimental settings. For example, one might consider shortening the period of tamoxifen activity by administering the drug already in its active form as 4-hydroxy-tamoxifen.

### 3.4.6. Later Staining Limits Lineage Dominance

The later the lineages are defined, the more the lineage dominance achieved is limited (**Figure S3**). While lineages fully dominating the GCs exist for stainings initiated at day 1–3 post GC onset, their frequency decreases. In stainings at day 4, the highest dominance is reduced to 60%. For late stainings, the identification of GCs dominated by single clones becomes rare based on tamoxifen-induced staining.

## 3.5. Colored GCs Are Predictive of Black GCs

Imposing a staining threshold in the range of 40% or higher turned out to be critical in order to ensure predictive power of the color dominance for the lineage dominance. This was tested for the GCs satisfying the staining threshold. It would be of particular interest, whether the statements on lineage dominance are not only valid for the highly stained GCs but apply to all GCs.

In order to test this, we compared the lineage dominance distribution for GCs above and below the staining threshold (**Figure 6**). There exists an optimal staining threshold of 45% for which the lineage dominance of the GCs kept (green bars) and deleted (red bars) from the analysis are widely identical (**Figure 6B**). With higher staining thresholds (**Figure 6C**), lineage dominance in the range of 30% are more frequent in the GC subset deleted from the analysis. Thus, the GC subset kept for analysis will underestimate the lineage dominance in this regime. For lower staining thresholds (**Figure 6A**), the situation is inverted. The difference between both subsets scales with the deviation of the staining threshold from 45%. The optimal staining threshold of 45%, shown in **Figure 6** for the case of decaying tamoxifen activity, equally holds true for one-shot stainings (data not shown). In conclusion, the staining threshold of 45% not only guarantees a fairly good correlation with lineage dominance with acceptable statistics. It also guarantees that the lineage dominance estimated with the subset of GCs stained to more than 45% remains valid for the whole set of GCs.

## 3.6. Impact of the Fraction of Stained Cells

The fraction of stained GC B cells induced by tamoxifen was in the range of 50% *in vivo* (7). It is not clear whether a different fraction of stained cells would improve the correlation between color and lineage dominance or reduce it. An increase of the stained fraction would allow to achieve better statistics. We varied the fraction of stained cells between 10 and 90% (**Figure 7**). Without imposing a staining threshold the intuitive result that staining more infers a better correlation of color and lineage dominance is confirmed (**Figure 7**, red lines).

This relationship is turned around for higher staining thresholds. The lower the stained fraction of GC B cells the better the color dominance informs about the lineage dominance. Compared to 50% stained cells with a staining threshold of 40%, the same correlation is found for 10% stained cells with a staining threshold of less than 20% (**Figure 7A**). There is a trade-off between less stained cells, which reduces the statistics, and a lower cut-off, which increases the statistics again. Experiments should be planned to stain a comparably low fraction of cells in order to facilitate the analysis and to improve the predictive power of the color distribution. Staining of lower fractions of cells requires less repetitive dosing of tamoxifen, such that the limitations due to extended staining periods (**Figure 5**) are also reduced.

The same trend holds true for a tamoxifen activity spread over 2 days. However, the overall level of correlation is lower (**Figure 7B**).

Tamoxifen-induced cell staining induces a color distribution that carries information on the lineage distribution but not on the clones. Information on the founder cells is widely lost. In the limit of low staining fractions with high staining thresholds it is possible to get a fair correlation of early one-shot induced color

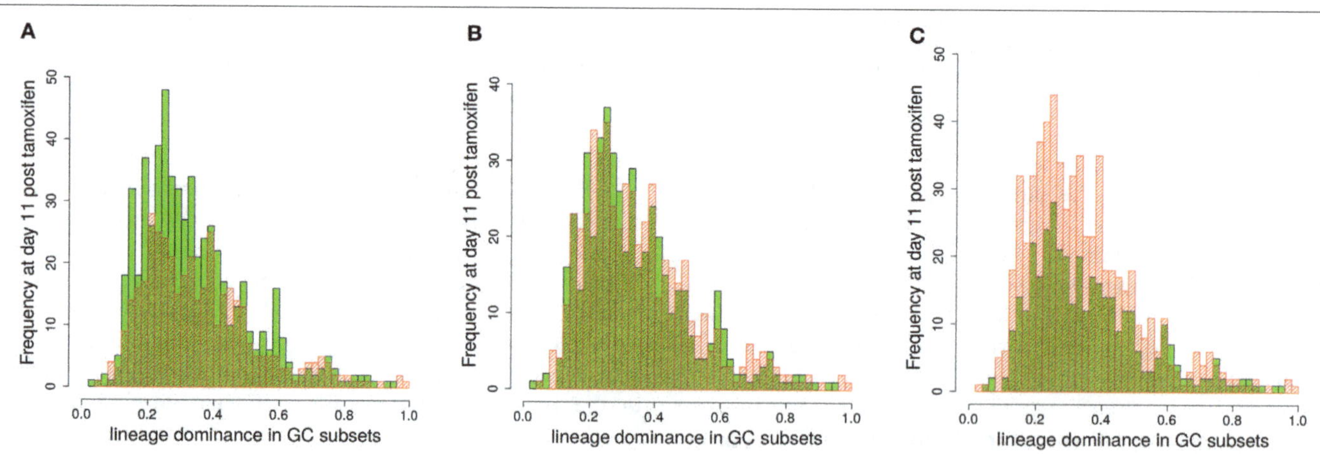


**FIGURE 6 |** Estimation of the lineage dominance of GCs below the staining threshold. The distribution of lineage dominance is shown for the GCs above (green) and below (red) the staining threshold separately. Data were derived from the 1,000 simulations with dynamic tamoxifen decay as described in **Figure 5** at day 11 post tamoxifen. The comparison of the GC subsets was repeated for staining thresholds of 40 **(A)**, 45 **(B)**, and 50% **(C)**.

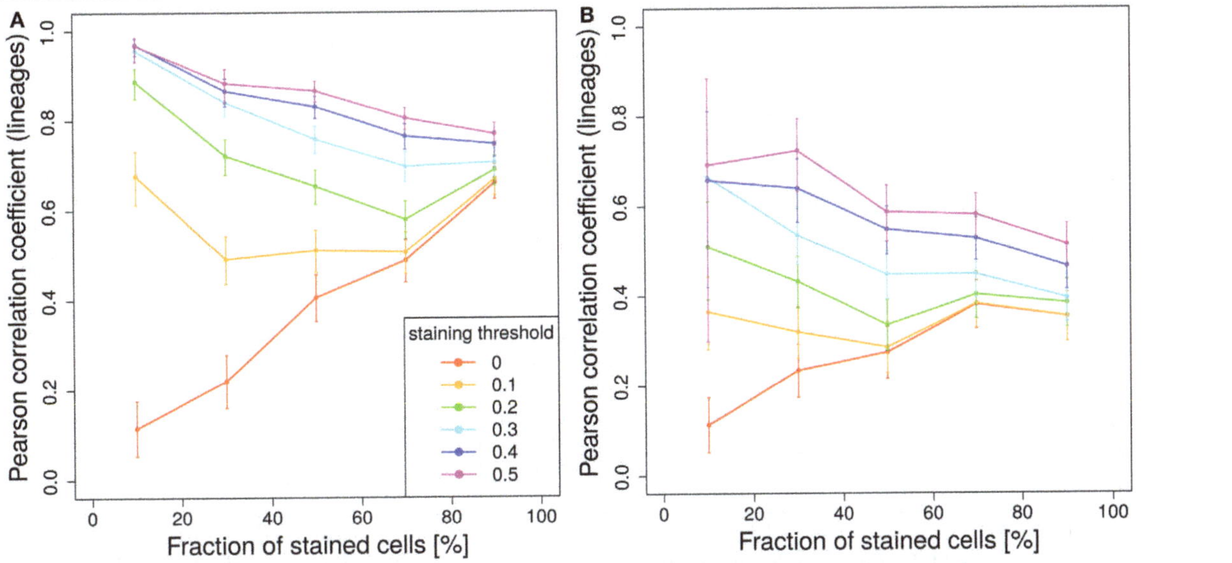


**FIGURE 7 |** Staining less cells improves predictive power. Correlation between lineage and the product of color dominance and color density in dependence on the fraction of stained cells. Simulations with single shot staining **(A)** or dynamic decay **(B)** with 10 colors (**Table 1**) at day 2 post GC onset. Pearson correlation coefficient from 1,000 *in silico* GCs at day 11 post tamoxifen with different staining thresholds (line colors). 95% approximate confidence intervals to the Pearson product moment correlation were computed using the Fisher transformation.

dominance and clonal dominance (**Figure S6**). However, already at day 2 the correlation becomes rather weak.

## 3.7. The Predictive Power of 4 and 10 Colors Is Similar

In experimental settings, the variety of colors is generated making use of the so-called brainbow allele (1), which was implemented in the Rosa26$^{Confetti}$ mice (5). The random Cre-recombination of the color segments is induced by injection of tamoxifen and generates cells with 4 different colors. When the brainbow staining is implemented on both alleles, the diversity of colors is enhanced to 10 colors (7). Here we investigated, whether 10 colors are more predictive for the lineage dominance in GCs than single allele Confetti mice. It turns out that the correlation of lineage dominance and the product of color dominance and stained fraction of cells is rather similar with 4 or 10 colors (compare **Figure 8** to **Figures 5A,B** and **Figure 7**). In particular, in one-shot stainings it is found that the predictive power of 4 colors is even better than with 10 colors for early stainings and low fractions of stained cells (**Figures 8A,C**). Further, for simulations with decaying tamoxifen-activity, the optimal time point (day 3 post GC onset) for the initiation of staining is the same as for 10 colors and the overall correlation is reduced to a similar degree (**Figure 8B**). This can be rescued by reducing the fraction of intially stained cells (**Figure 8D**).

The unexpected result that 10 colors would not be substantially better predictors than 4 colors prompted us to test whether the reason for this lack of improvement by more colors would be related to the rather inhomogeneous probability of activation of the different colors (**Table 1**). Indeed, when assuming equal probabilities for all 10 colors, the predictive power is better than for 4 colors and also better than for 10 colors based on real activation probabilities in **Table 1** (compare **Figure 8B**, dashed and full lines).

# 4. DISCUSSION

The present analysis supports that the Brainbow construct is suitable for the analysis of an evolutionary system like the evolution of GC B cells in the context of an immune response. When all germline B cells are stained before the GC reaction, the color distribution during and at the end of the evolutionary process in the GC reaction is predictive of the clonal distribution. Thus, staining and fate monitoring of colors is a good approximation for the analysis of clonal evolution. Sequencing of B cells is only necessary to account for specific clones, but the clonal dominance is well evaluated based on the colors alone.

When the Cre-dependent recombination is employed to stain the B cells in the course of a GC reaction, the color is predictive of the clonal composition provided the staining is limited to a rather short time interval. The longer the staining progresses, the weaker the correlation to the clonal distribution. With a prolonged staining procedure, staining ambiguities like staining of two lineages with the same color, is aggravated by the variability of initial states of the color distributions. A lineage is defined at the beginning of the staining procedure, such that a late staining event leads to a few stained cells in comparison to an early staining event, where the whole lineage branch would be stained. For that reason, it is recommended to limit the action of tamoxifen to a short time period.

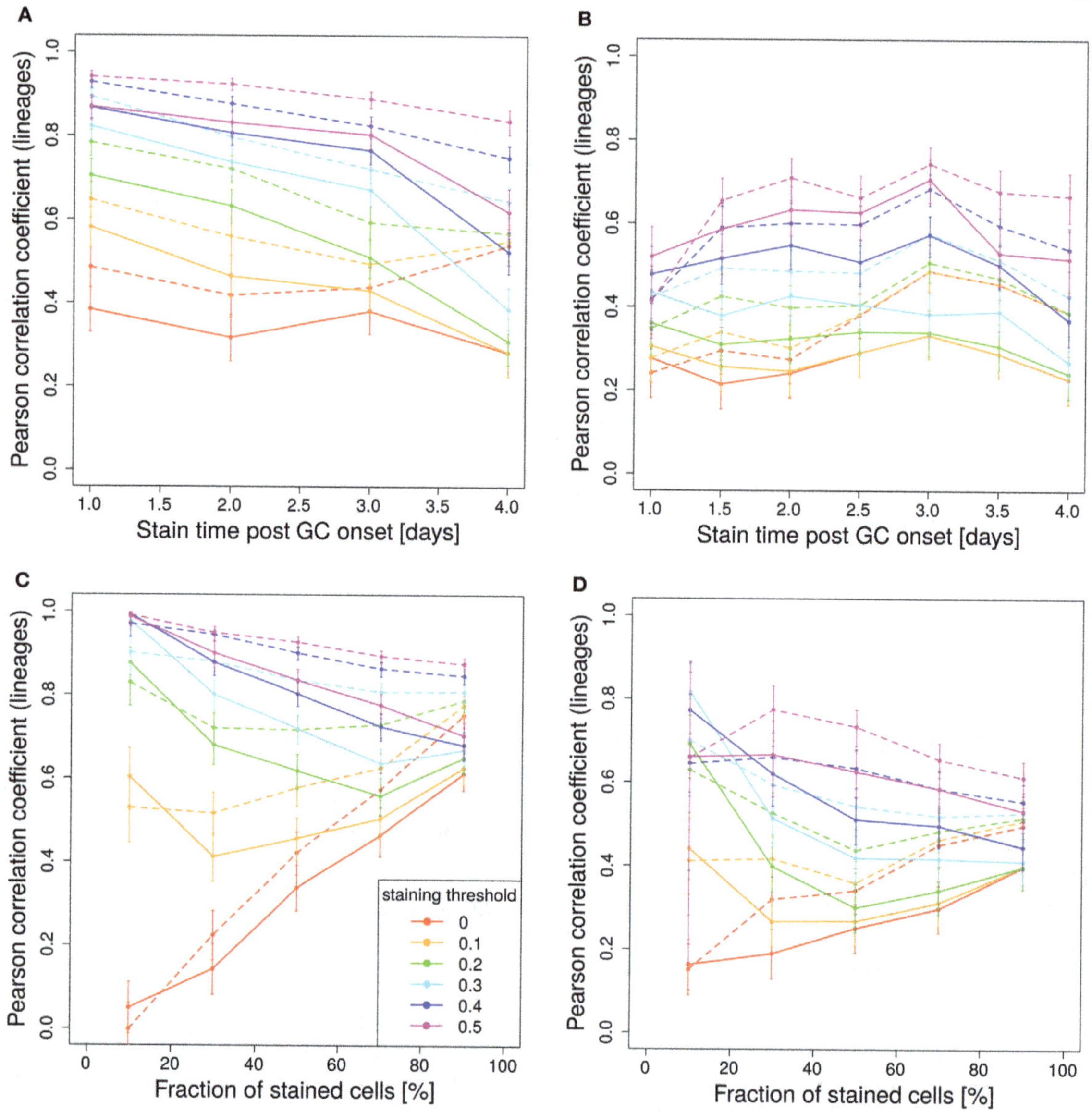


**FIGURE 8 |** Four colors have similar predictive power than 10 colors. Correlation between lineage and the product of color dominance and density in dependence on the time point of staining **(A,B)** or the fraction of stained cells **(C,D)**. Simulations with single shot **(A,C)** or dynamic decay **(B,D)** of tamoxifen-induced staining with 4 colors (**Table 1**) (full lines) or with 10 colors with equal probabilities (dashed lines). For dynamic tamoxifen decay, a half life of $\tau_{\text{tamoxifen}} = 24$ h was assumed in Equation (3). Lineages were defined by the cells present at the time of tamoxifen injection. Pearson correlation coefficient from 1,000 *in silico* GCs at day 11 post tamoxifen with different staining thresholds (line colors). 95% approximate confidence intervals to the Pearson product moment correlation were computed using the Fisher transformation.

An important source of ambiguity is that there is only a fraction of cells stained by tamoxifen-induced recombination. This implies that there is a proportion of GCs in which the unstained B cells would become dominant. A good predictive power relies on the elimination of black-dominated GCs, which can be achieved by imposing a staining threshold. This threshold eliminates all poorly stained GCs from the analysis. A suitable staining threshold is in the range of 40%. With longer staining periods, 50% leads to better results. A staining threshold of 45% was identified that allows to extrapolate the lineage dominance derived from the subset of GCs above the staining threshold to the whole set of measured GCs, including the GCs left out from the analysis.

Intuitively, one would expect that staining more B cells would improve the predictive power. This is only true without a staining threshold, thus, including all GCs irrespective how strongly they are stained. However, together with imposing a staining threshold, the relationship is inverted. Low staining fractions are substantially more predictive of clonal dominance than high staining fractions. At the same time, the total number of GCs eliminated by the threshold increases if only a small fraction of B cells per GC is stained. Thus, in the future design of such experiments it is important to find the right balance between statistical significance and low staining. Staining of 30% of the GC B cells appears as a good starting point from the point of view of *in silico* GCs.

The time point of staining is an important parameter. The general tendency is the earlier the better. At later time points, a pre-selected set of B cells is stained, which increases errors of staining different lineages with the same color, thus, further over-estimating the clonal dominance by the color dominance. This happens because the pre-selected B cells are more likely to both survive and persist in the continuation of the GC reaction. However, at very early time points, the set of different lineages is limited. Physiologically, it might make sense to wait until a minimum of B cell diversity was achieved. Otherwise, it would make more sense to use the Mx1-Cre system, in which founder GC B cells carry a color already when they start the GC reaction.

Depending on the question under consideration, one might want to analyse the set of cells present in the GC at the particular time point at which staining is induced, or of all cells getting stained in the course of the GC reaction. In the latter case, earlier staining increases predictive power. In the former case, earlier staining reduces predictive power. This is due to late founder cells that enter the *in silico* GC reaction and still get stained. Colored B cells exist without any lineage counterpart in the analysis. If lineages defined at a particular time point are in the focus of the research, there exists a time point of inducing the staining between day 2 and 3 post GC onset, which is optimal for the analysis of lineage dominance.

The analysis is based on a set of 1,000 *in silico* GC simulations in agreement with data from two-photon imaging (22–24) and anti-DEC205-OVA experiments (15). This set of GC simulations was used to interpret the data in Tas et al. (7) and correlates well with the results therein. Clonal and color dominance are likely depending on model parameters like affinity of founder cells to the antigen, division rate, selection pressure, strength of antibody feedback, etc. A different set of simulations might well quantitatively shift one or the other result, provided the change would influence the timing of selection or the number of mutations in the GC reaction. For example, the quality of the GC founder cells might vary depending on the type of immunization and the existence of transgenic B cells with a particular affinity to the immunizing antigen. This implies that the planning of new experiments would ideally go hand-in-hand with a specifically adapted set of simulations.

## AUTHOR CONTRIBUTIONS

MM-H and GV initiated the study. MM-H designed the C++ code and performed the analysis. SB contributed to R-coding and to the strategy of the data analysis. MM-H wrote the manuscript. All authors contributed to the scientific content and interpretation and revised the manuscript.

## FUNDING

MM-H was supported by the Human Frontier Science Program (RGP0033/2015). He was further supported by the Helmholtz Initiative on Personalized Medicine–iMed, and Helmholtz Association, Zukunftsthemen Aging and Metabolic Programming (AMPro) as well as Immunology and Inflammation (ZT-0027). SB was supported by the German Federal Ministry of Education and Research within the Measures for the Establishment of Systems Medicine, project SYSIMIT (BMBF eMed project SYSIMIT, FKZ: 01ZX1308B). SB and MM-H were supported by the pilot project Information & Data Science of the Helmholtz Association, project Reduced Complexity Models.

## REFERENCES

1. Livet J, Weissman T, Kang H, Draft R, Lu J, Bennis R, et al. Transgenic strategies for combinatorial expression of fluorescent proteins in the nervous system. *Nature* (2007) 450:56–62. doi: 10.1038/nature06293
2. Singh S, LaSarge C, An A, McAuliffe J, Danzer S. Clonal analysis of newborn hippocampal dentate granule cell proliferation and development in temporal lobe epilepsy. *eNeuro* (2015) 2:e0087–15. doi: 10.1523/ENEURO.0087-15.2015
3. Wang J, O'Sullivan M, Mukherjee D, Punal V, Farsiu S, Kay J. Anatomy and spatial organization of Mueller glia in mouse retina. *J Comp Neurol.* (2017) 525:1759–77. doi: 10.1002/cne.24153
4. Roossien D, Cai D. Imaging neural architecture in Brainbow samples. *Methods Mol Biol.* (2017) 1642:211–28. doi: 10.1007/978-1-4939-7169-5_14
5. Snippert H, van der Flier L, Sato T, van Es J, van den Born M, Kroon-Veenboer C, et al. Intestinal crypt homeostasis results from neutral competition between symmetrically dividing Lgr5 stem cells. *Cell* (2010) 143:134–44. doi: 10.1016/j.cell.2010.09.016
6. Henninger J, Santoso B, Hans S, Durand E, Moore J, Mosimann C, et al. Clonal fate mapping quantifies the number of haematopoietic stem cells that arise during development. *Nat Cell Biol.* (2017) 19:17–27. doi: 10.1038/ncb3444
7. Tas J, Mesin L, Pasqual G, Targ S, Jacobsen J, Mano Y, et al. Visualizing antibody affinity maturation in germinal centres. *Science* (2016) 351:1048–54. doi: 10.1126/science.aad3439
8. MacLennan ICM. Germinal centers. *Annu Rev Immunol.* (1994) 12:117–39. doi: 10.1146/annurev.iy.12.040194.001001
9. Victora G, Dominguez-Sola D, Holmes A, Deroubaix S, Dalla-Favera R, Nussenzweig M. Identification of human germinal center light and dark zone cells and their relationship to human B-cell lymphomas. *Blood* (2012) 120:2240–8. doi: 10.1182/blood-2012-03-415380
10. Firl D, Degn S, Padera T, Carroll M. Capturing change in clonal composition amongst single mouse germinal centers. *eLife* (2018) 7:e33051. doi: 10.7554/eLife.33051

11. Berek C, Milstein C. Mutation drift and repertoire shift in the maturation of the immune response. *Immunol Rev.* (1987) 96:23–41. doi: 10.1111/j.1600-065X.1987.tb00507.x
12. Küppers R, Zhao M, Hansmann ML, Rajewsky K. Tracing B cell development in human germinal centers by molecular analysis of single cells picked from histological sections. *EMBO J.* (1993) 12:4955–67.
13. Amitai A, Mesin L, Victora G, Kardar M, Chakraborty A. A population dynamics model for clonal diversity in a germinal center. *Front Microbiol.* (2017) 8:1693. doi: 10.3389/fmicb.2017.01693
14. Kepler TB, Perelson AS. Cyclic re-entry of germinal center B cells and the efficiency of affinity maturation. *Immunol Today* (1993) 14:412–5. doi: 10.1016/0167-5699(93)90145-B
15. Victora GD, Schwickert TA, Fooksman DR, Kamphorst AO, Meyer-Hermann M, Dustin ML, et al. Germinal center dynamics revealed by multiphoton microscopy with a photoactivatable fluorescent reporter. *Cell* (2010) 143:592–605. doi: 10.1016/j.cell.2010.10.032
16. Meyer-Hermann M, Mohr E, Pelletier N, Zhang Y, Victora GD, Toellner KM. A theory of germinal center B cell selection, division, and exit. *Cell Rep.* (2012) 2:162–74. doi: 10.1016/j.celrep.2012.05.010
17. Meyer-Hermann M. Overcoming the dichotomy of quantity and quality in antibody responses. *J Immunol.* (2014) 193:5414–9. doi: 10.4049/jimmunol.1401828
18. Gitlin AD, Shulman Z, Nussenzweig MC. Clonal selection in the germinal centre by regulated proliferation and hypermutation. *Nature* (2014) 509:637–40. doi: 10.1038/nature13300
19. Kroese FG, Wubbena AS, Seijen HG, Nieuwenhuis P. Germinal centers develop oligoclonally. *Eur J Immunol.* (1987) 17:1069–72. doi: 10.1002/eji.1830170726
20. Binder S, Meyer-Hermann M. Implications of intravital imaging of murine germinal centers on the control of B cell selection and division. *Front Immunol.* (2016) 7:593. doi: 10.3389/fimmu.2016.00593
21. Jacob J, Przylepa J, Miller C, Kelsoe G. *In situ* studies of the primary response to (4-hydroxy-3-nitrophenyl)acetyl. III. The kinetics of V region mutation and selection in germinal center B cells. *J Exp Med.* (1993) 178:1293–307. doi: 10.1084/jem.178.4.1293
22. Allen CD, Okada T, Tang HL, Cyster JG. Imaging of germinal center selection events during affinity maturation. *Science* (2007) 315:528–31. doi: 10.1126/science.1136736
23. Schwickert TA, Lindquist RL, Schakhar G, Livshits G, Skokos D, Kosco-Vilbois MH, et al. *In vivo* imaging of germinal centres reveals a dynamic open structure. *Nature* (2007) 446:83–7. doi: 10.1038/nature05573
24. Hauser AE, Junt T, Mempel TR, Sneddon MW, Keinstein SH, Henrickson SE, et al. Definition of germinal-center B cell migration *in vivo* reveals predominant intrazonal circulation patterns. *Immunity* (2007) 26:655–67. doi: 10.1016/j.immuni.2007.04.008

17

# Tracing Antibody Repertoire Evolution by Systems Phylogeny

*Alexander Dimitri Yermanos*[1,2], *Andreas Kevin Dounas*[3], *Tanja Stadler*[1], *Annette Oxenius*[2] *and Sai T. Reddy*[1*]

[1] *Department of Biosystems Science and Engineering, ETH Zurich, Basel, Switzerland,* [2] *Department of Biology, Institute of Microbiology, ETH Zurich, Zurich, Switzerland,* [3] *Department of Chemistry and Applied Biosciences, ETH Zurich, Zurich, Switzerland*

***Correspondence:**
*Sai T. Reddy*
*sai.reddy@ethz.ch*

Antibody evolution studies have been traditionally limited to either tracing a single clonal lineage (B cells derived from a single V-(D)-J recombination) over time or examining bulk functionality changes (e.g., tracing serum polyclonal antibody proteins). Studying a single B cell disregards the majority of the humoral immune response, whereas bulk functional studies lack the necessary resolution to analyze the co-existing clonal diversity. Recent advances in high-throughput sequencing (HTS) technologies and bioinformatics have made it possible to examine multiple co-evolving antibody monoclonal lineages within the context of a single repertoire. A plethora of accompanying methods and tools have been introduced in hopes of better understanding how pathogen presence dictates the global evolution of the antibody repertoire. Here, we provide a comprehensive summary of the tremendous progress of this newly emerging field of systems phylogeny of antibody responses. We present an overview encompassing the historical developments of repertoire phylogenetics, state-of-the-art tools, and an outlook on the future directions of this fast-advancing and promising field.

**Keywords: systems immunology, phylogenetics, antibody lineage, B cell evolution, Ig-Seq**

## INTRODUCTION

B cells are the foundation of humoral immunity and are defined by their characteristic B cell receptors (BCR, or secreted version: antibodies), which bind foreign pathogens and initiate effector functions, such as pathogen opsonization, neutralization, complement activation, and cellular cytotoxic and phagocytosis signaling (1). Antibodies are composed of two identical heavy chains and two identical light chains, where each chain consists of a variable region and a constant region. The variable regions dictate antigen-binding specificity (2), whereas the constant regions enable interactions with other molecular and cellular components of the immune system (1). Initial variable region diversity is encoded in the organism's genome through the presence of multiple V-, D- (heavy chain only), and J-gene segments, which pseudo-randomly recombine in both the heavy and light chain loci (3, 4). During somatic recombination, the variable regions can undergo further diversification due to deletions or insertions at the V-D and J-D junctions, rendering a potential theoretical amino acid diversity in humans and mice of $>10^{13}$ (5–7). The region encompassing the last few nucleotides of the V-gene segment, the entire D-gene segment (in the case of heavy chain rearrangement), and the start of the J-gene segment is known as the complementary determining region 3 (CDR3), and has been shown to largely dictate antigen specificity (2).

Selective pressures are present during early B cell development to ensure binding specificity is not directed toward self-antigens through interactions with stromal cells in the bone marrow. This is done via deletion or induction of anergy in B cells expressing BCRs exhibiting self-reactivity. B cells surviving this selection emigrate from the bone marrow and enter the circulating population of mature B cells. These newly produced B cells circulate between blood and secondary lymphoid organs until encountering their respective antigen. The BCRs which bind their respective target can subsequently engulf the foreign antigen via receptor-mediated endocytosis and display these pathogen-derived peptides on the cell surface using major histocompatibility class (MHC)-II proteins (8, 9). This prepares the B cell for further differentiation via binding of CD4+ T cells, which interact specifically with the foreign peptides displayed on the B cell's MHC-II molecules. Both the strength and duration of this interaction between B and T cells have been implicated in dictating the fate of the B cell (10). Longer conjugate interactions may preferentially lead to a germinal center (GC) reaction, where affinity maturation and class switching occur (11, 12).

GCs are structurally divided into a dark zone, where B cells rapidly proliferate while mutations are selectively introduced into the antibody locus, initially via the enzyme activation-induced cytidine deaminase (AID) and the upregulation of the error-prone DNA polymerase eta (13–15), a process referred to as somatic hypermutation (SHM) (16). A number of reviews exist describing the complex biochemistry underlying SHM and are available for further reading (17, 18). The light zone in GCs is where T follicular helper (TFH) cells mediate the selection of B cell clones with higher antigen affinity and their differentiation into plasma cells (**Figure 1A**) (12, 19, 20). B cell clones incurring SHM that increase the strength of the antibody-antigen binding interaction will subsequently receive more survival signals, such as ICOS, CD40, and interleukin-21 (IL-21) (11, 21, 22).

It has been shown that antibodies surviving the selective pressures faced during affinity maturation are capable of producing high affinity antibodies with binding disassociation constants (Kds) hundreds to thousands of times higher than their germline progenitor (23). Furthermore, recent work in mouse models of chronic viral infection have revealed that the continued presence of TFH cells is crucial for the development of neutralizing antibodies (24). While it is intuitive that affinity maturation holds an essential role to improve the specificity and affinity of B cells against complex antigens (such as pathogens and their proteins), a recent study has questioned this, as it was proposed that there is a continuous recruitment of naïve or memory B cells equipped with high affinity BCRs into an ongoing humoral immune response (25). This suggests that SHM might play a prominent role in broadening the antibody response with respect to its ability to recognize antigenic variants (26, 27). Despite these recent findings, the exact nature regarding whether and how affinity maturation instructs antibody evolution remains at the forefront of contemporary antibody repertoire research. What recent studies have made abundantly clear, however, is that B cells with unique V-(D)-J rearrangements exist contemporarily, both within an organism and even within a single germinal center (**Figure 1B**) (27, 28). The utilization of new experimental techniques (e.g., multiphoton microscopy, confetti mice, and bone marrow chimeras) in concert with sequencing technologies have provided an unprecedented insight into how biological factors such as BCR affinity or clonal diversity can influence the evolutionary landscape.

Over the past decade, many fields of research have leveraged the increased resolution and decreased cost of high throughput sequencing (HTS) to better understand genomic diversity and evolution. Similarly, the field of immunology has employed HTS to investigate the genetic diversity of antibody variable regions, also referred to as immunoglobulin sequencing or Ig-Seq. This application has been instrumental in providing a quantitative description and profile of antibody repertoires (29–31). Ig-Seq experiments capture the diversity found in the variable regions of co-existing antibodies, enabling the reconstruction of multiple antibody lineages within a single host over time (32–34). Given the immense wealth of sequencing data arising from Ig-Seq, phylogenetic inference is a well-suited methodology to better understand clonal selection and expansion mechanisms that drive B cell evolution.

The standard evolutionary analysis of a B cell involves the reconstruction of a phylogenetic tree, in which the temporal relationships between recovered antibody sequences are modeled. The phylogenetic tree is often referred to as a clonal lineage, whereas a "phylogenetic lineage" represents a branch in the tree. In the case of antibody repertoire phylogenetics, each phylogenetic tree represents a clonal lineage descending from an independent V-(D)-J recombination event. From a single Ig-Seq experiment, a multitude of phylogenetic trees can be inferred, demanding a novel analysis pipeline not typically required in conventional phylogenetic studies examining species or viral evolution. The sequencing reads covering the full V-(D)-J region (~350–400 base pairs) are represented as nodes in the tree, while the edges indicate the relationship between the tips, and the edge lengths represent the time between branching events. These representations provide valuable information regarding the evolutionary history of a given antibody or B cell clone and can be employed to understand the selective pressures experienced during affinity maturation.

Studying how antibodies evolve in the context of pathogen neutralization has the potential to both answer basic biological questions pertaining to clonal selection and to aid in the development of precision vaccines or discovery of therapeutic monoclonal antibodies. Extensive research efforts have already been dedicated to better comprehend a subset of antibodies capable of neutralizing the infectious potential of multiple strains of HIV-1 (broadly neutralizing antibodies, bNAbs) (35–38). A prominent example involves the VRC01 bNAb lineage, originally identified from B cells of an HIV-1 patient, which has been shown to neutralize 90% of HIV-1 strains after undergoing extensive SHM (39). Using traditional phylogenetic methods, the evolutionary steps preceding virus-neutralizing capability were inferred, enabling the inference of both ancestral and intermediate sequences (38, 39). Further work has attempted to design vaccine immunogens that target these intermediate progenitor sequences in hopes of directing the subsequent evolution of antibodies toward

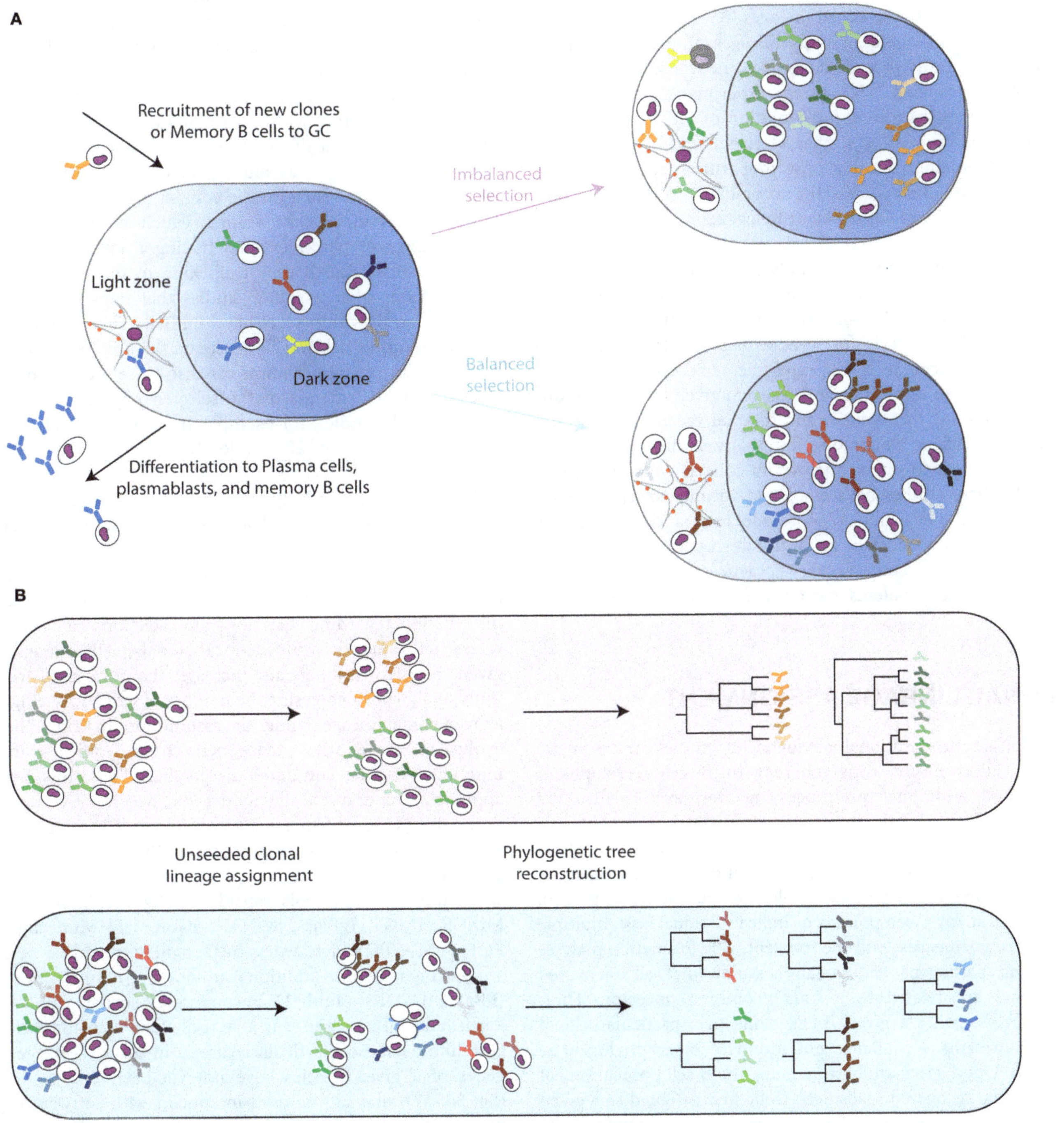


**FIGURE 1** | Evolutionary dynamics of the Germinal center reaction. **(A)** Naïve and memory B cells are recruited into germinal center reactions where they undergo subsequent rounds of somatic hypermutation in the dark zone and selection via follicular dendritic cells in the light zone. This leads to successive rounds of division and mutations (shown by colored antibody receptors) or apoptosis (shown by gray cells). Different selection pressures can lead to either balanced selection, in which multiple independent clones expand and undergo SHM, or imbalanced selection where a few clones dominate the GC reaction and undergo many rounds of SHM. **(B)** Ig-Seq can capture the sequence diversity within populations of B cells. Systems phylogeny aims to assign the recovered sequences into clonal families, followed by the inference of evolutionary histories. The resulting phylogenetic trees can then be compared both within one host and between hosts.

the broadly neutralizing phenotype (40, 41). Additionally, how affinity, avidity, and the initial concentration of these progenitor BCRs influence the subsequent GC reactions and incurred mutations was recently described, providing further insight about the appearance and propagation of bNAbs (42).

While the various HIV-1 bNAbs have ignited hopes of utilizing phylogenetics to design vaccines for rapidly mutating viruses, most research employing antibody phylogenetics has been confined to single clonal lineages (35–37, 43, 44). Despite the emphasis on single antibody lineages, the majority of the sequencing data used to describe these neutralizing antibodies has been recovered via Ig-Seq experiments. Thus, while individual trees describing the evolution of HIV-1-neutralizing antibodies have been well characterized, several unanswered questions remain regarding how to partition the sequencing reads into the individual V-(D)-J recombination trees, and how this antibody "forest" of distinct phylogenetic trees evolves as a system.

The unique opportunity to apply sequencing technologies to the study of B cells has led to the development of several tools and practices specifically tailored to the investigation of antibody evolution (45–47). It is foreseeable that this trend will only continue to increase as Ig-Seq experiments become increasingly commonplace in immunological research given the applications both to antibody therapeutics and rational vaccine design (48). Despite the lack of standardization, many studies have already incorporated phylogenetic analyses in concert with Ig-Seq (34, 38, 49). These studies have employed various tools, inference methods, and heuristics. We provide here a comprehensive review tailored specifically to antibody repertoire phylogeny. We outline both contemporary practices and software, in addition to the problems currently faced by this promising field.

## CLONAL LINEAGE ASSIGNMENT

As opposed to traditional phylogenetic studies, the somatic diversification mechanisms inherent to B cell development present an additional pre-processing step even before the selection of a tree-inference method. V-(D)-J recombination creates an immense starting pool of roots, each of which has the potential to encounter its cognate antigen and subsequently undergo clonal expansion and evolution (polyclonal response). Therefore, at any given point in a single individual host, multiple co-evolving lineages will be present. Phylogenetic analyses involving pathogens traditionally assume that all recovered sequences are related to a single common ancestor. Thus, correctly assigning a given B cell clone to a particular clonal lineage presents a challenge not found in other phylogenetic analyses. Upon successfully sequencing the B cell populations of interest, the recovered reads need to be first assigned to a given phylogenetic tree, representing a group of clones expanded from a single V-(D)-J recombination event (**Figure 1B**). A given Ig-Seq experiment can produce millions of sequencing reads per sample (4, 29, 50), rendering it difficult to disentangle the simultaneous, independently co-evolving lineages. Several strategies and tools have been recently developed in response to this problem and are outlined below.

A common starting approach is to initially cluster sequences by their germline genes, and subsequently infer an individual tree for each cluster. Based on the number of possible combinations of V-, D-, and J-genes, this implies that thousands of phylogenetic trees could be inferred within a single individual. In practice, not all germline genes and combinations thereof are used at the same frequency, which dramatically reduces the number of actual trees produced within one host (4, 51). Additionally, low alignment accuracy of the D-gene segment has led many studies to only consider the V- and J-gene segments during clustering. The number of trees within a single individual can be further reduced by setting a threshold for a number of sequences per tree. Unfortunately, the value to define the threshold is less clear and often depends on the context of biological questions. For example, there exist studies which have set thresholds of 10 sequences per tree when tracing B cells across various compartments (e.g., B cells trafficking to the central nervous system) (52), whereas other studies that depict differentiated memory B cells within a tree have omitted a threshold altogether (49). In addition to lower limits set on the number of sequences required per tree, upper limits can also be set depending on the computational demands of the selected phylogenetic method. Multiple HIV studies, for example, have restricted each lineage tree to a maximum of 200 randomly sampled sequences for the root of interest (36, 43).

The challenge of assigning reads to a clonal lineage can be addressed by taking advantage of the nature of SHM to preferentially introduce nucleotide substitutions during GC reactions (53). This implies that insertions and deletions are mainly introduced via V-(D)-J recombination. Therefore, information regarding insertions and deletions can be utilized to restrict sequences with identical clonal (CDR3) lengths to a given tree. This dramatically increases the number of trees per individual, while decreasing the number of sequences assigned to a given clonal lineage. Under the assumption that clonal lineages evolve independently, phylogenetic trees from a particular individual can be computed in parallel. Thus, this heuristic approach can dramatically reduce the necessary computation time while incorporating relevant biological insight regarding a constant CDR3 length throughout the affinity maturation process.

Commonly used tools capable of aligning Ig-Seq data are MiXCR, IMGT, IgBlast, SONAR, IGoR, iHMMunealign, and Partis (54–60), which work by assigning germline genes to sequencing reads and additional annotation [Framework regions (FRs) and CDRs] (**Table 1**). In some cases, such as with MiXCR, Partis, and IgBlast, a user is able to include a custom reference germline database (particularly useful in cases where germline genes of a given species have not yet been fully annotated) (54, 56, 57); this can be used in concert with software capable of predicting germline alleles from Ig-Seq data. While Partis has this capability built in (61), other standalone software includes IgDiscover and TigGER (62, 63). Additionally, one can extract germline information from whole genome shotgun sequencing, as performed by VGeneRepertoire (64). One of the major drawbacks of the previously mentioned lineage assignment is the large reliance on an initial alignment of recovered reads to the germline. Furthermore, any rare insertions or deletions introduced during SHM will be excluded due to restricting trees to an identical clonal (CDR3) length.

Several methods have been developed to circumvent problems arising during alignment-based lineage assignment. These

**TABLE 1** | Comparison of tools and methods used for clonal lineage assignment and phylogenetic inference.

| | Attributes (+) | Notes (–) |
|---|---|---|
| **Clonal LINEAGE ASSIGNMENT** | | |
| Alignment based<br>(Mixcr, IMGT, IgBlast, IGoR, IHMMunealign) | • Potentially fast run time (depends on the tool)<br>• Can often supply own germline genes | • Often arbitrary thresholds for clonal relatedness (e.g., 80% CDR3 similarity) |
| Partis<br>(https://github.com/psathyrella/partis) | • Human, mouse and macaque germline built in<br>• Germline inference possible<br>• Docker image available<br>• Good documentation | • Large datasets may require subsampling due to computational demands |
| Clonify<br>(https://github.com/briney/clonify-python) | • Antibody specific edit distance<br>• Explicit incorporation of shared mutational histories | • Limited to unseeded alignment |
| SONAR<br>(https://github.com/scharch/SONAR) | • Multiple seeded lineage assignment algorithms<br>• Easy export to other phylogenetic software<br>• Docker image available | • Limited to Human germlines |
| **PHYLOGENETIC METHOD** | | |
| Distance based<br>(ape, ClustalOmega, EBI, phangorn, FastML) | • Computational speed<br>• Multiple distance metrics possible | • Difficult to calculate distances for sequences with large divergence and alignment gaps<br>• Less sophisticated than probabilistic methods |
| Maximum parsimony<br>(PHYLIP, Rphylip, GCTree, phangorn, IgTree) | • Intuitive algorithm<br>• Clonal frequency incorporation (GCTree)<br>• Polytomies and internal nodes (IgTree) | • Ignores antibody specific properties (hotspots, transversions, transitions)<br>• Long-branch attraction problem |
| Maximum likelihood<br>(FastML, MEGA, IQ-TREE, dnaml, IgPhyML) | • Complex substitution models<br>• Hotspot specific codon models (IgPhyML) | • Computationally demanding<br>• Sensitive to model misspecification |
| Bayesian<br>(BEAST, Mr. Bayes, ImmuniTree) | • Complex substitution models<br>• Can produce rooted trees without explicit outgroup<br>• Possible to incorporate biological knowledge with priors<br>• Mutation rate returned in calendar time (BEAST) | • Sensitive to model misspecification<br>• Highest computational demands due to Markov chain Monte Carlo algorithm |

methods include both seeded and unseeded lineage assignment. Seeded lineage assignment aims to extract all clonally-related transcripts to an input antibody sequence. Conversely, unseeded lineage assignment attempts to decompose the entirety of input sequences into their constitutive clonal families. Three prominent tools specifically tailored to clonal lineage determination are Partis, Clonify, and SONAR (57, 58, 65). Partis models B cell evolution with a likelihood function that avoids the need to strictly define rooting assumptions, such as an arbitrarily defined percentage of CDR3 sequence homology (57). This tool can perform both unseeded and seeded lineage assignment, with input sizes reaching hundreds of thousands and millions of sequences, respectively. Another tool, Clonify, uses hierarchical clustering based on an antibody specific edit distance to determine clonal lineage inclusion (65). One benefit of this proposed algorithm relative to the aforementioned alignment tools is that neither CDR3 lengths nor germline alignments explicitly define a clonal lineage. Instead, CDR3 similarity, germline alignment scores, and information regarding shared mutational histories are included in the clonal assignment. Finally, SONAR first aligns reads to germlines provided by IMGT and can subsequently perform either seeded or unseeded lineage assignment (58). Their unseeded alignment relies upon first separating transcripts into groups based on V- and J- genes, with subsequent clustering based on CDR3 sequence similarity. Multiple algorithms for seeded lineage assignment are available, in addition to functions which allow visualization of homology to germline genes and other known antibodies (58). While the subsequent phylogenetic tree inference is possible with SONAR, clonal lineages can also be easily exported to formats compatible with other commonly used tree inference software. Finally, both Partis and SONAR are available as Docker containers, which can dramatically simplify the installation process. While these methods are a promising step to improve the delineation of independent V-(D)-J recombination events from bulk sequencing data, further benchmarking studies are still required to illustrate how clonal lineage assignment algorithms influence the downstream evolutionary conclusions. Such studies, for example, could examine how the amount, topologies, and sizes of lineage trees from a single repertoire change based on preprocessing and lineage assignment pipelines.

## STRUCTURE OF THE B CELL TREE

Phylogenetic trees are commonly defined such that each node represents a recovered B cell sequence (or clone), whereas the branches represent the relationship between sequences. However, there exist several important differences between traditional phylogenetic trees and models specifically tailored to describe B cell evolution (**Figure 2**). One important characteristic of B cell maturation is clonal selection during expansion, which results in multiple B cells that have identical BCR sequences. Therefore, Ig-Seq can return identical reads corresponding to different B cells, adding a frequency attribute to each recovered sequence. The most common method currently employed by repertoire studies has been to remove replicate sequences, producing a phylogenetic tree entirely composed of unique sequences. However, this approach is inherently biased given the disregard for clonal expansion, a biological phenomenon seminal to B cell immunity. In particular, evolutionary rates are over-estimated as the periods without mutation during clonal expansion are disregarded.

Furthermore, it has been recently shown that the starting amount of antigen-specific memory (precursor) B cells (i.e., ancestral sequences) in a given lineage directly impacts the ability to engage in GC reactions and undergo further mutations (42). This stresses the importance of implementing phylogenetic methods that can incorporate clonal frequencies into the tree reconstruction calculation. To account for clonal expansion, antibody studies have displayed phylogenetic trees where the size of the node refers to the number of identical sequences (**Figure 2A**). While this leads to a visual representation of clonal abundance, this information does not contribute to the phylogenetic inference, thereby ignoring valuable information describing the evolutionary processes underlying clonal selection. Therefore, recent progress has been made to combine traditional phylogenetic inference methods with this clonal abundance data (66). In what are referred to as GCTrees, clonal abundance information was explicitly modeled into the phylogenetic inference process, leading to increased accuracy based on simulated trees (66). Furthermore, this reconstruction method allows for the inclusion of recovered sequences to serve as internal nodes (for the rationale, see section The Mutation Process Along the Tree) (66). This methodology highlights the progress toward integrating the biologically relevant information recovered from Ig-Seq experiments into the reconstruction of antibody phylogenies.

The traditional phylogenetic framework produces trees where the recovered sequences are positioned as leaves of the trees. However, there are several antibody evolution studies that have conceptualized the internal structure of the phylogenetic tree to better suit B cell evolution and selection. This involves the allowance of polytomies (more than two descendants from a single internal node) and intermediate sequences serving as internal nodes (**Figures 2B,C**). The underlying logic behind this dramatic shift from traditional evolutionary studies relies on the assumption that a given B cell clone can produce multiple distinct offspring (somatic variants), each of which may be separated by only a single mutation. Furthermore, this same ancestral B cell may persist long after giving rise to progenitor cells without incurring further mutations (**Figure 2D**). To account for both of these biological considerations, antibody-specific phylogenetic tools such as IgTree and ImmuniTree allow for both the presence of polytomies and the presence of recovered sequences as internal nodes in the resulting lineage tree. While these topological frameworks diverge from traditional phylogenetic analyses, they introduce a flexibility that allows for the incorporation of antibody-relevant information. However, it remains unknown how these adjustments to the phylogenetic model tree impact the biological conclusions such as tree shape and mutation rates. It would be interesting to investigate into how the tree structure of HIV neutralizing antibodies, for example, would change if polytomies were allowed in the phylogenetic reconstruction.

## THE MUTATION PROCESS ALONG THE TREE

The enzymatic nature of how AID induces mutations during affinity maturation dictates the evolutionary trajectories possible for a given B cell. AID introduces mutations by preferentially targeting the immunoglobulin locus via the deamination of deoxycytidine residues into deoxyuridines. This newly introduced deoxyuridine results in a mismatch pairing in the DNA and is subsequently corrected by either MMR or BER. The majority of mutations introduced after these nucleotide repair pathways are in the form of point mutations, although there are occasional deletions or insertions present (67, 68). These substitutions must not only maintain stability of the BCR, but also provide a functional antibody capable of surviving antigen selection imposed during GC reactions (**Figure 1A**). This selection has been implicated in improving binding affinity, broadening of antigen recognition and the development of specific effector functions such as pathogen neutralization (24, 39). Interestingly, the shift from pathogen binding to pathogen neutralizing is not always associated with a large increase in binding affinity, suggesting a more nuanced role of affinity maturation than solely promoting high affinity antibodies (69).

Given that mutations are introduced through enzyme-mediated mechanisms, it is somewhat intuitive that particular patterns in the genome would be preferentially targeted. Even before the advent of HTS, certain nucleotide motifs, termed "hotspots," have been demonstrated to incur point mutations at greater than average frequency (70). One initial example supporting this neighbor-dependent model of SHM was the discovery of the RGYW motif (where W = A/T, R = A/G, Y = C/T), where the adjacent nucleotides influence the mutability of the central G nucleotide (70). Subsequent experiments uncovered additional motifs targeted by AID, albeit at low numbers due to limitations arising from low-throughput experimental settings (71–73). However, recent studies employing Ig-Seq have provided a thorough analysis of how neighboring nucleotides influence the probabilities of

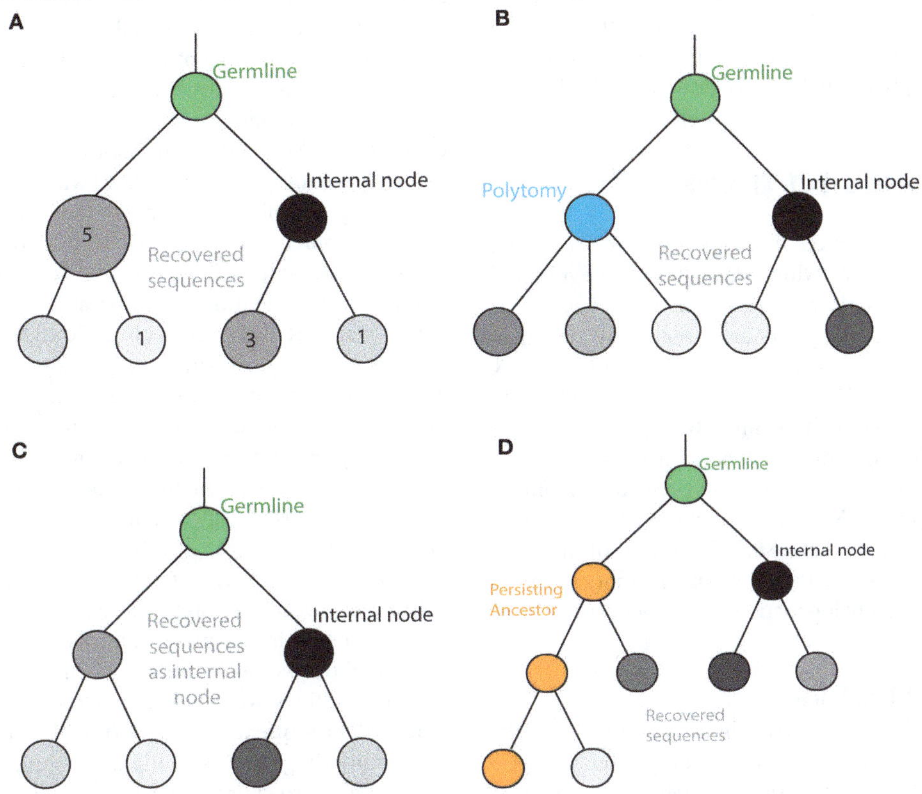


**FIGURE 2 |** Tree topologies for B cells. **(A)** The inclusion of polytomies in the phylogenetic tree allows a B cell to produce more than two distinct offspring at a given internal node. **(B)** Experimentally recovered sequences can be inferred as either internal nodes or tips in the phylogenetic tree. **(C)** Persisting ancestral sequences can be sampled at multiple time points while also producing distinct offspring. **(D)** Clonal frequencies have often been illustrated by the size of the nodes. Therefore, information regarding clonal expansion can be incorporated into the resulting topologies.

point mutations (74, 75). One prominent example compared synonymous and non-synonymous mutations across multiple Ig-Seq datasets to infer mutational probabilities for 5mers (nucleotide sequences with length 5), termed the "S5F" model (74). This substitution model contains inferred transition probabilities for the middle nucleotide of all possible 5mers, both verifying historical, low-throughput experimental data, and discovering novel motifs. In subsequent work, similar models were developed to describe the specific mutational properties of the 5mer motifs found in light chains arising from human and mouse data, providing a wealth of pertinent information to the mutational landscape of SHM (75). The refinement of distinct hotspot models for heavy and light chain evolution is crucial because the inference of heavy and light chain phylogenies can be performed separately, as performed in studies comparing the evolution of heavy and light chains in the context of HIV infection (38). However, when the pairing of heavy and light chains is known, the loci can be combined (concatenated to each other) and treated as a single evolving entity. This can increase the information used when inferring evolutionary parameters such as mutation rates and tree structure, given that both loci must share the same tree topology. Despite these findings describing the neighbor-dependent nature of AID, most modern phylogenetic methods rely on the assumption of site-independent substitution models, in which the neighboring nucleotides play no role in the evolutionary inference calculation. Thus, current studies analyzing B cell lineages typically do not account for this well-established biological phenomenon that may also have evolutionary ramifications.

One promising step to incorporate the properties of SHM hotspot motifs into the phylogenetic inference process has been demonstrated by the implementation of the HLP17 codon substitution model, which accounts for neighbor-dependent hotspot mutations, germline sequence knowledge, and irreversible evolution (76). This substitution model (available in the IgPhyML program) has been shown to perform better on Ig-Seq data than conventional phylogenetic substitution models because of the inclusion of phylogenetic inference parameters that describe the WRC hotspot (76). Specifically, it could be observed that the use of this codon model reduced bias in evolutionary parameters such as tree length (76), which has been previously shown to be difficult to estimate for multiple bNAb lineages with traditional substitution models (38). Their model allows for any motifs of length three nucleotides to be incorporated while still assuming that these hotspot motifs (i.e., codons) evolve independently to maintain computational feasibility (76). While all motifs cannot yet be explicitly accounted for simultaneously due to computational limitations, this work represents important progress toward incorporated motif-specific properties of SHM. One additional drawback remains that this substitution model is not yet available in many commonly used phylogenetic tools, potentially limiting its application.

## FROM SEQUENCES TO TREES

Multiple phylogenetic inference methods exist to construct the antibody lineages, each of which have their strengths and weaknesses (**Table 1**). A variety of these methods have been employed for the analysis of Ig-Seq data, including distance-based methods (44, 45, 77), maximum parsimony (36, 52, 78, 79), maximum likelihood (37, 43, 44, 80, 81), and Bayesian inference (38, 47, 82). Most methods initially require a multiple sequence alignment (MSA), which allows for lists of sequences with varying lengths to be compared in a site-dependent manner. Some common examples of MSA tools include ClustalOmega, Kalign, MUSCLE, and T-coffee (83–86). The output of the MSA file will usually be in fasta, nexus, or phylip format, which is easily integrated with the phylogenetic reconstruction methods described below.

### Distance-Based Methods

Distance-based methods involve first filling a matrix by an all-against-all calculation of a given metric comparing pairwise sequence similarity (87). The distances between sequences are often calculated using a substitution model. This allows for the incorporation of certain characteristics of sequence evolution, such as indicating different rates of evolution for transitions (purine <-> purine, pyrimidine <-> pyrimidine), and transversions (purine <-> pyrimidine), as well as taking into account the possibility of hidden mutations (such as backward mutations). A neighbor-joining algorithm is utilized to produce the tree, which involves successively joining two sequences together with newly created internal nodes (88, 89). One major advantage of this method is that tree inference is very fast. Therefore, this method can be especially useful for exploring large Ig-Seq data sets, particularly when there are many sequences in each lineage tree. A noteworthy example of this implementation was seen when examining the evolution of HIV-1 bNAbs, in which the neighbor-joining method was used exclusively for large datasets (45). There exist many tools that can produce neighbor-joining trees, either found online with ClustalOmega or EBI bioinformatics server, in addition to R packages such as phangorn or ape (84, 90, 91). One notable example of a distance metric that does not require a MSA is the Levenshtein distance. The Levenshtein distance describes the number of changes (mutations, insertions, or deletions) required to change one string into another, and has been used extensively in Ig-Seq experiments in the past (4, 92).

### Maximum Parismony

Another non-parametric method of inferring antibody evolution involves the use of maximum parsimony, in which the output phylogeny is the tree that can explain the evolution with the least amount of mutations (93, 94). This method does not allow for the incorporation of parameters specific to antibody evolution, which can be a disadvantage when there is abundant background knowledge of the experimental system. Conversely, the lack of assumptions regarding the substitution process may prevent model misspecification and thereby erroneous conclusions. Maximum parsimony has been used in multiple studies pertaining to Ig-Seq data, with some notable examples, examining B cell migration to the cervical lymph node or the development of neutralizing antibodies against West Nile virus (4, 74). Several tools exist to create maximum parsimony trees, although the most common among them is PHYLIP (95). Additionally, R packages such as Rphylip and phangorn have both incorporated maximum parsimony, allowing one to work within the R framework (91, 96). Finally, as previously stated, the GCTree utilizes a modified maximum parsimony to allow for clonal frequencies to influence the phylogenetic inference (67).

One of the earliest methods specifically tailored to inferring antibody evolution, IgTree, utilized a customized parsimony metric to produce lineage trees (45). This tool additionally introduced the concept of inferred intermediate sequences, in which all direct ancestral sequences were restricted to the separation of a single mutation (46). For example, two "inferred" internal nodes would be created when two sequences differing by three nucleotides are in the same clonal family. Thus, even if an intermediate sequence was not explicitly sampled, there would be a corresponding internal node in the output phylogeny. IgTree has been used to characterize how B cells evolve under a variety of selective pressures, such as lymphomas, multiple sclerosis, and autoimmunity (33, 77, 97).

### Maximum Likelihood

Another method applied to study antibody evolution is maximum likelihood, which relies on the optimization of a likelihood function. This parametric method incorporates a substitution model that can dictate parameters such as nucleotide/amino acid frequencies and allow for different substitution rates for transitions and transversions. Thus, maximum likelihood can utilize evolutionary models that may better describe antibody evolution than the neutral assumption that all nucleotides are the same. Some of these models include the HKY, GTR gamma, and JC69 (98–100), which allow for nucleotide specific behavior (e.g., *A* mutating to *C* can have a different rate as *C* mutating to *G*). It may not be immediately apparent which substitution model best fits the data at hand, whereby tools that include model selection capabilities may be useful. Notable programs utilized in the context of Ig-Seq data include FastML, MEGA, IQ-TREE, and Phylip's dnaml (33, 90, 94–96, 98, 101–103). As mentioned above, one notable limitation of these substitution models is that the transition probability of a given site is independent to the neighboring nucleotides. Thus, building upon models which incorporate information regarding hotspot mutability represents a cornerstone of contemporary systems phylogenetics research (76).

A multitude of studies have employed the maximum likelihood method to analyze Ig-Seq data, with many focusing on the evolution of HIV-neutralizing antibodies (35, 37, 39, 43, 44, 80, 104, 105). Despite most maximum likelihood programs producing a "traditional" phylogenetic tree, where recovered sequences cannot serve as intermediate nodes and polytomies are absent, the biological relevance of these maximum likelihood trees has been proven by the inference and production of intermediate and ancestral germline sequences which possessed virus-binding capabilities (36, 40).

## Bayesian Inference

The final considered method of phylogenetic inference relies upon Bayesian statistics, which is thus capable of incorporating prior biological information (known as priors) into the inference process. This includes information regarding the evolution of the B cells, in particular the mutation rate, and the replication of the B cells generating the tree, in particular B cell duplication and death rates. The most commonly used tool is BEAST (106, 107), which has many learning resources and user-contributed modules that are available for download. This method involves the largest computational demands compared to other phylogenetic methods both in terms of memory and calculation time (87). This largely is due to the inference process, which utilizes a Markov chain Monte Carlo (MCMC) algorithm to explore parameter space. This provides a sample from the posterior probability distribution, i.e., the output consists of millions of trees, which are a sample of the probability distribution. One can summarize this distribution into a single tree, termed as the most credible clade (MCC) tree, allowing for an easier comparison between multiple trees.

One further advantage of BEAST is that one can easily specify the time at which sequences were sampled, and that the output consists of trees with branch lengths in calendar time units (rather than number of substitutions as in all methods above). This kinetic information restricts the position of the sequence in the tree, in addition to inferring mutation rates in calendar time units. Thus, Bayesian methods present a strong advantage when time-resolved Ig-Seq data is available. One major drawback is the limited number of sequences that can be included in each phylogenetic tree, as trees with more than ~500 antibody sequences often require substantial computation time (e.g., months on a server) and do not always converge to the posterior distribution. Furthermore, if many lineage trees are desired, running the MCMCs in parallel is essential given the slow computation time. BEAST has been used to infer mutation rates of neutralizing antibodies and subsequently compared to viral evolution (39). An interesting result from this analysis was that the heavy and light chains evolved at similar rates for this particular bNAb. Furthermore, it was shown that different neutralizing antibody lineages evolve at different rates, suggesting multiple mechanisms underlying the maturation of bNAbs.

An antibody-specific tool, ImmuniTree, has been developed that incorporates a Bayesian framework into the inference of lineage trees (48). ImmuniTree allows for recovered sequences to be placed at internal nodes, polytomies, and accounts for spurious diversity arising from sequencing errors. Furthermore, the trees produced by ImmuniTree can depict the percentage of mutations a given immunoglobulin sequence has, thereby incorporating information not included in most other inference methods. Practically, this tool has been used to reconstruct lineages of bNAbs and to infer ancestral intermediates of these antibodies (47, 82). The phylogenetic data was subsequently used to direct experiments which displayed that the neutralizing breadth of these intermediate antibodies was still present, despite a lesser extent of SHM (48).

## Rooting the Phylogenetic Tree

The presented phylogenetic methods (with the Bayesian methods as exceptions) return trees without a root, i.e., the tree does not consist of information regarding on which branch the clonal expansion process started. Thus, these unrooted trees need to be rooted, which is typically done using an outgroup (for example, when inferring an ape tree, one can use a-non-ape primate sequence as an outgroup for rooting). For B cell phylogenies, we have knowledge regarding the underlying V-(D)-J recombination, meaning that unmutated V-(D)-J germline sequence can be incorporated into the tree reconstruction process as the outgroup. One major assumption of this strategy is that there is sufficient confidence in the germline annotations. This assumption may increase the information present during the phylogenetic analysis for inbred model organisms, such as mice or zebrafish. However, when the exact genomic composition of the V-(D)-J germline segments is unknown (e.g., in humans, where there are slight allelic changes in the germline between individuals), this discrepancy could alter the inferred mutation rate.

BEAST produces rooted trees even without explicitly designating any germline sequences as the outgroup. This can be advantageous when an exact annotation of the germline genes is lacking. While it is possible in BEAST to explicitly specify the root of a tree, it is not immediately straightforward due to the nature of the software. In the case where no germline sequences are supplied as a root, there exists an additional tool in the program that allows for the user to infer the sequence at the root (in addition to sequences at internal nodes). Important to note, however, is that the accuracy of this method has not yet been explicitly validated for antibody evolution (i.e., compared unmutated ancestors inferred from BEAST to the known germline sequences). Further benchmarking on both simulated data and experimental data is required to better understand how rooting with the germline segments influences the subsequent biological conclusions, for example mutation rates and topology metrics.

## Simulations

Simulations of antibody evolution represents a powerful approach to validate and explore the consequences of various phylogenetic tools and heuristic strategies. Initial antibody repertoire simulation frameworks did not possess a temporal component (i.e., no explicit rate at which sequences change in regard to time), hence preventing the investigation of how traditional phylogenetic methods perform on Ig-Seq data (108). Recently, multiple tools have been developed to account for evolutionary properties specific to B cell evolution. Elements such as hotspot motifs, clonal abundances, and mutation rates can be defined to produce an output phylogenetic tree along with the accompanying mutated sequences. These sequences can then be fed as input into various phylogenetic inference methods to validate tree reconstruction accuracy. Tree accuracy is validated by comparing the inferred to the simulated tree, e.g., via the Robinson Foulds distance, clade accuracy, and treescape metrics (46, 109, 110). While simulations are commonly incorporated in Ig-Seq experiments, these are largely in-house and not always publically available. An important step to improve benchmarking tools and strategies for Ig-Seq experiments includes making these simulation platforms publicly available to increase their use.

## DOWNSTREAM ANALYSIS

One of the difficulties of including phylogenetic trees into Ig-Seq studies is the extraction and interpretation of biologically relevant conclusions. An emerging trend has been to focus on a few select lineages and leave the majority of the repertoire unanalyzed. Thus, major questions regarding how the entirety of the antibody repertoire evolves remain unanswered. The hurdles of inferring potentially hundreds to thousands of phylogenetic trees per individual is daunting both due to the computational demands and the subsequent analysis. Furthermore, comparing trees within a single host, and to other organisms introduces a further layer of complexity.

One of the most immediate results of phylogenetic inference is the output of a phylogenetic tree. The topology of these trees provides a visualization of the evolutionary relationship between a set of antibodies, which can be both qualitatively understood and quantitatively compared. Qualitatively, an imbalanced tree (defined as the two daughter lineages of a node have very different numbers of descending nodes) can be interpreted in that a single progenitor clone continuously out-survives the other clones. Thus, tree imbalance may describe the breadth of underlying selection pressures. This selective pressure where a single clone outcompetes the remaining population has been seen in other infectious species, for example influenza between hosts or HIV within a host (111). Conversely, when selection occurs evenly throughout a lineage, many clones may simultaneously proliferate, which can be observed as a balanced structure of the tree (**Figure 1**). Balanced trees have e.g., been observed for HIV between hosts (111). While Ig-Seq papers have mentioned these topological characteristics, few have thoroughly analyzed these phylogenetic structures. There exist metrics arising from the evolutionary biology field capable of describing tree topology in a way that allows comparison of the lineage trees both from within a single host and across individuals. Metrics such as the Colless number, the Sackin index, and the average number of ladders characterize tree "imbalance" (112, 113). Mathematically, these metrics account for the number of descendant sequences in right and left sub-trees at all internal nodes, producing a single value for the entire tree. This value can then be directly compared to other clonal lineage trees, providing a framework for a systems analysis of lineages. This concept of analyzing tree shape and imbalance has been implemented in the comparison of vaccine-responsive lineages to persistent lineages (highly abundant lineages that did not change in response to vaccination) (114). Lineages that were unresponsive to vaccination showed a more balanced evolution, whereas the vaccine-enriched lineages often had a focus on multiple positively selected subclones (114).

While the metrics above have not often been applied to Ig-Seq experiments, other topological metrics have been used to quantify clonal selection. For example, clonal lineage trees were produced to better understand the diversification processes underlying a subset of B cells residing in the bone marrow of human patients suffering from light chain amyloidosis (115). The downstream analysis described structural properties of the phylogenetic trees, such as the number of sequences per tree, the length of the trunk (distance from root to first branching event), pass-through nodes (internal nodes with a single offspring), the distance to the nearest branching event (thus quantifying how mutations separate a sequence's direct ancestor), and tree branching (determined by the outgoing number of internal nodes). Similarly, another study found that during gastric lymphomas, B cell evolution results in trees with longer trunks and path lengths when compared to gastritis, correlating with a higher initial affinity and a higher selection threshold (34).

While these structural motifs and tree-imbalance metrics provide a natural analysis of phylogenetic trees in biological terms, there additionally exist less intuitive metrics yet to be applied to Ig-Seq data. Phylogenetic trees are essentially acyclic graphs (graphs = networks), suggesting that novel methods in graph theory may potentially find their use in Ig-Seq studies. One potential example of utilizing graph theory arises from examining the Laplacian spectra of the many trees within an individual. This approach was suggested recently to possess a multitude of parameters describing individual tree shape and branch length in the context of eigenvector distributions (116). However, few studies have leveraged such topological analyses of unlabeled antibody trees, thus, the extent to which meaningful biological conclusions can be drawn remains unseen.

In contrast to qualitative topological analysis, statistically derived parameters may be of further interest to provide a quantitative description of the evolutionary process of antibody lineages. Traditionally, repertoire studies have been interested in counting the number of mutations found at a given time point, however, leveraging phylogenetics, one can quantify how often a given lineage accumulates mutations in a time-resolved fashion. As previously stated, Bayesian phylogenetics has already been utilized to calculate the mutation rates of heavy and light chain lineages of HIV-neutralizing antibodies (39). Furthermore, parameters describing population size, the speciation and extinction of species, and tree age can be further inferred, providing a set of parameters that lends itself easily to the comparison both within a single host and across different individuals.

### Toward Systems Phylogeny of Antibody Repertoires

The aforementioned metrics to quantify phylogenetic trees require just a single phylogenetic tree as input. The values arising from multiple trees can then be collectively analyzed to describe the selective pressure exerted upon the antibody repertoire as a whole. This traditional manner of studying the collection of antibody lineages, however, assumes a significant degree of independence between each phylogenetic tree. In an attempt to describe the population of antibody lineage trees, the UniFrac metric was applied to quantify the divergent evolution of immune systems arising during aging (35). The UniFrac metric was originally developed to measure the distance between microbial communities based on which branches are present in each sample, presenting a community-based statistic that can be easily adapted to Ig-Seq data (117). Another recent study aiming to characterize the dynamics of BCR evolution during HIV infection developed statistical models to describe clonal competition across multiple antibody lineages (118). Taken in concert, these studies represent important steps in the direction of statistics and analyses capable of describing the dynamic nature and evolution of antibody repertoire forests.

## CONCLUSION

Quantifying how antibody repertoires change over time represents an emerging field only possible due to the increased resolution of HTS and Ig-Seq. While the earliest phylogenetic metrics specifically tailored to antibody repertoire evolution were developed over a decade ago, more work remains necessary to comprehensively incorporate our experimental knowledge of antibodies into clonal lineage assignment, phylogenetic tree inference, and downstream analyses. Furthermore, benchmarking the aforementioned tools and strategies on both Ig-Seq data and multiple simulation frameworks can identify biases arising from the currently employed methodologies. The usage of lineage trees has immediate applications with medicinal relevance, such as vaccine design by targeting intermediate sequences or the discovery of therapeutic monoclonal antibodies. Furthermore, phylogenetics provides a unique opportunity to describe the clonal selection and competition underlying the pathogen-driven evolution of B cells. While phylogenetics has long held a role in the field of antibody research, the full potential of systems phylogenetics to delineate the complex co-evolving landscape between several independent lineages has not been realized. Other research fields such as machine learning, statistical entropy, and network analysis are becoming integral in antibody repertoire analysis, reinforcing the potential for phylogenetics to similarly take the stage to help delineate the complex picture of the B cell immunity.

## AUTHOR CONTRIBUTIONS

AY and SR conceived and designed the review. All authors wrote the review.

## FUNDING

This work was funded by the Swiss National Science Foundation (Project #: 31003A_170110, to SR), SystemsX.ch—antibody RTD project (to SR); European Research Council Starting Grant (Project #: 679403 to SR); and ETH Zurich (Research Grants). The professorship of SR is made possible by the generous endowment of the S. Leslie Misrock Foundation.

## REFERENCES


1. Lu LL, Suscovich TJ, Fortune SM, Alter G. Beyond binding: antibody effector functions in infectious diseases. *Nat Rev Immunol.* (2017) 18:46–61. doi: 10.1038/nri.2017.106
2. Xu JL, Davis MM. Diversity in the CDR3 region of VH is sufficient for most antibody specificities. *Immunity* (2000) 13:37–45. doi: 10.1016/S1074-7613(00)00006-6
3. Tonegawa S. Somatic generation of antibody diversity. *Nature* (1983) 302:575–81. doi: 10.1038/302575a0
4. Greiff V, Menzel U, Miho E, Weber C, Riedel R, Cook SC, et al. Systems analysis reveals high genetic and antigen-driven predetermination of antibody repertoires throughout B-cell development. *Cell Rep.* (2017) 19:1467–78. doi: 10.1016/j.celrep.2017.04.054
5. Elhanati Y, Sethna Z, Marcou Q, Callan CG, Mora T, Walczak AM. Inferring processes underlying B-cell repertoire diversity. *Phil Trans R Soc B* (2015) 370:20140243. doi: 10.1098/rstb.2014.0243
6. Nadel B, Feeney AJ. Nucleotide deletion and P addition in V (D) J recombination: a determinant role of the coding-end sequence. *Mol Cell Biol.* (1997) 17:3768–78. doi: 10.1128/MCB.17.7.3768
7. Glanville J, Zhai W, Berka J, Telman D, Huerta G, Mehta GR, et al. Precise determination of the diversity of a combinatorial antibody library gives insight into the human immunoglobulin repertoire. *Proc Natl Acad Sci USA.* (2009) 106:20216–21. doi: 10.1073/pnas.0909775106
8. Lanzavecchia A. Receptor-mediated antigen uptake and its effect on antigen presentation to class II-restricted T lymphocytes. *Annu Rev Immunol.* (1990) 8:773–93. doi: 10.1146/annurev.iy.08.040190.004013
9. Hou P, Araujo E, Zhao T, Zhang M, Massenburg D, Veselits M, et al. B cell antigen receptor signaling and internalization are mutually exclusive events. *PLoS Biol.* (2006) 4:e200. doi: 10.1371/journal.pbio.0040200
10. Zaretsky I, Atrakchi O, Mazor RD, Stoler-Barak L, Biram A, Feigelson SW, et al. ICAMs support B cell interactions with T follicular helper cells and promote clonal selection. *J Exp Med.* (2017) 214:3435–48. doi: 10.1084/jem.20171129
11. Mesin L, Ersching J, Victora GD. Germinal center B cell dynamics. *Immunity* (2016) 45:471–82. doi: 10.1016/j.immuni.2016.09.001
12. Allen CDC, Okada T, Cyster JG. Germinal-Center Organization and cellular dynamics. *Immunity* (2007) 27:190–202. doi: 10.1016/j.immuni.2007.07.009
13. Cattoretti G, Buettner M, Shaknovich R, Kremmer E, Alobeid B, Niedobitek G. Nuclear and cytoplasmic AID in extrafollicular and germinal center B cells. *Blood* (2006) 107:3967–75. doi: 10.1182/blood-2005-10-4170
14. Greeve J, Philipsen A, Krause K, Klapper W, Heidorn K, Castle BE, et al. Expression of activation-induced cytidine deaminase in human B-cell non-Hodgkin lymphomas. *Blood* (2003) 101:3574–80. doi: 10.1182/blood-2002-08-2424
15. McHeyzer-Williams LJ, Milpied PJ, Okitsu SL, McHeyzer-Williams MG. Class-switched memory B cells remodel BCRs within secondary germinal centers. *Nat Immunol.* (2015) 16:296–305. doi: 10.1038/ni.3095
16. Di Noia JM, Neuberger MS. Molecular mechanisms of antibody somatic hypermutation. *Annu Rev Biochem.* (2007) 76:1–22. doi: 10.1146/annurev.biochem.76.061705.090740
17. Methot SP, Di Noia JM. Molecular mechanisms of somatic hypermutation and class switch recombination. *Adv Immunol.* (2017) 133:37–87. doi: 10.1016/bs.ai.2016.11.002
18. Peled JU, Kuang FL, Iglesias-Ussel MD, Roa S, Kalis SL, Goodman MF, et al. The biochemistry of somatic hypermutation. *Annu Rev*

*Immunol.* (2008) 26:481–511. doi: 10.1146/annurev.immunol.26.021607.090236

19. Meyer-Hermann ME, Maini PK, Iber D. An analysis of B cell selection mechanisms in germinal centers. *Math Med Biol.* (2006) 23:255–77. doi: 10.1093/imammb/dql012
20. Victora GD, Schwickert TA, Fooksman DR, Kamphorst AO, Meyer-Hermann M, Dustin ML, et al. Germinal center dynamics revealed by multiphoton microscopy with a photoactivatable fluorescent reporter. *Cell* (2010) 143:592–605. doi: 10.1016/j.cell.2010.10.032
21. Liu D, Xu H, Shih C, Wan Z, Ma X, Ma W, et al. T–B-cell entanglement and ICOSL-driven feed-forward regulation of germinal centre reaction. *Nature* (2015) 517:214–18. doi: 10.1038/nature13803
22. Shulman Z, Gitlin AD, Weinstein JS, Lainez B, Esplugues E, Flavell RA, et al. Dynamic signaling by T follicular helper cells during germinal center B cell selection. *Science* (2014) 345:1058–62. doi: 10.1126/science.1257861
23. Wang Y, Keck Z, Saha A, Xia J, Conrad F, Lou J, et al. Affinity maturation to improve human monoclonal antibody neutralization potency and breadth against hepatitis C virus. *J Biol Chem.* (2011) 286:44218–33. doi: 10.1074/jbc.M111.290783
24. Greczmiel U, Kräutler NJ, Pedrioli A, Bartsch I, Agnellini P, Bedenikovic G, et al. Sustained T follicular helper cell response is essential for control of chronic viral infection. *Sci Immunol.* (2017) 2:eaam8686. doi: 10.1126/sciimmunol.aam8686
25. Murugan R, Buchauer L, Triller G, Kreschel C, Costa G, Pidelaserra Martí G, et al. Clonal selection drives protective memory B cell responses in controlled human malaria infection. *Sci Immunol.* (2018) 3:eaap8029. doi: 10.1126/sciimmunol.aap8029
26. Pappas L, Foglierini M, Piccoli L, Kallewaard NL, Turrini F, Silacci C, et al. Rapid development of broadly influenza neutralizing antibodies through redundant mutations. *Nature* (2014) 516:418–22. doi: 10.1038/nature13764
27. Kuraoka M, Schmidt AG, Nojima T, Feng F, Watanabe A, Kitamura D, et al. Complex antigens drive permissive clonal selection in germinal centers. *Immunity* (2016) 44:542–52. doi: 10.1016/j.immuni.2016.02.010
28. Tas JM, Mesin L, Pasqual G, Targ S, Jacobsen JT, Mano YM, et al. Visualizing antibody affinity maturation in germinal centers. *Science* (2016) 351:1048–54. doi: 10.1126/science.aad3439
29. Greiff V, Miho E, Menzel U, Reddy ST. Bioinformatic and statistical analysis of adaptive immune repertoires. *Trends Immunol.* (2015) 36:738–49. doi: 10.1016/j.it.2015.09.006
30. Georgiou G, Ippolito GC, Beausang J, Busse CE, Wardemann H, Quake SR. The promise and challenge of high-throughput sequencing of the antibody repertoire. *Nat Biotechnol.* (2014) 32:158–68. doi: 10.1038/nbt.2782
31. Yaari G, Kleinstein SH. Practical guidelines for B-cell receptor repertoire sequencing analysis. *Genome Med.* (2015) 7:121. doi: 10.1186/s13073-015-0243-2
32. Galson JD, Trück J, Clutterbuck EA, Fowler A, Cerundolo V, Pollard AJ, et al. B-cell repertoire dynamics after sequential hepatitis B vaccination and evidence for cross-reactive B-cell activation. *Genome Med.* (2016) 8:68. doi: 10.1186/s13073-016-0322-z
33. Michaeli M, Tabibian-Keissar H, Schiby G, Shahaf G, Pickman Y, Hazanov L, et al. Immunoglobulin gene repertoire diversification and selection in the stomach – from gastritis to gastric lymphomas. *Front Immunol.* (2014) 5:264. doi: 10.3389/fimmu.2014.00264
34. de Bourcy CF, Angel CJ, Vollmers C, Dekker CL, Davis MM, Quake SR. Phylogenetic analysis of the human antibody repertoire reveals quantitative signatures of immune senescence and aging. *Proc Natl Acad Sci USA.* (2017) 114:1105–10. doi: 10.1073/pnas.1617959114
35. Bonsignori M, Zhou T, Sheng Z, Chen L, Gao F, Joyce MG, et al. Maturation pathway from germline to broad HIV-1 neutralizer of a CD4-mimic antibody. *Cell* (2016) 165:449–63. doi: 10.1016/j.cell.2016.02.022
36. Banerjee S, Shi H, Banasik M, Moon H, Lees W, Qin Y, et al. Evaluation of a novel multi-immunogen vaccine strategy for targeting 4E10/10E8 neutralizing epitopes on HIV-1 gp41 membrane proximal external region. *Virology* (2017) 505:113–26. doi: 10.1016/j.virol.2017.02.015
37. Doria-Rose NA, Schramm CA, Gorman J, Moore PL, Bhiman JN, DeKosky BJ, et al. Developmental pathway for potent V1V2-directed HIV-neutralizing antibodies. *Nature* (2014) 509:55–62. doi: 10.1038/nature13036
38. Wu X, Zhang Z, Schramm CA, Joyce MG, Do Kwon Y, Zhou T, et al. Maturation and diversity of the VRC01-antibody lineage over 15 years of chronic HIV-1 infection. *Cell* (2015) 161:470–85. doi: 10.1016/j.cell.2015.03.004
39. Wu X, Zhou T, Zhu J, Zhang B, Georgiev I, Wang C, et al. Focused evolution of HIV-1 neutralizing antibodies revealed by structures and deep sequencing. *Science* (2011) 333:1593–602. doi: 10.1126/science.1207532
40. Jardine JG, Kulp DW, Havenar-Daughton C, Sarkar A, Briney B, Sok D, et al. HIV-1 broadly neutralizing antibody precursor B cells revealed by germline-targeting immunogen. *Science* (2016) 351:1458–63. doi: 10.1126/science.aad9195
41. Correia BE, Bates JT, Loomis RJ, Baneyx G, Carrico C, Jardine JG, et al. Proof of principle for epitope-focused vaccine design. *Nature* (2014) 507:201–6. doi: 10.1038/nature12966
42. Abbott RK, Lee JH, Menis S, Skog P, Rossi M, Ota T, et al. Precursor frequency and affinity determine B cell competitive fitness in germinal centers, tested with germline-targeting HIV vaccine immunogens. *Immunity* (2018) 48:133–46.e6. doi: 10.1016/j.immuni.2017.11.023
43. Bhiman JN, Anthony C, Doria-Rose NA, Karimanzira O, Schramm CA, Khoza T, et al. Viral variants that initiate and drive maturation of V1V2-directed HIV-1 broadly neutralizing antibodies. *Nat Med.* (2015) 21:1332–6. doi: 10.1038/nm.3963
44. Liao HX, Lynch R, Zhou T, Gao F, Alam SM, Boyd SD, et al. Co-evolution of a broadly neutralizing HIV-1 antibody and founder virus. *Nature* (2013) 494:476–96. doi: 10.1038/nature12053
45. Barak M, Zuckerman NS, Edelman H, Unger R, Mehr R. IgTree©: creating immunoglobulin variable region gene lineage trees. *J Immunol Methods* (2008) 338:67–74. doi: 10.1016/j.jim.2008.06.006
46. Yermanos A, Greiff V, Krautler NJ, Menzel U, Dounas A, Miho E, et al. Comparison of methods for phylogenetic B-cell lineage inference using time-resolved antibody repertoire simulations (AbSim). *Bioinformatics* (2017) 33:3938–46. doi: 10.1093/bioinformatics/btx533
47. Sok D, Laserson U, Laserson J, Liu Y, Vigneault F, Julien JP, et al. The effects of somatic hypermutation on neutralization and binding in the PGT121 family of broadly neutralizing HIV antibodies. *PLoS Pathog.* (2013) 9:e1003754. doi: 10.1371/journal.ppat.1003754
48. Parola C, Neumeier D, Reddy ST. Integrating high-throughput screening and sequencing for monoclonal antibody discovery and engineering. *Immunology* (2018) 153:31–41. doi: 10.1111/imm.12838
49. Andrews SF, Huang Y, Kaur K, Popova LI, Ho IY, Pauli NT, et al. Immune history profoundly affects broadly protective B cell responses to influenza. *Sci Transl Med.* (2015) 7:316ra192. doi: 10.1126/scitranslmed.aad0522
50. DeWitt WS, Lindau P, Snyder TM, Sherwood AM, Vignali M, Carlson CS, et al. A public database of memory and naive B-cell receptor sequences. *PLoS ONE* (2016) 11:e0160853. doi: 10.1371/journal.pone.0160853
51. Rettig TA, Ward C, Bye BA, Pecaut MJ, Chapes SK. Characterization of the naive murine antibody repertoire using unamplified high-throughput sequencing. *PLoS ONE* (2018) 13:e0190982. doi: 10.1371/journal.pone.0190982
52. Stern JN, Yaari G, Heiden JA, Church G, Donahue WF, Hintzen RQ, et al. B cells populating the multiple sclerosis brain mature in the draining cervical lymph nodes. *Sci Transl Med.* (2014) 6:248ra107. doi: 10.1126/scitranslmed.3008879
53. Smith DS, Creadon G, Jena PK, Portanova JP, Kotzin BL, Wysocki LJ. Di- and trinucleotide target preferences of somatic mutagenesis in normal and autoreactive B cells. *J Immunol.* (1996) 156:2642–52.
54. Bolotin DA, Poslavsky S, Mitrophanov I, Shugay M, Mamedov IZ, Putintseva EV, et al. MiXCR: software for comprehensive adaptive immunity profiling. *Nat Methods* (2015) 12:380–1. doi: 10.1038/nmeth.3364
55. Aouinti S, Malouche D, Giudicelli V, Kossida S, Lefranc MP. IMGT/HighV-QUEST statistical significance of IMGT clonotype (AA) diversity per gene for standardized comparisons of next generation sequencing immunoprofiles of immunoglobulins and T cell receptors. *PLoS ONE* (2015) 10:e0142353. doi: 10.1371/journal.pone.0142353
56. Ye J, Ma N, Madden TL, Ostell JM. IgBLAST: an immunoglobulin variable domain sequence analysis tool. *Nucleic Acids Res.* (2013) 41:W34–40. doi: 10.1093/nar/gkt382

57. Ralph DK, Matsen FA IV. Likelihood-based inference of B cell clonal families. *PLoS Comput Biol.* (2016) 12:e1005086. doi: 10.1371/journal.pcbi.1005086
58. Schramm CA, Sheng Z, Zhang Z, Mascola JR, Kwong PD, Shapiro L. SONAR: a high-throughput pipeline for inferring antibody ontogenies from longitudinal sequencing of B cell transcripts. *Front Immunol.* (2016) 7:372. doi: 10.3389/fimmu.2016.00372
59. Marcou Q, Mora T, Walczak AM. High-throughput immune repertoire analysis with IGoR. *Nat Commun.* (2018) 9:561. doi: 10.1038/s41467-018-02832-w
60. Gaëta BA, Malming HR, Jackson KJ, Bain ME, Wilson P, Collins AM. iHMMune-align: hidden Markov model-based alignment and identification of germline genes in rearranged immunoglobulin gene sequences. *Bioinformatics* (2007) 23:1580–7. doi: 10.1093/bioinformatics/btm147
61. Ralph DK, Matsen FA IV. Per-sample immunoglobulin germline inference from B cell receptor deep sequencing data. *ArXiv*:171105843[Preprint] (2017). Available online at: http://arxiv.org/abs/1711.05843 (Accessed July 12, 2018).
62. Corcoran MM, Phad GE, Bernat NV, Stahl-Hennig C, Sumida N, Persson MAA, et al. Production of individualized V gene databases reveals high levels of immunoglobulin genetic diversity. *Nat Commun.* (2016) 7:13642. doi: 10.1038/ncomms13642
63. Gadala-Maria D, Yaari G, Uduman M, Kleinstein SH. Automated analysis of high-throughput B-cell sequencing data reveals a high frequency of novel immunoglobulin V gene segment alleles. *Proc Natl Acad Sci USA.* (2015) 112:E862–70. doi: 10.1073/pnas.1417683112
64. Olivieri DN, von Haeften B, Sánchez-Espinel C, Faro J, Gambón-Deza F. Genomic V exons from whole genome shotgun data in reptiles. *Immunogenetics* (2014) 66:479–92. doi: 10.1007/s00251-014-0784-3
65. Briney B, Le K, Zhu J, Burton DR. Clonify: unseeded antibody lineage assignment from next-generation sequencing data. *Sci Rep.* (2016) 6:23901. doi: 10.1038/srep23901
66. DeWitt WS III, Mesin L, Victora GD, Minin VN, Matsen FA IV. Using genotype abundance to improve phylogenetic inference. *ArXiv*:170808944[Preprint] Q-Bio (2017). Available online at: http://arxiv.org/abs/1708.08944 (Accessed September 21, 2017).
67. Odegard VH, Schatz DG. Targeting of somatic hypermutation. *Nat Rev Immunol.* (2006) 6:573–83. doi: 10.1038/nri1896
68. Goossens T, Klein U, Küppers R. Frequent occurrence of deletions and duplications during somatic hypermutation: implications for oncogene translocations and heavy chain disease. *Proc Natl Acad Sci USA.* (1998) 95:2463–8. doi: 10.1073/pnas.95.5.2463
69. Simonich CA, Williams KL, Verkerke HP, Williams JA, Nduati R, Lee KK, et al. HIV-1 neutralizing antibodies with limited hypermutation from an infant. *Cell* (2016) 166:77–87. doi: 10.1016/j.cell.2016.05.055
70. Rogozin IB, Kolchanov NA. Somatic hypermutagenesis in immunoglobulin genes: II. Influence of neighbouring base sequences on mutagenesis. *Biochim Biophys Acta* (1992) 1171:11–8. doi: 10.1016/0167-4781(92)90134-L
71. Betz AG, Neuberger MS, Milstein C. Discriminating intrinsic and actigen-selected mutational hotspots in immunoglobulin V genes. *Immunol Today* (1993) 14:405–11. doi: 10.1016/0167-5699(93)90144-A
72. Betz AG, Rada C, Pannell R, Milstein C, Neuberger MS. Passenger transgenes reveal intrinsic specificity of the antibody hypermutation mechanism: clustering, polarity, and specific hot spots. *Proc Natl Acad Sci USA.* (1993) 90:2385–8. doi: 10.1073/pnas.90.6.2385
73. Shapiro GS, Aviszus K, Ikle D, Wysocki LJ. Predicting regional mutability in antibody V genes based solely on di- and trinucleotide sequence composition. *J Immunol.* (1999) 163:259–68.
74. Yaari G, Heiden JV, Uduman M, Gadala-Maria D, Gupta N, Stern JN, et al. Models of somatic hypermutation targeting and substitution based on synonymous mutations from high-throughput Immunoglobulin sequencing data. *Front B Cell Biol.* (2013) 4:358. doi: 10.3389/fimmu.2013.00358
75. Cui A, Niro RD, Vander Heiden JA, Briggs AW, Adams K, Gilbert T, et al. A model of somatic hypermutation targeting in mice based on high-throughput Ig sequencing data. *J Immunol.* (2016) 197:3566–74. doi: 10.4049/jimmunol.1502263
76. Hoehn KB, Lunter G, Pybus OG. A phylogenetic codon substitution model for antibody lineages. *Genetics* (2017) 206:417–27. doi: 10.1534/genetics.116.196303
77. Tipton CM, Fucile CF, Darce J, Chida A, Ichikawa T, Gregoretti I, et al. Diversity, cellular origin and autoreactivity of antibody-secreting cell population expansions in acute systemic lupus erythematosus. *Nat Immunol.* (2015) 16:755–65. doi: 10.1038/ni.3175
78. Bashford-Rogers RJ, Palser AL, Huntly BJ, Rance R, Vassiliou GS, Follows GA, et al. Network properties derived from deep sequencing of human B-cell receptor repertoires delineate B-cell populations. *Genome Res.* (2013) 23:1874–84. doi: 10.1101/gr.154815.113
79. Tsioris K, Gupta NT, Ogunniyi AO, Zimnisky RM, Qian F, Yao Y, et al. Neutralizing antibodies against West Nile virus identified directly from human B cells by single-cell analysis and next generation sequencing. *Integr Biol.* (2015) 7:1587–97. doi: 10.1039/C5IB00169B
80. Soto C, Ofek G, Joyce MG, Zhang B, McKee K, Longo NS, et al. Developmental pathway of the MPER-directed HIV-1-neutralizing antibody 10E8. *PLoS ONE* (2016) 11:e0157409. doi: 10.1371/journal.pone.0157409
81. Zhou T, Zhu J, Wu X, Moquin S, Zhang B, Acharya P, et al. Multidonor analysis reveals structural elements, genetic determinants, and maturation pathway for HIV-1 neutralization by VRC01-class antibodies. *Immunity* (2013) 39:245–58. doi: 10.1016/j.immuni.2013.04.012
82. Wang C, Liu Y, Xu LT, Jackson KJ, Roskin KM, Pham TD, et al. Effects of aging, cytomegalovirus infection, and EBV infection on human B cell repertoires. *J Immunol.* (2014) 192:603–11. doi: 10.4049/jimmunol.1301384
83. Di Tommaso P, Moretti S, Xenarios I, Orobitg M, Montanyola A, Chang JM, et al. T-Coffee: a web server for the multiple sequence alignment of protein and RNA sequences using structural information and homology extension. *Nucleic Acids Res.* (2011) 39:W13–7. doi: 10.1093/nar/gkr245
84. Sievers F, Wilm A, Dineen D, Gibson TJ, Karplus K, Li W, et al. Fast, scalable generation of high-quality protein multiple sequence alignments using Clustal Omega. *Mol Syst Biol.* (2014) 7:539. doi: 10.1038/msb.2011.75
85. Edgar RC. MUSCLE: multiple sequence alignment with high accuracy and high throughput. *Nucleic Acids Res.* (2004) 32:1792–7. doi: 10.1093/nar/gkh340
86. Lassmann T, Sonnhammer EL. Kalign – an accurate and fast multiple sequence alignment algorithm. *BMC Bioinformatics* (2005) 6:298. doi: 10.1186/1471-2105-6-298
87. Yang Z, Rannala B. Molecular phylogenetics: principles and practice. *Nat Rev Genet.* (2012) 13:303–14. doi: 10.1038/nrg3186
88. Gascuel O, Steel M. Neighbor-joining revealed. *Mol Biol Evol.* (2006) 23:1997–2000. doi: 10.1093/molbev/msl072
89. Saitou N, Nei M. The neighbor-joining method: a new method for reconstructing phylogenetic trees. *Mol Biol Evol.* (1987) 4:406–25.
90. Paradis E, Claude J, Strimmer K. APE: analyses of phylogenetics and evolution in R language. *Bioinformatics* (2004) 20:289–90. doi: 10.1093/bioinformatics/btg412
91. Schliep KP. phangorn: phylogenetic analysis in R. *Bioinformatics* (2011) 27:592–3. doi: 10.1093/bioinformatics/btq706
92. Wendel BS, He C, Qu M, Wu D, Hernandez SM, Ma KY, et al. Accurate immune repertoire sequencing reveals malaria infection driven antibody lineage diversification in young children. *Nat Commun.* (2017) 8:531. doi: 10.1038/s41467-017-00645-x
93. Fitch WM. Toward defining the course of evolution: minimum change for a specific tree topology. *Syst Zool.* (1971) 20:406–16. doi: 10.2307/2412116
94. Farris JS. Methods for computing Wagner Trees. *Syst Zool.* (1970) 19:83–92. doi: 10.2307/2412028
95. Felsenstein J. PHYLIP - Phylogeny Inference Package (Version 3.2). *Cladistics* (1989) 5:164–6.
96. Revell LJ, Chamberlain SA. Rphylip: an R interface for PHYLIP. *Methods Ecol Evol.* (2014) 5:976–81. doi: 10.1111/2041-210X.12233
97. Palanichamy A, Apeltsin L, Kuo TC, Sirota M, Wang S, Pitts SJ, et al. Immunoglobulin class-switched B cells form an active immune axis between CNS and periphery in multiple sclerosis. *Sci Transl Med.* (2014) 6:248ra106. doi: 10.1126/scitranslmed.3008930
98. Jukes T, Cantor C. *Evolution of Protein Molecules*. New York, NY Academic Press (1969). p. 121–32.

99. Hasegawa M, Kishino H, Yano T. Dating of the human-ape splitting by a molecular clock of mitochondrial DNA. *J Mol Evol.* (1985) 22:160–74. doi: 10.1007/BF02101694
100. Tavaré S. Some probabilistic and statistical problems in the analysis of DNA sequences. *Lect Math Life Sci.* (1986) 17:57–86.
101. Hall BG. Building phylogenetic trees from molecular data with MEGA. *Mol Biol Evol.* (2013) 30:1229–35. doi: 10.1093/molbev/mst012
102. Ashkenazy H, Penn O, Doron-Faigenboim A, Cohen O, Cannarozzi G, Zomer O, et al. FastML: a web server for probabilistic reconstruction of ancestral sequences. *Nucleic Acids Res.* (2012) 40:W580–4. doi: 10.1093/nar/gks498
103. Nguyen LT, Schmidt HA, von Haeseler A, Minh BQ. IQ-TREE: a fast and effective stochastic algorithm for estimating maximum-likelihood phylogenies. *Mol Biol Evol.* (2015) 32:268–74. doi: 10.1093/molbev/msu300
104. Doria-Rose NA, Bhiman JN, Roark RS, Schramm CA, Gorman J, Chuang GY, et al. New member of the V1V2-directed CAP256-VRC26 lineage that shows increased breadth and exceptional potency. *J Virol.* (2016) 90:76–91. doi: 10.1128/JVI.01791-15
105. Joyce MG, Wheatley AK, Thomas PV, Chuang GY, Soto C, Bailer RT, et al. Vaccine-induced antibodies that neutralize group 1 and group 2 influenza A viruses. *Cell* (2016) 166:609–23. doi: 10.1016/j.cell.2016.06.043
106. Drummond AJ, Rambaut A. BEAST: Bayesian evolutionary analysis by sampling trees. *BMC Evol Biol.* (2007) 7:214. doi: 10.1186/1471-2148-7-214
107. Bouckaert R, Heled J, Kühnert D, Vaughan T, Wu CH, Xie D, et al. BEAST 2: a software platform for Bayesian evolutionary analysis. *PLOS Comput Biol.* (2014) 10:e1003537. doi: 10.1371/journal.pcbi.1003537
108. Safonova Y, Lapidus A, Lill J. IgSimulator: a versatile immunosequencing simulator. *Bioinformatics* (2015) 1:3213–5. doi: 10.1093/bioinformatics/btv326
109. Robinson DF, Foulds LR. Comparison of phylogenetic trees. *Math Biosci.* (1981) 53:131–47. doi: 10.1016/0025-5564(81)90043-2
110. Kendall M, Colijn C. Mapping phylogenetic trees to reveal distinct patterns of evolution. *Mol Biol Evol.* (2016) 33:2735–43. doi: 10.1093/molbev/msw124
111. Grenfell BT, Pybus OG, Gog JR, Wood JL, Daly JM, Mumford JA, et al. Unifying the epidemiological and evolutionary dynamics of pathogens. *Science* (2004) 303:327–32. doi: 10.1126/science.1090727
112. Colless DH. Phylogenetics: The theory and practice of phylogenetic systematics. *Syst Zool.* (1982) 31:100–4. doi: 10.2307/2413420
113. Sackin MJ. "Good" and "Bad" phenograms. *Syst Zool.* (1972) 21:225–6. doi: 10.2307/2412292
114. Horns F, Vollmers C, Dekker CL, Quake SR. Signatures of selection in the human antibody repertoire: selective sweeps, competing subclones, and neutral drift. *bioRxiv* (2017) 111:145052. doi: 10.1101/145052
115. Manske MK, Zuckerman NS, Timm MM, Maiden S, Edelman H, Shahaf G, et al. Quantitative analysis of clonal bone marrow CD19+ B cells: use of B cell lineage trees to delineate their role in the pathogenesis of light chain amyloidosis. *Clin Immunol.* (2006) 120:106–20. doi: 10.1016/j.clim.2006.01.008
116. Lewitus E, Morlon H. Characterizing and comparing phylogenies from their Laplacian spectrum. *Syst Biol.* (2016) 65:495–507. doi: 10.1093/sysbio/syv116
117. Lozupone C, Knight R. UniFrac: a new phylogenetic method for comparing microbial communities. *Appl Environ Microbiol.* (2005) 71:8228–35. doi: 10.1128/AEM.71.12.8228-8235.2005
118. Nourmohammad A, Otwinowski J, Luksza M, Mora T, Walczak AM. Clonal competition in B-cell repertoires during chronic HIV-1 infection. (2018) *ArXiv*:1802.08841[Preprint]. doi: 10.1101/271130

# 18

# InterCells: A Generic Monte-Carlo Simulation of Intercellular Interfaces Captures Nanoscale Patterning at the Immune Synapse

*Yair Neve-Oz, Julia Sajman, Yair Razvag and Eilon Sherman**

*Racah Institute of Physics, The Hebrew University, Jerusalem, Israel*

***Correspondence:**
*Eilon Sherman*
*sherman@phys.huji.ac.il*

Molecular interactions across intercellular interfaces serve to convey information between cells and to trigger appropriate cell functions. Examples include cell development and growth in tissues, neuronal and immune synapses (ISs). Here, we introduce an agent-based Monte-Carlo simulation of user-defined cellular interfaces. The simulation allows for membrane molecules, embedded at intercellular contacts, to diffuse and interact, while capturing the topography and energetics of the plasma membranes of the interface. We provide a detailed example related to pattern formation in the early IS. Using simulation predictions and three-color single molecule localization microscopy (SMLM), we detected the intricate mutual patterning of T cell antigen receptors (TCRs), integrins and glycoproteins in early T cell contacts with stimulating coverslips. The simulation further captures the dynamics of the patterning under the experimental conditions and at the IS with antigen presenting cells (APCs). Thus, we provide a generic tool for simulating realistic cell-cell interfaces, which can be used for critical hypothesis testing and experimental design in an iterative manner.

**Keywords: cell signaling, T cell activation, kinetic segregation model, single molecule localization microscopy, photoactivated localization microscopy, direct STORM, microvilli, agent based Monte-Carlo simulation**

## INTRODUCTION

Cells associate and form functional interfaces to create tissues, to exchange molecular content and to convey information. Such interfaces form in multicellular organisms between adherent and developing cells in tissues (1), between neurons (2) and immune cells (3). Cell contacts can also occur in unicellular organisms, e.g., between bacteria in biofilms and between bacteria and their host cells (4).

A wide range of physical structures appear in intercellular interfaces, including junctions (e.g., plasmodesmata and gap junctions, tight junctions, and desmosomes) (5), neuronal synapses and immune synapses (IS). The dynamics of the interfaces may vary widely, from seconds to days. For instance, neuronal synapses may persist over much longer times, but still show surprising remodeling dynamics (6, 7).

In this study, we focus on the IS between $CD4^{+}$ T Cells and antigen presenting cells (APCs) as an example of a dynamic intercellular interface of outstanding importance and interest (**Figures 1A,B**). This synapse serves T cells to probe the outer surface of APCs for cognate antigens, and to mount an appropriate immune response (8). Advancements in microscopy have

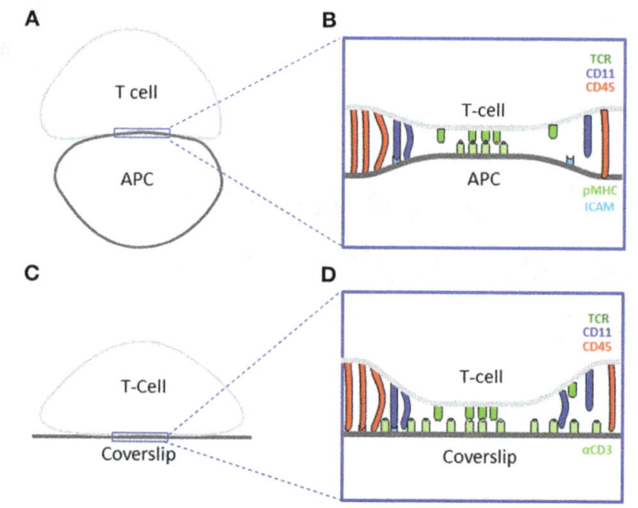


**FIGURE 1 |** Cell interfaces of the immune synapse. **(A)** A scheme of a physiological interface between a T cell and an antigen presenting cell (APC). **(B)** A physical model of the interface in panel **(A)**. **(C)** A scheme of an experimental interface between a T cell and a coverslip. **(D)** A physical model of the interface in panel **(C)**.

shown that such structures demonstrate complex levels of dynamic organization (9). The IS starts with early contacts that mature within a few minutes to form molecular segregation into supramolecular activating clusters (SMACs) (10). Such experiments often turn to artificial mimics of the APC for high resolution microscopy. Examples include coverslips coated with antibodies (11) (**Figures 1C,D**) or with lipid bilayers that include molecules of interest (12).

Recently, super-resolution cell imaging, and especially single molecule localization microscopy, has allowed to resolve the organization of molecules in live cells with resolution down to ~20 nm (13). Such methods include Photoactivated Localization Microscopy (PALM) (14) and direct Stochastic Optical Reconstruction Microscopy (dSTORM) (15). Through these techniques, whole (or a large part of) molecular populations of specific protein species can be directly visualized with such resolution. For instance, imaging of signaling molecules in $CD4^+$ T cells has shown surprising nanoscale patterning of proteins, in the form of hierarchical and functional clusters (16, 17). Specifically, the nanoscale segregation of the TCRs from bulky glycoproteins, such as CD45, has been detected (18). Still, the latter patterns of kinetic segregation in early contacts (18–20) have not been related to the hierarchical ordering of TCRs, integrins and glycoproteins into central, proximal and distal SMACs (c-, p- and d-SMACs; known also as the "bull's eye" pattern) that has been detected at the mature IS (10, 21, 22).

For gaining further insight on the structure, dynamics and functional role of interfaces, experimental techniques can be complemented with computational cell modeling and simulations. Indeed, multiple computational simulations have been developed and employed for studying cells (23). Such methods may vary widely in their details, from atoms to entire cells, time-scale, from microseconds to minutes and length-scales, from angstroms to microns and more.

Here, we introduce an agent-based Monte-Carlo simulation of user-defined cellular interfaces. The simulation, called InterCells, is based on detailed physical modeling of the interface and embedded molecules within. The simulation allows for the molecules to diffuse and interact, while capturing the topography and energetics of the interacting plasma membranes (PMs). It relies on simple and inexpensive computation that is still complex enough to capture realistic complexity and dynamics of the interfaces. Recently, similar modeling and simulations have served to resolve possible mechanisms of cooperativity and localized activation in TCR clusters (24) and to identify kinetic segregation of TCR and glycoproteins at the engaged tips of microvilli (18).

A special emphasis in our simulation is its easy operation by non-experts. For that, we provide a friendly graphical user interface (GUI) for rapid configuration and deployment of the simulation. Multiple analytical tools are provided for data analysis and interpretation. A key property of the simulation is its ability to confront the results and predictions of realistic simulations with experimental data, acquired by single molecule localization microscopy. We provide a detailed example related to pattern formation in intercellular contacts that characterize the early IS between $CD4^+$ T cells and antigen presenting cells (APCs) (18, 20). Specifically, our simulation results predict a new feature of pattern formation—the intricate mutual patterning of T cell antigen receptors (TCRs), integrins and glycoproteins in the early contacts. We confirm this patterning by SMLM imaging of T cells on functionally-coated coverslips. Thus, we provide a generic tool for simulating cell-cell interfaces, which can be used for critical hypothesis testing and experimental design in an iterative manner.

# RESULTS

## Intricate Patterning of Membrane Proteins at the IS

To study molecular patterning at the IS, we imaged Jurakt E6.1 $CD4^+$ T cells, as they adhered and spread on functionally coated coverslips (11) (see details in Materials and Methods). Anti-CD3-coated coverslips result in direct TCR stimulation, T cell activation and spreading. In contrast, coverslips coated with poly-L-lysine (PLL) show reduced levels of TCR stimulation and smaller cell footprints (25). For imaging, we used three-color single molecule localization microscopy (SMLM) in total internal reflection (TIRF; **Figure 2**). Our SMLM approach included PALM imaging of TCRζ-Dronpa, stably expressed by the cells. CD11 and CD45 molecules were immunostained using an anti-CD11-Alexa568 and anti-CD45-Alexa647, respectively (see Materials and Methods) and imaged by two-color dSTORM.

Our images showed a striking patterning of molecules where CD11 clusters (blue) localized in between TCR clusters

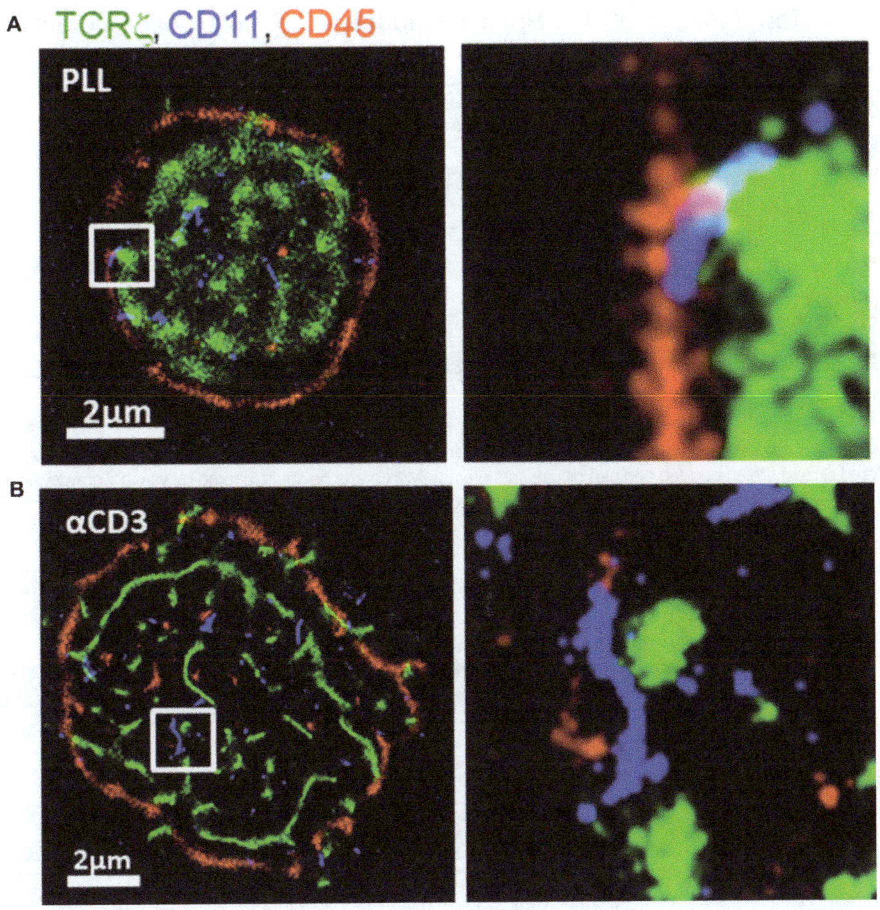


**FIGURE 2 |** Intricate molecular patterning at the immune synapse. Three-color PALM/dSTORM imaging of fixed E6.1 Jurkat cells expressing TCRζ-Dronpa (green) and stained for CD45 (red) and CD11 (blue). The cells were dropped on coverslips coated with either **(A)** poly-L-lysine (PLL; top raw) or **(B)** αCD3 (bottom raw). Cells were let spread on the coverslip for 1.5 min before fixation. Shown are representative cells ($N = 40$ cells on PLL and 31 cells on αCD3). Bars–2 μm.

(green) and CD45 clusters (red) on either TCR-stimulating and non-stimulating conditions. On PLL-coated coverslips, TCR clusters occupied the center of the interface, while CD45 showed an outer ring. CD11 clusters localized outside TCR clusters and in the formed gaps between TCRs and CD45. On αCD3-coated coverslips, CD11 also localized in between TCR and CD45. However, on these coverslips, the cells formed larger footprints and TCR was more clustered.

The segregation of TCRs from CD45 has been shown by diffraction limited microscopy, and more recently, in early contact (18). Also, the localization of CD11 was shown before in the pSMAC while CD45 localized to the dSMAC (22). However, such mutual patterning has not been resolved in early ISs and at the nanoscale. Thus, our imaging captured an intricate mutual patterning of TCRs, integrins and glycoproteins in the early contacts. The occurrence of the mutual patterning on coverslips coated with either αCD3 or PLL indicates that this patterning is caused by the physical contact of the cell with the opposing interface of the coverslip.

## Modeling and Simulation of Molecular Patterning Under the Experimental Conditions

For testing the robustness and dynamics of the patterns that we have detected, we turned to the modeling and simulation of the cell interfaces. The simulation is described in details in the Materials and Methods and in the User's Guide (provided in the **Supplemental Information**). Briefly, the simulation employs physical modeling of the PM of the interacting cells and of the molecular interactions (**Figure 3**, and below). The simulation structure is described in **Figure 4**, the simulation process is described in **Figure 5** and its GUI is shown in **Figure 6**.

An important feature of our agent-based Monte-Carlo simulation, is its ability to integrate experimental measurements at the single molecule level (as in **Figure 2**). Such data can be integrated as initial conditions for the simulation, or as dynamic physical constraints [as previously demonstrated (18)]. Here, we demonstrate the setting of initial conditions by cropped data from the footprints of cells, imaged by SMLM (**Figure 2**).

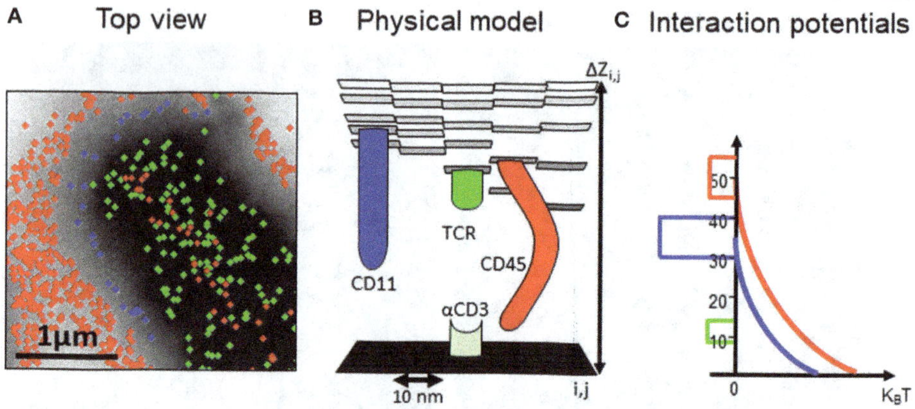


**FIGURE 3 |** A computational model of the intercellular interface between T cells and a coverslip. **(A)** A top view of a simulated membrane. The membrane is shown as a grid, where molecules (colored circles) are embedded and can diffuse and interact. Membrane height is marked by variable gray levels. **(B)** A 3D view of the simulated membrane. **(C)** The interaction potential between molecules embedded in the simulated membrane.

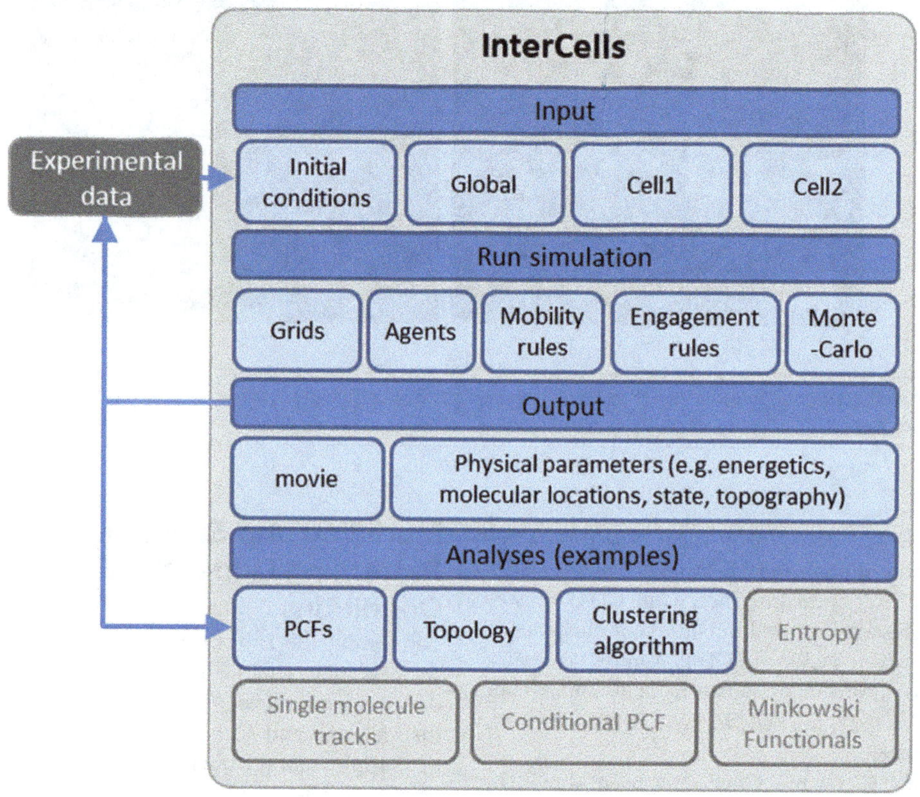


**FIGURE 4 |** A schematic description of the cell interface simulation. A detailed account of the simulation, its structure and interface are provided as a User's Guide in the **Supplemental Information**.

Specifically, coordinates were taken for TCRζ molecules (in green). To complete the initial conditions, the initial coordinates of CD11 and CD45 molecules were manually determined via the available tools of the simulation in the GUI.

In our simulation, the plasma membrane of the interacting cells are modeled as grids where molecules, modeled as agents, diffuse and interact within and across the grids (**Figures 3A,B**). The simulation included a model that captured the energetic of the PMs of interacting T cell and APC (26) (**Figure 3C**). Specifically, the simulation balanced forces due to attractive and repulsive interactions. Specific attraction occurred between the TCR and αCD3 and self-clustering of CD11 and TCR molecules.

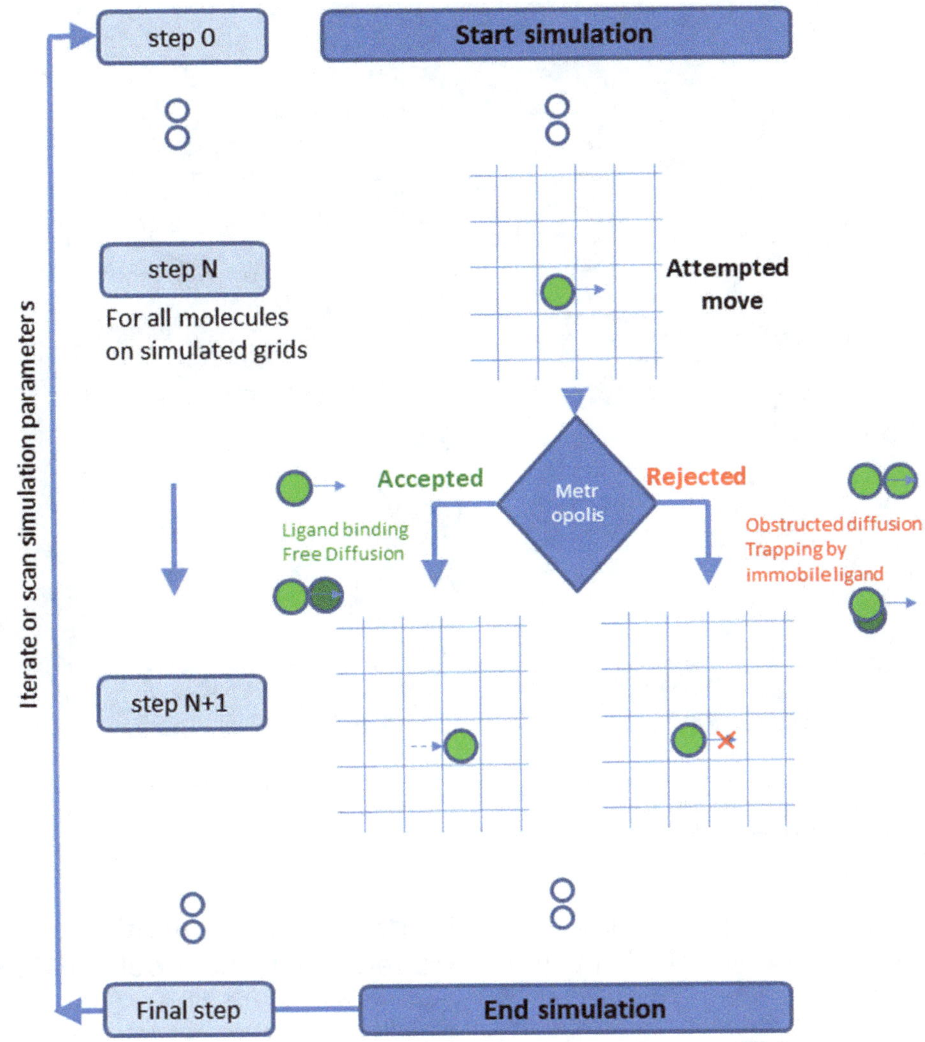


**FIGURE 5** | A schematic description of the simulation process.

Non-specific attraction affected the molecules at the T cell PM by the PLL. Repulsive interactions occurred between the molecule (and esp. for the bulky glycoprotein) and the coverslip (**Figure 3C**). The PM underwent thermal fluctuations during the simulation. The positions of the molecules were updated in each step of the simulation. The simulations included 10,000 steps of 400 × 400 pixels of 10 nm each and took ~5 min (~100 s in cell time) each, using a PC (i7 quad processor). Simulated parameters are detailed for the interacting molecules (**Table S1**).

The simulation resulted in a redistributed pattern of molecules that was embedded within the interface, and evolved over time (**Figures 7A,B, Movies M1, M2**). Strikingly, the simulations could recreate realistic patterning of CD45 molecules around the evolving TCR clusters. CD11 molecules were distributed in between TCR clusters and CD45. These results correlated well with experimentally imaged positions of these molecules on either PLL- or αCD3-coated coverslips (compare left and right columns in **Figures 7A,B** with **Figures 2A,B**).

## The Effect of Simulation Parameters on the Molecular Patterning

Multiple parameters could affect the resultant molecular patterns that we observed. Such parameters include the initial conditions of molecular placement (e.g., in **Figure 7** at $t = 0$); the density of the molecules; their diffusion coefficient and their interaction potential. Thus, we repeated the simulations shown in **Figure 7**, yet with modifying one of the described parameters in each simulation. Recent publications showed that TCRs are clustered in microvilli (27) that form early contacts (18, 28). Hence, we started with changing the initial placement of CD11 and CD45 molecules in relation to TCR clusters. The cells were attached to a coverslip coated with PLL and αCD3, for engaging the TCRs. **Figure S1** shows the results for applying the initial conditions as in **Figure 7B** (**Figures S1A–C**), a diffused pattern of CD45 (**Figures S1D–F**) or a diffused pattern of both CD45 and CD11 (**Figures S1G–I**). The variability in initial conditions was applied to simulations that either included molecular self-clustering of

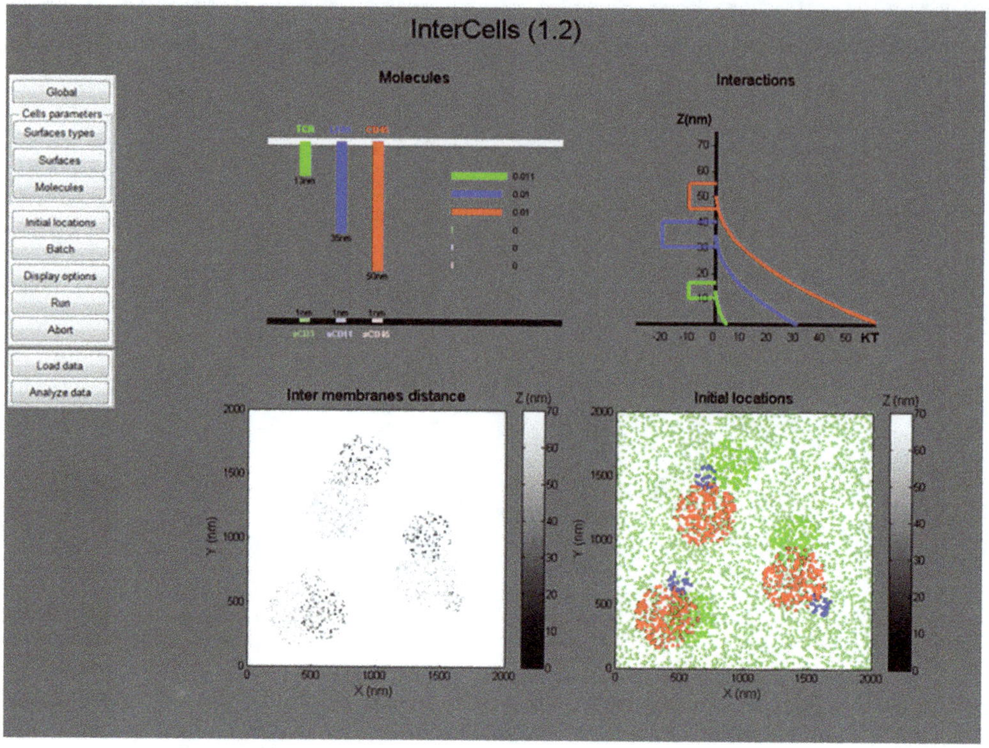


**FIGURE 6 |** The graphical user interface. A snapshot of the graphical user interface (GUI) of the simulation. The GUI includes dynamic menus for setting all simulation parameters and a live interface for presenting the simulated parameters (top) and initial conditions (bottom). All menus, parameters and operation instructions are provided in the User's Manual in the **Supplemental Information**.

TCR and CD11 (**Figures S1B,E,H**) or did not include such self-clustering (**Figures S1C,E,I**). Strikingly, the molecular patterning under all conditions showed the mutual patterning of TCRs, CD11 and CD45, as in **Figure 7B** an in our experiments (**Figure 2B**). As expected, TCR and CD11 were more diffused within these mutual patterns when the simulations did not include self-clustering of these molecules (**Figures S1C,E,I**). Our results indicate the robustness of the mutual patterning of TCR, CD11 and CD45 to variations in initial molecular placements and to their self-clustering.

We next conducted a sensitivity analysis of molecular patterning to variations in the density of CD45 (**Figure S2A**), the diffusion coefficient of the molecules (namely, TCR, CD11 and CD45; **Figure S2B**), and the interaction potential of CD45 (**Figure S2C**). Parameter values were taken as half, equal or twice the values that were chosen in the simulation shown in **Figure S1B**. The mutual patterning of TCR, CD11 and CD45 was robust to most of the conditions. Still, the following differences can be observed for the different conditions. For instance, the CD45 outer ring became relatively thicker with the increase of CD45 concentration (**Figure S2A**). The mutual shape of the TCR, CD11 and CD45 became more diffused and occupied a bigger area with the increase in the diffusion coefficients of the molecules (**Figure S2B**). Last, we observed a less diffused pattern of CD45 when its spring constant became stronger (**Figure S2C**).

## Modeling and Simulation of Molecular Patterning at the T cell-APC IS

Next, we studied the effects of the patterning in simulated physiological interface between T cells and APCs. Nanoscale imaging of T cells and APCs is technically complicated, yet is readily accessible to our modeling and simulation. Here, we included mobile ligands at the PM of the APC, namely pMHC and ICAM. These molecules exerted specific attraction forces on the TCR and CD11 molecules (respectively) as they diffused at the PM of the opposing T cell. The PM of the APC was given similar physical properties to the PM of the T cell (as detailed in **Table S2**). The molecular positions at the T cell PM were set manually as initial conditions, and were kept identical for the simulations on APCs (**Figures 8C,D**) and on coverslips coated with either PLL (**Figure 8A**) or αCD3 (**Figure 8B**). In this way, results could be directly compared across different interfaces.

Our simulations showed that the mutual patterning of CD11, TCRs and CD45 occurred not only on coverslips, but also at the PM of T cells conjugated to APCs (**Figures 8C,D**). Corresponding patterning of pMHC and of ICAM molecules appeared at the PM of the APCs (**Figure 8C**). Interestingly, CD11 was less self-clustered in such interfaces in comparison to the cell interface with αCD3-coated coverslips (**Figure 8B**).

Under physiological conditions, APCs typically carry only a small fraction of cognate peptides. Thus, we repeated our simulations for interface of T cells with APCs, while considering

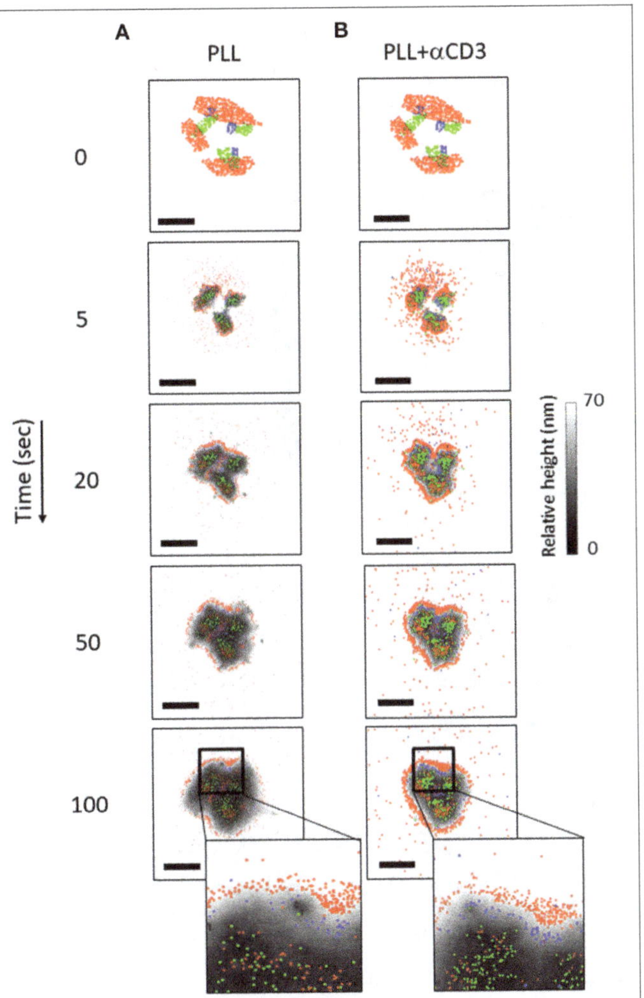


**FIGURE 7 |** The dynamics of molecular patterning in simulations. The dynamic evolution of molecular patterning of TCRs (green), CD11 (blue) and CD45 (red) at the cell interface. Simulated results are shown as a function of time for individual cells on either a PLL-coated coverslip **(A)** or on an αCD3-coated coverslip **(B)** along time. The simulations start from user-defined initial conditions (top raw) that are set for the simulated molecules. Membrane height is marked by variable gray levels. Bars–1 μm.

only 1% of cognate peptides (**Figures S3A,B**). As expected, the interface was not as tight as for the previous simulation (compare height levels with **Figures 8C,D**). Importantly, the molecular patterning of TCR, CD11 and CD45 seemed more diffused and their segregation was less pronounced.

Another important physiological condition is the translocation of TCR molecules toward the center of the IS 21 (29, 30). To simulate this process, we created an interactive tool within the software. Using this tool, we set a target coordinate for TCRs translocation at the center of the interface and set a constant velocity of 19 nm/s (29) toward the center to all TCRs. Along with translocation, we assumed TCR diffusion but no self-clustering, in order not to hinder its mobility further. Expectedly, the TCRs concentrated at the center of the IS, while a relatively pronounced and well-segregated CD45 ring formed at the periphery (**Figures S3C,D**). As before, CD11 molecules localized between the segregated TCRs and CD45 molecular patterns.

To quantitatively assess the mutual patterns of TCR, CD11 and CD45, we introduced a topological analysis (see details in the Materials and Methods and in **Figure 9A**). This analysis related the density of CD11 and CD45 molecules to individual TCR clusters. The density of the molecules as a function of the distance from TCR clusters is shown in **Figures 9B–E**. The results of the topological analysis of our experimental results (in **Figure 2**) clearly show the hierarchical ordering of TCR clusters at the center, surrounded consecutively by CD11 and CD45 molecules (**Figures 8B,C**). Moreover, the evolution of this pattern could now be captured using our simulated results on either PLL- or αCD3-coated coverslips (**Figures 9D,E**). As expected, the self-clustering of TCRs (the peak height of the green manifold) was higher, and more persistent for αCD3-coated coverslips relative to PLL-coated coverslips. Strikingly, the mutual patterning of TCR, CD11 and CD45 occurred within a few 10 s of seconds from the start of the simulations. The mutual patterning of CD11 and CD45 from TCR can be further compared between the experimental data and the simulated results (**Figures 9F,G**). Our simulations captured the shift in the peak of the molecular distributions of CD45 relative to the TCRs on both PLL (**Figure 9F**, red lines), and on αCD3 coated coverslips (**Figure 9G**, red lines). The separation of CD11 was captured more accurately on PLL-coated coverslips than on aCD3-coated coverslips (**Figures 9F,G**, blue lines). Thus, our simulations now set the stage for seeking parameters that would minimize the differences between the density distributions of the molecules under study (18).

## DISCUSSION

In this work, we introduce "InterCells"—a generic agent-based Monte-Carlo simulation of intercellular interfaces in molecular detail. Our study focused on dynamic molecular patterning at the early IS, as an important example of a dynamic intercellular interface. The study combined three-color SMLM imaging of fixed $CD4^+$ T cells on functionally coated coverslips, as well as modeling and simulations of the IS of such $CD4^+$ T cells with APCs. Our imaging and simulation showed an intricate patterning of TCRs, glycoproteins (e.g., CD45) and integrins (e.g., CD11) at the PM of the interacting T cells. In the detected patterns, clusters of CD11 localized in between segregated clusters of TCR and of CD45. Such patterning has been instructed by diffraction limited microscopy (12), recent detection of segregation of TCRs and CD45 molecules in early contacts (18), and by preliminary simulations. To our knowledge, such mutual patterns have not been observed at the nanoscale before and thus, have not been related to the macroscopic "bull's eye" patterns detected at the IS (10, 21).

To test the robustness of the detected pattern, we simulated a range of relevant interfaces, including coverslips with different coatings, different sets of initial conditions, and ISs with APCs. Varying such conditions in the simulation can be readily achieved

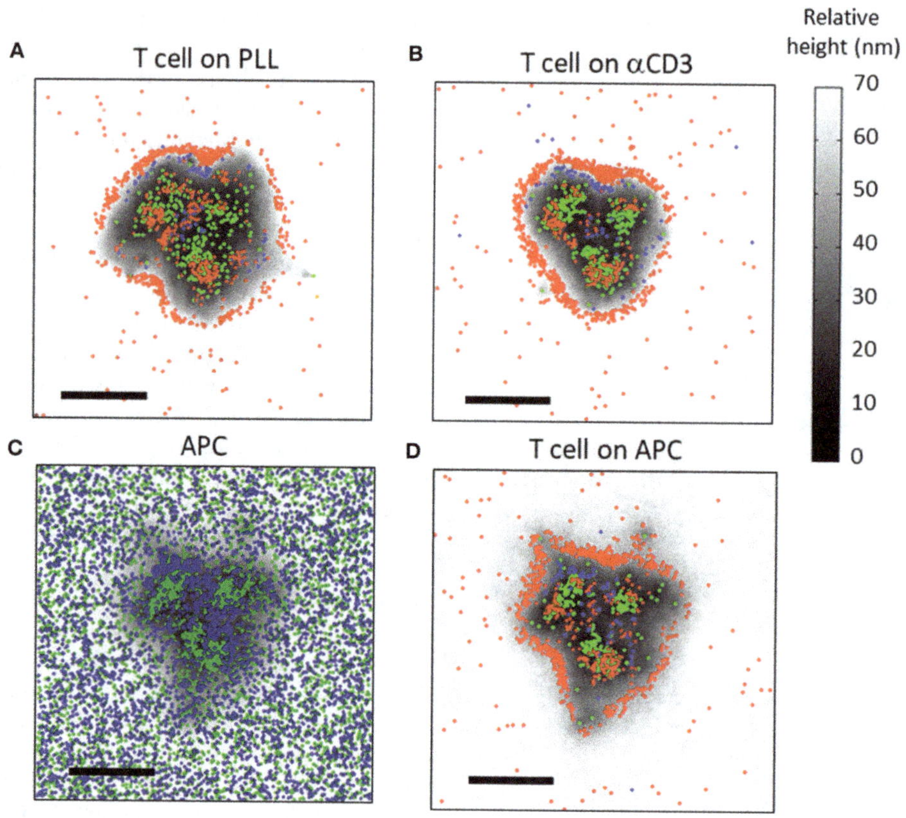


**FIGURE 8 |** Simulation results of molecular patterning at the immune synapse **(A,B)** The molecular patterning of TCRs (green), CD11 (blue) and CD45 (red) at the cell interface, on either **(A)** a PLL-coated or **(B)** an αCD3-coated coverslip. **(C,D)** The molecular patterning at the T cell-APC immune synapse. **(C)** ICAM (blue) and pMHC (green) molecules are shown at the PM of the APC. **(D)** TCRs (green), CD11 (blue) and CD45 (red) are shown at the PM of the T cell. Membrane height in panels **(C,D)** is marked by variable gray levels. Bars–1 μm.

through the design and the GUI of the simulation. Notably, our agent based simulation allows for the seamless integration of experimental data at the single molecule level, as captured by PALM and dSTORM. We have previously demonstrated the use of SMLM data as constrains for setting hybrid simulations (18). The results of such simulations can be directly compared to experimental results (18). The robustness of the molecular segregation between TCR, CD11 and CD45 clusters, which persisted in all simulations, indicates that it is driven by mechanical forces acting between molecules and the opposing surfaces of the IS. Notably, our simulation did not include translocation of molecules, such as TCRs or integrins, across the IS (31). Such translocation plays a role in the spatial sorting of newly appearing clusters at the cell periphery in the mature IS, while our simulation and imaging focused on relatively less mature ISs.

Multiple simulation tools have been developed to study molecular interactions in the cell, such as signaling pathways and enzymatic reactions. Such modeling often assumes complete molecular mixing via ordinary differential equations (ODEs) (32), or the use of cell automata with cell compartmentation that could average out critical spatial variations in local concentration of signaling proteins. The virtual cell [Vcell; (33)] allows for solving partial differential equations (PDEs) and ODEs, and the integration of spatial constraints from 2D and 3D optical microscopy. Still, such simulations cannot account for molecular heterogeneities and non-synchrony that are inherent to stochastic processes of molecular diffusion and interaction within cells. Such heterogeneities can be captured by Monte Carlo simulations of finite numbers of interacting molecules that are embedded in realistic models of cellular compartments [e.g., Smoldyn (34) and MCell (35)]. Specifically, MCell contains extensive simulation tools, including the generation of arbitrary meshes through integration with a powerful graphical package (Blender), the simulation of cytosolic proteins, allowing stochastic state transitions of molecules, various mobility states including diffusion and drift and running batches for scanning parameters. Notably, MCell is not designed to account for dynamically changing meshes. In contrast to MCell, InterCells is currently more modest in its flexibility and in its integration of advanced features and tools. For instance, multiple dynamic processes, such as molecular endocytosis and recycling are currently lacking and will become available in an upcoming update of the simulation. Also, it is currently limited to simulating membrane proteins, while cytosolic proteins will be integrated, but will

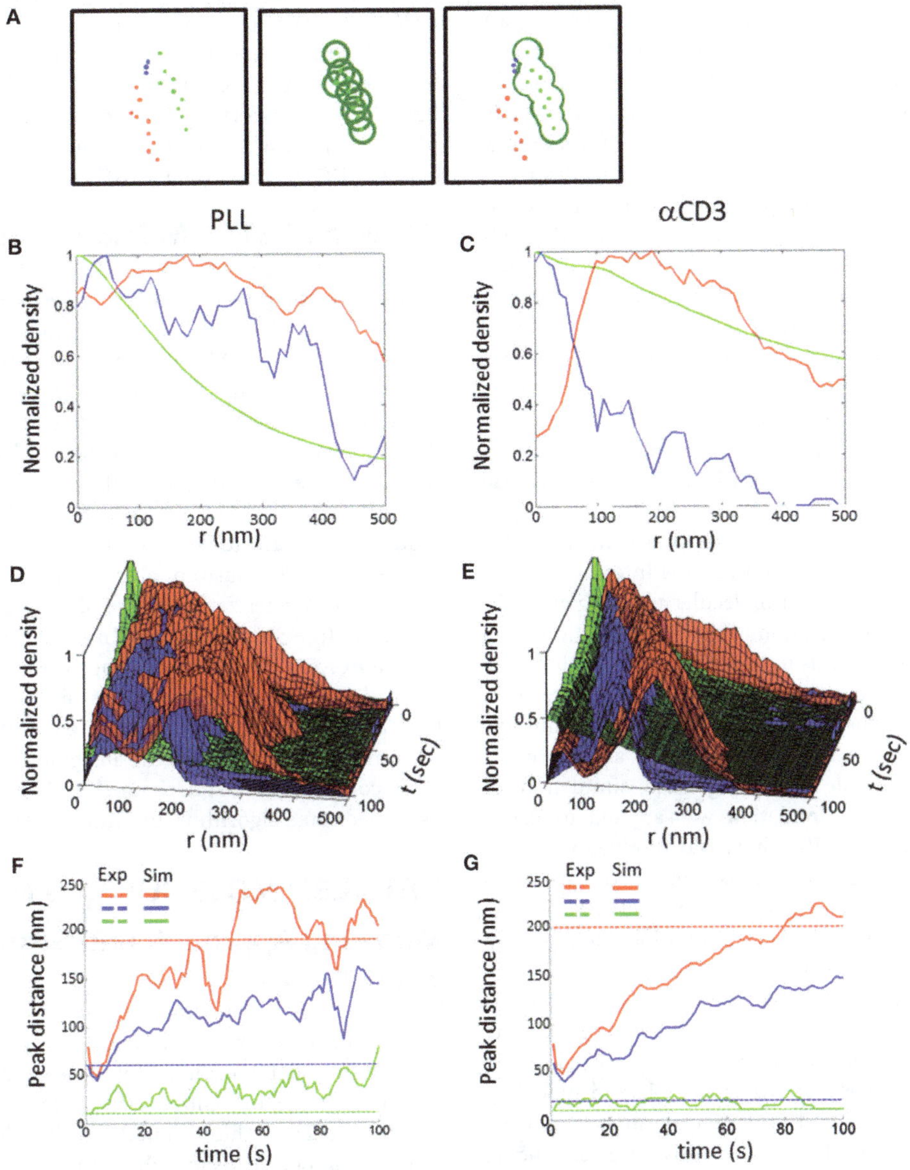


**FIGURE 9 |** Topology analysis of molecular patterning in experiments and simulations. **(A)** Topology analysis of molecular densities of different species (red and blue dots) relative to a cluster of reference (green dots). The cluster perimeter is defined by consecutive dilations. **(B,C)** Results of the analysis of molecular patterning in experimental results on either **(B)** a PLL-coated coverslip or **(C)** on an αCD3-coated coverslip. **(D,E)** Results of the analysis of molecular patterning in simulated results, on either **(D)** a PLL-coated coverslip or **(D)** on an αCD3-coated coverslip. **(F,G)** The shift in the peak of the molecular distributions of the topology analyses, on either **(F)** a PLL-coated coverslip or **(G)** on an αCD3-coated coverslip. Experimental results are shown as dashed colored lines while simulated results are shown as continuous colored lines.

not be explicitly simulated as diffusing agents in the 3D environment of the cytosol. Still, our simulation specializes in capturing complex and dynamic interactions and pattern formation in intercellular interfaces. It focuses on surface molecules interacting in a dynamic, fluctuating surfaces. To our knowledge, the integration of SMLM data into cell simulations and the effects of embedded molecules on the cells' surface are important features that have not been attempted in current simulations.

Our simulation has been designed as an accessible tool to non-experts. It operates on a PC with a standard (i7 quad) processor. It is coded in Matlab, in a modular structure that can be easily expanded to include additional membrane and cortical structures, such as cortical cytoskeleton, membrane bound proteins, channels, etc. Still, expansion of the simulation to whole cells will require much stronger computational power than is currently employed. It integrates a wide range of physical parameters of simulated entities (membranes, molecules) that are accessible via an intuitive GUI. We provide multiple analysis tools, including univariate and bivariate PCFs (36), clustering algorithms and the topological analysis demonstrated here (**Figure 9**). Additional analyses of relevance may include Minkowski functionals (37), conditional second order PCFs (13), and more. Our simulation enable batch runs for scanning systematically values of parameters of choice. The results of such batch simulations can be presented graphically using our statistical analyses tools. The user can then quantitatively compare the results of such statistics to experimental results, for further refinement of the simulation. We have recently demonstrated this approach to study inaccessible properties of the PM (e.g., its rigidity and its ligand density) (18). The further integration of iterative simulations with sensitivity analyses such as the Sobol method could enable more systematic evaluation of the wide parameter space of our agent-based simulation.

We believe that InterCells, esp. with its upcoming tools, will allow the study of molecular patterning at cell surfaces and interfaces in a wide range of cases. We provided in the User's Manual a second example, demonstrating how InterCells can be employed to quantify the effects of molecular trapping and self-clustering on molecular organization at the PM. Additional cell interfaces that can be studied using InterCells may include cell junctions between cells in a tissue, the evolution of interfaces in development, neuronal synapses, immune synapses of multiple types, and under various experimental conditions, and more.

To conclude, we provide here a generic simulation of intercellular interfaces. The simulation was applied to nano-scale pattern formation at the IS, which was resolved by three-color SMLM. The detailed simulations combined data from SMLM imaging, coarse-grained physical model PM of the interacting cells, and simulative data from multiple Monte-Carlo simulations. During this process, the simulation has proved to be an invaluable predictive and hypothesis generating tool. It further provided an elaborate test of our physical understanding of molecular patterning at the IS and of the forces behind it. The iterative application of novel experimental tools and modeling could provide critical feedback to future experiments and the adaptation of working models; thus, in this case, enhancing our mechanistic understanding of early T cell activation. Our simulations are modular, flexible and accessible, such that they can be employed for studying a wide range of intercellular interfaces and molecular interactions within.

# METHODS

## Sample Preparation

Jurkat E6.1 cells and such cells stably expressing TCRζ-Dronpa were available for this study from a previously published work (16). Positive expression was routinely monitored using fluorescence microscopy. For three-color, SMLM TCRζ-Dronpa were immunostained with antibodies: 1. αCD45-Alexa647 conjugated (BioLegend, 304056); 2. αCD11 (LFA1) primary (BD Pharmingen, 555378) and αMouse secondary antibody labbled with Alexa568.

Cells were dropped onto glass coverslips coated with 0.01% poly-L-lysine (Sigma) with or without following coating αCD3 (UCHT1, eBioscience 16-0038-85). The cells were incubated at 37°C for a specific spreading time on the coverslips of 1.5 min. After this time the cells were fixed with 2.4% Paraformaldehyde for 30 min at 37°C. Combined SMLM (PALM-dSTORM) imaging was performed in a dSTORM buffer (50 mM TRIS pH = 8, 10 mM NaCl, 0.5 mg/ml glucose oxidase, 40 μg/ml catalase, 10% glucose, 10 mM MEA).

## PALM and STORM Microscopy

Three-color SMLM (combined PALM/dSTORM) imaging was performed using a total internal reflection (TIRF) microscope (TI-E, Nikon). Imaging in TIRF mode served to visualize molecules at the PM of spreading cells in close proximity to the coverslip (up to ~100–200 nm). PALM images were analyzed using the N-STORM module in NIS-Elements (Nikon) or a previously described algorithm (ThunderSTORM) (38) to identify peaks and group them into functions that reflect the positions of single molecules (14). PALM acquisition sequence typically took ~5 min for three channel imaging at 50–100 frame/s. Custom algorithms were then applied for statistical characterization of the SMLM images of the detected molecules (see **Supplementary Information** for further details). The fluorescent proteins were imaged sequentially in the different channels using dedicated emission filters that minimized cross talk between the channels. Photoactivation illumination at 405 nm was changed over the imaging sequence of fixed cells. Drift compensation and channel registration were performed using dedicated algorithms in ThunderSTORM.

# DETAILED MOLECULAR SIMULATION

## Modeling Approach and Structure of the Simulation

Here, we take a reductionist approach for modeling, aiming to explain complex spatio-temporal patterns of molecular organization at intercellular interfaces. All simulation files are available online on Github (https://github.com/ShermanLab/InterCells). These files should be downloaded to the User's computer under a directory that can be accessed by Matlab.

### Requirements

For ease of use, the simulation Basic computational power, employing a standard PC (with an i7 processor). It is coded in Matlab (MathWorks). The structure of the simulation is depicted in **Figures 4,5** and is explained in detail in the User's Manual (provided in the **Supplemental Information**).

### Input

Input parameters include parameters that describe the physical properties of the interacting surfaces and of the molecules that interact within and across the interfaces. The parameters are typically extracted from experimental measurements, on molecular interactions that govern the signaling cascade (39, 40). In the case of hybrid simulations, initial conditions are set by single molecule data on molecular positions and their state from SMLM imaging (see User's Manual). Benchmark runs for testing a range of predetermined parameters. Such benchmark runs have previously served for critical evaluation of mechanistic models of T cell activation (24) and for studying the effects of variations in critical physical parameters on molecular patterning at the IS (18).

### Simulation Core

The simulation includes detailed models of relevant stochastic processes, including reaction-diffusion processes and relevant force fields. The details of the simulation algorithm are provided in separate sections below. Briefly, in our simulation we assume specific Hamiltonians of a quasi-equilibrium system and with mean-field approximations. The simulation relies on hierarchical levels of simplification. Continuous entities that are not the focus of the simulations are "coarse-grained." Such entities include lipids in the PM and water molecules, and are not specifically described in the simulation. In contrast, protein molecules of interest are described individually. The simulation algorithms is realized using "importance sampling" Monte-Carlo simulations (41). Molecular identities are maintained for the reactant molecules of interest. Metropolis criterion is applied to determine the transition probability between consecutive configurations.

### Outputs

Quantifiable readouts of the numeric simulations include the position and state of individual proteins, the morphology of the PM and their energetics. Visualization tools are provided for showing the simulation results. For instance, live evolution of molecular patterning is provided during the simulation run. The patterns can then be shown for each step individually, or as a movie.

### Analyses

Here we integrated multiple statistical tools for quantitative analyses and interpretation of the results. Our tools include clustering algorithms and second-order statistics (16, 36), and the topology analysis (**Figure 3**). These tools are important for the quantitative comparison between results from experiments and from simulations. Moreover, the analyses provide a critical feedback for generating experimentally testable hypotheses and the adaptation of working models in an iterative way. In fact, our imaging in this study was instructed by early simulative results that indicated the mutual patterning of TCR, CD11 and CD45.

### Simulation Setup

The simulations are based on a rectangular grid, of a size of few microns. The array is made of square 10 nm pixels. We used periodic boundary conditions (molecules that exit on one side appear on the opposite side). The initial height ($z$) of the membrane is set to 70 nm. The PM height in pixels that accommodate either TCR or CD11 molecules are set to the molecular height. The $z$-value of each pixel changes randomly at every iteration by $\Delta z$ that has a normal distribution with $\sigma = 1$ nm, according to the Metropolis criterion.

A specific limitation of our simulation to the number of simulated molecules originates from the occupancy of only one molecule (regardless of its species) in a single pixel. Thus, considering a pixel size of 10 nm and a rectangular grid of 1 × 1 $\mu m^2$, a limit of 10 K molecules can be simulated. Larger grids are often needed to show complex molecular patterns within a cell footprint. Thus, we often simulated tens of thousands of molecules within grids of 400 × 400 pixels. Such grids were chosen to include a region of interest of a cell footprint with an area of 4 × 4 $\mu m^2$ (i.e., each pixel representing an area of 10 × 10 nm). Such a size should leave a wide enough margin (e.g., ~50–100 pixels), such that boundary effects are minimized. Such simulations took ~15 min using a PC with a standard (i7 quad) processor. Acceleration of the simulation can be improved via operating parallel computing, computation via GPUs and more. A bigger grid size minimizes the effect of the boundary, yet requires longer (actual) simulation time, computational power and memory. Similar consideration may restrict the iteration time, overall simulation time, the save rate and the number of runs (**Table S3**). While other simulations, such as MCell, can accommodate millions of molecules and states, they require compartmentation of the simulated space for efficiently running.

We simulated multiple different types of proteins, as follows. TCRs behave as binding proteins to immobile ligands (αCD3) on a coverslip or to mobile pMHC molecules at the PM of APCs. CD11 may bind ICAM at the PM of APCs. The $z$ coordinates of the TCRs and CD11 are kept at 13 nm and at 35 nm, respectively, throughout the simulation runtime. The molecules, and esp. bulky CD45 molecules, act as repulsive springs. Non-specific binding occurs between all molecules and the PLL coating of coverslips. The numbers of simulated molecules remains constant throughout the simulation. All simulated parameters are detailed in **Tables S1–S3**.

## Monte Carlo Simulations

### Simulation Energetics

In the simulations we used the Hamiltonian $H = H_{int} + H_{el}$, to calculate the energetics of the overall interactions between the T cell membrane and the coverslip (represented by the term $H_{int}$) and the elasticity of the T cell membrane (represented by the term $H_{el}$). The interaction part, $H_{int}$, is defined as:

$$H_{int} = \sum_i (\delta_{1,mol_i}\delta_{1,lig_i})V_{mol-lig}(z_i) + \delta_{1,mol_i}V_{mol}(z_i) \quad (1)$$

where,

$$\delta_{1,X_i} = \begin{cases} 1, & \textit{if a molecule of type X exists in pixel i} \\ 0, & \textit{otherwise} \end{cases} \quad (2)$$

Single pixels from any surface (i.e., either a PM or a coverslip) can accommodate only one molecule at a time. The interaction potential of the molecule with its ligand, $V_{mol-lig}$, is defined as:

$$V_{mol-lig}(z_i) = \begin{cases} U_{mol-lig}, & |z_i - l_{mol-lig}| < \textit{Interaction range} \\ 0, & \textit{elsewhere} \end{cases} \quad (3)$$

where $U_{mol-lig}$ is the interaction strength of a molecule and its ligand, $l_{mol-lig}$ is the length of an engaged molecule-ligand conplex. $z_i$ is the inter surface distance at pixel $i$. The width of the molecule-ligand potential is set and its depth are set according to published results (see **Table S3**). The repulsion potential of the molecule is defined as:

$$V_{mol}(z_i) = \begin{cases} k_{mol}(z_i - l_{mol})^2, & z_i < l_{mol} \\ 0, & z_i > l_{mol} \end{cases} \quad (4)$$

The physical parameters of $k_{mol,}$ the compressional stiffness of the molecule and $l_{mol}$, the length of the uncompressed molecules, are detailed in **Table S1**.

The elastic part of the Hamiltonian, *Hel*, is defined as:

$$H_{el} = \sum_i \frac{\kappa}{2a^2} (\Delta_d z_i)^2 \quad (5)$$

where $\kappa = \kappa_1 \cdot \kappa_2 / (\kappa_1 + \kappa_2)$, is the general effective bending rigidity of two membranes. In this case, the bending rigidity is effectively $\kappa \approx \kappa_1$, since $\kappa_2 >> \kappa_1$ and is simulated at different values. The lattice constant, a, is 10 nm and $_dz_i = z_{i1} + z_{i2} + z_{i3} + z_{i4} - 4z_i$, (where $i1$, $i2$, $i3$, $i4$ are the indices of the four nearest neighbors of pixel $i$).

### Simulations Dynamics

The simulation propagates in time by iterations of 0.01 s. In every iteration all molecules attempt to hop to one of the neighboring pixels according to their diffusion coefficient. The hopping attempts of the molecules are accepted or rejected according to the following rules:

1. The target pixel is not occupied.
2. The probability of acceptance is according to Metropolis criterion is:

at an old pixel:

$$P(old\ state \rightarrow free) = \begin{cases} 1 \Delta E < 0 \\ \exp(-\Delta E)\ \Delta E > 0 \end{cases} \quad (6)$$

and at a new pixel:

$$P(free \rightarrow new\ state) = \begin{cases} 1 \Delta E < 0 \\ \exp(-\Delta E)\ \Delta E > 0 \end{cases} \quad (7)$$

While

$$P(attempt\ accepted) = P\left(old\ state \rightarrow free\right) \times P(free \rightarrow new\ state) \quad (8)$$

3. If more than one molecule attempted to hop to the same pixel, the molecule with the highest energy gain will hop.
4. The height, $z$, of each pixel of the surface is changed randomly by $\Delta z$, that has a normal distribution with $\sigma = 1$ nm and according to Metropolis criterion. The value of $\sigma$ is set by receiving 40–50% of acceptance of the membrane attempts 27.

### Topology Analyses

The topology analysis measures the conditional density of molecules from a spatial reference set by clusters of a chosen molecular type. In the example presented in **Figure 9A**, the cluster of reference is set by green molecules. Next, circles are placed around each green molecule (middle panel), and we consider the perimeter of their unified area. The densities of the other molecules (namely, red or blue points in our example) can now be calculated on this perimeter. The consecutive operation of these steps with growing radii from the molecules yields the Minkowski perimeter functional (37). The conditional densities of the molecules are then calculated for the growing perimeters, as shown in **Figures 9B–E**. Last, the density of the molecules of reference (here, green dots) is determined and presented by its univariate PCF as a function of the perimeter radius.

## AUTHOR CONTRIBUTIONS

ES supervised research; ES, YN-O designed research; YN-O developed and performed simulations; YR and JS developed reagents and performed imaging experiments research; ES, YN-O wrote the paper.

## FUNDING

This research was supported by Grant no. 321993 from the Marie Skłodowska-Curie actions of the European Commission, the Lejwa Fund, and Grants no.1417/13 and no. 1937/13 from the Israeli Science Foundation.

## REFERENCES

1. Chan CJ, Heisenberg CP, Hiiragi T. Coordination of morphogenesis and cell-fate specification in development. *Curr Biol.* (2017) 27:R1024–35. doi: 10.1016/j.cub.2017.07.010
2. Nicholls, J. G. *From Neuron To Brain. 5th edn.* Sunderland, MA: Sinauer Associates (2012).
3. Trautmann A, Valitutti S. The diversity of immunological synapses. *Curr Opin Immunol.* (2003) 15:249–54. doi: 10.1016/S0952-7915(03)00040-2
4. Flemming HC, Wingender J, Szewzyk U, Steinberg P, Rice SA, Kjelleberg S. Biofilms: an emergent form of bacterial life. *Nat Rev Microbiol.* (2016) 14:563–75. doi: 10.1038/nrmicro.2016.94
5. Cavey M, Lecuit T. Molecular bases of cell-cell junctions stability and dynamics. *Cold Spring Harb Perspect Biol.* (2009) 1:a002998. doi: 10.1101/cshperspect.a002998
6. Choquet D, Triller A. The dynamic synapse. *Neuron* (2013) 80:691–703. doi: 10.1016/j.neuron.2013.10.013
7. Sudhof TC, Malenka RC. Understanding synapses: past, present, and future. *Neuron* (2008) 60:469–76. doi: 10.1016/j.neuron.2008.10.011
8. Chakraborty AK, Weiss A. Insights into the initiation of TCR signaling. *Nat Immunol.* (2014) 15:798–807. doi: 10.1038/ni.2940
9. Balagopalan L, Sherman E, Barr VA, Samelson LE. Imaging techniques for assaying lymphocyte activation in action. *Nat Rev Immunol.* (2011) 11:21–33. doi: 10.1038/nri2903

10. Monks CR, Freiberg BA, Kupfer H, Sciaky N, Kupfer A. Three-dimensional segregation of supramolecular activation clusters in T cells. *Nature* (1998) 395:82–6. doi: 10.1038/25764
11. Bunnell SC, Barr VA, Fuller CL, Samelson LE. High-resolution multicolor imaging of dynamic signaling complexes in t cells stimulated by planar substrates. *Sci STKE* (2003):pl8. doi: 10.1126/stke.2003.177.pl8
12. Grakoui A, Bromley SK, Sumen C, Davis MM, Shaw AS, Allen PM, et al. The immunological synapse: a molecular machine controlling T cell activation. *Science* (1999) 285:221–27. doi: 10.1126/science.285.5425.221
13. Patterson G, Davidson M, Manley S, Lippincott-Schwartz J. Superresolution imaging using single-molecule localization. *Annu Rev Phys Chem.* (2010) 61:345–67. doi: 10.1146/annurev.physchem.012809.103444
14. Betzig E, Patterson GH, Sougrat R, Lindwasser OW, Olenych S, Bonifacino JS, et al. Imaging intracellular fluorescent proteins at nanometer resolution. *Science* (2006) 313:1642–5. doi: 10.1126/science.1127344
15. van de Linde S, Loschberger A, Klein T, eidbreder M, Wolter S, Heilemann M, et al. Direct stochastic optical reconstruction microscopy with standard fluorescent probes. *Nat Protoc.* (2011) 6:991–1009. doi: 10.1038/nprot.2011.336
16. Sherman E, Barr V, Manley S, Patterson G, Balagopalan L, Akpan I, et al. Functional nanoscale organization of signaling molecules downstream of the T cell antigen receptor. *Immunity* (2011) 35:705–20. doi: 10.1016/j.immuni.2011.10.004
17. Sherman E, Barr VA, Merrill RK, Regan CK, Sommers CL, Samelson LE. Hierarchical nanostructure and synergy of multimolecular signalling complexes. *Nat Commun.* (2016) 7:12161. doi: 10.1038/ncomms 12161
18. Razvag Y, Neve-Oz Y, Sajman J, Reches M, Sherman E. Nanoscale kinetic segregation of TCR and CD45 in engaged microvilli facilitates early T cell activation. *Nat Commun.* (2018) 9:732. doi: 10.1038/s41467-018-03127-w
19. Allard JF, Dushek O, Coombs D, van der Merwe PA. Mechanical modulation of receptor-ligand interactions at cell-cell interfaces. *Biophys J.* (2012) 102:1265–73. doi: 10.1016/j.bpj.2012.02.006
20. Chang VT, Fernandes RA, Ganzinger KA, Lee SF, Siebold C, McColl J, et al. Initiation of T cell signaling by CD45 segregation at 'close contacts'. *Nat Immunol.* (2016) 17:574–82. doi: 10.1038/ni.3392
21. Varma R, Campi G, Yokosuka T, Saito T, Dustin ML. T cell receptor-proximal signals are sustained in peripheral microclusters and terminated in the central supramolecular activation cluster. *Immunity* (2006) 25:117–27. doi: 10.1016/j.immuni.2006.04.010
22. Dustin ML, Chakraborty AK, Shaw AS. understanding the structure and function of the immunological synapse. *Cold Spring Harb Perspect Biol.* (2010) 2:a002311. doi: 10.1101/cshperspect.a002311
23. Alves R, Antunes F, Salvador A. Tools for kinetic modeling of biochemical networks. *Nat Biotechnol.* (2006) 24:667–72. doi: 10.1038/nbt06 06-667
24. Neve-Oz Y, Razvag Y, Sajman J, Sherman E. Mechanisms of localized activation of the T cell antigen receptor inside clusters. *Biochim Biophys Acta* (2015) 1853:810–21. doi: 10.1016/j.bbamcr.2014.09.025
25. Santos AM, Ponjavic A, Fritzsche M, Fernandes RA, de la Serna, JB, Wilcock MJ, et al. Capturing resting T cells: the perils of PLL. *Nat Immunol.* (2018) 19:203–05. doi: 10.1038/s41590-018-0048-8
26. Weikl TR, Lipowsky R. Pattern formation during T-cell adhesion. *Biophys J.* (2004) 87:3665–78. doi: 10.1529/biophysj.104.045609
27. Jung Y, Riven I, Feigelson SW, Kartvelishvily E, Tohya K, Miyasaka M, et al. Three-dimensional localization of T-cell receptors in relation to microvilli using a combination of superresolution microscopies. *Proc Natl Acad Sci USA.* (2016) 113:E5916–24. doi: 10.1073/pnas.1605399113
28. Cai E, Marchuk K, Beemiller P, Beppler C, Rubashkin MG, Weaver, VM, et al. Visualizing dynamic microvillar search and stabilization during ligand detection by T cells. *Science* (2017) 356:eaal3118. doi: 10.1126/science.aa l3118
29. Yokosuka T, Sakata-Sogawa K, Kobayashi W, Hiroshima M, Hashimoto-Tane A, Tokunaga M, et al. Newly generated T cell receptor microclusters initiate and sustain T cell activation by recruitment of Zap70 and SLP-76. *Nat Immunol.* (2005) 6:1253–62. doi: 10.1038/ni1272
30. Campi G, Varma R, Dustin ML. Actin and agonist MHC-peptide complex-dependent T cell receptor microclusters as scaffolds for signaling. *J Exp Med.* (2005) 202:1031–6. doi: 10.1084/jem.20051182
31. Kaizuka Y, Douglass AD, Varma R, Dustin ML, Vale RD. Mechanisms for segregating T cell receptor and adhesion molecules during immunological synapse formation in Jurkat T cells. *Proc Natl Acad Sci USA.* (2007) 104:20296–301. doi: 10.1073/pnas.0710258105
32. Bergmann FT, Hoops S, Klahn B, Kummer U, Mendes P, Pahle J, et al. COPASI and its applications in biotechnology. *J Biotechnol.* (2017) 261:215–20. doi: 10.1016/j.jbiotec.2017.06.1200
33. Slepchenko BM, Schaff JC, Macara I, Loew LM. Quantitative cell biology with the virtual cell. *Trends Cell Biol.* (2003) 13:570–6. doi: 10.1016/j.tcb.2003.09.002
34. Andrews SS, Addy NJ, Brent R, Arkin AP. Detailed simulations of cell biology with smoldyn 2.1. *Plos Comput Biol.* (2010) 6:e1000705. doi: 10.1371/journal.pcbi.1000705
35. Kerr RA, Bartol TM, Kaminsky B, Dittrich M, Chang JCJ, Baden SB, et al. Fast monte carlo simulation methods for biological reaction-diffusion systems in solution and on surfaces. *Siam J Sci Comput.* (2008) 30:3126–49. doi: 10.1137/070692017
36. Sherman E, Barr VA, Samelson LE. Resolving multi-molecular protein interactions by photoactivated localization microscopy. *Methods* (2013) 59:261–69. doi: 10.1016/j.ymeth.2012.12.002
37. Parker J, Sherman E, van de Raa M, van der Meer D, Samelson LE, Losert, W. Automatic sorting of point pattern sets using Minkowski functionals. *Phys Rev E Stat. Nonlin Soft Matter Phys.* (2013) 88:022720. doi: 10.1103/PhysRevE.88.022720
38. Ovesny M, Krizek P, Borkovec J, Svindrych ZK, Hagen GM. ThunderSTORM: a comprehensive ImageJ plug-in for PALM and STORM data analysis and super-resolution imaging. *Bioinformatics* (2014) 30:2389–90. doi: 10.1093/bioinformatics/btu202
39. van der Merwe PA, Dushek O. Mechanisms for T cell receptor triggering. *Nat Rev Immunol.* (2011) 11:47–55. doi: 10.1038/nri2887
40. Balagopalan L, Coussens NP, Sherman E, Samelson LE, Sommers, CL. The LAT story: a tale of cooperativity, coordination, and choreography. *Cold Spring Harb Perspect Biol.* (2010) 2:a005512. doi: 10.1101/cshperspect.a005512
41. Rubinstein RY, Kroese DP (editors). *Simulation And The Monte Carlo Method. 3rd edn.* Hoboken, NJ: John Wiley & Sons, Inc.

# 19

# Immunoglobulin Light Chain Gene Rearrangements, Receptor Editing and the Development of a Self-Tolerant Antibody Repertoire

*Andrew M. Collins [1]* and Corey T. Watson [2]*

[1] School of Biotechnology and Biomolecular Sciences, University of New South Wales, Sydney, NSW, Australia, [2] Department of Biochemistry and Molecular Genetics, University of Louisville School of Medicine, Louisville, KY, United States

***Correspondence:**
Andrew M. Collins
a.collins@unsw.edu.au

Discussion of the antibody repertoire usually emphasizes diversity, but a conspicuous feature of the light chain repertoire is its lack of diversity. The diversity of reported allelic variants of germline light chain genes is also limited, even in well-studied species. In this review, the implications of this lack of diversity are considered. We explore germline and rearranged light chain genes in a variety of species, with a particular focus on human and mouse genes. The importance of the number, organization and orientation of the genes for the control of repertoire development is discussed, and we consider how primary rearrangements and receptor editing together shape the expressed light chain repertoire. The resulting repertoire is dominated by just a handful of IGKV and IGLV genes. It has been hypothesized that an important function of the light chain is to guard against self-reactivity, and the role of secondary rearrangements in this process could explain the genomic organization of the light chain genes. It could also explain why the light chain repertoire is so limited. Heavy and light chain genes may have co-evolved to ensure that suitable light chain partners are usually available for each heavy chain that forms early in B cell development. We suggest that the co-evolved loci of the house mouse often became separated during the inbreeding of laboratory mice, resulting in new pairings of loci that are derived from different sub-species of the house mouse. A resulting vulnerability to self-reactivity could explain at least some mouse models of autoimmune disease.

**Keywords: immunoglobulin light chain, receptor editing, self-tolerance, antibody repertoire, V(D)J rearrangement, models of autoimmune disease, sub-species of the house mouse**

## INTRODUCTION

The success of the humoral arm of the adaptive immune system depends upon a diversity of antibody specificities within an individual's population of circulating B cells. This diversity is made possible by the process of gene recombination that takes place during B cell development, creating functional antibody heavy and light chain V(D)J transcripts from relatively small sets of Variable (V), Diversity (D), and Joining (J) genes. The basic processes underlying V(D)J recombination are now well understood (1, 2) and recently, thanks to advances in sequencing technologies that allow millions of different V(D)J gene rearrangements to be explored in a single individual, much has been learnt about the nature of the expressed antibody repertoire (3–8). Most repertoire studies, however, have focused upon the heavy chain repertoire. The nature of the light chain repertoire is less clear.

The diversity of the antibody repertoire is a consequence of the permutations of heavy chain V, D, and J genes, and light chain V and J genes, that are possible given the size of these sets of genes within the genome, and of the permutations of heavy and light chain pairings. This component of the overall diversity is referred to as combinatorial diversity, and is a simple reflection of the number of available heavy chain genes and κ and λ light chain genes. Additional diversity is generated during the recombination processes by imprecise joining at the V(D)J junctions. This is referred to as junctional diversity, and is principally determined by the extent to which random nucleotides are inserted between joining genes (4, 6).

In this review, we highlight important consequences for repertoire development that result from the organization of light chain genes within the mammalian genome. In particular, this organization facilitates repeated rounds of light chain gene rearrangement through the process of receptor editing. This helps to ensure that virtually all developing B cells successfully generate productive light chain rearrangements.

A number of biases and constraints are discussed which lead to substantially less diversity in the light chain repertoire than is usually calculated, and this limited diversity appears to be present in a wide range of species. We conclude that diversity is not the raison d'être of the light chain repertoire. In light of substantial evidence for a special role for light chains in autoimmune reactivity, we propose that the co-evolution of heavy and light chain genes has resulted in a limited light chain repertoire that usually serves to avoid self-reactivity. This hypothesis is explored through an examination of the generation of light chain repertoires in inbred mouse strains that are widely used in models of autoimmune disease.

## THE NUMBER AND ORGANIZATION OF LIGHT CHAIN GENES WITHIN THE MAMMALIAN GENOME

To properly understand how the heavy and light chain repertoires are generated, it is essential to have a detailed knowledge of the number of rearranging germline genes that give rise to these repertoires, and of their organization within the genome. The number of genes per species is highly variable as a result of dynamic evolutionary processes in these complex gene families. This can be appreciated by examining the phylogenetic relationships among genes within and between species, and is demonstrated in a phylogeny of functional human and mouse heavy and light chain variable genes (**Figure S1**). However, our understanding of the precise evolutionary histories of these genes across a larger range of species remains limited, largely due to a paucity of available genomic data.

The organization of the light chain genes is particularly complex, and quite different to that of the heavy chain genes. Heavy chain genes are found within a single gene locus (IGH), while light chain genes are generally found as two separate gene loci-the κ locus (IGK) and the λ locus (IGL). These two loci are found in virtually all mammalian species, while loci for these and other light chain variants are found in bony and even cartilaginous fish (9, 10). Such a general distribution of light chain genes between separate loci is intriguing, and suggests that this genomic organization may carry evolutionary advantages.

Within the κ chain loci of humans, mice and most other species, genes are organized in a similar fashion to the genes of the heavy chain locus (11–15). That is, a cluster of IGKV genes are found 5′ of a small number of IGKJ genes, with the IGKJ gene cluster located 5′ of a single IGKC gene. The dog genome is unusual in that half the canine IGKV genes are located upstream, and half are located downstream of the IGKJ and IGKC genes (16).

The number of functional IGKV genes varies widely between species, and this number may have some relationship to species size (**Figure S1**). We have argued that small species may require more germline genes because of the small burst size of the germinal center reaction in those species (17). As the number of cells responding to antigen is limited in small species, there is less chance for important higher affinity antibodies to emerge from the germinal center through the process of somatic point mutation. Critical specificities must therefore be encoded in the germline.

Sequencing of the human κ locus has identified 44 functional IGKV genes and open reading frames, which are found in two clusters that arose through segmental duplication (18, 19). An additional three functional IGKV sequences may be present in some haplotypes (20). A comparable number of functional IGKV genes ($n = 54$) was recently characterized in genomic sequences from the rhesus macaque, a commonly used non-human primate model (21). In contrast, studies of the horse genome reference sequence identified only 19 apparently functional IGKV genes (22), while 111 and 135 potentially functional IGKV genes have been found in the guinea pig and rat genome reference sequences, respectively (23, 24). Among mammalian species studied to date, the microbat (*Myotis lucifugis*) is unique in that it lacks a κ locus (25). It has been suggested that this may be part of a general simplification of immune function in a species that has met the weight to muscle challenge that is necessary for flight capability (26). This hypothesis is indirectly supported by the fact that the κ locus is also absent from the genome of chickens (25) and zebra finches (27), and it may have been lost from the genomes of all bird species.

In line with numbers reported in the small rodent species mentioned above, the genome of C57BL/6 mice carries around 101 functional IGKV genes (28). This number may, however, not be accurate for other inbred mouse strains. We recently reported that the heavy chain loci of different inbred strains of mice are derived from different sub-species of the house mouse. As a result, the C57BL/6 strain carries 99 functional IGHV genes, but the BALB/c strain carries 163 functional IGHV genes (29). We have also noted that based on available whole-genome SNP data (30), almost all inbred strains carry κ chain loci that appear to be derived from the *Mus musculus domesticus* sub-species (17). NOD/ShiLtJ mice are unusual in that they carry a *M. m. castaneus*-derived κ locus (17). Interestingly, many of the distinct κ genes of this diabetes-prone strain are identical to κ genes of the Systemic Lupus Erythematosis (SLE)-prone (NZB × NZW)F1 and MRL strains (31). SNP analysis shows that parts of the IGKV loci of NZB and MRL mice are also derived from the *M. m. castaneus* sub-species (**Figure 1**). This confirms an observation from a very early study of BALB/c and NZB-derived myeloma proteins. It was reported that NZB and BALB/c mice share some κ light chain sequences, but that other κ genes differ markedly between the strains (32). SNP analysis shows that the chr6:67.5m−68.2m region of the κ locus of the NZB strain is of *M. m. castaneus* origin. The chr6:68.2m−68.5m region is of uncertain origin, and the remainder of the NZB κ locus is *M. m. domesticus*-derived. Genes of *M. m. castaneus* origin are also found in the MRL strain, in the region chr6:68.8m−70.7m (see **Figure 1**).

The λ locus of most species investigated to date includes a set of IGLV genes that are located 5′ from a variable number of tandem cassettes, each made up of an IGLJ gene and an IGLC gene. The human locus includes as many as 38 functional IGLV genes and Open Reading Frames (18) and five functional J-C gene pairs (34). In the rhesus macaque, 47 IGLV genes are predicted to be functional based on genomic data (21), and in the pig, there are nine functional IGLV genes (35). In these species too, the IGKV genes are located 5′ of functional J-C pairs, but this organization is not invariant. 144 IGLV genes of uncertain functionality have been identified in the horse, with 110 genes being located upstream and 34 being located downstream of the IGLJ/IGLC cluster (22, 36). The locus of the mouse is also differently organized.

The C57BL/6 genome includes just three IGLV genes (**Figure S1**), and there has been speculation that IGLV genes might have been lost during the inbreeding of laboratory strains. In fact, diversity is lacking in wild mice of all three *Mus musculus* subspecies (37). Two of the C57BL/6 IGLV genes are associated with one functional J-C gene pair, while the third IGLV gene is associated with a second J-C pair. Lambda rearrangement in the mouse takes place within each of the two VJC units, with little or no recombination between the units (38).

The genes of both the human and mouse λ IGLV loci are all in the same transcriptional orientation as the λ J-C gene clusters (18, 39). The V, D, and J genes of the heavy chain loci of mammalian species are also found in the same orientation as their associated constant region genes (40–42). The κ chain locus of these species, on the other hand, includes many IGKV genes that are found in the opposite orientation to their associated IGKJ and IGKC genes. In the human, the orientation of the distal κ gene cluster is opposite to that of the IGKJ genes and IGKC gene, while all but the two most 3′ genes of the proximal gene cluster share their orientation with the IGKJ and IGKC genes (20). The κ locus of the mouse also includes IGKV genes in both the same and the opposite orientation to their respective IGKJ and IGKC genes (13). Such variable orientations of IGKV genes have also been reported in other species including the elephant (43), horse (22), pig (14), dog (16), and rhesus macaque (21).

In the horse, which is a species with a λ -dominant repertoire, IGLV genes are found both upstream and downstream of the λ J-C gene clusters. Many of these sequences are pseudogenes, but the few functional genes in the downstream cluster are found in the opposite orientation to that of the horse J-C genes, thereby allowing the genes to recombine (36).

The orientation of genes has other consequences for the generation of diversity. The opposite orientation of many IGKV genes within the murine and human κ loci means that primary rearrangements of such genes do not lead to deletion of the genes that are located between recombining IGKV and IGKJ genes (see **Figure 2**). This retention of genes becomes important if a rearrangement results in a non-productive chain or a self-reactive B cell receptor (BCR). In such situations, all other IGKV and IGKJ germline genes remain available for secondary rearrangements (see discussion below). In any cell that experiences such successive rounds of recombination, the order and orientation of the genes within the locus will be subject to complex changes, and this will have consequences for the repertoire that is generated by secondary rearrangements (**Figure 2**).

The frequencies with which different V, D, and J genes are utilized in gene rearrangements vary by many orders of magnitude. This appears to reflect, at least in part, the accessibility of genes, and their positions within the genome (28, 44, 45). Dramatic changes in the order of genes and in the distances between IGKV and IGKJ genes, arising from a primary rearrangement of genes, should therefore lead to changes to gene accessibility. This may mean that the utilization frequency of a gene can vary between primary, secondary and subsequent rearrangements. Complex changes could therefore compromise the tight regulation that otherwise appears to guide the generation of the antibody repertoire. In many species, this risk to the regulation of the repertoire may be mitigated by the action of Kappa Deleting Elements (KDE). The consecutive rearrangements that are possible within the κ locus can be terminated by KDE-mediated recombination, driving B cells to the expression of genes of the λ locus (46). This may also prevent or lead to the resolution of allelic inclusion, which can arise because of the orientation of IGKV genes within the locus (see **Figure 2**) (47).

Kappa Deleting Elements (KDE) are located downstream of IGKC genes, and they appear to be highly conserved within the mammalian genome (48). The mouse KDE is referred to as the Recombining Segment (RS), and it is distinct but very similar to the Recombination Signal Sequences (RSS) located adjacent to the 3′ ends of the IGKV genes and the 5′ ends of the IGKJ genes (49). KDEs of all species studied are made up of conserved heptamer and nonamer sequences separated by 23 base pair spacers (48). The KDEs function by allowing recombination between the KDEs and recombining elements that contain the palindromic heptamer CACAGTG. These are located within the IGKJ-IGKC intron and in the RSS at the 3′ ends of the IGKV genes. Such recombination effectively terminates the involvement of the rearranging locus in the generation of diversity. This will drive recombination from the first to the second κ locus (i.e., on the alternate chromosome), or from the second κ locus to the λ gene-bearing chromosomes (see

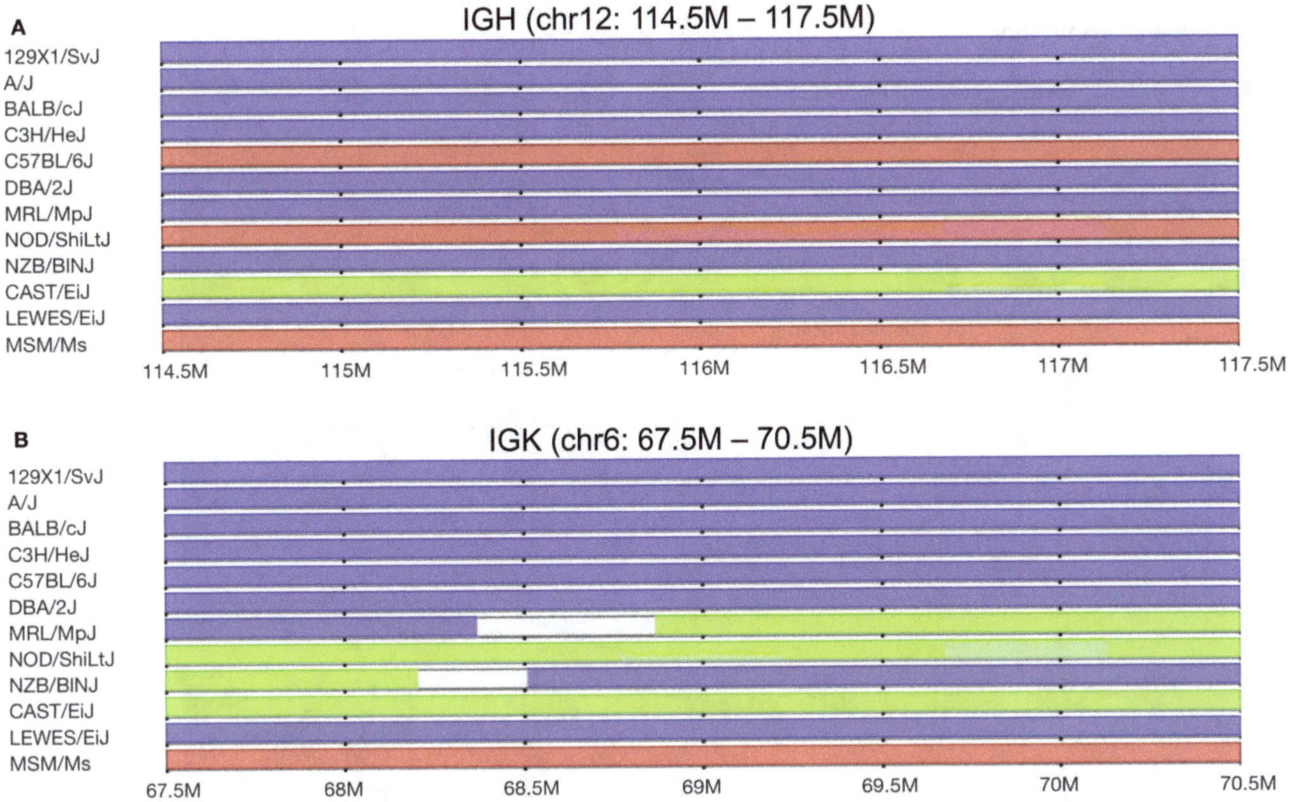


**FIGURE 1** | Predicted sub-specific origins of germline haplotypes found in the **(A)** immunoglobulin IGHV and **(B)** immunoglobulin IGKV loci among selected classical inbred and wild-derived mouse strains. The MRL/MpJ strain is the parental strain of the MRL/lpr strain, and although MRL/MpJ mice carry a normal Fas gene, they are also prone to autoimmunity. The lowest three strains shown are wild-derived, with genomes that are representative of the three major subspecies. *M. m. domesticus*-derived sequences are shown in blue, *M. m. musculus*-derived sequences are shown in red, and *M. m. castaneus*-derived sequences are shown in green. Data from Yang et al. (30). Graphics by Mouse Phylogeny Viewer (33).

**Figures 2, 3**). It is likely that despite the conservation of this element within the κ locus, the strength of action of the elements varies between species. The preponderance of κ chains in the expressed antibody repertoire of the mouse, for example, suggests that the mouse RS usually fails to drive rearrangement to the λ locus. Instead, each murine κ locus will likely be rearranged to exhaustion, and this will prevent the overexpression of the handful of λ genes that remain in the mouse genome. The activities of RS in different sub-species of the house mouse have not been explored.

## Gene Rearrangement of the Light Chain Loci

The light chain repertoire is shaped by the order of gene rearrangement, and early studies in the mouse and human showed that rearrangement begins with the κ locus (34, 50). This may not be true for all species. It has recently been shown that the λ locus rearranges first in the fetal and neonatal pig (51, 52). Timing therefore requires further investigation, particularly in species with repertoires that are dominated by the λ light chain, for regulation of the expressed repertoire could be more difficult if the minor locus was to rearrange first. If a species had just a handful of functional κ genes, and abundant functional λ genes, initial rearrangements of the κ locus would risk over-expression of the few available IGKV genes.

In the mouse and human, if an initial κ rearrangement is unproductive or self-reactive, additional rounds of secondary rearrangement can proceed, in a process known as receptor editing (53–55). Receptor editing is usually discussed as a pathway to resolution of auto-reactivity, either in developing B cells in which self-reactivity is generated by primary rearrangements (56), or in mature antigen-selected B cells where self-reactivity may result from somatic point mutations (57). Less attention has been paid to the more general role that receptor editing plays in shaping the formation of the repertoire.

The organization of genes within the light chain loci facilitates receptor editing, and this increases the likelihood that each B cell will form an in-frame light chain rearrangement (58). As long as unrearranged V genes remain 5′ of a VJ rearrangement, and unrearranged J genes remain 3′ of the rearrangement, receptor editing can continue (see **Figure 2**). In the mouse, the potential of κ chain receptor editing is maximized by a bias toward rearrangement of the 5′ IGKJ1 gene (59), and this targeting

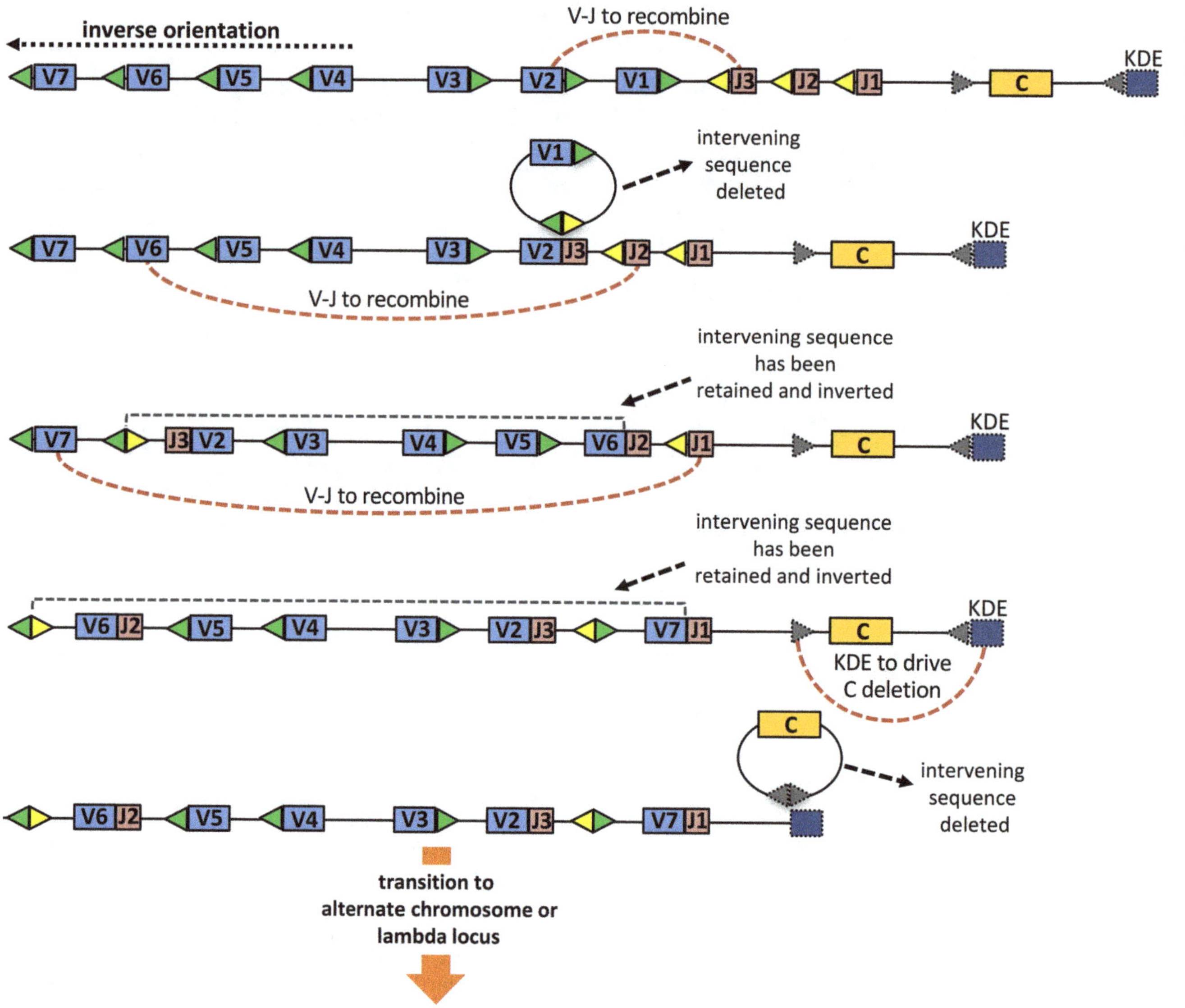


**FIGURE 2 |** Three rounds of VJ rearrangement of the κ locus, that might result from non-productive rearrangements or rearrangements resulting in self-reactive BCR. The initial configuration of genes **(top)** shows four IGKV genes in the reverse orientation to the IGKJ and IGKC genes, and 3 IGKV genes in the orientation shared with those genes. Gene loss, as well as the changing order and orientation of genes is highlighted through successive rounds of rearrangement. Expression of the final configuration (shown in row 4), which threatens allelic inclusion and possible continuing auto-reactivity, is terminated through the action of the Kappa Deleting Element **(bottom)**.

results from the action of the proximal IGKJ germline transcript promoter (60).

A process of serial rearrangement of the κ chain locus may continue on one chromosome until all possibilities of recombination have been exhausted. Recombination will then proceed on the second κ chromosome (**Figure 3**). A failure to produce a productive, self-tolerant rearrangement on the second chromosome, after multiple rounds of rearrangement, will be followed by rearrangement of the λ loci.

The human λ locus also seems permissive of receptor editing (61), and the absence of deletional elements in the λ locus should maximize the potential of serial λ recombination in the human. This should ensure that relatively few human B cells fail to make a suitable productive light chain rearrangement that is self-tolerant when expressed in association with the cell's heavy chain rearrangement. The possibility of repeated rounds of λ rearrangement could be particularly important for the avoidance of self-reactivity, for it has been suggested that λ - bearing human B cells are less prone to self-reactivity than κ-bearing B cells (61). The λ chains of these cells may also provide stability during an ongoing immune response, for it has been shown that the codon usage of λ genes reduces the likelihood of structural changes arising from accumulating somatic point mutations (62).

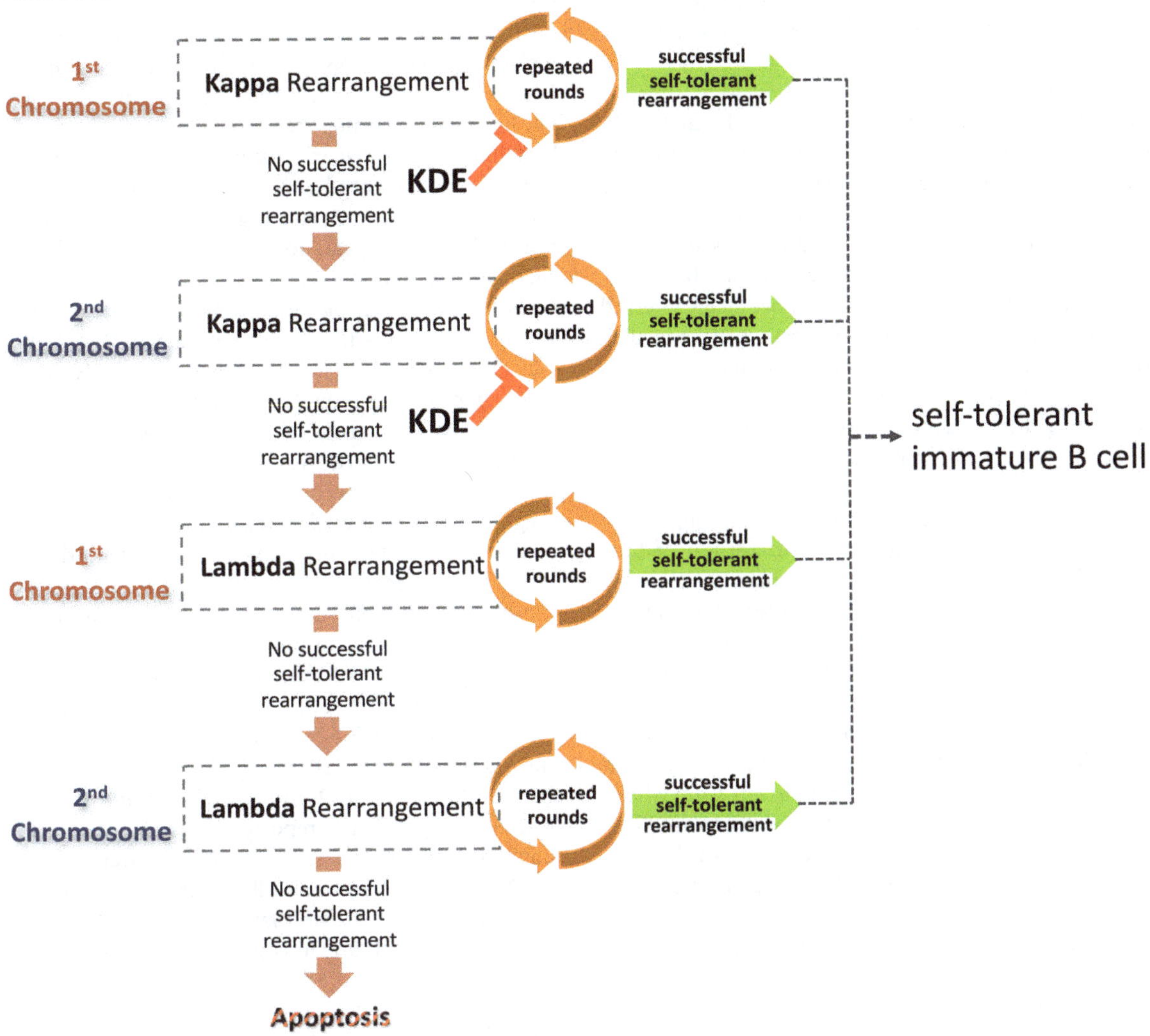


**FIGURE 3 |** Light chain rearrangements provide multiple pathways to the production of self-tolerant B cells. Alternative pathways are a consequence of rearrangements of the light chain loci that result in non-productive or auto-reactive BCR. Beginning with rearrangements of the κ locus on the first selected chromosome, a succession of light chains can be paired with an existing heavy chain that is already expressed on the surface of the pre-B cell. Each resulting BCR is assessed for affinity to self-antigen. Cells expressing autoreactive antibodies can be rescued via further rounds of receptor editing. If repeated rounds of rearrangements of a locus fail to generate a functional, self-tolerant antibody, and the possibilities of rearrangement are exhausted, the process may continue on other chromosomes. Rounds of κ rearrangement may be prematurely curtailed by the action of the kappa deleting element. B cells unable to generate self-tolerant antibodies despite multiple rounds of receptor editing will ultimately be deleted or rendered anergic. In contrast, B cells that generate successful light chain rearrangements that result in self-tolerant antibodies will go on to develop further into immature B cells.

## Population Variation in the κ and λ Gene Loci

Combinatorial diversity is expanded by heterozygous gene loci, and such diversity appears to be of functional significance (63). It is therefore important that repertoire studies include a focus on alleles and gene heterozygosity. Although a few new allelic variants of human IGKV genes have recently been reported (19), the reported IGKV germline gene repertoire appears to be relatively complete (64). According to the IMGT reference directory, 26 IGKV genes have no known allelic variants, while 15 IGKV genes have only one reported variant and five have two known variants. The extent of allelic variation within the κ light chain locus could be even less than is indicated in the IMGT reference directory, for some of the reported variants are likely to be artifacts arising from sequencing errors. This is certainly the case for many reported IGHV alleles that were identified in early sequencing studies (65).

The reported human IGLV germline gene repertoire may also be relatively complete, for only five new alleles have been reported since 1997. These sequences are more varied than genes and allelic variants of the IGH and κ loci (66), but like the IGKV repertoire, there appears to be relatively little allelic variation amongst the IGLV genes. Functional and ORF allelic variants have been reported for 24 IGLV genes, but not for 15 other

IGLV genes. No more than four alleles are identified in the IMGT reference directory for any IGLV gene (http://www.imgt.org/vquest/refseqh.html).

In contrast to the genes of the κ and λ loci, there is just a single functional IGHV gene (IGHV3-NL1) that lacks reported allelic variants in the IMGT reference directory or in the IgPdb database (https://cgi.cse.unsw.edu.au/~ihmmune/IgPdb/). So many common variants are known for some genes that heterozygosity in any individual is almost assured. For example there are 16 *IGHV1-69* gene sequences in the IMGT reference directory, and a further 13 alleles have been inferred from analysis of high throughput genomic and AIRR-seq data (67, 68). Although the larger number of IGHV allelic variants could reflect the greater attention that has been given to defining this set of germline genes, there is additional evidence that points to a lack of diversity in the light chain gene repertoire.

A lack of allelic variation in the human κ locus is supported by AIRR-seq studies of κ rearrangements. In a study of four individuals, involving the dominant three human IGKV gene families (IGKV1, IGKV2 and IGKV3), VJ rearrangements were seen involving between 20 and 25 genes (69). One individual was homozygous at all gene loci. In the three other individuals, heterozygosity was only seen at 1 or 2 of the IGKV loci (69). The contrast with the heavy chain locus is striking. A recent AIRR-seq study of 95 individuals explored heterozygosity at 50 heavy chain IGHV gene loci (70). Other than in three individuals from whom relatively few sequences were generated, study participants were shown to be heterozygous at between 20% and 40% of the loci. Six gene loci were heterozygous in over 50% of study participants. Only six genes that were relatively abundantly present in the datasets showed homozygosity in all individuals (70). Similar patterns of heterozygosity within IGHV coding segments have also been noted from targeted genomic sequencing data (67).

In addition to allelic variation, gene copy number variation is also enriched in the IGHV locus, relative to IGLV and IGKV. Greater than half of the known human functional/ORF IGHV genes have evidence of copy number variation (45, 67, 70–75), compared to only one and three IGLV and IGKV genes, respectively (76–78).

Additional albeit indirect evidence for an evolutionary drive to conserve rather than diversify the human κ locus comes from the similarity of the genes in the proximal and distal IGKV clusters. The large segmental duplication that gave rise to the human κ locus appears to have occurred since the divergence of the human lineage from the most recent shared ancestor with other great apes (11). There are 23 functional IGKV genes and ORFs in the proximal cluster, and 22 in the distal cluster. Eighteen paired sequences are found in both clusters, and no coding changes have evolved at eight of these paired gene loci. In addition, one sequence in each of two other sequence pairs are now non-expressible pseudogenes. Expressed variation is therefore concentrated in just 8 of the 18 sequences. Furthermore, comparisons of nucleotide variation across the entirety of the sequence comprising the large proximal and distal gene clusters reveal strong similarity. Diversity within the large segmental duplications harboring these gene clusters appears to be much lower on average (>6 fold less) than that observed within segmental duplications found in the IGHV locus (19). We have speculated that this lack of diversity in IGKV may be the result of homogenizing effects of gene conversion events between the proximal and distal regions, as such events have been explicitly documented (19). We also reported that locus-wide IGHV diversity is ~3-fold higher than IGLV diversity; in fact, IGHV diversity appears to be generally higher than the genome average (19). Earlier analyses based on limited datasets have suggested that nucleotide and amino acid substitution patterns within V segments may differ between IGHV, IGKV, and IGLV loci (79); specifically, and consistent with decreased genomic diversity in κ locus haplotypes, Schwartz and Hershberg showed that, relative to κ chain V segments, heavy and λ chain genes exhibit greater amino acid diversity in both framework and complementarity determining regions (66). Together, these data suggest contrasting evolutionary histories that have resulted in different genetic features being associated with the human heavy and light chain loci.

The κ locus of the mouse seems to display the same lack of variation that is seen in the human locus. The IGKV locus was first mapped using YACs and BACs derived largely from C57BL/6 and C3H mice (12, 80, 81), and these sequences dominate the IMGT mouse IGKV database. An alternative assembly of the mouse κ locus was later produced based upon data from the C57BL/6, A/J, 129 and DBA/2 strains (82). Each of the IGKV genes previously reported by Zachau and colleagues were mapped to this new assembly, and they were all found to have >99% identity. Not a single allelic variant was reported from this study, although it is true that their approach means that some highly similar but previously unreported polymorphisms may have been overlooked (82).

Evidence of a lack of allelic variation amongst germline genes within mouse strains also comes from analysis of the IMGT database. Studies of light chain germline genes have included a sampling of a wide variety of inbred strains, and from wild-derived *M. m. musculus* and *M. m. castaneus* mice (83–85). Yet the IMGT database includes allelic variants for just 11 functional IGKV genes, and when analysis is confined to reports from studies of strains appearing to carry *M. m. domesticus*-derived genes, variants have only been seen for 6 IGKV genes. Confirmation that the apparent lack of variation is genuine, rather than reflecting insufficient investigation of mouse light chain genes, needs to be pursued through more comprehensive surveys of variation across wild mice from each of the sub-species.

## The Diversity of the Expressed Light Chain Repertoire

It is generally held that a stupendous diversity is the defining characteristic of the antibody repertories of all species. This was famously expressed by Peter Medawar as the miracle of immunology: "that a rabbit yet unborn will be able to make antibodies to an antigen not yet synthesized" (86). We have recently argued that the production of antibodies that target molecules never before seen, and unlikely to be seen, could be a costly investment for many species (17). The immune repertoires of different species may have developed varying levels of diversity in response to the quite differing evolutionary pressures faced by each species. Some of the most significant pressures may result from basic aspects of the biology of species, including their differing reproductive strategies and longevity, and especially from their varying sizes. The antibody repertoires of small species are necessarily small, and there is therefore a greater need for regulatory processes to steer the development of their repertoires toward specificities that target key pathogens (17). This may explain why in comparison to the human antibody repertoire, the murine repertoire includes more heavy chain clonotypes that are shared by many individuals of the species (6, 17, 87).

Public clonotypes may be rare in the human heavy chain repertoire, but there is a surprising lack of diversity in the human light chain repertoire, and public clonotypes account for about 60% of the human κ (69) and λ (88) light chain repertoires. This is in part a consequence of very strong biases in light chain gene usage. Six IGKV sequences dominate reported human IGK rearrangements: IGKV3-20*01, IGKV3-15*01, IGKV3-11*01, IGKV1-5*01, IGKV2-30*01, and IGKV1-39*01/IGKV1D-39*01 (69). The IGKV3-20*01 gene alone is seen in over 30% of rearrangements in some individuals (69). On the other hand, some genes are utilized at very low frequencies. In fact, amongst 22,193 rearrangements analyzed from four individuals, we saw no sequences that utilized eight reportedly functional IGKV genes (69).

Similarly, while the mouse may have over 100 available IGKV genes, just seven genes are responsible for over 40% of rearrangements, and the utilization frequencies of some IGKV genes are as low as 0.001% (28).

Biased usage of λ IGLV genes is also seen. Three IGLV genes account for more than 50% of human rearrangements, and individual IGLV genes are used at frequencies that range from 0.02 to 27% (89). In the neonatal pig, biases are even more extreme, with three IGLV genes accounting for 70% of rearrangements (51). The utilization of the four functional human IGLJ genes are also affected by biases, with frequencies varying from just 5% for IGLJ1 to almost 55% for IGLJ7 (90, 91).

The lack of D genes in light chain rearrangements limits their diversity. Diversity is further limited by the fact that relatively few nucleotides are lost from κ and λ V and J gene ends by exonuclease removals and few N nucleotides are added to the junction of the joining genes. Public human κ clonotypes have on average just 0.4 added N nucleotides, while even private clonotypes have an average of only 2.5 N additions (69). Similarly, on average, public λ VJ junctions include a single N addition, and private junctions average around two additions (88). There is even less N addition in the mouse (92), and interestingly, this is also true in the humanized mouse (88). This severely limits junctional diversity of the complementarity determining region 3 (CDR3) of light chains in the mouse. Together with the lack of combinatorial diversity, this ensures that the light chain repertoire of the mouse and human are highly constrained. In an analysis of over 250,000 mouse κ chain VJ rearrangements from 59 mice, over 90% of the sequences encoded just 1000 amino acid sequences (28). A similar number of amino acid sequences dominate the human κ chain repertoire (69).

## LIGHT CHAINS AND THE CONTROL OF SELF-REACTIVITY

The light chain repertoire is constrained, and there is an extensive body of research that suggests that an important factor that constrains the repertoire is the need for light chain rearrangements to minimize BCR self-reactivity. Human antibodies formed with κ chains may have a greater tendency toward self-reactivity (61), but through repeated rounds of κ rearrangement, and through similar rounds of λ rearrangement, much self-reactivity seems to be avoided. This may explain the recent observations that reduced light chain editing is associated with several autoimmune conditions in the human, including Systemic Lupus Erythematosis (SLE), type 1 diabetes (T1D), and myasthenia gravis (47, 93). This has also been observed in several mouse models of autoimmunity (47). It has also been shown that reduced KDE rearrangements can lead to dual κ and λ chain expression, through a failure to delete κ rearrangements in λ-switched cells, and this disturbance of light chain editing is associated with SLE (94).

The study of cells in which both κ and λ rearrangements are present has highlighted the fact that certain IGKV genes may be prone to self-reactivity. Biases in IGKV gene expression are seen when productive κ rearrangements are studied in λ-bearing B cells, and compared with κ rearrangements from κ-bearing cells (95). This comparison is possible because of the persistence of κ VJ rearrangements in cells that have switched to a λ light chain rearrangement as a consequence of the earlier generation of a self-reactive κ positive BCR. The biased gene expression therefore points to a tendency of some genes to mediate self-reactivity.

Some heavy chain IGHV genes are also associated with autoreactivity, and human *IGHV4-34* in particular has been implicated in anti-red blood cell autoimmune responses (96). It may be, however, that this association should be seen as resulting from a difficulty in finding a suitable light chain partner for *IGHV4-34*. The persistence of *IGHV4-34* in the human population, and its expression at relatively high frequency within the antibody repertoire, points to the value of *IGHV4-34* heavy chains when a self-tolerant light chain partner is found.

Evidence in support of a special role for light chains in the etiology of autoimmune diseases also comes from a consideration of mouse disease models. There are several types of mouse model of autoimmune disease (97). Autoimmunity can be induced by challenging animals with self-antigen in the presence of powerful adjuvants. An example is the Experimental Allergic Encephalitis (EAE) model that involves the challenge of SJL mice with spinal cord homogenate (97). Other models of autoimmune disease involve the spontaneous development of disease. This is the case with the NOD Type 1 Diabetes model and models of SLE using MRL/lpr mice and (NZB × NZM)F1 mice (97). These spontaneous models may more closely approximate human disease than the antigen challenge models.

A third kind of model relies upon genetic manipulation of animals using gene knockout and transgenic techniques. These models have been particularly important for the study of self-reactive B and T cells, and how they are deleted or otherwise controlled. Some of these models involve the use of transgenic antigen and antibody pairs (eg HEL/anti-HEL) (98). Other models use transgenic immunoglobulin chains derived from autoreactive B cells arising in autoimmune-prone mice. For example, Andrews and colleagues recently published a study exploring receptor editing in mice that carry an IGKV4-IGKJ4 anti-DNA transgene (99). Although more self-reactive cells were seen when the transgene was expressed in autoimmune-prone MRL/lpr mice, self-reactive B cells were also generated when the transgene was expressed in C57BL/6 mice (99).

This IGKV4-IGKJ4 anti-DNA transgene sequence is derived from a monoclonal antibody that was first isolated from an MRL/lpr mouse in 1987 (100, 101). In describing this and other anti-DNA antibodies, the authors acknowledged their lack of knowledge of the germline genes in MRL/lpr mice, but concluded that the mAb antibody gene sequences were relatively unmutated, based upon a consensus sequence created from both the anti-DNA and other non-DNA-specific antibodies. The apparent presence of some somatic point mutations was, however, deemed to be highly significant. In fact studies describing these antibodies stand as the first evidence for the possibility that self-reactive B cells can arise from self-tolerant B cells by the accumulation of somatic point mutations within the germinal center reaction (100, 101).

Thirty years later, our understanding of MRL/lpr germline genes is still far from complete, but comparisons can now be made between the anti-DNA antibodies and the complete repertoire of C57BL/6 IGKV genes and other murine IGKV genes. This includes sequences that are likely to be NOD IGKV germline genes, many of which are identical to MPL-derived IGKV sequences in GenBank (31). The IGKV sequence in the transgene includes 18 nucleotide differences with respect to the nearest reported IGKV gene (*IGKV4-81*) in the IMGT reference directory. The sequence is, however, much more similar to a NOD sequence reported by Henry and colleagues, differing only within the CDR3 region of the sequence (31). We believe that the many differences with respect to C57BL/6 IGKV genes are a consequence of the separate evolutionary origins of the IGKV loci of the C57BL/6 and MRL/lpr mouse strains. Based upon the haplotype analysis depicted in **Figure 1**, the MRL/MpJ-derived transgene appears to be of *M. m. castaneus* origin. In the absence of further information about the MRL/lpr IGK locus, there can now be no certainty regarding the presence or absence of somatic point mutations in the anti-DNA sequences reported in 1987. Only when the germline IGKV genes of MRL mice have been properly documented will it be possible to say whether or not these anti-DNA antibodies arose through an accumulation of point mutations in previously self-tolerant cells.

We believe that the autoreactivity of the light chain product of the IGKV4-IGKJ4 transgene may be the result of its *M. m. castaneus* origin, and of its association with *M. m. domesticus* and *M. m. musculus*-derived heavy chains. We also believe that *M. m. castaneus* genes may also explain the spontaneous autoreactivity that is seen in NOD and other inbred mice. The complete κ light chain locus of the NOD strain, and portions of the loci of the MRL/lpr and NZB strains, are derived from the *M. m. castaneus* sub-species of the house mouse (**Figure 1**). The heavy chain locus of the NOD mouse, on the other hand, comes from the *M. m. musculus* sub-species, while the MRL/lpr and NZB strains appear to carry IGH loci that are *M. m. domesticus*-derived.

The three major sub-species of the house mouse emerged from a common ancestor about 350,000 years ago (102), and it is reasonable to assume that their heavy and light chain genes co-evolved as the sub-species diverged. This co-evolution would be required to minimize self-reactivity, and to ensure that each heavy chain could successfully partner with light chains encoded by at least a subset of the IGKV genes. It appears, however, that the breeding histories of many laboratory mice have resulted in heavy and light chain gene sets that did not evolve together being found in their genomes. A few common laboratory strains, including BALB/c and 129 mice, carry matching *M. m. domesticus*-derived IGH and IGK loci, whereas others like the AEJ, C57BL/6, C57BL/10, and SJL strains carry a *M. m. domesticus*-derived IGH locus but a *M. m. musculus*-derived κ locus (**Figure 1**).

Not all inbred mice that have been reported to be prone to autoimmunity harbor obviously mismatched loci. For example, C57BLKS/J mice are diabetes-prone, but have heavy and light chain loci that appear to be derived from *M. m. domesticus* (103). DBA mice are used in a collagen-induced arthritis model of rheumatoid arthritis (104), and both their heavy and light chain loci also appear to be *M. m. domesticus*-derived. It is also true that not all strains that carry mismatched loci have been reported to be susceptible to autoimmunity. An example is the RF/J strain, which appears to have a *M. m. domesticus* IGH locus and a *M. m. castaneus* IGK locus. However, it is striking how many models of autoimmunity involve mismatched heavy and light chain gene loci. In addition to the NOD, MRL/lpr, and NZB models, SJL mice that are used in the EAE model of multiple sclerosis (97) appear to have a *M. m. musculus* IGH locus and a *M. m. domesticus* IGK locus. A model of autoreactivity to matrix collagen uses a C57BL/6-derived IGKV3 transgene in C57BL/6 hosts (105). In this strain, the IGH locus seems to be *M. m. musculus*-derived, while the IGK locus is *M. m. domesticus*-derived. Hybrid (129 × C57BL/6) mice spontaneously develop an SLE-like condition (106), and these mice express *M. m. domesticus* heavy chains in association with both *M. m. domesticus* and *M. m. musculus*-derived κ chains. Finally, the BXSB mouse spontaneously develops lupus-like pathology (107). SNP analysis suggests that it has a *M. m. domesticus* IGH locus and a *M. m. musculus* κ locus (**Figure 1**).

For over 30 years, mouse models have provided profound insights into the nature of autoreactivity and self-tolerance. It may be though that an ignorance of the makeup of the immunoglobulin gene loci has kept hidden a key genetic contributor to autoimmunity. To determine if this may be the case, the repertoires of laboratory mice will need to be compared to repertoires generated in animals in which the heavy and light chain loci and all critical regulatory elements, as well as self-antigens, are all derived from the same sub-species of the house mouse. The immunoglobulin genes of the different strains will also need to be properly characterized. It is possible that this may reveal that the apparently matched loci of some autoimmune-prone strains are derived from disparate sources. SNP analysis at present characterizes mouse strains with respect to the three major sub-species of the house mouse, but other minor sub-species may also have contributed genes to the laboratory mouse. We believe that such a focus on heavy and light chain pairings, in mouse models and in human studies, may help explain some of the mysteries that still surround autoimmune diseases.

## AUTHOR CONTRIBUTIONS

All authors listed have made a substantial, direct and intellectual contribution to the work, and approved it for publication.

## REFERENCES


1. Schatz DG. V(D)J recombination. *Immunol Rev.* (2004) 200:5–11. doi: 10.1111/j.0105-2896.2004.00173.x
2. Schatz DG, Swanson PC. V(D)J recombination: mechanisms of initiation. *Annu Rev Genet.* (2011) 45:167–202. doi: 10.1146/annurev-genet-110410-132552
3. Ellebedy AH, Jackson KJ, Kissick HT, Nakaya HI, Davis CW, Roskin KM, et al. Defining antigen-specific plasmablast and memory B cell subsets in human blood after viral infection or vaccination. *Nat Immunol.* (2016) 17:1226–34. doi: 10.1038/ni.3533
4. Jackson KJ, Kidd MJ, Wang Y, Collins AM. The shape of the Lymphocyte receptor repertoire: lessons from the B cell receptor. *Front Immunol* .(2013) 4:263. doi: 10.3389/fimmu.2013.00263
5. Georgiou G, Ippolito GC, Beausang J, Busse CE, Wardemann H, Quake SR. The promise and challenge of high-throughput sequencing of the antibody repertoire. *Nat Biotechnol.* (2014) 32:158–68. doi: 10.1038/nbt.2782
6. Greiff V, Menzel U, Miho E, Weber C, Riedel R, Cook S, et al. Systems Analysis reveals high genetic and antigen-driven predetermination of antibody repertoires throughout b cell development. *Cell Rep.* (2017) 19:1467–78. doi: 10.1016/j.celrep.2017.04.054
7. Kirik U, Persson H, Levander F, Greiff L, Ohlin M. Antibody heavy chain variable domains of different germline gene origins diversify through different paths. *Front Immunol.* (2017) 8:1433. doi: 10.3389/fimmu.2017.01433
8. Rettig TA, Ward C, Bye BA, Pecaut MJ, Chapes SK. Characterization of the naive murine antibody repertoire using unamplified high-throughput sequencing. *PloS ONE* (2018) 13:e0190982. doi: 10.1371/journal.pone.0190982
9. Sun Y, Wei Z, Li N, Zhao Y. A comparative overview of immunoglobulin genes and the generation of their diversity in tetrapods. *Dev Comp Immunol.* (2013) 39:103–9. doi: 10.1016/j.dci.2012.02.008
10. Mashoof S, Criscitiello MF. Fish immunoglobulins. *Biology* (2016) 5:E45. doe: 10.3390/biology5040045
11. Ermert K, Mitlohner H, Schempp W, Zachau HG. The immunoglobulin kappa locus of primates. *Genomics* (1995) 25:623–9. doi: 10.1016/0888-7543(95)80003-5
12. Kirschbaum T, Pourrajabi S, Zocher I, Schwendinger J, Heim V, Roschenthaler F, et al. The 3' part of the immunoglobulin kappa locus of the mouse. *Eur J Immunol.* (1998) 28:1458–66. doi: 10.1002/(SICI)1521-4141(199805)28:05<1458::AID-IMMU1458>3.0.CO;2-5
13. Martinez-Jean C, Folch G, Lefranc MP. Nomenclature and overview of the mouse (*Mus musculus* and Mus sp.) immunoglobulin kappa (IGK) genes. *Exp Clin Immunogenet.* (2001) 18:255–79. doi: 10.1159/000049204
14. Schwartz JC, Lefranc MP, Murtaugh MP. Evolution of the porcine (Sus scrofa domestica) immunoglobulin kappa locus through germline gene conversion. *Immunogenetics* (2012) 64:303–11. doi: 10.1007/s00251-011-0589-6
15. Schwartz JC, Philp RL, Bickhart DM, Smith TPL, Hammond JA. The antibody loci of the domestic goat (*Capra hircus*). *Immunogenetics* (2018) 70:317–26. doi: 10.1007/s00251-017-1033-3
16. Martin J, Ponstingl H, Lefranc MP, Archer J, Sargan D, Bradley A. Comprehensive annotation and evolutionary insights into the canine (*Canis lupus familiaris*) antigen receptor loci. *Immunogenetics* (2018) 70:223–36. doi: 10.1007/s00251-017-1028-0
17. Collins AM, Jackson KJL. On being the right size: antibody repertoire formation in the mouse and human. *Immunogenetics* (2018) 70:143–58. doi: 10.1007/s00251-017-1049-8
18. Kawasaki K, Minoshima S, Nakato E, Shibuya K, Shintani A, Schmeits JL, et al. One-megabase sequence analysis of the human immunoglobulin lambda gene locus. *Genome Res.* (1997) 7:250–61. doi: 10.1101/gr.7.3.250
19. Watson CT, Steinberg KM, Graves TA, Warren RL, Malig M, Schein J, et al. Sequencing of the human IG light chain loci from a hydatidiform mole BAC library reveals locus-specific signatures of genetic diversity. *Genes Immun.* (2015) 16:24–34. doi: 10.1038/gene.2014.56
20. Lefranc MP. Nomenclature of the human immunoglobulin kappa (IGK) genes. *Exp Clin Immunogenet.* (2001) 18:161–74. doi: 10.1159/000049195
21. Ramesh A, Darko S, Hua A, Overman G, Ransier A, Francica JR, et al. Structure and diversity of the *Rhesus macaque* immunoglobulin loci through multiple *de novo* genome assemblies. *Front Immunol.* (2017) 8:1407. doi: 10.3389/fimmu.2017.01407
22. Sun Y, Wang C, Wang Y, Zhang T, Ren L, Hu X, et al. A comprehensive analysis of germline and expressed immunoglobulin repertoire in the horse. *Dev Comp Immunol* .(2010) 34:1009–20. doi: 10.1016/j.dci.2010.05.003
23. Guo Y, Bao Y, Meng Q, Hu X, Meng Q, Ren L, et al. Immunoglobulin genomics in the guinea pig (*Cavia porcellus*). *PLoS ONE* (2012) 7:e39298. doi: 10.1371/journal.pone.0039298
24. Dammers PM, Hendricks J, Terpstra P, Bos NA, Kroese FG. The organization of the immunoglobulin heavy- and light-chain loci in the rat. In: Kaushik AKaP, Y, editor. *Comparative Immunoglobulin Genetics.* Boca Raton, FL: CRC Press (2014). 107–30.
25. Das S, Nikolaidis N, Klein J, Nei M. Evolutionary redefinition of immunoglobulin light chain isotypes in tetrapods using molecular markers. *Proc Natl Acad Sci USA.* (2008) 105:16647–52. doi: 10.1073/pnas.0808800105
26. Butler JE, Wertz N, Baker ML. The immunoglobulin genes of bats. In: Kaushil AK, Pasman Y, editors. *Comparative Immunoglobulin Genetics.* Toronto, ON: Apple Academic Press (2014). 53–84.
27. Das S, Mohamedy U, Hirano M, Nei M, Nikolaidis N. Analysis of the immunoglobulin light chain genes in zebra finch: evolutionary implications. *Mol Biol Evol.* (2010) 27:113–20. doi: 10.1093/molbev/msp212
28. Aoki-Ota M, Torkamani A, Ota T, Schork N, Nemazee D. Skewed primary Igkappa repertoire and V-J joining in C57BL/6 mice: implications for recombination accessibility and receptor editing. *J Immunol.* (2012) 188:2305–15. doi: 10.4049/jimmunol.1103484
29. Collins AM, Wang Y, Roskin KM, Marquis CP, Jackson KJ. The mouse antibody heavy chain repertoire is germline-focused and highly variable between inbred strains. *Philos Trans R Soc Lond B Biol Sci.* (2015) 370:20140236. doi: 10.1098/rstb.2014.0236
30. Yang H, Wang JR, Didion JP, Buus RJ, Bell TA, Welsh CE, et al. Subspecific origin and haplotype diversity in the laboratory mouse. *Nat Genet.* (2011) 43:648–55. doi: 10.1038/ng.847
31. Henry RA, Kendall PL, Woodward EJ, Hulbert C, Thomas JW. Vkappa polymorphisms in NOD mice are spread throughout the entire immunoglobulin kappa locus and are shared by other autoimmune strains. *Immunogenetics* (2010) 62:507–20. doi: 10.1007/s00251-010-0457-9
32. Loh E, Black B, Riblet R, Weigert M, Hood JM, Hood L. Myeloma proteins from NZB and BALB/c mice: structural and functional differences. *Proc Natl Acad Sci USA.* (1979) 76:1395–9. doi: 10.1073/pnas.76.3.1395

33. Wang JR, de Villena FP, McMillan L. Comparative analysis and visualization of multiple collinear genomes. *BMC Bioinf.* (2012) 13(Suppl. 3):S13. doi: 10.1186/1471-2105-13-S3-S13
34. Hieter PA, Korsmeyer SJ, Waldmann TA, Leder P. Human immunoglobulin kappa light-chain genes are deleted or rearranged in lambda-producing B cells. *Nature* (1981) 290:368–72. doi: 10.1038/290368a0
35. Schwartz JC, Lefranc MP, Murtaugh MP. Organization, complexity and allelic diversity of the porcine (*Sus scrofa domestica*) immunoglobulin lambda locus. *Immunogenetics* (2012) 64:399–407. doi: 10.1007/s00251-011-0594-9
36. Walther S, Rusitzka TV, Diesterbeck US, Czerny CP. Equine immunoglobulins and organization of immunoglobulin genes. *Dev Comp Immunol.* (2015) 53:303–19. doi: 10.1016/j.dci.2015.07.017
37. Scott CL, Potter M. Variation in V lambda genes in the genus Mus. *J Immunol.* (1984) 132:2638–43.
38. Sanchez P, Nadel B, Cazenave PA. V lambda-J lambda rearrangements are restricted within a V-J-C recombination unit in the mouse. *Eur J Immunol.* (1991) 21: 907–11. doi: 10.1002/eji.1830210408
39. Lefranc MP, LeFranc G. Immunoglobulin lambda (IGL) genes of human and mouse. In: Honjo T, Alt FW, Neuberger MS, editors. *Molecular Biology of B cells.* London: Elsevier Academic Press (2004). 37–59.
40. Matsuda F, Ishii K, Bourvagnet P, Kuma K, Hayashida H, Miyata T, et al. The complete nucleotide sequence of the human immunoglobulin heavy chain variable region locus. *J Exp Med.* (1998) 188:2151–62. doi: 10.1084/jem.188.11.2151
41. Riblet R. Immunoglobulin heavy chain genes in the mouse. In: Honjo T, Alt FW, Neuberger M, editors. *Molecular Biology of B cells.* London: Elsevier Academic Press (2004). p 19–26. doi: 10.1016/B978-012053641-2/50003-4
42. Ma L, Qin T, Chu D, Cheng X, Wang J, Wang X, et al. Internal duplications of DH, JH, and C region genes create an unusual IgH gene Locus in cattle. *J Immunol.* (2016) 196:4358–66. doi: 10.4049/jimmunol.1600158
43. Guo Y, Bao Y, Wang H, Hu X, Zhao Z, Li N, et al. A preliminary analysis of the immunoglobulin genes in the African elephant (*Loxodonta africana*). *PLoS ONE* (2011) 6:e16889. doi: 10.1371/journal.pone.0016889
44. Guo C, Gerasimova T, Hao H, Ivanova I, Chakraborty T, Selimyan R, et al. Two forms of loops generate the chromatin conformation of the immunoglobulin heavy-chain gene locus. *Cell* (2011) 147:332–43. doi: 10.1016/j.cell.2011.08.049
45. Kidd MJ, Jackson KJ, Boyd SD, Collins AM. DJ Pairing during VDJ recombination shows positional biases that vary among individuals with differing IGHD Locus immunogenotypes. *J Immunol.* (2016) 196:1158–64. doi: 10.4049/jimmunol.1501401
46. Langerak AW, Nadel B, De Torbal A, Wolvers-Tettero IL, van Gastel-Mol EJ, Verhaaf B, et al. Unraveling the consecutive recombination events in the human IGK locus. *J Immunol.* (2004) 173:3878–88. doi: 10.4049/jimmunol.173.6.3878
47. Panigrahi AK, Goodman NG, Eisenberg RA, Rickels MR, Naji A, Luning Prak ET. RS rearrangement frequency as a marker of receptor editing in lupus and type 1 diabetes. *J Exp Med.* (2008) 205:2985–94. doi: 10.1084/jem.20082053
48. Das S, Nikolaidis N, Nei M. Genomic organization and evolution of immunoglobulin kappa gene enhancers and kappa deleting element in mammals. *Mol Immunol.* (2009) 46:3171–7. doi: 10.1016/j.molimm.2009.05.180
49. Siminovitch KA, Moore MW, Durdik J, Selsing E. The human kappa deleting element and the mouse recombining segment share DNA sequence homology. *Nucleic Acids Res.* (1987) 15:2699–705. doi: 10.1093/nar/15.6.2699
50. Alt FW, Enea V, Bothwell AL, Baltimore D. Activity of multiple light chain genes in murine myeloma cells producing a single, functional light chain. *Cell* (1980) 21:1–12. doi: 10.1016/0092-8674(80)90109-9
51. Butler JE, Wertz N. The porcine antibody repertoire: variations on the textbook theme. *Front Immunol.* (2012) 3:153. doi: 10.3389/fimmu.2012.00153
52. Wertz N, Vazquez J, Wells K, Sun J, Butler JE. Antibody repertoire development in fetal and neonatal piglets. XII. Three IGLV genes comprise 70% of the pre-immune repertoire and there is little junctional diversity. *Mol Immunol.* (2013) 55:319–28. doi: 10.1016/j.molimm.2013.03.012
53. Prak EL, Weigert M. Light chain replacement: a new model for antibody gene rearrangement. *J Exp Med.* (1995) 182:541–8. doi: 10.1084/jem.182.2.541
54. Retter MW, Nemazee D. Receptor editing occurs frequently during normal B cell development. *J Exp Med.* (1998) 188:1231–8. doi: 10.1084/jem.188.7.1231
55. Halverson R, Torres RM, Pelanda R. Receptor editing is the main mechanism of B cell tolerance toward membrane antigens. *Nat Immunol.* (2004) 5:645–50. doi: 10.1038/ni1076
56. Lang J, Ota T, Kelly M, Strauch P, Freed BM, Torres RM, et al. Receptor editing and genetic variability in human autoreactive B cells. *J Exp Med.* (2016) 213:93–108. doi: 10.1084/jem.20151039
57. Detanico T, St Clair JB, Aviszus K, Kirchenbaum G, Guo W, Wysocki LJ. Somatic mutagenesis in autoimmunity. *Autoimmunity* (2013) 46:102–14. doi: 10.3109/08916934.2012.757597
58. Li S, Liu W, Li Y, Zhao S, Liu C, Hu M, et al. Contribution of secondary Igkappa rearrangement to primary immunoglobulin repertoire diversification. *Mol Immunol.* (2016) 78:193–206. doi: 10.1016/j.molimm.2016.09.006
59. Yamagami T, ten Boekel E, Andersson J, Rolink A, Melchers F. Frequencies of multiple IgL chain gene rearrangements in single normal or kappaL chain-deficient B lineage cells. *Immunity* (1999) 11:317–27. doi: 10.1016/S1074-7613(00)80107-7
60. Vettermann C, Timblin GA, Lim V, Lai EC, Schlissel MS. The proximal J kappa germline-transcript promoter facilitates receptor editing through control of ordered recombination. *PLoS ONE* (2015) 10:e0113824. doi: 10.1371/journal.pone.0113824
61. Wardemann H, Hammersen J, Nussenzweig MC. Human autoantibody silencing by immunoglobulin light chains. *J Exp Med.* (2004) 200:191–9. doi: 10.1084/jem.20040818
62. Hershberg U, Shlomchik MJ. Differences in potential for amino acid change after mutation reveals distinct strategies for kappa and lambda light-chain variation. *Proc Natl Acad Sci USA.* (2006) 103:15963–8. doi: 10.1073/pnas.0607581103
63. Avnir Y, Watson CT, Glanville J, Peterson EC, Tallarico AS, Bennett AS, et al. IGHV1-69 polymorphism modulates anti-influenza antibody repertoires, correlates with IGHV utilization shifts and varies by ethnicity. *Sci Rep.* (2016) 6:20842. doi: 10.1038/srep20842
64. Collins AM, Wang Y, Singh V, Yu P, Jackson KJ, Sewell WA. The reported germline repertoire of human immunoglobulin kappa chain genes is relatively complete and accurate. *Immunogenetics* (2008) 60:669–76. doi: 10.1007/s00251-008-0325-z
65. Wang Y, Jackson KJ, Sewell WA, Collins AM. Many human immunoglobulin heavy-chain IGHV gene polymorphisms have been reported in error. *Immunol Cell Biol.* (2008) 86:111–5. doi: 10.1038/sj.icb.7100144
66. Schwartz GW, Hershberg U. Conserved variation: identifying patterns of stability and variability in BCR and TCR V genes with different diversity and richness metrics. *Phys Biol.* (2013) 10:035005. doi: 10.1088/1478-3975/10/3/035005
67. Scheepers C, Shrestha RK, Lambson BE, Jackson KJ, Wright IA, Naicker D, et al. Ability to develop broadly neutralizing HIV-1 antibodies is not restricted by the germline Ig gene repertoire. *J Immunol.* (2015) 194:4371–8. doi: 10.4049/jimmunol.1500118
68. Sheng Z, Schramm CA, Kong R, Program NCS, Mullikin JC, Mascola JR, et al. Gene-specific substitution profiles describe the types and frequencies of amino acid changes during antibody somatic hypermutation. *Front Immunol.* (2017) 8:537. doi: 10.3389/fimmu.2017.00537
69. Jackson KJ, Wang Y, Gaeta BA, Pomat W, Siba P, Rimmer J, et al. Divergent human populations show extensive shared IGK rearrangements in peripheral blood B cells. *Immunogenetics* (2012) 64:3–14. doi: 10.1007/s00251-011-0559-z
70. Gidoni M, Snir O, Peres A, Polak P, Lindeman I, Clouser C, et al. Mosaic deletion patterns of the human antibody heavy chain gene locus. (2018) *BioRxiv. [Preprint].* doi: 10.1101/314476
71. Boyd SD, Gaeta BA, Jackson KJ, Fire AZ, Marshall EL, Merker JD, et al. Individual variation in the germline Ig gene repertoire inferred from variable region gene rearrangements. *J Immunol.* (2010) 184:6986–92. doi: 10.4049/jimmunol.1000445

72. Chimge NO, Pramanik S, Hu G, Lin Y, Gao R, Shen L, et al. Determination of gene organization in the human IGHV region on single chromosomes. *Genes Immun.* (2005) 6:186–93. doi: 10.1038/sj.gene.6364176
73. Watson CT, Breden F. The immunoglobulin heavy chain locus: genetic variation, missing data, and implications for human disease. *Genes Immun.* (2012) 13:363–73. doi: 10.1038/gene.2012.12
74. Watson CT, Steinberg KM, Huddleston J, Warren RL, Malig M, Schein J, et al. Complete haplotype sequence of the human immunoglobulin heavy-chain variable, diversity, and joining genes and characterization of allelic and copy-number variation. *Am J Hum Genet.* (2013) 92:530–46. doi: 10.1016/j.ajhg.2013.03.004
75. Milner EC, Hufnagle WO, Glas AM, Suzuki I, Alexander C. Polymorphism and utilization of human VH Genes. *Ann N Y Acad Sci.* (1995) 764:50–61. doi: 10.1111/j.1749-6632.1995.tb55806.x
76. Juul L, Hougs L, Barington T. A new apparently functional IGVK gene (VkLa) present in some individuals only. *Immunogenetics* (1998) 48:40–6. doi: 10.1007/s002510050398
77. Lefranc MP, Pallares N, Frippiat JP. Allelic polymorphisms and RFLP in the human immunoglobulin lambda light chain locus. *Hum Genet.* (1999) 104:361–9. doi: 10.1007/s004390050969
78. Moraes Junta C, Passos GA. Genomic EcoRI polymorphism and cosmid sequencing reveal an insertion/deletion and a new IGLV5 allele in the human immunoglobulin lambda variable locus (22q11.2/IGLV). *Immunogenetics* (2003) 55:10–5. doi: 10.1007/s00251-003-0549-x
79. Romo-Gonzalez T, Vargas-Madrazo E. Substitution patterns in alleles of immunoglobulin V genes in humans and mice. *Mol Immunol.* (2006) 43:731–44. doi: 10.1016/j.molimm.2005.03.018
80. Kirschbaum T, Roschenthaler F, Bensch A, Holscher B, Lautner-Rieske A, Ohnrich M, et al. The central part of the mouse immunoglobulin kappa locus. *Eur J Immunol.* (1999) 29:2057–64. doi: 10.1002/(SICI)1521-4141(199907)29:07<2057::AID-IMMU2057>3.0.CO;2-P
81. Roschenthaler F, Kirschbaum T, Heim V, Kirschbaum V, Schable KF, Schwendinger J, et al. The 5′ part of the mouse immunoglobulin kappa locus. *Eur J Immunol.* (1999) 29:2065–71. doi: 10.1002/1521-4141(2000012)30:123.0.CO;2-G
82. Brekke KM, Garrard WT. Assembly and analysis of the mouse immunoglobulin kappa gene sequence. *Immunogenetics* (2004) 56:490–505. doi: 10.1007/s00251-004-0659-0
83. Fitzsimmons SP, Clark KJ, Shapiro MA. Evolutionary relationships and polymorphisms among V kappa 10 genes from inbred and wild-derived inbred mice. *Immunogenetics* (2002) 54:9–19. doi: 10.1007/s00251-002-0438-8
84. Henderson TJ, Rudikoff S. Characterization of a V kappa family in Mus musculus castaneus: sequence analysis. *Immunogenetics* (1993) 37:426–36.
85. Kim SO, Sanz I, Williams C, Capra JD, Gottlieb PD. Polymorphism in V kappa 10 genes encoding L chains of antibodies bearing the Ars-A and A48 cross-reactive idiotypes. *Immunogenetics* (1991) 34:231–41. doi: 10.1007/BF00215258
86. Good RA. Contempo ’81. Immunology. *JAMA* (1981) 245:2197–8. doi: 10.1001/jama.1981.03310460049021
87. Greiff V, Weber CR, Palme J, Bodenhofer U, Miho E, Menzel U, et al. Learning the high-dimensional immunogenomic features that predict public and private antibody repertoires. *J Immunol.* (2017) 199:2985–97. doi: 10.4049/jimmunol.1700594
88. Hoi KH, Ippolito GC. Intrinsic bias and public rearrangements in the human immunoglobulin Vlambda light chain repertoire. *Genes Immun.* (2013) 14:271–6. doi: 10.1038/gene.2013.10
89. Ignatovich O, Tomlinson IM, Jones PT, Winter G. The creation of diversity in the human immunoglobulin V(lambda) repertoire. *J Mol Biol.* (1997) 268:69–77. doi: 10.1006/jmbi.1997.0956
90. Vasicek TJ, Leder P. Structure and expression of the human immunoglobulin lambda genes. *J Exp Med.* (1990) 172: 609–20. doi: 10.1084/jem.172.2.609
91. Farner NL, Dorner T, Lipsky PE. Molecular mechanisms and selection influence the generation of the human V lambda J lambda repertoire. *J Immunol.* (1999) 162:2137–45.
92. Longo NS, Rogosch T, Zemlin M, Zouali M, Lipsky PE. Mechanisms that shape human antibody repertoire development in mice transgenic for human Ig H and L chain Loci. *J Immunol.* (2017) 198:3963–77. doi: 10.4049/jimmunol.1700133
93. Vander Heiden JA, Stathopoulos P, Zhou JQ, Chen L, Gilbert TJ, Bolen CR, et al. Dysregulation of B cell repertoire formation in *Myasthenia Gravis* patients revealed through deep sequencing. *J Immunol.* (2017) 198:1460–73. doi: 10.4049/jimmunol.1601415
94. Fraser LD, Zhao Y, Lutalo PM, D’Cruz DP, Cason J, Silva JS, et al. Immunoglobulin light chain allelic inclusion in systemic lupus erythematosus. *Eur J Immunol.* (2015) 45:2409–19. doi: 10.1002/eji.201545599
95. Hehle V, Fraser LD, Tahir R, Kipling D, Wu YC, Lutalo PM, et al. Immunoglobulin kappa variable region gene selection during early human B cell development in health and systemic *Lupus erythematosus*. *Mol Immunol.* (2015) 65:215–23. doi: 10.1016/j.molimm.2015.01.017
96. Li Y, Spellerberg MB, Stevenson FK, Capra JD, Potter KN. The I binding specificity of human VH 4-34 (VH 4-21) encoded antibodies is determined by both VH framework region 1 and complementarity determining region 3. *J Mol Biol.* (1996) 256:577–89. doi: 10.1006/jmbi.1996.0110
97. Morel L. Mouse models of human autoimmune diseases: essential tools that require the proper controls. *PLoS Biol.* (2004) 2:E241. doi: 10.1371/journal.pbio.0020241
98. Burnett DL, Langley DB, Schofield P, Hermes JR, Chan TD, Jackson J, et al. Germinal center antibody mutation trajectories are determined by rapid self/foreign discrimination. *Science* (2018) 360:223–6. doi: 10.1126/science.aao3859
99. Andrews SF, Zhang Q, Lim S, Li L, Lee JH, Zheng NY, et al. Global analysis of B cell selection using an immunoglobulin light chain-mediated model of autoreactivity. *J Exp Med.* (2013) 210:125–42. doi: 10.1084/jem.20120525
100. Shlomchik MJ, Aucoin AH, Pisetsky DS, Weigert MG. Structure and function of anti-DNA autoantibodies derived from a single autoimmune mouse. *Proc Natl Acad Sci USA.* (1987) 84:9150–4. doi: 10.1073/pnas.84.24.9150
101. Shlomchik MJ, Marshak-Rothstein A, Wolfowicz CB, Rothstein TL, Weigert MG. The role of clonal selection and somatic mutation in autoimmunity. *Nature* (1987) 328:805–11. doi: 10.1038/328805a0
102. Geraldes A, Basset P, Smith KL, Nachman MW. Higher differentiation among subspecies of the house mouse (Mus musculus) in genomic regions with low recombination. *Mol Ecol.* (2011) 20:4722–36. doi: 10.1111/j.1365-294X.2011.05285.x
103. Mao HZ, Roussos ET, Peterfy M. Genetic analysis of the diabetes-prone C57BLKS/J mouse strain reveals genetic contribution from multiple strains. *Biochim Biophys Acta* (2006) 1762:440–6. doi: 10.1016/j.bbadis.2006.01.002
104. Joosten LA, Helsen MM, van de Loo FA, van den Berg WB. Anticytokine treatment of established type II collagen-induced arthritis in DBA/1 mice. A comparative study using anti-TNFα, anti-IL-1α/β, and IL-1Ra. *Arthritis Rheum.* (1996) 39:797–809. doi: 10.1002/art.23363
105. Clark AG, Worni-Schudel IM, Korte FM, Foster MH. A murine Ig light chain transgene reveals IGKV3 gene contributions to anti-collagen types IV and II specificities. *Mol Immunol.* (2017) 91:49–56. doi: 10.1016/j.molimm.2017.08.015
106. Bygrave AE, Rose KL, Cortes-Hernandez J, Warren J, Rigby RJ, Cook HT, et al. Spontaneous autoimmunity in 129 and C57BL/6 mice-implications for autoimmunity described in gene-targeted mice. *PLoS Biol.* (2004) 2:E243. doi: 10.1371/journal.pbio.0020243
107. Bubier JA, Sproule TJ, Foreman O, Spolski R, Shaffer DJ, Morse HC, III, et al. A critical role for IL-21 receptor signaling in the pathogenesis of systemic lupus erythematosus in BXSB-Yaa mice. *Proc Natl Acad Sci USA.* (2009) 106:1518–23. doi: 10.1073/pnas.0807309106

# Permissions

All chapters in this book were first published by Frontiers; hereby published with permission under the Creative Commons Attribution License or equivalent. Every chapter published in this book has been scrutinized by our experts. Their significance has been extensively debated. The topics covered herein carry significant findings which will fuel the growth of the discipline. They may even be implemented as practical applications or may be referred to as a beginning point for another development.

The contributors of this book come from diverse backgrounds, making this book a truly international effort. This book will bring forth new frontiers with its revolutionizing research information and detailed analysis of the nascent developments around the world.

We would like to thank all the contributing authors for lending their expertise to make the book truly unique. They have played a crucial role in the development of this book. Without their invaluable contributions this book wouldn't have been possible. They have made vital efforts to compile up to date information on the varied aspects of this subject to make this book a valuable addition to the collection of many professionals and students.

This book was conceptualized with the vision of imparting up-to-date information and advanced data in this field. To ensure the same, a matchless editorial board was set up. Every individual on the board went through rigorous rounds of assessment to prove their worth. After which they invested a large part of their time researching and compiling the most relevant data for our readers.

The editorial board has been involved in producing this book since its inception. They have spent rigorous hours researching and exploring the diverse topics which have resulted in the successful publishing of this book. They have passed on their knowledge of decades through this book. To expedite this challenging task, the publisher supported the team at every step. A small team of assistant editors was also appointed to further simplify the editing procedure and attain best results for the readers.

Apart from the editorial board, the designing team has also invested a significant amount of their time in understanding the subject and creating the most relevant covers. They scrutinized every image to scout for the most suitable representation of the subject and create an appropriate cover for the book.

The publishing team has been an ardent support to the editorial, designing and production team. Their endless efforts to recruit the best for this project, has resulted in the accomplishment of this book. They are a veteran in the field of academics and their pool of knowledge is as vast as their experience in printing. Their expertise and guidance has proved useful at every step. Their uncompromising quality standards have made this book an exceptional effort. Their encouragement from time to time has been an inspiration for everyone.

The publisher and the editorial board hope that this book will prove to be a valuable piece of knowledge for researchers, students, practitioners and scholars across the globe.

# List of Contributors

**Adar Toledano, Jennifer I. C. Benichou and Yoram Louzoun**
Department of Mathematics, Gonda Brain Research Center, Bar Ilan University, Ramat Gan, Israel

**Yuval Elhanati**
Joseph Henry Laboratories, Princeton University, Princeton, NJ, United States

**Aleksandra M. Walczak**
Laboratoire de Physique Théorique, UMR8549, CNRS and Ecole Normale Supérieure, Paris, France

**Thierry Mora**
Laboratoire de physique statistique, UMR8550, CNRS, UPMC and Ecole normale supérieure, Paris, France

**David Gfeller**
Department of Oncology, Ludwig Institute for Cancer Research, University of Lausanne, Lausanne, Switzerland
Swiss Institute of Bioinformatics (SIB), Lausanne, Switzerland

**Michal Bassani-Sternberg**
Department of Oncology, Ludwig Institute for Cancer Research, University of Lausanne, Lausanne, Switzerland
Department of Oncology, Ludwig Institute for Cancer Research, University Hospital of Lausanne, Lausanne, Switzerland

**Oren Avram, Anna Vaisman-Mentesh, Dror Yehezkel, Haim Ashkenazy, Tal Pupko and Yariv Wine**
George S. Wise Faculty of Life Sciences, School of Molecular Cell Biology and Biotechnology, Tel Aviv University, Ramat Aviv, Israel

**Ke-Yue Ma**
Institute for Cellular and Molecular Biology, The University of Texas at Austin, Austin, TX, United States

**Chenfeng He and Chad M. Williams**
Department of Biomedical Engineering, Cockrell School of Engineering, The University of Texas at Austin, Austin, TX, United States

**Ben S. Wendel**
McKetta Department of Chemical Engineering, Cockrell School of Engineering, The University of Texas at Austin, Austin, TX, United States

**Jun Xiao**
ImmuDX, LLC, Austin, TX, United States

**Hui Yang**
School of Life Sciences, Northwestern Polytechnical University, Xi'an, Shaanxi, China
Research Center of Special Environmental Biomechanics & Medical Engineering, Xi'an, Shaanxi, China

**Ning Jiang**
Institute for Cellular and Molecular Biology, The University of Texas at Austin, Austin, TX, United States
Department of Biomedical Engineering, Cockrell School of Engineering, The University of Texas at Austin, Austin, TX, United States

**Syed Ahmad Chan Bukhari**
Department of Pathology, Yale School of Medicine, Yale University, New Haven, CT, United States

**Martin J. O'Connor, Marcos Martínez-Romero, Attila L. Egyedi, Debra Willrett, John Graybeal and Mark A. Musen**
Stanford Center for Biomedical Informatics Research, Stanford University, Stanford, CA, United States

**Florian Rubelt**
Department of Microbiology and Immunology, Institute for Immunity, Transplantation and Infection, Stanford University School of Medicine, Stanford, CA, United States

**Kei-Hoi Cheung**
Department of Emergency Medicine, Yale School of Medicine, Yale University, New Haven, CT, United States
Yale Center for Medical Informatics, Yale School of Medicine, Yale University, New Haven, CT, United States
Interdepartmental Program in Computational Biology and Bioinformatics, Yale University, New Haven, CT, United States

**Steven H. Kleinstein**
Department of Pathology, Yale School of Medicine, Yale University, New Haven, CT, United States
Interdepartmental Program in Computational Biology and Bioinformatics, Yale University, New Haven, CT, United States

**Nima Nouri**
Department of Pathology, Yale School of Medicine, New Haven, CT, United States

**Steven H. Kleinstein**
Department of Pathology, Yale School of Medicine, New Haven, CT, United States
Interdepartmental Program in Computational Biology and Bioinformatics, Yale University, New Haven, CT, United States

**Jie H. S. Zhou and Philip D. Hodgkin**
Immunology Division, The Walter and Eliza Hall Institute of Medical Research, Parkville, VIC, Australia
Department of Medical Biology, The University of Melbourne, Parkville, VIC, Australia

**John F. Markham**
Immunology Division, The Walter and Eliza Hall Institute of Medical Research, Parkville, VIC, Australia
Victoria Research Laboratory, National ICT Australia
The University of Melbourne, Parkville, VIC, Australia

**Ken R. Duffy**
Hamilton Institute, Maynooth University, Maynooth, Ireland

**Balachandran Manavalan**
Department of Physiology, Ajou University School of Medicine, Suwon, South Korea

**Rajiv Gandhi Govindaraj**
Department of Biological Sciences, Louisiana State University, Baton Rouge, LA, United States

**Tae Hwan Shin and Gwang Lee**
Department of Physiology, Ajou University School of Medicine, Suwon, South Korea
Institute of Molecular Science and Technology, Ajou University, Suwon, South Korea

**Myeong Ok Kim**
Division of Life Science and Applied Life Science (BK21 Plus), College of Natural Sciences, Gyeongsang National University, Jinju, South Korea

**Chaim A. Schramm and Daniel C. Douek**
Vaccine Research Center, National Institute of Allergy and Infectious Diseases, NIH, Bethesda, MD, United States

**Aaron M. Rosenfeld**
School of Biomedical Engineering Science and Health Systems, Drexel University, Philadelphia, PA, United States

**Sylvain Simon, J. Cruard, Agnes Fortun and Francois Lang**
CRCINA, INSERM, Université d'Angers, Université de Nantes, Nantes, France
LabEx IGO "Immunotherapy, Graft, Oncology," Nantes, France

**Wenzhao Meng and Eline T. Luning Prak**
Department of Pathology and Laboratory Medicine, Perelman School of Medicine, University of Pennsylvania, Philadelphia, PA, United States

**Uri Hershberg**
School of Biomedical Engineering Science and Health Systems, Drexel University, Philadelphia, PA, United States
Department of Microbiology and Immunology, College of Medicine, Drexel University, Philadelphia, PA, United States
Department of Human Biology, Faculty of Sciences, University of Haifa, Haifa, Israel

**Zhong Wu and Samuel J. Rulli**
Qiagen Sciences, Frederick, MD, United States

**Virginie Vignard and Nathalie Labarriere**
CRCINA, INSERM, Université d'Angers, Université de Nantes, Nantes, France
LabEx IGO "Immunotherapy, Graft, Oncology," Nantes, France
Centre Hospitalier Universitaire Nantes, Nantes, France

**Amir Khammari and Brigitte Dreno**
CRCINA, INSERM, Université d'Angers, Université de Nantes, Nantes, France
LabEx IGO "Immunotherapy, Graft, Oncology," Nantes, France
Department of Dermato-Cancerology of Nantes Hospital, Nantes, France

**Wahiba Chaara, Laura-Maria Florez, David Klatzmann, Encarnita Mariotti-Ferrandiz and Adrien Six**
Sorbonne Université, INSERM, UMR_S 959, Immunology-Immunopathology-Immunotherapy (i3), Paris, France
AP-HP, Hôpital Pitié-Salpêtrière, Biotherapy (CIC-BTi) and Inflammation-Immunopathology-Biotherapy Department (i2B), Paris, France

**Ariadna Gonzalez-Tort**
Sorbonne Université, INSERM, UMR_S 959, Immunology-Immunopathology-Immunotherapy (i3), Paris, France

**Mark R. Dowling, Andrey Kan, Susanne Heinzel, Julia M. Marchingo, Philip D. Hodgkin and Edwin D. Hawkins**
Immunology Division, The Walter and Eliza Hall Institute of Medical Research, Parkville, VIC, Australia
Department of Medical Biology, The University of Melbourne, Parkville, VIC, Australia

**V. Britanova**
Shemyakin and Ovchinnikov Institute of Bioorganic Chemistry, Moscow, Russia

**Evgeny S. Egorov, Vasiliy N. Zubov, Mark Izraelson, Tatiana O. Nakonechnaya, Ilgar Z. Mamedov, Mikhail V. Pogorelyy and Olga Sofya A. Kasatskaya**
Shemyakin and Ovchinnikov Institute of Bioorganic Chemistry, Moscow, Russia
Center of Life Sciences, Skolkovo Institute of Science and Technology, Moscow, Russia

**Andrea Angius and Francesco Cucca**
Istituto di Ricerca Genetica e Biomedica, Consiglio Nazionale delle Ricerche, Monserrato, Italy

**Elisa Rosati and Andre Franke**
Institute of Clinical Molecular Biology, Kiel University, Kiel, Germany

**Alexey N. Davydov**
Adaptive Immunity Group, Central European Institute of Technology, Brno, Czechia

**Anna S. Obraztsova**
Faculty of Bioengineering and Bioinformatics, Lomonosov Moscow State University, Moscow, Russia
Center of Life Sciences, Skolkovo Institute of Science and Technology, Moscow, Russia

**Mikhail Y. Lebedin**
Genomics of Adaptive Immunity Department, Shemyakin and Ovchinnikov Institute of Bioorganic Chemistry, Moscow, Russia

**Maria A. Turchaninova and Olga V. Britanova**
Genomics of Adaptive Immunity Department, Shemyakin and Ovchinnikov Institute of Bioorganic Chemistry, Moscow, Russia
Department of Molecular Technologies, Pirogov Russian National Research Medical University, Moscow, Russia
Laboratory of Genomics of Antitumor Adaptive Immunity, Privolzhsky Research Medical University, Nizhny Novgorod, Russia

**Ekaterina M. Merzlyak**
Genomics of Adaptive Immunity Department, Shemyakin and Ovchinnikov Institute of Bioorganic Chemistry, Moscow, Russia
Department of Molecular Technologies, Pirogov Russian National Research Medical University, Moscow, Russia

**George V. Sharonov**
Genomics of Adaptive Immunity Department, Shemyakin and Ovchinnikov Institute of Bioorganic Chemistry, Moscow, Russia
Laboratory of Genomics of Antitumor Adaptive Immunity, Privolzhsky Research Medical University, Nizhny Novgorod, Russia

**Olga Kladova**
Department of Molecular Technologies, Pirogov Russian National Research Medical University, Moscow, Russia

**Mikhail Shugay**
Center of Life Sciences, Skolkovo Institute of Science and Technology, Moscow, Russia
Genomics of Adaptive Immunity Department, Shemyakin and Ovchinnikov Institute of Bioorganic Chemistry, Moscow, Russia
Department of Molecular Technologies, Pirogov Russian National Research Medical University, Moscow, Russia
Laboratory of Genomics of Antitumor Adaptive Immunity, Privolzhsky Research Medical University, Nizhny Novgorod, Russia

**Dmitriy M. Chudakov**
Adaptive Immunity Group, Central European Institute of Technology, Brno, Czechia
Center of Life Sciences, Skolkovo Institute of Science and Technology, Moscow, Russia
Genomics of Adaptive Immunity Department, Shemyakin and Ovchinnikov Institute of Bioorganic Chemistry, Moscow, Russia
Department of Molecular Technologies, Pirogov Russian National Research Medical University, Moscow, Russia
Laboratory of Genomics of Antitumor Adaptive Immunity, Privolzhsky Research Medical University, Nizhny Novgorod, Russia

**Michael Meyer-Hermann**
Department of Systems Immunology, Braunschweig Integrated Centre of Systems Biology, Helmholtz Centre for Infection Research, Braunschweig, Germany
Institute for Biochemistry, Biotechnology and Bioinformatics, Technische Universität Braunschweig, Braunschweig, Germany
Centre for Individualised Infection Medicine, Hanover, Germany

**Sebastian C. Binder**
Department of Systems Immunology, Braunschweig Integrated Centre of Systems Biology, Helmholtz Centre for Infection Research, Braunschweig, Germany
Institute for Biochemistry, Biotechnology and Bioinformatics, Technische Universität Braunschweig, Braunschweig, Germany

**Alexander Dimitri Yermanos**
Department of Biosystems Science and Engineering, ETH Zurich, Basel, Switzerland
Department of Biology, Institute of Microbiology, ETH Zurich, Zurich, Switzerland

**Dmitriy B. Staroverov**
Center of Life Sciences, Skolkovo Institute of Science and Technology, Moscow, Russia
Genomics of Adaptive Immunity Department, Shemyakin and Ovchinnikov Institute of Bioorganic Chemistry, Moscow, Russia
Department of Molecular Technologies, Pirogov Russian National Research Medical University, Moscow, Russia

**Luka Mesin and Gabriel D. Victora**
Laboratory of Lymphocyte Dynamics, The Rockefeller University, New York, NY, United States

**Andreas Kevin Dounas**
Department of Chemistry and Applied Biosciences, ETH Zurich, Zurich, Switzerland

**Tanja Stadler and Sai T. Reddy**
Department of Biosystems Science and Engineering, ETH Zurich, Basel, Switzerland

**Annette Oxenius**
Department of Biology, Institute of Microbiology, ETH Zurich, Zurich, Switzerland

**Yair Neve-Oz, Julia Sajman, Yair Razvag and Eilon Sherman**
Racah Institute of Physics, The Hebrew University, Jerusalem, Israel

**Andrew M. Collins**
School of Biotechnology and Biomolecular Sciences, University of New South Wales, Sydney, NSW, Australia

**Corey T. Watson**
Department of Biochemistry and Molecular Genetics, University of Louisville School of Medicine, Louisville, KY, United States

# Index

www.ingramcontent.com/pod-product-compliance
Lightning Source LLC
LaVergne TN
LVHW082202200926
848484LV00008B/2199